Genomics Protocols

METHODS IN MOLECULAR BIOLOGY™

John M. Walker, SERIES EDITOR

METHODS IN MOLECULAR BIOLOGY™

Genomics Protocols

Edited by

Michael P. Starkey

and

Ramnath Elaswarapu

*UK Human Genome Mapping Project Resource Centre,
Cambridge, UK*

Humana Press ✳ Totowa, New Jersey

Library of Congress Cataloging in Publication Data

Genomics protocols / edited by Michael P. Starkey and Ramnath Elaswarapu.
    p. ; cm.—(Methods in molecular biology ; 175)
    Includes bibliographical references and index.
    ISBN 0-89603-774-6 (hardcover ; alk. paper)--ISBN 0-89603-708-8 (comb ; alk. paper)
    1. Molecular genetics—Laboratory manuals. 2. Genomics–Laboratory manuals. I. Starkey, Michael P. II. Elaswarapu, Ramnath. III. Series QH440.5 G46 2001]
    572.8—dc21

                                                                                    00-046106

Preface

We must unashamedly admit that a large part of the motivation for editing *Genomics Protocols* was selfish. The possibility of assembling in a single volume a unique and comprehensive collection of complete protocols, relevant to our work and the work of our colleagues, was too good an opportunity to miss. We are pleased to report, however, that the outcome is something of use not only to those who are experienced practitioners in the genomics field, but is also valuable to the larger community of researchers who have recognized the potential of genomics research and may themselves be beginning to explore the technologies involved.

Some of the techniques described in *Genomics Protocols* are clearly not restricted to the genomics field; indeed, a prerequisite for many procedures in this discipline is that they require an extremely high throughput, beyond the scope of the average investigator. However, what we have endeavored here to achieve is both to compile a collection of procedures concerned with genome-scale investigations and to incorporate the key components of "bottom-up" and "top-down" approaches to gene finding. The technologies described extend from those traditionally recognized as coming under the genomics umbrella, touch on proteomics (the study of the expressed protein complement of the genome), through to early therapeutic approaches utilizing the potential of genome programs via gene therapy (Chapters 27–30).

Although a number of the procedures described represent the tried and trusted, we have striven to include new variants on existing technologies in addition to exciting new approaches. Where there are alternative approaches to achieving a particular goal, we have sought assistance from an expert in the field to identify the most reliable technique, one suitable for a beginner in the field. Unique to the Methods in Molecular Biology series is the "Notes" section at the end of each chapter. This is a veritable Aladdin's cave of information in which an investigator describes the quirks in a procedure and the little tricks that make all the difference to a successful outcome.

The first section of the volume deals with the traditional positional cloning approach to gene identification and isolation. The construction of a high-resolution genetic map (Chapter 1) to facilitate the mapping of monogenic traits and approaches to the analysis of polygenic traits (Chapter 2) are described. Identification of large numbers of single-nucleotide polymorphisms (Chapter 3) will pave the way for the construction of the next generation of genetic maps. Also described are such comparatively new technologies as genomic mismatch scanning (Chapter 4), for the mapping of genetic traits, and comparative genomic hybridization (Chapter 5), for the identification of gross differences between genomes.

Such studies are a prelude to the screening of large genomic clones, or clone contigs (Chapter 7). These transitions are made possible by the localization of genomic clones (Chapter 8) and the integration of the genetic and physical maps (Chapter 9) achieved by STS mapping. Identification of cDNAs mapping to the genomic clones implicated (Chapters 12–14) is the next step toward candidate gene identification. With the desire to acquire cDNAs capable of expressing authentic proteins, the emphasis in cDNA library construction is placed on a technology capable of delivering full-length cDNAs (Chapter 10).

One of the consequences of genome-scale sequencing programs has been the need to annotate large stretches of anonymous sequence data, and this has been the impetus for an explosion of bioinformatics programs targeted at gene prediction (Chapter 16). The use of model organisms (Chapter 17) to expedite gene discovery, on the basis of coding sequence similarites between genes with similiar functions, is another tool accessible to the gene hunter.

As an alternative to genetic studies, expression profiling seeks to identify candidate genes on the basis of their differential patterns of expression, either at the level of transcription or translation. A number of technologies, based on subtractive hybridization, differential display, and high throughput *in situ* hybridization are thus described (Chapters 18–22).

Functional characterization of isolated cDNAs is the next stage in establishing the likely candidature and thus potential utility of genes isolated as targets for therapeutic intervention. Predictions of protein structure and function (Chapter 23), mutagenesis (Chapter 24), or knockout studies (Chapter 25) can enable predictions of gene function. The yeast two-hybrid system (Chapter 26) is described at the level of monitoring interaction between individual proteins, but also on a potential genome scale.

In compiling *Genomics Protocols,* the aim—as with all other volumes in the Methods in Molecular Biology series—has been to produce a self-contained laboratory manual useful to both experienced practitioners and beginners in the field. We trust that we have been at least moderately successful. We must conclude by giving a vote of thanks to all the contributing authors, and to John Walker and the staff at Humana Press for seeing this project through.

Michael P. Starkey
Ramnath Elaswarapu

Contents

Contributors

TERRY J. AMISS • *Gene Therapy Center, University of North Carolina at Chapel Hill, Chapel Hill, NC*

DONALD S. ANSON • *Women's and Children's Hospital, North Adelaide, South Australia, Australia*

JAN P. A. BAAK • *Department of Pathology, Free University Hospital Amsterdam, Amsterdam, The Netherlands*

SIMON M. BROCKLEHURST • *Cambridge Antibody Technology, Melbourn, UK*

STEPHEN P. BRYANT • *Gemini Research Ltd., Cambridge, UK*

MATHIAS N. CHIANO • *Gemini Research Ltd., Cambridge, UK*

SANGDUN CHOI • *Division of Biology, California Institute of Technology, Pasadena, CA*

AMANDA COTTAGE • *Department of Pathology, Cambridge University, Cambridge, UK*

RONALD W. DAVIS • *Department of Biochemistry, Beckman Center, Stanford University School of Medicine, Stanford, CA*

PANAGIOTIS DELOUKAS • *The Sanger Centre, Cambridge, UK*

JOHAN T. DEN DUNNEN • *MGC-Department of Human and Clinical Genetics, Leiden University Medical Center, Leiden, The Netherlands*

YVONNE J. K. EDWARDS • *UK Human Genome Mapping Project Resource Centre, Cambridge, UK*

RAMNATH ELASWARAPU • *UK Human Genome Mapping Project Resource Centre, Cambridge, UK*

GREG ELGAR • *UK Human Genome Mapping Project Resource Centre, Cambridge, UK*

RUSSELL L. FINLEY, JR. • *Center for Molecular Medicine and Genetics, Wayne State University School of Medicine, Detroit, MI*

RUTH GJERSET • *Sidney Kimmel Cancer Center, San Diego, CA*

ERICA A. GOLEMIS • *Division of Basic Science, Fox Chase Cancer Center, Philadelphia, PA*

THOMAS M. GRESS • *Department of Internal Medicine I, University of Ulm, Ulm, Germany*

ALI HAGHIGHI • *Sidney Kimmel Cancer Center, San Diego, CA*

DAVID E. HARRIS • *The Sanger Centre, Cambridge, UK*

MARIO A. J. A. HERMSEN • *Department of Pathology, Free University Hospital Amsterdam, Amsterdam, The Netherlands*

FRANK T. HORRIGAN • *Department of Physiology, University of Pennsylvania School of Medicine, Philadelphia, PA*

SEAN J. HUMPHRAY • *The Sanger Centre, Cambridge, UK*

UNG-JIN KIM • *Division of Biology, California Institute of Technology, Pasadena, CA*

SUSAN J. KNAGGS • *Genomics Laboratory, Division of Medical and Molecular Genetics, UMDS, Guy's Hospital, London, UK*

NATALI KOLKER • *Department of Molecular Biotechnology, University of Washington, Seattle, WA*

RICHARD M. LAWN • *Falk Cardiovascular Research Center, Stanford University School of Medicine, Stanford, CA*

SVETLANA LEBEDEVA • *Sidney Kimmel Cancer Center, San Diego, CA*

MARGARET A. LEVERSHA • *Roy Castle International Centre for Lung Cancer Research, Liverpool, UK*

XING JIAN LOU • *Moleular Biology Systems Analysis, LumiCyte, Inc., Fremont, CA*

PAUL A. LYONS • *Department of Medical Genetics, Wellcome Trust Centre for Molecular Mechanisms in Disease, University of Cambridge, Cambridge, UK*

AHMED MANSOURI • *Department of Molecular and Cell Biology, Max-Planck-Institute for Biophysical Chemistry, Göttingen, Germany*

GERRIT A. MEIJER • *Department of Pathology, Free University Hospital Amsterdam, Amsterdam, The Netherlands*

DAN MERCOLA • *Sidney Kimmel Cancer Center, San Diego, CA; Cancer Center, University of California at San Diego, La Jolla, CA*

FARIDEH MIRZAYANS • *Department of Ophthalmology, Ocular Genetics Laboratory, University of Alberta, Edmonton, Alberta, Canada*

LEE MURPHY • *The Sanger Centre, Cambridge, UK*

DEBORAH A. NICKERSON • *Department of Molecular Biology, University of Washington, Seattle, WA*

CHRISTOF NIEHRS • *Division of Molecular Embryology, Deutsches Krebsforschungszentrum, Heidelberg, Germany*

MARIA PACK • *RZPD Deutsches Resourcenzentrum für Genomforschung GmbH, Berlin, Germany*

LEONIDAS A. PHYLACTOU • *Cyprus Institute of Neurology and Genetics, Nicosia, Cyprus*

NICOLAS POLLET • *Division of Molecular Embryology, Deutsches Krebsforschungszentrum, Heidelberg, Germany*

IOANNIS RAGOUSSIS • *Genomics Laboratory, Division of Medical and Molecular Genetics, UMDS, Guy's Hospital, London, UK*

MARK J. RIEDER • *Department of Molecular Biology, University of Washington, Seattle, WA*

RICHARD JUDE SAMULSKI • *Gene Therapy Center, University of North Carolina at Chapel Hill, Chapel Hill, NC*

KATJA SCHÄFER • *RZPD Deutsches Resourcenzentrum für Genomforschung GmbH, Berlin, Germany*

MARK SCHENA • *Department of Biochemistry, Beckman Center, Stanford University School of Medicine, Stanford, CA*

ILYA G. SEREBRIISKII • *Division of Basic Science, Fox Chase Cancer Center, Philadelphia, PA*

MICHAEL P. STARKEY • *UK Human Genome Mapping Project Resource Centre, Hinxton, Cambridge, UK*

SUMIO SUGANO • *Department of Virology, The Institute of Medical Sciences, University of Tokyo, Tokyo, Japan*

YUTAKA SUZUKI • *Department of Virology, The Institute of Medical Sciences, University of Tokyo, Tokyo, Japan*

SCOTT L. TAYLOR • *Division of Development and Neurobiology, Walter and Eliza Hall Institute of Medical Research, Melbourne, Australia*

TIM THOMAS • *Department of Molecular and Cell Biology, Max-Planck-Institute for Biophysical Chemistry, Göttingen, Germany*

GARABET G. TOBY • *Division of Basic Science, Fox Chase Cancer Center, Philadelphia, PA, and Cell and Molecular Biology Graduate Group, University of Pennsylvania, Philadelphia, PA*

DANIELA TONIOLO • *Institute of Genetics, Biochemistry, and Evolution, CNR, Pavia, Italy*

OLIVER DORIAN VON STEIN • *InDex Pharmaceuticals AB, Stockholm, Sweden*

ANNE K. VOSS • *Division of Development and Neurobiology, Walter and Eliza Hall Institute of Medical Research, Melbourne, Australia*

CHRISTINE WALLRAPP • *Department of Internal Medicine I, University of Ulm, Ulm, Germany*

MICHAEL A. WALTER • *Department of Ophthalmology, Ocular Genetics Laboratory, University of Alberta, Edmonton, Alberta, Canada*

MARTIN C. WAPENAAR • *MGC-Department of Human and Clinical Genetics, Leiden University Medical Center, Leiden, The Netherlands*

MARJAN M. WEISS • *Department of Gastroenterology, Free University Hospital Amsterdam, Amsterdam, The Netherlands*

GÜNTHER ZEHETNER • *Max-Planck-Institut für Molekulare Genetik, Berlin, Germany*

1

Construction of Microsatellite-Based, High-Resolution Genetic Maps in the Mouse

Paul A. Lyons

1. Introduction

The mapping of genes underlying either simple mendelian or complex traits can be broken down into a number of distinct stages—initial detection of the locus in a genome scan, determination of the most likely map location for the gene, and finally fine mapping of the locus. A number of experimental strategies for mapping genes in experimental organisms are available and their relative merits have been reviewed recently *(1)*. Whatever strategy is chosen, an essential prerequisite for any gene identification project is the ability to construct a high resolution genetic map around the locus of interest.

The focus of this chapter is the construction of such genetic maps using microsatellite markers in the mouse, however, the methodology described here is applicable to most experimental organisms for which microsatellite markers are available. The mapping process can be broken down into a number of discrete steps. The first step is selecting the experimental strategy and determining the numbers of mice required to give the desired resolution. For the purpose of this chapter it is assumed that a suitable experimental strategy has been chosen and the requisite number of mice have been bred. The next step is selection and polymerase chain reaction (PCR) optimization of a panel of microsatellite markers from the region of interest that are variant between the mouse strains being used. **Subheading 3.1.** of this chapter discusses criteria for selecting markers and provides sources of microsatellite markers available in the public databases. In **Subheading 3.2.** protocols are provided for the PCR optimization of selected microsatellite markers. The next step in the procedure is the preparation of DNA from samples for genotyping. **Subheading 3.3.**

From: *Methods in Molecular Biology, vol. 175: Genomics Protocols*
Edited by: M. P. Starkey and R. Elaswarapu © Humana Press Inc., Totowa, NJ

describes a protocol for the rapid extraction of DNA from mouse tails that is of a suitable quality for PCR analysis. **Sections 3.4.–3.6.** describe protocols for genotyping these DNA samples using either fluorescent or nonfluorescent-based approaches. The final step in the procedure, as outlined in **Subheading 3.7.**, is the construction of a genetic map from the genotyping data that has been obtained.

2. Materials

1. Tail buffer: 50 mM Tris-HCl, pH 8.0, 100 mM ethylenediaminetetraacetic acid (EDTA), 100 mM NaCl and 1% (w/v) sodium dodecyl sulfate (SDS).
2. Proteinase K solution (10 mg/mL). Store in aliquots at –20°C.
3. Saturated NaCl solution.
4. 1X TE$_{0.1}$: 10 mM Tris-HCl, pH 8.0, 0.1 mM EDTA.
5. 4 mM deoxyribonucleoside triphosphate (dNTPs).
6. Thermocycler (MJ Research, Watertown, MA).
7. PCR mix: Make 2000 reaction batches of PCR mix as follows. To 9.5 mL of dH$_2$O add 3 mL of 10X TaqGold buffer (PE Biosystems, Warrington, UK) and 1.5 mL of 4 mM dNTPs. Mix and store at 4°C.
8. TaqGold DNA polymerase (PE Biosystems).
9. Nusieve agarose (Flowgen, Lichfield, UK).
10. Agarose loading buffer: 10 mM Tris-HCl, pH 8.0, 1 mM EDTA, 1% (w/v) SDS, 40% (w/v) sucrose, xylene cyanol, and bromophenol blue.
11. GS500 tamra-size standards (PE Biosystems).
12. Long-Ranger acrylamide/urea sequencing gel mix (Flowgen).
13. Acrylamide loading buffer: 90% (v/v) deionized formamide, 50 mM EDTA, pH 8.0, and dextran blue.
14. Deep-well titer plates (Beckman, High Wycombe, UK, cat. no. 267004).
15. Genescan and genotyper software (PE Biosystems).
16. ABI 377 Automated Sequencer (PE Biosystems).

3. Methods

Microsatellites are regions of DNA made up of repeating blocks of nucleotides where the length of the repeated unit is either 2 bp (dinucleotide repeats), 3 bp (trinucleotide repeats), or 4 bp (tetranucleotide repeats). Microsatellites are widely distributed throughout the mouse genome with the (CA)n dinucleotide repeat estimated as occurring 100,000 times *(2)*. In addition to being widely distributed, the number of repeat units, and hence the size of the microsatellite, varies between mouse strains, even among closely related inbred mouse strains. This variation in size can be readily followed by PCR amplification and gel electrophoresis, which makes microsatellites an ideal source of markers for genetic map construction *(3)*.

3.1. Microsatellite Marker Selection

1. Sources of microsatellite markers: Over the past decade a large effort has gone into generating, characterizing, and mapping microsatellite markers. The largest effort has come from Eric Lander and colleagues at the Whitehead Institute in Cambridge, MA, who have generated a map of over 6000 markers, with an average spacing of one every 0.2 c*M*, throughout the mouse genome *(4)*. Information regarding microsatellite markers developed at the Whitehead Institute, including primer sequences, chromosomal location, and allele sizes in a panel of inbred strains is readily accessible via the Internet *(5)*. Another major source of marker information is the Mouse Genome Database, which is maintained by the Jackson Laboratories *(6)*. This database acts as a central repository for mouse genetic mapping data, including marker information, and is updated on a regular basis.

2. Marker selection: An important consideration when selecting microsatellite markers for use is how the genotyping will be performed, that is, whether markers will be analyzed using fluorescence-based gel systems or nonfluorescence-based systems. For nonfluorescence-based genotyping analyzed on agarose gels, the allele sizes need to vary by at least 10% to be resolvable. For fluorescence based gel systems, this is not a consideration, as differences as small as 2 bp can be resolved. Another consideration is whether or not markers will be pooled for gel electrophoresis in which case markers with nonoverlapping allele size ranges should be chosen.

3.2. PCR Optimization of Microsatellite Markers

1. Prepare 10X working dilutions of each microsatellite primer pair as follows: Dilute the forward and reverse stock primers together in a single tube to a final concentration of 25 µg/mL of each primer.

2. For each microsatellite primer pair being titrated, prepare a master mix as follows:
   a. Aliquot 105 µL of PCR mix into a microfuge tube.
   b. Add 22.5 µL of 10X primer dilution and 1.5 µL of TaqGold polymerase.
   c. Mix by vortexing briefly and place on ice.

3. Set up PCR reactions in three microtiter plates as follows at room temperature: For each primer pair being titrated, aliquot 5 µL of mouse genomic DNA (8 µg/mL) into four wells of the microtiter plate. To each well add 1.5 µL of either 10 m*M*, 20 m*M*, 30 m*M*, or 40 m*M* MgCl$_2$ solution and 8.5 µL of master mix (final reaction volume 15 µL). If appropriate, overlay with one drop of mineral oil.

4. Centrifuge the microtiter plates briefly and place on a thermocycler.

5. PCR the first microtiter plate as follows: 94°C 10 min followed by 36 cycles of 94°C for 10 s, 55°C for 20 s, and 72°C for 20 s. For the two subsequent PCR plates, adjust the 55°C annealing temperature to 53°C and 50°C, respectively (*see* **Note 1**).

6. Prepare a 2% (w/v) agarose gel in 1X TBE buffer.

7. Add 1.5 µL of agarose loading buffer to the samples in each microtiter plate and centrifuge briefly to mix. Load 10 µL of sample onto a 2% agarose gel and electrophorese until the xylene cyanol dye has migrated approx 2 cm.

8. Determine the optimal PCR conditions by visualizing the PCR products on a UV-transilluminator. Select the Mg^{2+} concentration and annealing temperature that gives a strong, discrete band of the expected size PCR product (*see* **Note 2** and **Fig. 1A**).

3.3. DNA Extraction from Mouse Tails

1. Cut 1 cm of tail and place in a 1.5-mL microfuge tube on ice (*see* **Note 3**).
2. To each tail sample add 400 μL of tail buffer and 10 μL of proteinase K solution.
3. Incubate at 42°C overnight in a shaking incubator.
4. To each sample add 200 μL of saturated NaC1 solution. Mix well by shaking for 30 s, do not vortex.
5. Centrifuge at 18,000g for 20 min at room temperature in a benchtop centrifuge.
6. Transfer the DNA containing supernatant to a fresh 1.5-mL microfuge tube being careful not to disturb the pellet.
7. Add 800 μL of 100% ethanol to each sample and mix by gentle inversion (*see* **Note 4**).
8. Pellet the DNA precipitate by centrifuging at 18,000g for 3 min at room temperature.
9. Remove the supernatant and wash the pellet with 500 μL of 70% ethanol to remove excess salt.
10. Centrifuge at 18,000*g* for 1 min, carefully remove the supernatant and allow the DNA pellet to air dry briefly.
11. Gently resuspend the DNA pellet in 200 μL of 1X $TE_{0.1}$ (*see* **Note 5**).
12. Measure the DNA concentration of each stock solution at OD_{260} with a spectrophotometer.
13. Prepare a working dilution (8 μg/mL) of each sample by diluting in 1X $TE_{0.1}$. To facilitate downstream sample processing, prepare the dilutions in 96-well format deep-well titer plates.
14. Store the working dilutions at 4°C and the stock DNAs at –20°C.

3.4. PCR Amplification

1. For each microsatellite to be genotyped, prepare a master mix as follows: For each DNA sample add 7 μL of PCR mix, 1.5 μL of 10X $MgCl_2$ (as previously determined in **Subheading 3.2.**), 1.5 μL of 10X primer dilution and 0.1 μL of TaqGold polymerase. Mix by vortexing.
2. Aliquot 5 μL of genomic DNA (8 μg/mL) into a microtiter plate, add 10 μL of master mix and overlay with a drop of mineral oil, if necessary.
3. Centrifuge briefly and place on a thermocycler.
4. Perform PCR as follows: 94°C for 10 min followed by 36 cycles of 94°C for 10 s, X°C for 20 s and 72°C for 20 s, where X equals the optimal annealing temperature determined in **Subheading 3.2.** (*see* **Note 1**).
5. Store PCR products at –20°C prior to analysis.

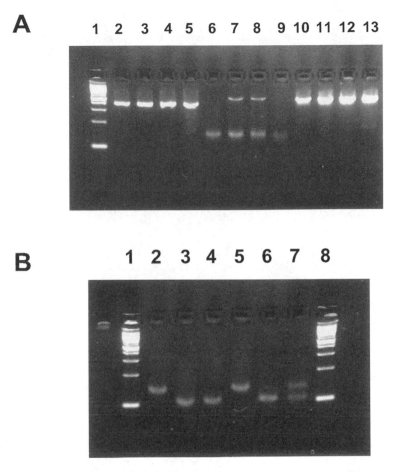

Fig. 1. PCR optimization of microsatellite markers. (**A**) Magnesium titrations of *DlNds31* (lanes 2–5), *DlNds32* (lanes 6–9), and *D4Nds26* (lanes 10–13) at 1 mM Mg^{2+} (lanes 2, 6, and 10), 2 mM Mg^{2+} (lanes 3, 7, and 11), 3 mM Mg^{2+} (lanes 4, 8, and 12), and 4 mM Mg^{2+} (lanes 5, 9, and 13). Lane 1 molecular-weight markers. (**B**) Amplification of C57BL/10 (lanes 2 and 5), NOD (lanes 3 and 6), and (NODxC57BL/10)F1 (lanes 4 and 7) DNA with *D3Nds6* using TaqGold (lanes 2-4) or Amplitaq (lanes 5–7) DNA polymerase. Lanes 1 and 8 are molecular-weight markers.

3.5. Analysis of PCR Products by Gel Electrophoresis

3.5.1. Agarose-Resolvable PCR Products

1. Prepare a 3% (w/v) Nusieve agarose/1% (w/v) agarose gel in 1X TBE.
2. Using a multichannel pipet add 1.5 µL of agarose loading buffer to each sample and centrifuge briefly to mix.

3. Load 10 µL of sample using a multichannel pipet onto the 3% Nusieve agarose/ 1% agarose gel and run until the xylene cyanol band has migrated approximately 2 cm from the well (*see* **Note 6**).
4. Visualize the PCR products on a UV-transilluminator and photograph.

3.5.2. Acrylamide-Resolvable PCR Products

1. Prepare a 2% agarose gel in 1X TBE.
2. For each microtiter plate of PCR products to be analyzed transfer 5 µL of four random samples into a fresh microtiter plate. Add 1 µL of agarose loading dye, mix by pipetting up and down, and load onto the 2% agarose gel.
3. Electrophorese samples until the xylene cyanol band has migrated 2 cm from the wells and check the presence and yield of PCR product on a UV-transilluminator.
4. Prepare a 4.75% Long-Ranger acrylamide/6 *M* urea ABI 377 sequencing gel in 1X TBE.
5. Pool compatible PCR products together as follows (*see* **Note 7**). Mix 3 µL of PCR products labeled with 6-carboxyfluorescein (FAM), 6 µL of 6-carboxy-tetrachlorofluorescein (TET)-labeled PCR products and 9 µL of 6-carboxy-hexachlorofluorescein (HEX)-labeled PCR products and make up to a final volume of 60 µL with dH$_2$O. Mix by centrifugation.
6. Prerun sequencing gel at 1000 V, 400 mA, and 30 W until it reaches 51°C.
7. Aliquot 2.5 µL of pooled samples into a fresh microtiter plate, add 0.5 µL GS500 Tamra standards and 2 µL of acrylamide loading dye. Mix by centrifugation. Denature by incubating at 95°C for 3 min, and place denatured PCR products on ice.
8. Pause sequencing gel and flush wells with 1X TBE to remove free urea. Load 2 µL of denatured, pooled sample into alternate wells and resume prerun.
9. Electrophorese samples for 3 min, pause gel and reflush all the wells with 1X TBE. Load 2 µL of each remaining sample into the intervening wells.
10. Run gel at 3000 V, 400 mA, and 30 W until the 500-bp size standard has passed the read window. Stop gel, track the lanes, and extract data using the Genescan software.

3.6. Genotyping

1. Create a Map Manager database to store the genotype data for each microsatellite marker being analyzed (*see* **Note 8**).
2. For agarose-resolvable markers, the genotype of each mouse at each marker can be assigned by eye from the photograph of the gel. Mice are scored as homozygous if a single PCR product is present or heterozygous if two PCR products are present (*see* **Note 9**).
3. Enter assigned genotypes into the Map Manager database.
4. For acrylamide-resolvable microsatellite markers the genotype is assigned using the Genotyper software as follows.
   a. Create a Genotyper template file containing allele size information for each marker used.

    b. Import data files for each gel lane to be genotyped (*see* **Subheading 3.5.**).

    c. Use the "label peaks" command to automatically assign a size to every PCR product in each lane.

    d. Use the "filter labels" command to remove size information from stutter bands.

    e. Using the "add rows to table" command, create a data table containing allele size information for each marker in each lane.

    f. Manually check and edit each assigned size using the "view plot" command and then recreate the data table with the corrected data.

    g. Export the allele size data to a file.

    h. Convert the allele size data into genotype data as described for agarose resolvable markers in **Subheading 3.6., step 1**.

    i. Enter the assigned genotypes into the Map Manager database.

5. In Map Manager, order the microsatellite markers such that the number of recombinants between adjacent markers is minimized.

6. Check genotyping data to identify potential double recombinants (*see* **Note 10**).

3.7. Genetic Map Construction

1. Export the genotyping data from the Map Manager database in Mapmaker format (*see* **Note 11**).

2. Run Mapmaker and parse the genotyping data using the Mapmaker "prepare data" command.

3. Select all of the markers for analysis using the Mapmaker "sequence" command. To speed the mapping process, turn on three-point analysis using the "use three-point" command.

4. Map the microsatellite markers relative to each other using the Mapmaker "orders" command.

5. To view the map on the screen, use the Mapmaker "map" command. To save the map to file for subsequent printing, use the "draw map" command, which draws the calculated map as a PostScript graphic file.

4. Notes

1. These cycling conditions have been optimized for hot start PCR reactions performed on a Tetrad thermocycler using TaqGold polymerase. It may be necessary to adjust the lengths of the individual steps when using alternative thermocyclers or polymerases.

2. In the case of most microsatellite primer pairs, these conditions will yield an optimal annealing temperature and magnesium concentration (*see* **Fig. 1A**). However, for some primer pairs it may be necessary to try different conditions or PCR protocols, such as touchdown PCR, to obtain optimal reaction conditions. Once optimal PCR reaction conditions have been determined for a microsatellite primer pair, it is essential to perform a test amplification on each of the parental strains together with an F1 mouse produced from the two parental strains. It is important to verify that the microsatellite marker is indeed polymorphic between the strains

of interest, as some groups have reported differences between expected and observed microsatellite allele sizes *(7)*. The inclusion of an F1 mouse is important, as some microsatellite markers show preferential amplification of one allele. In extreme cases, preferential amplification may result in the complete absence of one parental allele in the F1 mouse (*see* **Fig. 1B**, lanes 4 and 7). It has been found that, in many cases, substituting Amplitaq for TaqGold in the PCR reaction and reoptimizing the PCR conditions eliminates the problem of preferential amplification.

3. If not being processed immediately, tail biopsies should be stored at −80°C.
4. The DNA should form a clearly visible precipitate following addition of ethanol. The lack of an obvious precipitate is usually an indication of degraded DNA. Partially degraded DNA may still be suitable for PCR amplification and can be recovered as follows: precipitate the DNA by centrifugation at 18,000g for 15 min and then proceed with **step 9**.
5. To ensure the DNA pellet is completely in solution it may be necessary to leave at 4°C overnight.
6. The use of gel systems that allow loading with a multichannel pipet and that allow up to six microtiter plates worth of samples to be run on a single gel, such as the Bio-Rad Sub-Cell Model 192 (Bio Rad, Hemel Hempstead, UK), is highly recommended to facilitate the processing of large sample numbers. Samples are loaded into alternate wells and following genotyping the scores are rearranged into their original order.
7. Microsatellite markers with nonoverlapping allele size ranges can be pooled and run together. It is possible to mix up to 12 markers in any one pool. By using primers labeled with different fluorescent dyes, the size interval between adjacent markers can be reduced. Because the available fluorescent dyes have different intensities, it is necessary to pool varying amounts of the differently labeled PCR products to ensure equal loading. Assuming equivalent amplification, pool 3 µL of FAM-labeled products, 6 µL of TET-labeled products, and 9 µL of HEX-labeled products. However, these volumes will need to be adjusted accordingly where amplification is not equivalent.
8. Map Manager is a specialized database program for handling mouse genetic mapping data. It was written by Ken Manley and colleagues at the Roswell Park Cancer Institute in Buffalo, NY. It is available at the following web site: http://mcbio.med.buffalo.edu/mapmgr.html.
9. For backcross progeny only two possible genotypes exist. The mouse is either homozygous for the recurrent parent or heterozygous. For intercross progeny three possible genotypes exist, the mouse can be homozygous for either parental allele or heterozygous.
10. A mouse that has been incorrectly genotyped at a marker will appear to recombine on either side of that marker, such double recombinants artificially increase the map distance between adjacent markers. All such genotypes should be confirmed by checking the genotyping and, if necessary, repeating the PCR.

11. Mapmaker is a computer package for calculating genetic linkage maps written by Eric Lander. The program can be obtained from the following web site: http://www-genome.wi.mit.edu/ftp/distribution/software/.

References

1. Darvasi, A. (1998) Experimental strategies for the genetic dissection of complex traits in animal models. *Nature Genet.* **18,** 19–24.
2. Stallings, R. L., Ford, A. F., Nelson, D., Torney, D. C., Hildebrand, C. E., and Moyzis, R. K. (1991) Evolution and distribution of (GT)n repetitive sequences in mammalian genomes. *Genomics* **10,** 807–815.
3. Weber, J. L. and May, P. E. (1989) Abundant class of human DNA polymorphisms which can be typed using the polymerase chain reaction. *Am. J. Hum. Genet.* **44,** 388–396.
4. Dietrich, W. F., Miller, J., Steen, R., Merchant, M. A., Damron-Boles, D., Husain, Z., et al. (1996) A comprehensive genetic map of the mouse genome. *Nature* **380,** 149–152.
5. <http://www-genome.wi.mit.edu>.
6. <http://www.informaticsjax.org>.
7. Lord, C. J., Bohlander, S. K., Hopes, E. A., Montague, C. T., Hill, N. J., Prins, J. B., et al. (1995) Mapping the diabetes polygene Idd3 on mouse chromosome 3 by use of novel congenic strains. *Mamm. Genome* **6,** 563–570.

2

Genetic Analysis of Complex Traits

Stephen P. Bryant and Mathias N. Chiano

1. Introduction

The analysis of traits and disorders that exhibit a straightforward Mendelian genetics, based on the kind of major gene models that are easy to set up in computer programs such as LINKAGE *(1)*, has been enormously successful in facilitating identification of the genes responsible. These monogenic models typically use two alleles to represent the trait locus, one allele predisposing to development of the disease or disorder and the other allele showing a normal phenotype, with a penetrance parameter that is specified for each genotype (*see* **Table 1**). Family studies using these techniques have led to the localization of many hundreds of single gene disorders *(2)* and an appreciable fraction of those localized have been positionally cloned.

It is possible to easily model both dominant and recessive genetics using this approach (*see* **Table 2**) and to handle some of the uncertainty in the outcome by manipulating the values of the genotype penetrance parameters, thereby permitting the occurrence of phenocopies (cases not attributable to the locus) and partially penetrant individuals (gene carriers that do not manifest the disease). Although these approaches work best when the model specified accurately reflects the unknown real situation, they have been shown to be robust to model misspecification and can be used with care in situations where extended families with several affected individuals are employed in a genetic study and where inheritance is not straightforward. In this case, the most obvious effect is loss of statistical power. Refer to earlier reviews on the subject for workable protocols *(3,4)*.

The most usual strategy for isolating genes for Mendelian traits has been to concentrate linkage analysis on regions of the genome that are candidates for involvement. This evidence might come from cytogenetic observations,

From: *Methods in Molecular Biology, vol. 175: Genomics Protocols*
Edited by: M. P. Starkey and R. Elaswarapu © Humana Press Inc., Totowa, NJ

Table 1
Modeling the Expression of a Trait Phenotype

Parameter	Meaning
P_t	Trait allele frequency $= 1 - Pn$
f_{tt}	Penetrance of the t/t genotype $= p(T\|tt)$
f_{tn}	Penetrance of the t/n genotype $= p(T\|tn)$
f_{nn}	Penetrance of the n/n genotype $= p(T\|nn)$
f_t	Penetrance of the t allele $= p(T\|t)$
f_n	Penetrance of the n allele $= p(T\|n)$

animal studies, and so on. The systematic screening of the entire genome (genome scanning) using microsatellite markers is more recent and has found most application in the hunt for genes for complex disorders.

In a genome-wide linkage analysis, rare, single-gene disorders typically localize to a small region (say 5 Mb), which means that the positional cloning workload is not beyond the bounds of a modest laboratory collaboration.

With so much success in mapping single gene disorders, it is no surprise that many groups and consortia have adopted similar methodologies to map genes for those traits that are more complex. Although the principles and techniques of the genetic analysis of complex disorders are becoming mature and established and are subject to intense international collaborative research efforts, it is as well to note that successes, that is genes identified, isolated and functionally characterized as a direct result of applying these approaches, are minimal. Genome scans are typically difficult to replicate and often give multiple, poorly defined, broad peaks that are not optimal for candidate positional cloning work. However, it is the opinion of the authors that success in this regard is only a matter of time, with several recent factors contributing favorably to make the outcome more likely (such as the placement in the public domain of large numbers of mapped single nucleotide polymorphisms [SNPs]), and in this review we concentrate on those methodologies that we believe are more likely to yield results given the impetus of recent work.

For the purposes of this review, we define a complex trait as any that does not follow straightforward, Mendelian genetics. Complex traits are regarded as being the outcome of an interplay of multiple genetic, environmental, and chance factors. They encompass many of the disorders that are the most common and those in which an advance in understanding the underlying genetics would make the most difference to their management in people suffering from the disorder. These include Type II

Table 2
A Selection of Qualitative Trait Models,
Showing How Varying the Penetrance Parameters
Can Model the Segregation of the Phenotype

Name	P_t	f_{tt}	f_{tm}	f_{nn}	f_t	f_n	Examples
Fully penetrant autosomal dominant	0 001	1.0	1.0	0.0	—	—	Adenomatous polyposis coli (MIM # 175100); nonepidermolytic palmoplantar keratoderma (MIM# 600962)
Fully penetrant autosomal recessive	0 04	1.0	0.0	0.0	—	—	Muscular dystrophy with epidermolysis bullosa (MIM # 226670)
Fully penetrant X-linked recessive	0 04	1.0	0.0	0.0	1.0	0.0	Charcot-Marie-Tooth Neuropathy (MIM # 302800)
Partially penetrant autosomal dominant	0 003	0.4	0.4	0.02	—	—	Early-onset breast cancer (MIM # dominant 113705)

^{a}Parameters that are not used in the model are indicated by "—". MIM = Mendelian Inheritance in Man.

diabetes, cardiovascular disease, osteoarthritis, schizophrenia, obesity, and osteoporosis.

These disorders tend to be strongly age related, with the age of onset under genetic and/or environmental control. Furthermore, they are defined by a combination of quantitative risk factors that typically exhibit a statistically normal frequency distribution in the general population. It is as well to note that even traits that heretofore have been regarded as simple and monogenic are starting to reveal their complexity, with the discovery of "modifying" genes for several disorders.

Common, complex, age-related disorders are often the result of many genes (quantitative trait loci [QTL]) controlling quantitative physiological parameters that are themselves risk factors for the disease. Each of these risk factors may be controlled by several genes and are themselves affected by environment and chance events. Each gene may only contribute a small fraction of the final probability of outcome of disease, and this means that it is difficult to approach the genetics of a complex trait or disorder using the same methods that work for monogenic traits and at the same time expect the same degree of success. The traditional methods of analyzing these traits attempt to demonstrate a relationship between gene and disease, including the complexity as part of the statistical "noise." Affected sib–pair analyses are an example of this approach.

As an example, consider osteoporotic fracture. The most important risk factor influencing fracture outcome is the mineral density of the bone (BMD). Other factors include the quality of bone mineralization and the length of the hip-femur. Several genes have been shown to have an association with reduced BMD *(5,6)* and several environmental factors are known to be important, including exercise and diet.

The most striking known genetic effect in osteoporosis is from the *COLIA1* gene, where a polymorphism in an *SpI* binding site has been shown to increase the risk of hip fracture in low-BMD individuals to 30:1 compared with 5:1 for low BMD alone *(5)*.

It has been shown that the major risk factor—bone mineral density—is under the control of several genes, the effect of all of which have been defined by genetic association rather than linkage, with most of them being rational candidates for involvement, rather than being selected on the basis of a known linkage from a genome-scanning experiment. At the moment, whole-genome association experiments are prohibitive in terms of cost, and the gene discovery process is still required to start for the most part with microsatellite linkage scans. The protocols considered in the remainder of this chapter cover both the initial genome-scan analysis by linkage and subsequent positional-candidate analysis by association.

2. Materials

1. Software for performing linkage analysis: Mapmaker/Sibs (or GeneHunter) *(7)*.
2. A general statistical package for setting up association analyses (STATA).
3. A Unix workstation.

3. Methods

In this section, we explore common statistical methods for mapping complex disorders and QTLs.

There are two fundamental approaches:

1. Concentrate on individuals possessing the disorder or affected with the disease and perform a qualitative analysis on related individuals (usually pairs), optionally using a family member as an internal control for population stratification, or
2. Use unselected, related individuals and perform a quantitative analysis on a continuous trait known to affect the risk of developing the disorder.

Both approaches involve broadly similar genome-scanning protocols.

3.1. Genome Scanning

Genome scans of many common, complex disorders have been completed in recent years. These have yielded regions of genetic linkage that vary in size but are typically much larger than those that arise from genome scans of simpler, Mendelian traits. This is a simple outcome of the effect of polygenic inheritance confounded by environment and other modulating factors.

Dissecting the disease into underlying factors, that may be under simpler genetic control, prior to analyzing the genome scan, offers a rational route for increasing the precision of any linkage peaks uncovered by a scan and therefore decreasing the amount of fine mapping work required.

There are many strategies for exploiting DNA markers in mapping and char acterizing disease susceptibility loci that influence variation in quantitative traits. These methods depend on the design of the study and the proposed disease transmission model. However, there are a few basic concepts that are common to all disease mapping analysis strategies. These fundamental concepts bear on the need to correlate some measure of genotypic similarity at a particular locus or loci with a measure of phenotypic similarity among related or population-based individuals. If such a correlation exists, then it is possible that variation at the said locus, or another locus nearby, influences susceptibility to disease or variation in the phenotype under study. Although linkage tests for cosegregation of disease or trait with a locus assuming a model that explains the inheritance pattern between related individuals, association tests for correlation between genotype and phenotype across unrelated individuals. Linkage is, therefore, the method of choice for simple Mendelian traits because the admissible models are few and easily tested. However, application to complex traits is more complicated since it is difficult to find precise models that adequately explain inheritance patterns in complex traits.

As an alternative, the development of model-free methods of analysis that are based purely on a test of the degree to which related individuals, who are similar phenotypically, share parts of their genome identical by descent (IBD), that is, inherited from a common ancestor within a family, has been particularly useful. Implemented in software such as Mapmaker/Sibs *(7)*, GENEHUNTER *(8,9)*, and SPLINK *(10)*, they are based on comparing the likelihood assuming a gene effect with that under a null hypothesis of no involvement with the trait of interest. The affected sib–pair method initially proposed by Risch *(11,12)* has been developed to a significant extent *(13)* and has been used effectively in whole-genome studies of many complex traits.

Some work has been done on extending the sib–pair method to larger sibships *(14)* and even to extended multiplex families *(15)*, but they have been dogged by difficulty in interpretation of what is actually being tested *(16)*, and other approaches based on multivariate statistics have shown more promise *(17)*.

3.1.1. Regressive Models

The basic formulation for linkage analysis of QTL using sibling pairs was first outlined by Haseman and Elston more than 27 years ago *(18)*. This procedure involves regressing the squared intrapair difference in trait values, D, on the fraction of alleles shared IBD by the sibpair at the trait locus, π. Note that in this formulation, D and π are measures of similarity at the phenotype and at the trait locus, respectively. For example, if i indicates the ith sibling pair out of N sibpairs sampled, then a simple linear regressive model relating D to π can be constructed as follows

$$E(D_i | \pi_i) = \alpha + \beta \pi_i$$

Where β is the regression coefficient and α *is* the intercept term. Under certain assumptions, Haseman and Elston *(18)* showed that the regression equation also holds when IBD proportions are replaced by estimates. Specifically, $E(D_i | \pi_i) = \alpha + \beta \hat{\pi}_i$ where $\hat{\pi}_i$ is an estimate of the marker locus IBD proportions, $\beta \cong -2(1 - 2\theta)^2 \sigma_g^2$, θ the recombination fraction between the trait and marker loci, and σ_g^2 is the genetic variance of the trait. This simple technique has been extended to include IBD sharing proportions estimated from genotype data on multiple loci surrounding the locus of interest *(7,19)*. Usually, the regression coefficient and its standard error are estimated via least squares. Using standard asymptotic theory, one-sided t-tests are constructed to test for linkage H_O: $\beta = O$ against the alternative hypothesis H_1: $\beta < O$, as can nonparametric rank correlation tests *(18)*. This test has been implemented into the program GENEHUNTER *(9)*. Nonparametric tests, although slightly conservative, are robust against nonnormality assumptions. They are, therefore, well suited for traits with nonnormal distributions (e.g., many biochemical measurements, *see* **Note 1**).

3.1.2. The Variance Components Model

Given that measured trait values are distributed as normal, one can test for linkage by testing for differences in phenotypic covariation conditional on whether siblings share 0, 1, or 2 alleles identical by descent at a particular locus. Because the Haseman and Elston approach models intrapair differences as a measure of phenotypic similarity, this ignores information inherent in the multivariate distribution of individuals in the sibship. Recent work has shown that more extensive modeling of the complete multivariate distribution (bivariate normal if the sampling units are sibpairs) has enormous power advantages and flexibility *(20–22)*. The variance-components approach, therefore, has major advantages over the regressive model, allowing a more extensive separation of the observed phenotypic variance into estimable components characterizing gene-/locus-specific effects, additive genetic effects, shared environment and random effects. In addition, these models can accommodate covariates, environmental factors, and multilocus gene effects. These models are implemented in the current release of GENEHUNTER (version 2.0). Recent simulation studies have shown that variance components models are more powerful than the ordinary regressive models *(23,24)*. However, these models are more sensitive to distributional assumptions.

3.1.3. A Genome Scan Protocol

There are many analysis tools for genome scanning for quantitative trait loci, including Mapmaker/Sibs, particularly suited for QTL mapping in nuclear families *(7)*; GENEHUNTER for extended families *(8,9)*, and other more general modeling packages such as SAGE *(25)*, GAS *(26)*, SOLAR *(27)*, and Mx *(28)*. However, for the purposes of this illustration, we consider Mapmaker/Sibs.

To perform linkage analysis using Mapmaker/Sibs, three input files are required (*see* **Figs. 1–3**). Having created the input files using a standard text editor, performing the analysis is straightforward. The file shown in **Fig. 4** can be executed on most Unix systems with

```
sibs < myfile & [return]
```

The program first loads the locus, pedigree, and phenotype files, then specifies the density at which sharing probabilities would be estimated across the genome and how far beyond the most terminal markers the program should

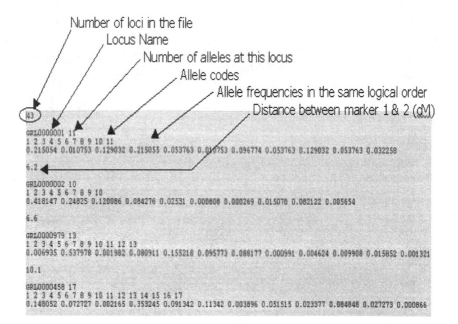

Fig. 1. A sample locus description file. This is the file specifying information about markers and mapping information. Mapmaker/Sibs would also accept locus files in standard LINKAGE format.

estimate these probabilities. Finally, the program fits the chosen model to the data and computes the appropriate linkage statistic.

The sharing probability at any point takes into account marker information at that point and all its neighbors. These are multipoint sharing probabilities. Alternatively, sharing at each locus may be restricted to the marker information at that locus and is called single-point linkage. Admittedly, multipoint linkage is much more powerful, as it uses as much linkage information in the data as possible. With the sharing probabilities estimated, we can fit various models to the data to determine evidence for linkage using either maximum likelihood (if the phenotypic data are reasonably normally distributed) or less powerful but more robust nonparametric methods if the data are nonnormally distributed. The output is a text file summarizing the likelihood for linkage at each scanned location and, if desired, a postscript file of the linkage results. Instead of running such analysis iteratively, especially when analyzing many phenotypes at the same time, the commands could be collated into a file and executed in batch mode. An example command file showing how this is done is shown in **Fig. 4** and a sample set of results in **Fig. 5**, with a corresponding graph in **Fig. 6**.

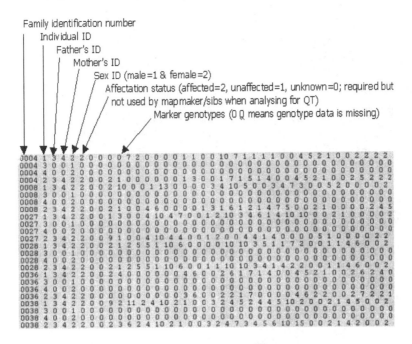

Fig. 2. A sample pedigree file. This file specifies the interrelationship between individuals in a sibship and their respective genotypic constitution for all the markers in the locus file. It is worth noting that this file has the same format as a linkage pedigree input file before further processing using MAKEPED.

3.2. Fine Mapping Strategies: Modeling Genotype/Phenotype Correlations

As stated in **Subheading 1.**, mapping diseases of complex etiology through conventional linkage approaches would often localize the disease susceptibility gene to quite a large region. Fine mapping and candidate gene association studies are then needed to further localize and isolate these genes. This involves testing the contribution of candidate polymorphisms to variation in trait values or susceptibility to disease. There are many methods for testing and quantifying the effect of candidate locus genotypes on a disease or quantitative trait. First, with properly designed case/control studies, we test whether or not a particular allele (or combination of alleles) at a candidate locus occur more or less frequently in cases than in the control group. Recent work has shown that testing for genotype-specific relative risks, whereas restricting the parameter space to the set of biologically plausible models increases statistical power and efficiency *(29)*.

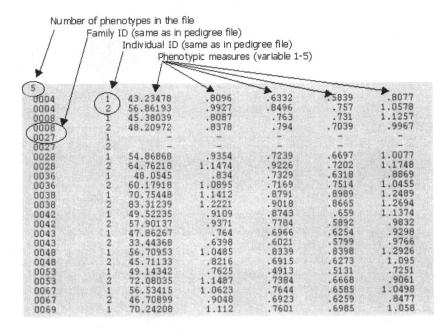

Fig. 3. A phenotype file. The phenotype file lists the quantitative phenotypic measures for all siblings, excluding parents. Family and individual ID in this file should correspond to those in the pedigree file. A phenotype file can have one or more phenotypes. Note that missing phenotypic measures are denoted by "–".

Second, with quantitative traits, especially in randomly ascertained family data, we estimate and test the equality of mean phenotype values associated with each genotype (*see* **Fig. 7**). This is analogous to an analysis of variance but allowing for within-family correlation using the generalized estimating equation (GEE) *(30,31)*. A positive finding for association is taken as evidence that the polymorphism is close to a disease or trait susceptibility gene or that it is the candidate gene itself. This approach is referred to as the "mean effects" model. Other investigators have shown, by simulation, that the mean effects model is superior to other variance component linkage models in sibpair studies with biallelic markers. With the proliferation of SNPs and SNP maps, this strategy is likely to make a significant contribution to QTL mapping.

3.2.1. A Protocol for Applying GEE Using the STATA Package

Suppose we have N independent observations for a response variable, Y, assumed to be distributed as normal with mean vector μ given by the regression model $\mu = \beta X$, β are the regression parameters to be estimated. The rela-

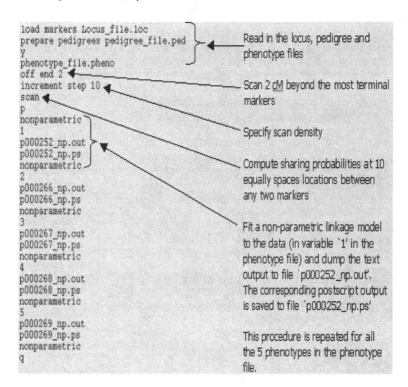

```
load markers Locus_file.loc
prepare pedigrees pedigree_file.ped
y
phenotype_file.pheno
off end 2
increment step 10
scan
p
nonparametric
1
p000252_np.out
p000252_np.ps
nonparametric
2
p000266_np.out
p000266_np.ps
nonparametric
3
p000267_np.out
p000267_np.ps
nonparametric
4
p000268_np.out
p000268_np.ps
nonparametric
5
p000269_np.out
p000269_np.ps
nonparametric
q
```

Read in the locus, pedigree and phenotype files

Scan 2 cM beyond the most terminal markers

Specify scan density

Compute sharing probabilities at 10 equally spaces locations between any two markers

Fit a non-parametric linkage model to the data (in variable `1' in the phenotype file) and dump the text output to file `p000252_np.out'. The corresponding postscript output is saved to file `p000252_np.ps'

This procedure is repeated for all the 5 phenotypes in the phenotype file.

Fig. 4. Sample mapmaker/sibs annotated command file. These analyses could be carried out interactively by typing in these commands or in noninteractive mode by typing "sibs< myfile &" at the Unix command line.

tionship between the mean vector and the linear part of the model, $g(\mu)$, is called the *link function*. For independent observations with variance v, the score function or estimating equation, $U(\beta)$, is calculated from independent contributions $U(\beta) = \Sigma u_i$, where $u_i = (1/v)(y_i - \mu)x$. The variance for U is estimated by $\text{var}(U) = U(u_i)^2$ and that of the regression coefficients, β, estimated as $(I)^{-2}\Sigma(u_i)^2$. This argument only holds when the score contributions, u_i, are independent, otherwise, $\Sigma(u_i)^2$ would not accurately estimate $\text{var}(U)$.

For clustered observations, we may use subscript t to denote the family to which each subject belongs. In this case:

1. $(y_i - \mu i)$ is a vector with elements $(Y_{it} - \mu_{it})$
2. x_i is a vector with elements x_{it}, and
3. v_i is a matrix with elements $v_i(st) = \text{Cov}(Y_{is}, Y_{it})$.

In vector and matrix notation, $U(\beta) = \Sigma(y_i - \mu_i)^{\text{T}} \cdot v_i^{-1} \cdot x_i$. In other words, if we redefine the covariance matrices, v_i, as sets of regression equations for each

```
pos      Z-score

 4.650   -0.175078
35.400   -0.121088
36.150   -0.066302
36.900   -0.011353
37.650    0.043118
38.400    0.096504
39.150    0.148260
39.900    0.197923
40.680    0.257036
41.460    0.317135
42.240    0.377253
43.020    0.436402
43.800    0.493641
44.580    0.548136
45.360    0.599200
46.140    0.646326
46.920    0.689191
47.700    0.727645
48.590    0.683388
49.480    0.634657
50.370    0.581815
51.260    0.525480
52.150    0.466513
53.040    0.405956
53.930    0.344946
54.820    0.284617
55.710    0.226004
56.600    0.169971
57.600    0.158029
58.600    0.145146
59.600    0.131316
60.600    0.116597
61.600    0.101126
```

Fig. 5. Sample output result file from a nonparametric analysis listing the Z score for each map location.

$(y_{it} - \mu_{it})$ on all the other $(y_{is} - \mu_{it})$, $s \neq t$, then, each observation which is largely predicted by other observations within the same family will, intuitively, make little or no contribution to the score function. Hence, using measurements on sibling data as though they were independent observations (e.g., $2N$) would yield wrong standard errors for the regression parameters. Often these standard errors are underestimated leading to exaggerated p-values.

In what follows, we assume that the reader has some elementary knowledge of data structures in STATA and how to read in such data. The two important commands here are xtgee and xtgls. The latter is most suitable for time series or longitudinal data with the number of time periods the *same* as the number of clusters (or siblings in the study). This type of well-balanced data are more common in model organisms but difficult to find in human genetic data. We therefore restrict our discussion here to the xtgee command.

Usually, STATA holds its data in virtual memory and variables are by default stored as categorical variables. Unfortunately, xtgee does not understand this. One has to explicitly "ask" STATA to expand a categorical variable

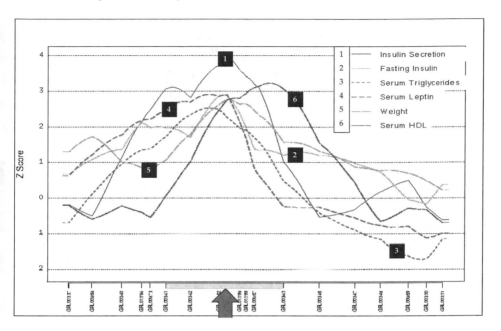

Fig. 6. Sample linkage trace plots for five physiologically related phenotypes show-ing subtle evidence for linkage clustering in these phenotypes, all related to the devel-opment of metabolic syndrome or "Syndrome X," a clustering of type 2 diabetes (insulin resistance and secretion are surrogate risk factors), hypertension, hyperlipi-demia, and obesity. This kind of localized clustering of linked regions for phenotypes that are not all highly statistically correlated demonstrates the value of broad phenotyping in the study of complex disease.

into dummy variables. This can be done either manually or by using the STATA command, *xi*.

Let us look at the xtgee command in some detail. At the STATA prompt, you may type the following:

```
STATA> Xtgee <depvar> <varlist>, <family>(<model>)
link(<link function>) corr(<correlation structure>)
                i(<family>) [robust]
```

where
- <depvar> is the dependent variable, e.g., body mass index and serum insulin levels.
- <varlist> are the independent variables or covariates, e.g., age, height, and genotypic information.
- family(<model>) specifies the assumed distribution for the dependent vari-able <depvar>, whereas <model> is one of the following:

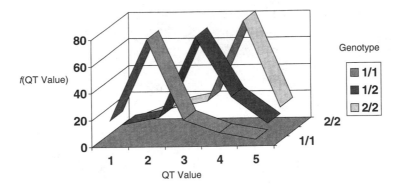

Fig. 7. The mean effects model (simplified). A typical SNP will partition into three distinct genotypes in the population. By comparing the three corresponding quantitative trait (QT) distributions using a test similar to an analysis of variance, it is possible to test the relationship between the SNP and the QT. In this example, it is clear by observation that a significant difference exists.

1. *Binomial:* If the disease endpoint is the dependent variable, i.e., affected/nonaffected.
2. *Gaussian or normal* (the default): This specifies that random errors are normally distributed. This is suitable for nearly all analysis of continuous response variables, but a gamma distribution is sometimes a more useful alternative.
3. *Gamma:* May be suitable for distributions that are clearly nonnormal, and
4. *Poisson:* Suitable for counted data, e.g., the number of fractures, number of cigarettes/packets smoked, and so on.

- `<link function>` specifies the relationship between the mean response and the independent variables, $g(\mu) = \beta X$.

- `corr(<correlation structure>)` Specifies a convenient working correlation structure within clusters or sibships, chosen from the following menu:

1. Independence (zero correlation)
2. Exchangeable (all within family correlations equal)
3. Unstructured (all within family correlations potentially different)
4. Stationary (all correlations with the same lag equal), and
5. Autoregressive (correlations of an ARn process, i.e., correlation goes down exponentially with separation in time).

Usually, assuming that the correlation within clusters is constant is probably sufficient.

- `i(<variable>)`: The dummy variable that identifies the family to which subject belongs, and

- The robust option is used if the data are clearly nonnormal. Although this option ensures convergence even if the data are clearly nonnormal, the parameter estimates might not be true maxima and the results should be interpreted with caution.

3.3. Haplotype Analysis

In the study of simple mendelian diseases—in particular, rare traits for which it is difficult to assemble a corroborative set of recombination events—haplotype analysis has often provided greater information for localization. For example, tracing the cosegregation of disease and marker haplotypes in families that independently support linkage can reveal key recombination events that may exclude those regions of the genome deemed to be incompatible with the known genetic model and would suggest flanking markers to the disease locus. However, common diseases are genetically heterogeneous with the same clinical manifestation under the influence of a combination of many small-effect genes. Clusters of high-risk families are therefore difficult to find. There are merits of being able to map multiple genes.

Although there is renewed interest in developing algorithms for haplotype reconstruction in the absence of phase information, haplotype analysis techniques in quantitative genetics research are still in their infancy, although with a lot of promise *(32–34)*.

4. Note

The regression technique has found great application in twin and sibling designs where the basic linear model is easily extended to test for measured environmental effects as well as gene/environmental effects.

Acknowledgments

The authors would like to thank Gemini Genomics for support during the preparation of this manuscript.

References

1. Lathrop, G. M. and Lalouel, J. M. (1984) Easy calculations of lod scores and genetic risks on small computers. *Am. J. Hum. Genet.* **36,** 460–465.
2. McKusick, V. A. (1994) Mendelian Inheritance in Man, in *Catalogs of Human Genes and Genetic Disorders,* 11th ed., John Hopkins University Press, Baltimore, MD.
3. Bryant, S. P. (1994) Genetic linkage analysis, in *Guide to Human Genome Computing* (Bishop, M. J. B., ed.), Academic Press, London, pp. 59–110.
4. Bryant, S. P. (1998) Constructing and using genetic maps, in *Handbook of Genome Analysis* (Spurr, N. K., Young, B. D., and Bryant, S. P., eds.), ICRF Blackwells, Oxford, UK, pp. 43–87.

5. Grant, S. F. A., Reid, D. M., Blake, G., Herd, R., Fogelman, I., and Ralston, S. H. (1996) Reduced bone density and osteoporosis associated with a polymorphic Spl binding site in the collagen type I-alpha 1 gene. *Nature Genet.* **14,** 203–305.
6. Masi, L., Becherini, L., Gennari, L., Colli, E., Mansani, R., Falchetti, A., et al. (1998) Allelic variants of human calcitonin receptor: distribution and association with bone mass in postmenopausal Italian women. *Biochem. Biophys. Res. Commun.* **245,** 622–626.
7. Kruglyak, L. and Lander, E. S. (1995) Complete multipoint sib-pair analysis of qualitative and quantitative traits. *Am. J. Hum. Genet.* **57,** 439–454.
8. Kruglyak, L. and Lander, E. S. (1995) High–resolution genetic mapping of complex traits. *Am. J. Hum. Genet.* **56,** 1212–1223.
9. Kruglyak, L., Daly, M. J., Reeve–Daly, M. P., and Lander, E. S. (1996) Parametric and nonparametric linkage analysis: a unified multipoint approach. *Am. J. Hum. Genet.* **58,** 1347–1363.
10. Holman, P. and Clayton, D. (1995) Efficiency of typing unaffected relatives in an affected-sib-pair linkage study with single-locus and multiple tightly linked markers. *Am. J. Hum. Genet.* **57,** 1221–1232.
11. Risch, N. (1990a) Linkage strategies for genetically complex traits: I. multilocus models. *Am. J. Hum. Genet.* **46,** 222–228.
12. Risch, N. (1990b) Linkage strategies for genetically complex traits: II. The power of affected relative pairs. *Am. J. Hum. Genet.* **46,** 229–241.
13. Holmans, P. (1993) Asymptotic properties of affected-sib-pair linkage analysis. *Am. J. Hum. Genet.* **52,** 362–374.
14. Lange, K. (1986a) A test statistic for the affected-sib-set method. *Ann. Hum. Genet.* **50,** 283–290.
15. Weeks, D. E. and Lange, K. (1988) The affected-pedigree-member method of linkage analysis. *Am. J. Hum. Genet.* **42,** 315–326.
16. Babron, M. C., Martinez, M., Bonaite-Pellie, C., and Clerget-Darpoux, F. (1993) Linkage detection by the affected-pedigree-member method: what is really tested? *Genet. Epidemiol.* **10,** 389–394.
17. Allison, D. B., Thiel, B., St Jean, P., Elston, R. C., Infante, M. C., and Schork, N. J. (1998) Multiple phenotype modelling in gene-mapping studies of quantitative traits: power advantages. *Am. J. Hum. Genet.* **63,** 1190–1201.
18. Haseman, J. K. and Elston, R. C. (1972) The investigation of linkage between a quantitative trait and a marker locus. *Behav. Genet.* **2,** 3–19.
19. Fulker, D. W. and Cardon, L. R. (1994) A sib-pair approach to interval mapping of quantitative trait loci. *Am. J. Hum. Genet.* **54,** 1092–1103.
20. Searle, S. R., Casella, G., and McCulloch, C. E. (1992) *Variance Components,* John Wiley and Sons, New York.
21. Schork, N. J., North, S. P., Lindpainter, K., and Jacob, H. J. (1996) Extensions to quantitative trait locus mapping in experimental organisms. *Hypertension* **28,** 1104–1111.
22. Amos, C. I. (1994) Robust variance-component approach for assessing genetic linkage pedigrees. *Am. J. Hum. Genet.* **54,** 535–543.

23. Goldgar, D. E. (1990) Multipoint analysis of human quantitative genetic variation. *Am. J. Hum. Genet.* **47,** 957–967.
24. Schork, N. J. (1993) Extended multipoint identity-by-descent analysis of human quantitative traits: efficiency, power and modelling considerations. *Am. J. Hum. Genet.* **53,** 1306–1319.
25. SAGE (1994) *Statistical Analysis for Genetic Epidemiology,* Computer package, available from the Department of Epidemiology and Biostatistics, Case Western Reserve University, Cleveland, OH.
26. GAS Package Version 2.0, available from Dr. Alan Young, Oxford University (http://users.ox.ac.uk/~ayoung/gas.html).
27. Blanjero, J. (1996) SOLAR: *Sequential Oligogenic Linkage Analysis Routines,* Population Genetics Lab Technical Report No. 6, Southwest Foundation for Biomedical Research, San Antonio, TX.
28. Neale, M. C. (1997) Mx: *Statistical Modelling,* 2nd ed., Box 980126 WCV, Richmond, VA 23298.
29. Chiano, M. N. and Clayton, D. G. (1998) Genotype relative risks under ordered restriction. *Genet. Epidemiol.* **15,** 135–146.
30. Zeger, S. L. and Liang, K. Y. (1986) Longitudinal data analysis for discrete and continuous outcomes. *Biometrics* **42,** 121–130.
31. Tregouet, D. A., Ducimetiere, P., and Tiret, L. (1997) Testing association in candidate-genes, markers and phenotype in related individuals, by use of estimating equations. *Am. J. Hum. Genet.* **61,** 189–199.
32. Excoffier, L. and Slatkin, M. (1995) Maximum-likelihood estimation of molecular haplotype frequencies in a diploid population. *Mol. Biol. Evol.* **12,** 921–927.
33. Chiano, M. N. and Clayton, D. G. (1998) Fine genetic mapping using haplotype analysis and the missing data problem. *Ann. Hum. Genet.* **62,** 55–60.
34. Martin, R. B., Maclean, C. J., Sham, P. C., Straub, R. E., and Kendler, K. S. (2000) The trimmed-haplotype test for linkage disequilibrium. *Am. J. Hum. Genet.* **66,** 1062–1075.

3

Sequence-Based Detection of Single Nucleotide Polymorphisms

Deborah A. Nickerson, Natali Kolker, Scott L. Taylor, and Mark J. Rieder

1. Introduction

One of the major tasks in human genome analysis is the identification and typing of DNA sequence variations (1). There are many types of sequence variations in the human genome. One type comprises sequences with variations in the number of repeat units such as short tandem repeat polymorphisms in the form of di-, tri, and tetranucleotide repeats; more complex sequence repeats such as variable number tandem repeats; or variations in the lengths of mononucleotide tracks such as A- or T-tracks in the genome. The other major type of variation in the genome arises from discrete changes in a specific DNA sequence such as small but unique base insertions or deletions, or more frequently as single nucleotide substitutions, also known as single nucleotide polymorphisms (SNPs). SNPs are the most abundant form of DNA sequence variation in the human genome (2). Based on their natural frequency and presence in both coding and noncoding regions, single nucleotide substitutions are probably the underlying cause of most phenotypic differences among humans. Therefore, the identification of SNPs in human genes will play an increasingly important role in analyzing genotype-phenotype correlations within and among human populations (2). Amplification of genomic DNA by the polymerase chain reaction (PCR) has greatly simplified the identification of SNPs by eliminating the need to clone and isolate regions of the genome from multiple individuals. Many approaches to find SNPs rely on first amplifying a specific region of the genome from several different individuals using PCR, and then comparing the properties or sequences of the amplified products to identify SNPs. Because of their biologic and medical importance, a wide array of

From: *Methods in Molecular Biology, vol. 175: Genomics Protocols*
Edited by: M. P. Starkey and R. Elaswarapu © Humana Press Inc., Totowa, NJ

methods have been developed to find single nucleotide substitutions including denaturing gradient analysis *(3,4)*, chemical or enzymatic cleavage *(5–7)*, heteroduplex or conformational analysis *(8,9)*, hybridization to oligonucleotide arrays *(10,11)* and DNA sequencing *(12,13)*. Direct sequence analysis has many advantages in variation analysis because it provides complete information about the nature and location of an SNP in a single pass, and it is amenable to automation, widely available, and simple to apply (only a single set of reagents and assay conditions is required). Additionally, rapid improvements in the sequencing chemistries *(14,15)*, instrumentation (high-throughput capillary-based systems *[16]*, and the development of automated analysis tools *(17–19)* have greatly enhanced the use of DNA sequencing in SNP detection. The following protocol provides an overview of the methods and computational tools that can be applied to find SNPs using fluorescence-based sequencing of PCR products.

2. Materials

1. Specific PCR primers to amplify a unique region of the genome for variation analysis.
2. 10X PCR buffer: 100 mM Tris-HCl, pH 8.3; 500 mM KCl, and 15 mM MgCl$_2$.
3. AmpliTaq DNA polymerase (Perkin-Elmer, Foster City, CA).
4. dNTPs (4 mM each).
5. Distilled H$_2$O.
6. Thermocycler.
7. PCR product presequencing kit; exonuclease I (10 U/µL) and shrimp alkaline phosphatase (SAP) (2 U/µL) (Amersham Life Sciences, Cleveland, OH).
8. Big-dye terminator sequence ready reaction kit (Perkin-Elmer).
9. 30% acrylamide stock: 37.5:1 acrylamide:N,N'-methylenbisacrylamide (Bio-Rad, Hercules, CA).
10. 377 DNA analyzer (Perkin Elmer Corporation).
11. 4% Denaturing polyacrylamide gel prepared and casted for sequence analysis by the 377 instrument directly according to the manufacturer's instructions (Perkin-Elmer).
12. 95% (v/v) Nondenaturing ethanol.
13. Loading buffer: 5:1 deionized formamide:50 mM EDTA, pH 8.0.
14. Sequence analysis tools: Phred, Phrap and Consed (*see* Tools/Protocols at http://www.genome.washington.edu/, and for PolyPhred *see* http://droog.mbt. washington.edu/).

3. Methods

3.1. PCR Amplification and Preparation Product for Sequencing

1. Amplify the genomic region of interest in 20-µL reactions containing 1X PCR buffer, 0.001% (w/v) gelatin, 0.4 mM dNTPs, 0.5 mM of each PCR primer, 0.5 U of AmpliTaq DNA polymerase, and 20 ng of genomic DNA (*see* **Note 1**).

2. Inactivate unincorporated PCR primers and deoxynucleotide triphosphates by combining 5 μL of the PCR product with 1 μL of 10 U/μL exonuclease and 1 μL of 2 U/μL SAP.
3. Incubate at 37°C for 30 min followed by 90°C for 15 min to inactivate the exonuclease and SAP enzymes prior to sequencing.

3.2. Sequencing of PCR Products

1. Assemble sequencing reactions by mixing 3.2 μL of the enzyme-treated PCR product; 4 pmol of sequencing primer (same as PCR primer) in 2.8 μL of dH_2O, 2 μL of 400 mM Tris-HCl, pH 9.0; 10 mM $MgCl_2$, and 2 μL of ready-reaction big-dye terminator mix (*see* **Note 2**).
2. Following a denaturation step at 95°C for 5 min, perform 30 thermocycles of the assembled sequencing reactions for 95°C for 30 s, 50°C for 10 s, and 60°C for 4 min.
3. Add 8 μL of deionized H_2O and 32 μL of nondenaturing 95% (v/v) ethanol and mix with a multichannel micropipettor.
4. Centrifuge at 3000g for 45 min.
5. Remove ethanol by inverting the microtray on a paper towel and centrifuging at 700g for 1 min.
6. Resuspend each sample in 3 μL of loading buffer.
7. Heat the samples for 2 min at 90°C and electrophorese through a prerun 4% (w/v) denaturing polyacrylamide gel using a 377 DNA analyzer (*see* **Note 3**).

3.3. Sequence Analysis SNP Identification

1. Following the sequencer run, verify lane tracking, and perform data extraction and first pass sequence analysis using the installed 377 software (*see* **Fig. 1** for an overview of the analysis events in SNP identification).
2. Transfer chromatogram files to a Unix or Linux workstation and reanalyze using the base-calling software Phred *(17,18)* (*see* **Note 4**).
3. Assemble the sequences using the Phrap program, which creates an ".ace" file.
4. Execute the program PolyPhred (*see* **Note 5**), using the ".ace" file as input, to identify heterozygous single nucleotide variants in fluorescence-based sequencing traces *(13)*. PolyPhred (*see* **Note 6**) reads the normalized peak information and quality values obtained by Phred for each position in a sequence. It then searches for reductions in peaks (*see* **Fig. 2**) across the contigs assembled by Phrap. If a peak drop and second base are detected by comparing the reads, PolyPhred calls the site a potential polymorphic site and tags the position in the sequence reads with their determined genotypes for later viewing with the Consed program *(19)* (*see* **Note 7**).
5. Using the Consed program, view the assembled sequence reads and mark polymorphic single nucleotide variants by color-coded tags for review and confirmation by an analyst.

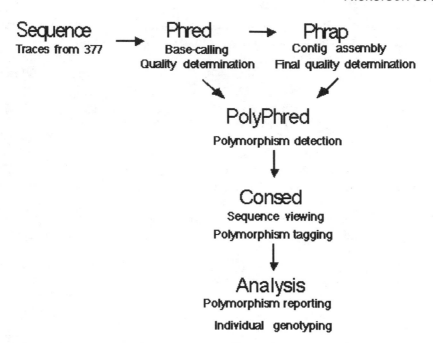

Fig. 1. An overview of the analysis tools used in SNP identification by fluorescence-based sequencing. PolyPhred, a polymorphism detection tool, is integrated with several other software tools, i.e., Phred, Phrap, and Consed, currently used in large-scale sequence analysis. Together these tools provide a system for genotyping SNPs in sequencing traces.

4. Notes

1. If a PCR product contains more than one band following DNA amplification, i.e., gives nonspecific products in addition to the specific product, then the PCR primer cannot be used as the sequencing primer after enzymatic treatment because it will yield low-quality sequences. In this case, several options are available. The most efficient option is to try to amplify the PCR product using a gradient thermocycler (e.g., Mastercycler gradient; Eppendorf, Westbury, NY). Using a gradient thermocycler, the conditions that optimize the specificity of the product can readily be determined. Another option is to purify the specific PCR product from the nonspecific ones by gel electrophoresis in 1% low-melting-point agarose *(12)*. The specific products are cut from the ethidium bromide–stained gel and purified using a Wizard PCR prep purification system (Promega, Madison, WI) according to the manufacturer's instructions. A final option, which is suggested if the region will be sequenced repeatedly and cannot be optimized for specificity, is to select and obtain a sequencing primer that is internal to the PCR primer(s), which will greatly improve the sequence quality obtained with enzymatically treated PCR products.

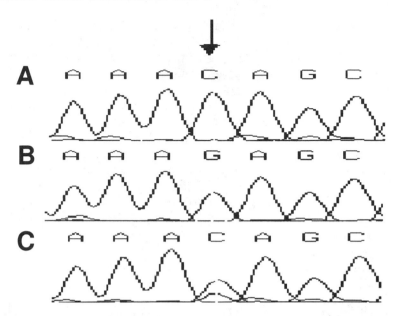

Fig. 2. An example of a single nucleotide substitution found in the human alpha T-cell receptor loci. (**A**) A portion of a sequencing trace from an individual homozygous for a C nucleotide at this polymorphic site (arrow); (**B**) an individual who is homozygous for the G allele; and (**C**) an individual heterozygous for this loci revealing both a C and G peak at the polymorphic position. Cases like this are often missed without programs such as PolyPhred because the heterozygous position is often called a homozygote if the two peaks do not overlap as shown in the example (**C**).

2. We recommend using a quarter of the sequence-ready big-dye terminator mix suggested by the manufacturer. This greatly reduces the amount of free dye associated with samples following ethanol precipitation. The presence of free dyes in the samples lowers the sequence quality and locally can affect the normalization process used by PolyPhred to identify SNPs.
3. It is important that the E-filter be used during data collection with the 377 sequencer. Failure to set this filter correctly will lead to the generation of low-quality sequence.
4. The Phred base-caller has been shown to have a lower error rate in base-calling than the 377 software *(17)*. Phred also provides an estimated error probability for each base-call, known as a quality score, which can be used to measure the success of the produced sequences *(18)*. Using this protocol, we routinely obtain at least 500 bp of sequence with an average Phred quality of 30. If lower sequence quality is obtained ensure that the samples are being mixed appropriately at the ethanol precipitation step and that the necessary rotation speed is being achieved during centrifugation, and check the purity of the PCR product either by using an internal primer or by isolating the product by band purification following gel electrophoresis *(12)*.

5. PolyPhred is integrated for use with Phred, Phrap, and Consed (**Fig. 1**) and cannot operate independently. PolyPhred detects the polymorphic site using a comparative approach, and, therefore, more than one trace across the same region is required for its detection of polymorphisms. This program is capable of detecting >99% of all potential heterozygotes using single-pass sequence data *(13)*. However, we have seen that there is a clear relationship between sequence quality (determined by Phred) and PolyPhred performance *(13)*. We have observed that higher sequence qualities yield greater specificity especially in heterozygote detection *(13)*.

6. Several command line parameters can be set in PolyPhred including the average sequence quality used to set the search limits in the sequence (default is quality of 30), peak drop ratio (default is 0.65), the background or second peak ratio (default is 0.25), the method of tagging polymorphisms on the sequence reads (polymorphism, genotype, or ranks; default is genotype tags), and the ranks of the polymorphic sites to be viewed in Consed (default shows ranks 1 to 3, highest likely polymorphic candidates). The default parameters are recommended for most situations and have been optimized by the analysis of more than 4 Mb of sequence. However, as the user gains more experience, variations in the command line parameters to increase the quality of the sequence examined and the ranks of the polymorphism viewed can be undertaken, and a simplified command line interface known as PolyTool provided with PolyPhred can help with this.

7. In analyzing specific regions of the genome, we have found that developing a set of highly annotated reference sequences and viewing these with Consed greatly simplifies data analysis *(20)*. We usually develop reference sequences containing information on the location of the PCR primers; coding, noncoding, repeat, or regulatory sequences; and known DNA variants. These reference sequences are assembled with the sequence trace data, and the information stored on the reference sequence provides a readily available visual database that can be accessed by Consed during the analysis phase of any project.

References

1. Lander, E. S. (1996) The new genomics: global views of biology. *Science* **264,** 536–539.
2. Collins, F. S., Guyer, M. S., and Chakravarti, A. (1997) Variations on a theme: Cataloging human DNA sequence variation. *Science* **278,** 1580, 1581.
3. Sheffield, V. C., Cox, D. R., Lerman, L. S., and Myers, R. M. (1989) Attachment of 40-base-pair G + C-rich sequence (GC-clamp) to genomic fragments by the polymerase chain reaction results in improved detection of single-base changes. *Proc. Natl. Acad. Sci. USA* **86,** 232–236.
4. Underhill, P. A., Jin, L., Lin, A. A., Mehdi, S. Q., Jenkins, T., Vollrath, R. W., Davis, R. W., Cavalli-Sforza, L. L., and Oefner, P. J. (1997) Detection of numerous Y chromosome biallelic polymorphisms by denaturing high-performance liquid chromatography. *Genome Res.* **7,** 996–1005.

5. Cotton, R. G., Rodrigues, N. R., and Campbell, R. D. (1988) Reactivity of cytosine and thymine in single-base-pair mismatches with hydroxylamine and osmium tetroxide and its application to the study of mutations. *Proc. Natl. Acad. Sci. USA* **85,** 4397–4401.
6. Myers, R. M., Larin, Z., and Maniatis, T. (1985) Detection of single base substitutions by ribonuclease cleavage at mismatches in RNA:DNA duplexes. *Science* **230,** 1242–1246.
7. Youil, R., Kemper, B. W., and Cotton, R. G. (1995) Screening for mutations by enzyme mismatch cleavage with T4 endonuclease VII. *Proc. Natl. Acad. Sci. USA* **92,** 87–91.
8. Keen, J., Lester, D., Inglehearn, C., Curtis, A., and Bhattacharya, S. (1991) Rapid detection of single-base mismatches as heteroduplexes on hydrolink gels. *Trends Genet.* **7,** 5.
9. Hayashi, K. (1991) PCR-SSCP: a simple and sensitive method for detection of mutations in genomic DNA. *Genomics* **5,** 874–879.
10. Hacia, J. G., Brody, L. C., Chee, M. S., Fodor, S. P. A., and Collins, F. S. (1996) Detection of heterozygous mutations in BRCA1 using high-density oligonucleotide arrays and two-colour fluorescence analysis. *Nature Genet.* **14,** 441–447.
11. Chee, M. S., Yang, R, Hubbell, E., Berno, A., Huang, X. C., Stern, D., Winlcler, J., Lockhart, D. J., Morris, M. S., and Fodor, S. P. (1996) Accessing genetic information with high-density DNA arrays. *Science* **274,** 610–614.
12. Kwok, P., Carlson, C., Yager, T. D., Ankener, W., and Nickerson, D. A. (1994) Comparative analysis of human DNA variations by fluorescence-based sequencing of PCR products. *Genomics* **23,** 138–144.
13. Nickerson, D. A., Tobe, V. O., and Taylor, S. L. (1997) PolyPhred: automating the detection of single nucleotide substitutions using fluorescence-based sequencing. *Nucleic Acids Res.* **14,** 2745–2751.
14. Ju, J., Glazer, A. N., and Mathies, R. A. (1996) Energy transfer primers: a new fluorescence labeling paradigm for DNA sequencing and analysis. *Nature Med.* **2,** 246–249
15. Rosenblum, B. B., Lee, L. G., Spurgeon, S. L., Khan, S. H., Menchen, S. M., Heiner, C. R., and Chen, S. M. (1997) New dye-labeled terminators for improved DNA sequencing patterns. *Nucleic Acids Res.* **25,** 4500–4504.
16. Mullikin, J. C. and McMurragy, A. A. (1999) Techview: DNA sequencing. Sequencing the genome, fast. *Science* **283,** 1867–1869.
17. Ewing, B., Hillier, L., Wendl, M. C., and Green, P. (1998) Base-calling of automated sequencer traces using Phred. I. Accuracy assessment. *Genome Res.* **8,** 175–185.
18. Ewing, B. and Green, P. (1998) Base-calling of automated sequencer traces using Phred. II. Error probabilities. *Genome Res.* **8,** 186–194.
19. Gordon, D., Abajian, C., and Green, P. (1998) Consed: a graphical interface tool for sequence finishing. *Genome Res.* **8,** 195–202.
20. Rieder, M. J., Taylor, S. L., Tobe, V. O., and Nickerson, D. A. (1998) Automating the identification of DNA variations using quality-based fluorescence-resequencing: analysis of the human mitochondrial genome. *Nucleic Acids Res.* **26,** 967–973.

4

Genomic Mismatch Scanning for the Mapping of Genetic Traits

Farideh Mirzayans and Michael A. Walter

1. Introduction

Genome mismatch scanning (GMS) is a rapid method of isolating regions of identity by descent (IBD) between two related individuals *(1–5)*. With the availability of simple PCR techniques, vast numbers of highly informative genomewide polymorphic markers, and more recently, radiation hybrid mapping, DNA microarrays, and gene chip technology (Research Genetics, AL), GMS is a very practical shortcut to conventional genetic linkage methods. The basic procedure (**Fig. 1**) involves the restriction enzyme digestion of each of the genomic DNA samples from two related individuals, yielding fragment sizes up to 20 kb, followed by the methylation of one genome. Hybridization of the two genomes (one fully methylated and one fully unmethylated) results in four possible DNA hybrid fragments. Through specific restriction enzyme digestions, the fully methylated and the fully unmethylated homohybrids (both strands from the same individual) are removed. The *E. coli* mismatch repair enzyme selection facilitates the removal of most of the mismatch-containing heterohybrids *(6,7)*, therefore, DNA fragments from all IBD regions are isolated on the basis of their ability to form extended mismatch-free heterohybrids (double-stranded DNA [dsDNA] molecules consisting of one strand from each of the individuals). These GMS-enriched mismatch-free heterohybrids are likely to include a disease gene locus inherited through a common ancestor. The heterohybrid DNA pool, recovered through the GMS process, can be subjected to polymerase chain reaction (PCR) using polymorphic markers for a genomewide scan. The GMS-selected DNA pool may also be subjected to whole-genome amplification techniques such as inter-alu PCR, to generate sufficient amounts of DNA for hybridizing to cDNA

From: *Methods in Molecular Biology, vol. 175: Genomics Protocols*
Edited by: M. P. Starkey and R. Elaswarapu © Humana Press Inc., Totowa, NJ

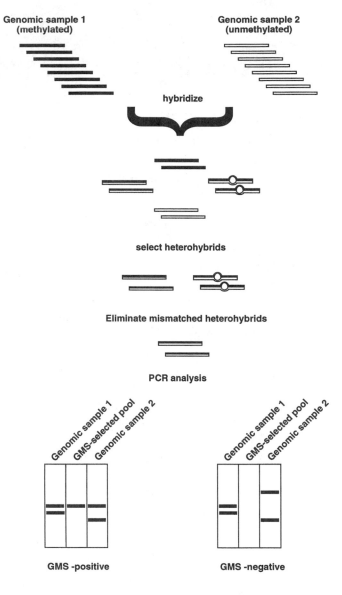

Fig. 1. A schematic outline of the GMS process.

microarray blots *(8,9)* or GeneFilters Microarrays (Research Genetics) to scan the human genome to identify genes that lie in the shared IBD regions. Although modifications can be made to improve the yield and sensitivity of this relatively new approach to genetic linkage analysis, GMS is still a sufficiently

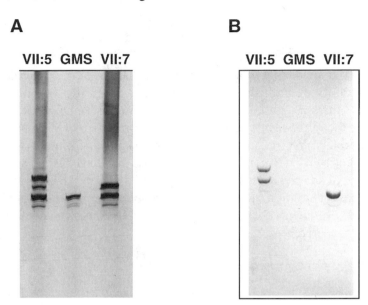

Fig. 2. Examples of results obtained from analysis of GMS-selected DNA pool. (**A**) Positive GMS results obtained with microsatellite marker D6S1281. A PCR product corresponding to one allele shared between the two individuals (pedigree numbers VII:5 and VII:7 *[3]*) is recovered in the GMS lane. (**B**) Negative results obtained with microsatellite marker D6S1040. No PCR product is recovered in the GMS pool when the two individuals do not share any alleles of this marker.

robust technique for identifying IBD regions for mapping complex human diseases *(3,4,10)*. We have successfully used GMS to identify the chromosomal region containing the iridogoniodysgenesis anomaly (IGDA) locus using DNA samples from two fifth-degree cousins from a large Canadian family *(3)*. IGDA is a rare autosomal dominant ocular neurocristopathy that involves hypoplasia of the iris stroma and iridocorneal angle defects leading to elevated intraocular pressure and glaucoma in more than 50% of affected individuals. Experiments in our laboratory using conventional linkage methods with this large family indicated that an 8.3-c*M* region of chromosome 6p25 contained the IGDA locus *(11)*. GMS-selected hybrid DNA and individual DNA samples from each of the two cousins used for GMS were subsequently typed for polymorphic markers on chromosome 6. PCR products indicating IBD regions were recovered in the GMS-enriched pool (**Fig. 2**), whereas control markers on a second chromosome (chromosome 12) were not recovered.

2. Materials

2.1. DNA Sample Selection

Detailed statistical analyses regarding the selection of the two related individuals for GMS are published elsewhere *(3,12)*. Basically, one is attempting to maximize the size of the IBD region containing the gene of interest, while minimizing the number of additional IBD regions shared by chance between these individuals. We recommend that DNA samples from fourth- or fifth-degree cousins be used to conduct GMS, because they have 89 and 86% chance, respectively, of sharing at least one marker residing in the IBD region containing the disease gene for a map density of 10 cM. The probability of sharing at least two IBD segments for fourth- or fifth-degree cousins is negligible—2.5 and 0.5%, respectively.

2.2. DNA Prepared from Blood

Approximately 20 mL of blood from each individual (**Subheading 2.1.**) is collected in EDTA tubes and DNA is extracted using conventional methods *(13,14)*.

2.3. Solutions and Reagents

1. 1 M Tris-HCl, pH 7.6; and 1 M Tris-HCl, pH 8.0. Autoclave and store at room temperature.
2. 0.5 M Disodium EDTA, pH 8.0. Sterilize by autoclaving and store at room temperature.
3. TE buffer: 10 mM Tris and 0.1 mM EDTA, pH 7.6. Autoclave and store at 4°C.
4. 4 M Ammonium acetate. Filter sterilize through a 0.22-μm membrane and store at 4°C.
5. 95% (v/v) Ethanol. Denatured ethanol is used to precipitate DNA in the presence of moderate concentrations of salt such as ammonium or sodium acetates. Store at –20°C.
6. 70% (v/v) Ethanol. Use to wash DNA precipitates and store at 4°C.
7. 5 M Sodium chloride. Sterilize by autoclaving and store at room temperature.
8. 1 M Magnesium chloride. Autoclave and store at room temperature.
9. Bovine serum albumin (BSA) 20 mg/mL (cat. no. 711 454; Roche, Laval, Québec, Canada). Store at –20°C.
10. Formamide, deionized. Store in a dark bottle at 4°C. Deionized formamide should be clear; if it is yellow, it must be deionized or a new batch obtained.
11. Buffer-saturated phenol. This reagent is used for DNA extractions. Store at 4°C.
12. Chloroform:isoamyl alcohol (24:1 [v/v]). Store in a dark bottle at room temperature.
13. Buffer-saturated phenol:chloroform/isoamyl alcohol (1:1).
14. Water-saturated phenol. This reagent is used to form an emulsion with the formamide phenol emulsion reassociation technique (FPERT) hybridization solution. Store at 4°C.

15. 3 *M* Sodium thiocyanate. Filter sterilize using a 0.45-µm filter and store at –80°C. Handle powdered sodium thiocyanate (highly poisonous) with extreme caution and only in a chemical fume hood carefully following the manufacturer's instructions.

16. FPERT hybridization solution: 2 *M* sodium thiocyanate; 10 m*M* Tris-HCl, pH 8.0; 0.1 m*M* EDTA; and 8% (v/v) formamide. Divide into 1-mL aliquots and store at –20°C.

17. 1 *M* Potassium chloride. Sterilize by autoclaving and store at room temperature.

18. 1 *M* HEPES-KOH, pH 8.0. Filter sterilize using a 0.22-µm syringe filter and store at –20°C.

19. Dithiothreitol (DTT) (500 m*M*). Filter sterilize (0.22-µm syringe filter) and store in 1-mL aliquots at –20°C.

20. 10X Mismatch repair enzyme buffer: 200 m*M* KCl; 500 m*M* HEPES-KOH, pH 8.0; 50 m*M* MgCl$_2$; 10 m*M* DTT; 500 µg/mL of BSA. Divide into 1-mL aliquots and store at –20°C. Prepare a 1X buffer just before use.

21. 50 m*M* Adenosine 5' triphosphate (ATP) (cat. no. A6419, Sigma-Aldrich Canada, Oakville, Ontario, Canada). Store in 1-mL aliquots at –20°C.

22. Benzolated naphthoylated DEAE cellulose (BNDC), medium mesh (cat. no. B6385; Sigma-Aldrich Canada). Equilibrate 500 mg of BNDC beads in 2.5 mL of 50 m*M* Tris-HCl (pH 8.0) and 1 *M* NaCl for 24–48 h on a rotary mixer (Hematology mixer, cat. no. 14-059-346, Fisher Scientific Ltd., Nepean, Ontario, Canada). We recommend that this equilibration step be done just before needed, at 4°C to prevent bacterial growth.

2.4. Restriction and Modifying Enzymes

All the restriction and modifying enzymes mentioned listed next were obtained from New England Biolabs (Mississauga, Ontario, Canada).

1. *Pst*I restriction endonuclease (20 U/µL) and 10X NEB buffer 3 (1 *M* NaCl; 500 m*M* Tris-HCl; 100 m*M* MgCl$_2$; 10 m*M* DTT, pH 7.9). Store at –20°C (*see* **Note 1**).

2. *Dpn*I restriction endonuclease (20 U/µL) and 10X NEB buffer 4 (500 mM potassium acetate; 200 m*M* Tris-acetate; 100 m*M* magnesium acetate; 1 m*M* DTT, pH 7.9). *Dpn*I recognizes and cleaves GA↓TC when the adenine residue is methylated. Store at –20°C (*see* **Notes 2** and **3**).

3. *Mbo*I restriction endonuclease (25 U/µL) and 10X NEB buffer 3. *Mbo*I recognizes and cleaves ↓GATC when the adenine residue is not methylated. Store at –20°C (*see* **Notes 2** and **3**).

4. *dam* Methylase (8 U/µL). This enzyme is supplied with 10X methylase buffer (500 m*M* Tris-HCl, pH 7.5; 100 m*M* EDTA; 50 m*M* 2-mercaptoethanol) and 32 m*M* *S*-adenosylmethionine (SAM). Store at –20°C. *dam* Methylase methylates the adenine residue within its GATC recognition site (*see* **Note 4**).

5. Exonuclease III (100 U/µL). Store at –20°C (*see* **Note 2**).

2.5. Mismatch Repair Enzymes

E. coli methyl-directed mismatch repair enzymes MutH (500 ng/µL; cat. no. 71432), MutL (0.28 µg/µL; cat. no. 71435), and MutS (2 U/µL; cat no.

71422, special lot no.200196) (Amersham Pharmacia Biotech, Piscataway, NJ). Store at –80°C (*see* **Note 5**).

2.6. Equipment

1. Polypropylene snap-cap culture tubes (5 mL) (cat. no. 2063, Falcon; Fisher).
2. Vortex mixer (cat. no. 12-812; Fisher).
3. Nalgene polypropylene tubes (30 mL) (cat. no. 05-529-1C; Fisher).
4. Beckman Avanti J-25I centrifuge (Beckman, Mississauga, Ontario, Canada).
5. DNA DipSticks (cat. no. K5632-01; Invitrogen, Carlsbad, CA).

2.7. Genomewide Polymorphic Marker Sets

Whole-genome screening sets and single chromosome scan sets that have been multiplexed by chromosome are available from Research Genetics. These primer sets are available unlabeled or fluorescently labeled for automated systems.

2.8. GeneFilters Microarrays

Several human GeneFilters Microarrays are available through Research Genetics. These consist of DNA from thousands of I.M.A.G.E. consortium cDNA clones arrayed on 5 × 7 cm membranes and permit a high-density expression scan of the human genome using radioactive or nonradioactive methods. Complete description of these microarrays can be obtained from the Research Genetics Web site (http://www.resgen.com).

3. Methods

Start with 100 μg of DNA resuspended in 100 μL of sterile ddH$_2$O (distilled and deionized water) from each of the two individuals selected for GMS (*[3,12]* also *see* **Subheading 2.1.**). It is recommended to start with a relatively large amount of genomic DNA (100 μg) from each individual because substantial loss of sample occurs in different selection steps of this procedure. Throughout this procedure, DNA concentrations should be measured as a guide for the researcher to adjust reagent volumes relative to the amount of DNA at each step.

1. Digest a 100-μg sample of DNA from each individual at 37°C with 200 U of *Pst*I in separate 300-μL overnight reactions (this will result in DNA fragment sizes of approx 20 kb and smaller (*see* **Note 1**).
2. To ensure that complete digestion of genomic DNA is achieved, take 6 μL (2 μg DNA) from each overnight digestion reaction and size separate by electrophoresis through a 0.8% (w/v) agarose gel. If digestion is not complete, add an additional 100 U of *Pst*I and continue digestion for several more hours.

3. Extract each digestion with an equal volume of 1:1 (v/v) phenol/chloroform. Precipitate the DNA from each upper aqueous phase by adding 2.5 vol of 95% (v/v) ethanol and $^1/_{10}$ vol of 4 M ammonium acetate. Resuspend each DNA sample in 98 μL of ddH$_2$O.

4. Methylate all 98 μg of DNA from one individual only using 240 U of *dam* methylase and 0.75 μL of SAM in a total volume of 300 μL. Add an additional 0.75 μL of SAM every 4 h if possible throughout the reaction, and continue methylation overnight (*see* **Note 4**).

5. The following day, inactivate *dam* methylase by incubating at 65°C for 15 min. Precipitate the DNA (as described in **step 3**) and resuspend in 98 μL of ddH$_2$O (final concentration of 1 μg/μL).

6. In 20-μL reactions, digest a 1-μg aliquot of each of the *Pst*I-digested, methylated and unmethylated DNA samples separately with 10 U of MboI and 20 U of *Dpn*I, respectively, at 37°C overnight. Analyze each digest by electrophoresis through a 1% (w/v) agarose gel (*see* **Note 3**).

7. Combine 97 μg of the *Pst*I-digested unmethylated DNA from one individual (from **step 3**) and 97 μg of the *Pst*I-digested methylated DNA from the second individual (from **step 5**) in a total volume of 194 μL and denature by heating at 95°C for 10 min. Centrifuge briefly and put on ice.

8. Add the DNA to 1 mL of FPERT hybridization mix in a 5-mL polypropylene snap-cap culture tube. Add 350 μL of water-saturated phenol to form an emulsion. Attach the reaction tube to a vortex mixer at a 30° angle and shake vigorously at three-quarter speed for 12–24 h at room temperature.

9. Extract the sample twice with equal volumes of chloroform and precipitate DNA from the upper aqueous phase with 10 vol of 95% (v/v) ethanol in a 30-mL polypropylene tube. Incubate at –80°C for at least 30 min. Centrifuge at 16,000*g* for 1 h at 4°C. Dissolve the pellet in 500 μL of TE buffer and precipitate again by adding 2.5 vol of 95% (v/v) ethanol and $^1/_{10}$ vol of 4 M ammonium acetate and incubating either at –20°C overnight or at –80°C for at least 30 min. Centrifuge at 16,000*g* for 1 h at 4°C, wash the pellet with 70% (v/v) ethanol, and resuspend in 200 μL of TE buffer.

10. To remove homohybrids of fully methylated or fully unmethylated DNA duplexes, double digest the hybridized DNA sample with *Mbo*I and *Dpn*I. Combine 200 μL of DNA mix, 40 μL of 10X NEB buffer 4, 10 μL of DpnI, 20 μL of MboI, and 130 μL of ddH$_2$O. Incubate overnight at 37°C (*see* **Note 2**).

11. Precipitate the DNA (as described in *step* 9) and resuspend the pellet in 100 μL of TE buffer.

12. Measure the concentration of the DNA in 1 μL of the sample using a DNA DipStick (*see* **Note 6**).

13. Set up the mismatch repair enzyme reaction by combining 100 μL ($\cong$60 μg) of DNA, 1.856 μL (930 μg) of MutH, 207.143 μL (60 μg) of MutL, 75 μL (150 U) of MutS, 835.4 μL of 10X mismatch repair enzyme buffer, 334.0 μL of 50 mM ATP, and 6.8006 mL of ddH$_2$O to bring the total reaction volume to 8.354 μL. Incubate at 37°C for 1 h and stop the reaction by heating at 65°C for 10 min (*see* **Note 5**).

14. Adjust the total volume of reaction mix to 9.28 mL by adding 926 µL of 10 m*M* MgCl$_2$, and 50 m*M* Tris-HCl, pH 8.0 (*see* **Note 7**) Add 200 U of exonuclease III and incubate for 15 min at 37°C (*see* **Note 8**).

15. Extract the sample once with an equal volume of phenol/chloroform. Add 2.4 mL of 5 *M* NaC1 to the aqueous phase to adjust the NaC1 concentration of the sample to 1 *M* NaCl, prior to BNDC treatment.

16. Centrifuge the equilibrated BNDC beads (**Subheading 2.3., item 22**) at 16,000*g* for 10 min and remove excess buffer. Add the GMS-selected DNA mix to the BNDC and mix on a rotary mixer for approx 4 h at either 4°C or at room temperature (*see* **Note 9**).

17. Centrifuge the BNDC-treated DNA sample at 16,000*g* for 10 min. Extract the supernatant containing the mismatch-free hemimethylated dsDNA with chloroform, and precipitate the DNA with 2.5 vol of 95% (v/v) ethanol and $^1/_{10}$ vol of 4 *M* ammonium acetate. Resuspend the DNA in 500 µL of TE.

18. Utilize the GMS product (GMS-selected DNA) in PCR reactions with multiplexed whole-genome markers to identify IBD regions in these related individuals. Alternatively, employ the GMS product to screen microarrays of known and unknown human genes.

4. Notes

1. *Pst*I restriction enzyme cleaves human genomic DNA, yielding fragment sizes of 2–20 kb with 3' overhangs, which protect these ends from being digested by exonuclease III at later stages of the procedure.

2. *Dpn*I and *Mbo*I cut the fully methylated and fully unmethylated duplexes, respectively, at GATC sites, leaving blunt ends *(Dpn*I*)* and 5' overhangs *(Mbo*I*)* sensitive to exonuclease III digestion.

3. Electrophoresis of these reactions through a 1% (w/v) agarose gel should reveal that the unmethylated DNA sample is digested by *Mbo*I but not *Dpn*I and that the methylated sample is digested by *Dpn*I but not *Mbo*I. Methylation must be complete before the two DNA samples are hybridized. If the methylated DNA sample is not fully methylated (i.e., there is partial *Mbo*I digestion), repeat the methylation step (**Subheading 3., step 4**), and ensure that complete methylation is achieved before proceeding to the next step.

4. SAM is unstable at 37°C and pH 7.5 and must be replenished if reactions are incubated for more than 4 h. It is important to use fresh SAM, because it is critical in achieving complete methylation.

5. The E. *coli* methyl-directed mismatch repair enzymes MutH, MutL, and MutS recognize and process seven of eight possible base-pair mismatches in a strand-specific manner. High concentrations of these proteins in the presence of ATP will cleave the unmethylated strand of a hemimethylated heterohybrid DNA molecule at the d(GATC) sequence located within 1 kb of the mismatched strands *(6,7)*.

6. It is reasonable to expect a total of 50–60 µg of DNA.

7. This renders the buffer suitable for supporting exonuclease III activity.

8. Exonuclease III will degrade dsDNA homohybrids 3' to 5' and can initiate digestion at the blunt end or the 5' overhang produced by *Dpn*I and *Mbo*I, respectively.
Exonuclease III will also recognize and initiate digestion at a nick caused by
mismatch repair enzymes and degrade one strand and produce single-stranded
DNA (ssDNA). These single strands are eliminated by binding to BNDC beads
(*see* **Subheading 3., step 17**).
9. At high salt concentrations, BNDC binds DNA containing ssDNA regions, separating them from the mismatch-free dsDNA.

Acknowledgments

We are grateful to the members of Ocular Genetics Laboratory for their
critical comments on the preparation of the manuscript. This research was
funded by Medical Research Council of Canada (MRC) grant MT12916. MAW
is an MRC and Alberta Heritage Fund for Medical Research (AHFMR) scholar.

References

1. Nelson, S. F., McCusker, J. H., Sander, M. A., Kee, Y., and Modrich, P. (1993)
Genomic mismatch scanning: a new approach to genetic linkage mapping. *Nature
Genet.* **4,** 11–18.
2. Brown, P. O. (1994) Genome scanning methods. *Curr. Opin. Genet. Dev.* **4,** 366–373.
3. Mirzayans, F., Mears, A. J., Guo, S.-W., Pearce, W. G., and Walter, M. A. (1997)
Identification of the human chromosomal region containing the iridogoniodysgenesis anomaly locus by genomic-mismatch scanning. *Am. J. Hum. Genet.*
61, 111–119.
4. Cheung, V. G. and Nelson, S. F. (1998) Genomic mismatch scanning identifies
human genomic DNA shared identical by descent. *Genomics* **47,** 1–6.
5. Cheung, V. G., Gregg, J. P., Goglin-Ewens, K. J., Bandong, J., Stanley, C. A.,
Baker, L., Higgins, M. J., Nowak, N. J., Shows, T. B., Ewens, W. J., Nelson, S. F.,
and Spielman, R. S. (1998) Linkage-disequilibrium mapping without genotyping.
Nature Genet. **18,** 225–230.
6. Lahue, R. S., Au, K. G., and Modrich, P. (1989) DNA mismatch correction in a
defined system. *Science* **245,** 160–164.
7. Learn, B. A. and Graistrom, R. H. (1989) Methyl-directed repair of frameshift
heteroduplexes in cell extracts from Escherichia coli. *J. Bact.* 171, 6473–6481.
8. Shalon, D., Smith, S. J., and Brown, P. O. (1996) A DNA microarray system for
analyzing complex DNA samples using two-color fluorescent probe hybridisation.
Genome Res. **6,** 639–645.
9. DeRisi, J., Penland, L., Brown, P. O., Bittner, M. L., Meltzer, P. S., Ray, M.,
Chen, Y., Su, Y. A., and Trent, J. M. (1996) Use of a cDNA microarray to analyze
gene expression patterns in human cancer. *Nature Genet.* **14,** 457–460.
10. McAllister, L., Penland, L., and Brown, P. O. (1998) Enrichment for loci
identical-by-descent between pairs of mouse or human genomes by genomic mismatch scanning. *Genomics* **47,** 7–11.

11. Mears, A. J., Mirzayans, F., Gould, D. B., Pearce, W. G., Walter, M. A. (1996) Autosomal dominant iridogoniodysgenesis maps to 6p25. *Am. J. Hum. Genet.* **59,** 1321–1327.

12. Guo, S.-W. (1995) Proportion of genome shared identical by descent by relatives: concept, computation, and applications. *Am. J. Hum. Genet.,* **56,** 1468–1476.

13. Kunkel, L., Smith, K., Boyer, S., Borgaorkar, D., Wachtel, S., Miller, O., Berg, W., Jones, H., and Rary, J. (1977) Analysis of human Y-chromosome-specific reiterated DNA in chromosome variants. *PNAS* **74,** 1245–1249.

14. Madisen, L., Hoar, D. I., Holroyd, C. D., Crisp, M., and Hodes. M. E. (1987) The effect of storage of blood and isolated DNA on the integrity of DNA. *Am. J. Med. Genet.* **27,** 379–390.

5

Detection of Chromosomal Abnormalities by Comparative Genomic Hybridization

Mario A. J. A. Hermsen, Marjan M. Weiss, Gerrit A. Meijer, and Jan P. A. Baak

1. Introduction

Comparative genomic hybridization (CGH) provides genome-scale over-views of chromosomal copy number changes in tumors (1). Unlike conventional cytogenetic analysis, it needs no cell culturing, making it applicable to practically any kind of clinical specimen from which DNA can be obtained, including archival paraffin-embedded material *(1)*. CGH maps the origins of amplified and deleted DNA sequences on normal chromosomes, thereby high-lighting locations of important genes. However, this technique cannot detect chromosomal translocations, inversions, or subchromosomal changes. By its nature, CGH is especially suitable for screening tumors in various stages of development, such as premalignant lesions and invasive carcinomas and metastases, pointing out the location of possible oncogenes or tumor suppressor genes that may play a role in the early onset of malignancy or in the process of metastasis. In addition, CGH can be used to compare different histologic components within one tumor, enabling a better understanding of the relation between phenotype and genotype, or to compare derivative cell lines with the original cell line.

The principle of CGH is shown in **Fig. 1**. Labeled tumor DNA competes with differentially labeled normal DNA for hybridization to normal human metaphase chromosomes. Using fluorescence microscopy and digital image processing, the ratio of the two is measured along the chromosomal axes. Deviations from the normal ratio of 1.0 at certain chromosome regions represent amplification or deletion of genetic material in the tumor and may sometimes already be seen in a green and red overlay image of the hybridized

From: *Methods in Molecular Biology, vol. 175: Genomics Protocols*
Edited by: M. P. Starkey and R. Elaswarapu © Humana Press Inc., Totowa, NJ

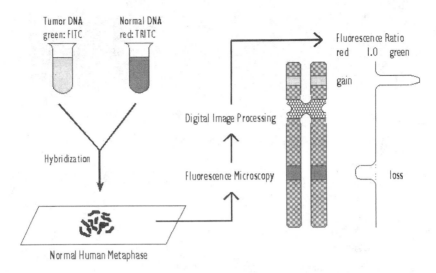

Fig. 1. Schematic overview of the CGH technique. Tumor and reference DNA are labeled with green and red fluorochromes, respectively, and hybridized to normal metaphase spreads. Images of the fluorescent signals are captured and the green-to-red signal ratios are digitally quantified for each chromosomal locus along the chromosomal axis. (Reprinted with permission from Human Pathology *[2]*.)

metaphase (**Fig. 2, top**). However, digital image processing is necessary for adequate evaluation. The final result is a so-called relative copy number karyotype (*see* **Fig. 2, bottom**) that shows an overview of chromosomal copy number changes in the tumor. The sensitivity of CGH depends on the purity of the tumor sample (*see* **Note 1**); admixture with normal cells will reduce it. For deletions the limit of detection is 10 Mb, which is about the size of an average chromosome band, but amplifications may be smaller (down to 250 kb) when the number of copies is high *(3)* (*see* **Fig. 3**). The following steps are required to perform CGH: preparation of normal metaphase chromosomes, DNA labeling, hybridization and washing, fluorescence microscopy, and capturing and analyzing of images with dedicated computer software including karyotyping.

2. Materials

1. Ham F10 culture medium (Gibco-BRL Life Technologies, Paisley, UK).
2. Fetal calf serum (FCS) (Gibco-BRL Life Technologies).
3. L-Glutamine (Gibco-BRL Life Technologies).
4. Penicillin, streptomycin (Gibco-BRL Life Technologies).
5. Phytohemagglutinin (Gibco-BRL Life Technologies).
6. Colchicine (Gibco-BRL Life Technologies).

7. Glass microscope slides.
8. Glass cover slips (18 × 18 mm and 24 × 50 mm).
9. Phase-contrast microscope.
10. Fluorescence microscope equipped with three single bandpass filters.
11. Charge-coupled device camera and dedicated CGH software (e.g., Applied Imaging, MetaSystems ISIS, Vysis, PSI PowerGene, Leica QCGH) that performs the following steps: background subtraction, segmentation of chromosomes and removal of nonchromosome objects, normalization of a fluorescein isothiocyanate (FITC) tetramethylenediamine isothiocyanate (TRITC) ratio for a whole metaphase spread, interactive karyotyping, and scaling of chromosomes to a standard length.
12. DNA polymerase I/DNase I (Gibco-BRL Life Technologies).
13. DNase I (Gibco-BRL Life Technologies).
14. dNTP reaction mixture: 0.2 mM dATP, dCTP, dGTP (Roche Lewes, East Sussex, UK), 500 mM Tris-HCl, pH 7.8; 50 mM MgCl$_2$; 100 µM dithiothreitol, 100 µg/mL of bovine serum albumin.
15. dTTP (0.2 mM) (Roche).
16. Biotin-16-dUTP (1 nmol/µL) (Roche).
17. Digoxigenin-11-dUTP (1 nmol/µL) (Roche).
18. Human Cot-1 DNA (Gibco-BRL Life Technologies).
19. Hybridization mixture: 50% (v/v) deionized formamide; 10% (w/v) dextran sulfate, 2X saline sodium citrate (SSC), pH 7.0.
20. 20X SSC: 0.3 M sodium citrate; 3 M sodium chloride, pH 7.0.
21. 10X TN: 1 M Tris-HCl, 1.5 M NaCl, pH 7.5.
22. TNT: 50 mL of 10X TN, 450 mL of H$_2$O, 1.25 mL of 20% (v/v) Tween-20.
23. TNB: 0.5% (w/v) blocking reagent (Roche) in 1X TN.
24. Avidin-FITC (12.5 µg/mL) (Sigma-Aldrich, Poole, Dorset, UK).
25. Sheep-antidigoxigenin (DIG)-TRITC (4.0 µg/mL) (Roche).
26. Antifade solution: Vectashield (Vector, Peterborough, Cambridgeshire, UK).
27. 4,6 Diamino-2-phenylindole) (DAPI) (350 ng/mL) in antifade solution.

3. Methods

3.1. Preparation of Metaphase Chromosomes

1. Incubate 1 mL of heparinized blood with 9 mL of Ham F10 culture medium containing 10% (v/v) FCS, 1% (w/v) L-glutamine, 1% (w/v) penicillin and streptomycin, and 1.5% (w/v) phytohemagglutinin at 37°C in an atmosphere of 5% (v/v) CO$_2$ for 72 h.
2. Arrest the cells in mitosis by adding colchicine to 0.1 µg/mL and incubating at 37°C for 30 min.
3. Spin down the cells at g for 10 min. Discard the supernatant.
4. Resuspend the pellet in 10 mL of hypotonic 0.075M KCl and incubate for 20 min at room temperature.
5. Spin down the cells at g for 10 min. Discard the supernatant.

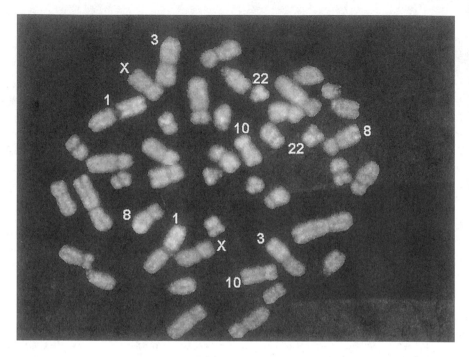

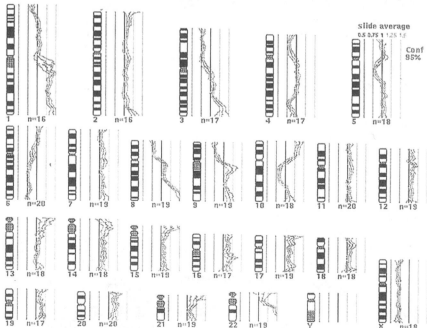

6. Fix the cells in 10 mL of 3:1 methanol:acetic acid by carefully adding small volumes with continuous mixing.
7. Spin down the cells at 150g for 10 min. Discard the supernatant. Repeat **step 6**.
8. Spin down the cells at 150g for 10 min. Discard the supernatant.
9. Resuspend the cells in approx 1 mL of 3:1 methanol:acetic acid.
10. Using a Pasteur pipet, mount one or two drops of the cell suspension onto ethanol-cleaned slides.
11. Postfix the slides immediately by adding several drops of 3:1 methanol:acetic acid.
12. Check the quality of the metaphase chromosomes with a phase-contrast microscope (*see* **Note 2**).
13. Air-dry the slides overnight at room temperature and store in dry conditions at −20°C.

3.2. DNA Labeling

1. Combine 1 μg of DNA, 3 μL of dNTPs, 0.5 μL of dTTP, 1 μL of DIG- or biotin-conjugated dUTP, 3 μL of DNA polymerase I/DNase I, and 0–1 μL of diluted DNase I (adjust this concentration to obtain the optimal fragment lengths). Add ddH$_2$O to adjust the volume to 30 μL.
2. Incubate for 1.5–2 h at 15°C.
3. Inactivate the enzymes at 70°C for 15 min.
4. Visualize 5 μL of labeled DNA by gel electrophoresis through an ethidium bromide stained 1% (w/v) agarose gel.
5. Inspect the DNA fragment lengths with an ultraviolet transilluminator; the optimum smear is between 500 and 1500 kb in length (*see* **Note 3**).

3.3. Hybridization and Washing

1. Mix 10 μL of labeled (usually with biotin) tumor DNA with 10 μL of labeled (usually with DIG) normal DNA and 40 μg of unlabeled Cot-1 DNA.
2. Ethanol precipitate the sample by adding 0.1 vol of 3 M sodium acetate and 2 vol of ethanol and centrifuging at 12,000g for 30 min.
3. Decant the supernatant and air-dry the pellet.
4. Dissolve the pellet in 6 μL of hybridization mixture.

Fig. 2. *(previous page)* **(Top)** Green and red overlay image of a representative metaphase spread after hybridization with tumor DNA from a laryngeal squamous cell carcinoma (green and normal DNA (red). Clearly visible amplifications are at chromosome arms 1q, 3q, 8q, 10p, and 22q, and clear losses can be seen at 3p, 4p+5q, 6q, 8p, 10q, and Xp+q. **(Bottom)** Relative copy number karyotype showing the quantitative analysis of the same tumor. The mean green-to-red fluorescence ratios of the chromosomes of multiple metaphase spreads are plotted in a graph corresponding to the chromosome ideograms, together with the 95% CI. The following chromosome abnormalities are now detected: gains at 1q, 1p, 2q, 3q, 7q, 8q, 9q, 10p, 14q, 15q, 16, 17, 19q, 20q, 21q, and 22q; and losses at 1p, 3p, 4p, 4q, 5q, 6q, 8p, 9p, 10q, and X.

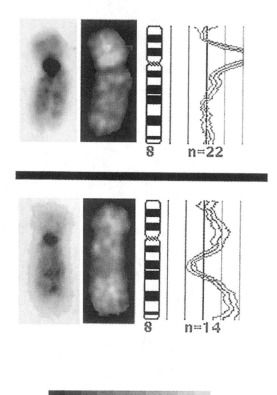

Fig. 3. **(Top)** Example of a small high-level amplification in chromosome band 8p11; **(bottom)** example of a small deletion (approx 10 Mb) in chromosome band 8q21.

5. Denature a metaphase chromosome slide at 72°C in a jar containing 70% (v/v) formamide and 2X SSC in a water bath for 6 min (*see* **Note 4**).
6. Dehydrate the slide in an ethanol series (70, 96, and 100%).
7. Denature the DNA probe mixture at 80°C for 10 min.
8. Mount the probe mixture immediately on the metaphase slide.
9. Cover with a cover slip (18 × 18 mm) and seal with rubber cement.
10. Hybridize for 3 d in a humid incubator at 40°C.
11. Remove the cover slip carefully.
12. Wash for 5 min in 2X SSC at room temperature.
13. Wash 3 times for 5 min in 0.1X SSC at 45°C.
14. Wash for 5 min in TNT at room temperature.
15. Preincubate for 10 min in 100 µL of TNB under a cover slip (24 × 50 mm).
16. Incubate for 60 min in 100 µL of TNB with avidine-FITC (1:200) and sheep-anti-DIG-TRITC (1 :50) under a cover slip (24 × 50 mm) in a humid chamber at 37°C (from now on keep the slide in the dark).

17. Wash 3 times for 5 min in TNT at room temperature.
18. Wash for 5 min in 2X SSC at room temperature.
19. Dehydrate the slide in an ethanol series (70, 96, and 100%).
20. Mount 20 μL of antifade containing DAPI, cover with a cover slip (24 × 50 mm), and seal with rubber cement.

3.4. Fluorescence Microscopy and Image Analysis

A fluorescence microscope equipped with three single bandpass filters is suitable for CGH. DAPI (blue) is used for chromosome identification, FITC (green) for the hybridized tumor DNA, and TRITC (red) for the hybridized normal DNA detection.

1. Screen the slide for well-spread metaphase chromosomes with a homogeneous green and red fluorescent signal and a low background (*see* **Note 5**). Capture three images (DAPI, FITC, TRITC) of each metaphase spread.
2. Plot the averaged ratios of several well-selected metaphases spreads along the corresponding chromosomes in a so-called relative copy number karyotype (**Fig. 2**). The significance of deviations from the 1.0 ratio can be evaluated with the help of the 95% confidence interval (CI), which can be plotted along with the averaged ratios (*see* **Note 6**).

4. Notes

1. When using tissue sections to isolate DNA from tumor cells, an admixture of normal cells (stroma or infiltrating lymphocytes) may present a problem. When a sample contains more than 50% normal cells, microdissection becomes necessary. This can be done manually *(4)* or using advanced laser microdissection equipment *(5)*. However, the latter yields only a limited number of cells (hence DNA), necessitating universal DNA amplification techniques *(6,7)*. These techniques are time consuming and expensive, and the user must perform good control experiments to ensure the reliability of CGH results. Another approach could be cell sorting (e.g., antibodies attached to magnetic beads, or flow cytometric sorting), which may enable selection (and extraction) of tumor cells, or elimination of inflammatory cells from a tissue sample.
2. High-quality metaphase preparations for CGH preferentially should contain an abundance of metaphase chromosomes and have little residual cytoplasm (too much cytoplasm causes background and may prevent optimal denaturation) and minimal overlapping of the chromosomes. In addition, the chromosomes should have adequate length (400–550 bands) and not contain separated chromatics. Finally, for good banding strength, chromosomes should appear dark, not shiny, when looking through a phase-contrast microscope *(8)*. It is important to test several batches of metaphase spreads from different donors when setting up CGH, because their behavior in hybridization can be quite different. Alternatively, fully prepared metaphase spread slides are commercially available. However, these

slides still need to be tested before use, and the quality is not necessarily better than that of slides produced in-house (prepared as described in **Subheading 3.1.**).

3. When biotinylated and DIG-conjugated deoxynucleotides (dUTPs) are incorporated into the DNA (indirect labeling), a detection step with fluorochrome-conjugated antibodies (avidin-FITC and sheep-anti-DIG-TRITC, respectively) is required after hybridization. Directly fluorochrome-conjugated deoxynucleotides render a smoother but weaker hybridization signal along the chromosomes. It is important that the labeled DNA fragments of both tumor and reference DNA be in the same range of lengths and are within the limits of 500–1500 bp.

4. The time of denaturation is a variable that should be adjusted to each new batch of metaphase preparations. When the metaphase spreads are denatured too long, the fluorescent signal probably will be strong, but the DAPI banding will be very bad, making karyotyping impossible; conversely, when the slides are not denatured sufficiently, there will be a nice, easy-to-recognize banding DAPI pattern, but the signal will be too low and granular. The art of CGH is to find a balance between these two scenarios.

5. The selection of good-quality metaphase spreads for digital image processing is crucial in the CGH. The fluorescent signal should be strong and homogeneous over the whole metaphase spread. The user should avoid metaphase spreads with many overlapping chromosomes or metaphase spreads with very small or very large chromosomes. The background should be low. Local high backgrounds are probably caused by residual cytoplasm. An even field illumination by the microscope is essential. Uneven illumination can cause gross artifacts. Furthermore, good-quality metaphases in CGH show dark centromeric regions as a sign of good blocking by Cot-1 DNA. Centromeres contain repetitive DNA sequences that are highly variable in length among individuals (and thus between tumor and reference DNA) and can therefore interfere with the CGH analysis. These repetitive sequences also occur in a lesser but nonetheless significant extent throughout the whole genome. Suboptimal blocking by Cot-1 DNA leads to reduced sensitivity.

6. There are two ways to interpret the relative copy number karyotypes. Some researchers use fixed limits, e.g., 0.85/1.15 or 0.75/1.25, depending on the quality of the hybridization. Others prefer to use the 95% CI, which takes into account the quality of the signal. According to the latter definition, an amplification or a deletion is present when the 95% confidence interval of the fluorescence does not contain 1.0.

References

1. Kallioniemi, A., Kallioniemi, O. P., Sudar, D., et al. (1992) Comparative genomic hybridization for molecular cytogenetic analysis of solid tumors. *Science* **258,** 818–821.
2. Hermsen, M. A. J. A., Meijer, G. A., Baak, J. P. A., Joenje, H., Walboomers, J. M. M. (1996) Comparative genomic hybridization: a new tool in cancer pathology. *Hum. Pathol.* **27,** 342–349.

3. Kallioniemi, O. P., Kallioniemi, A., Piper, J., et al. (1994) Optimizing comparative genomic hybridization for analysis of DNA sequence copy number changes in solid tumors. *Genes Chrom. Cancer* **10,** 231–243.
4. Weiss, M. M., Hermsen, M. A. J. A., Meijer, G. A., Van Grieken, N. C. T., Baak, J. P. A., Kuipers, E. J., and Van Diest, P. J. (1999) Comparative genomic hybridisation (CGH). *Mol. Pathol.* **52,** 243–251.
5. Zikelsberger, H., Kulka, U., Lehmann, L., et al. (1998) Genetic heterogeneity in a prostatic carcinoma and associated prostatic intraepithelial neoplasia as demonstrated by combined use of laser-microdissection, degenerate oligonucleotide primed PCR and comparative genomic hybridization. *Virchows Arch.* **433,** 297–304.
6. Kuukasjarvi, T., Tanner, M., Pennanen, S., et al. (1997) Optimizing DOP-PCR for universal amplification of small DNA samples in comparative genomic hybridization. *Genes Chrom. Cancer* **18,** 94–101.
7. Lucito, R., Nakimura, M., West, J. A., et al. (1998) Genetic analysis using genomic representations. *Proc. Natl. Acad. Sci. USA* **95,** 4487–4492.
8. Karhu, R., Kahkonen, M., Kuukasjarvi, T., et al. (1997) Quality control of CGH: impact of metaphase chromosomes and the dynamic range of hybridization. *Cytometry* **28,** 198–205.

6

Construction of a Bacterial Artificial Chromosome Library

Sangdun Choi and Ung-Jin Kim

1. Introduction

1.1. Bacterial Artificial Chromosome Cloning System

Bacterial artificial chromosomes (BACs) represent a very useful cloning system for large DNA fragments and utilize the *Escherichia coli* F factor as their backbone. *E. coli* F factor allows strict copy number control of the clones so that they are stably maintained at one to two copies per cell (*1*). The stability of the cloned DNA during propagation in *E. coli* host is substantially higher in lower copy number vectors than in multi-copy counterparts.

The BAC vector permits the cloning of DNA up to 350 kb in *E. coli* (*2*). Because of its clone stability and ease of use, the BAC cloning system has emerged as the system of choice for the construction of large-insert genomic DNA libraries for humans, animals, and plants (*3–5*). However, BAC libraries have been difficult to construct with average insert sizes >150 kb (*6*). By using more reproducible megabase-size DNA preparations, and sizing and eluting procedures, we have constructed BAC libraries from human DNA with an average insert size of 202 kb and from *Arabidopsis* DNA with an average insert size of 190 kb (*7*). In this chapter, we describe advanced methodologies for generating larger insert BAC libraries from animals, plants, and bacteria.

1.2. BAC Vectors

The pBAC108L vector is the first version of a BAC vector (*2*). After transformation, clones carrying the human DNA insert had to be selected by colony hybridization with labeled human DNA. The next version, pBeloBAC11 (**Fig. 1**), allows lacZ-based positive color selection of the BAC clones that

From: *Methods in Molecular Biology, vol. 175: Genomics Protocols*
Edited by: M. P. Starkey and R. Elaswarapu © Humana Press Inc., Totowa, NJ

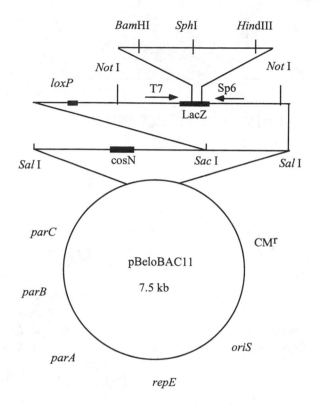

Fig. 1. Diagram of pBeloBAC11 vector. CM^r, chloramphenicol resistance.

have insert DNA in the cloning sites *(3)*. The nucleotide sequence of pBeloBACll is available from GenBank (accession no. U51113).

Additional BAC vectors have been derived from pBAC108L or pBeloBAC11. pECSBAC4 *(8)* and pIndigoBAC536 (Shizuya, H. et al., unpublished data) have a unique *Eco*RI cloning site and pBACwich *(9)* has been designed for plant transformation using biolistic bombardment. BIBAC2 is designed for Agrobacterium-mediated plant transformation *(10)*. pBACe3.6 allows positive selection for insert-containing BAC clones through inclusion of the *sacBII* gene (de Jong, P. J. et al., unpublished data).

2. Materials

1. LB medium: 1% tryptone, 0.5% yeast extract, 1% NaCl.
2. QIAGEN Plasmid Maxi Kit (Qiagen).
3. Plasmid-Safe ATP-dependent DNase (Epicentre).
4. QIAquick PCR Purification Kit (Qiagen).

5. Spermidine (Sigma).
6. Shrimp alkaline phosphatase (SAP) (USB).
7. TE: 10 mM Tris-HCl; 1 mM EDTA, pH 8.0.
8. InCert agarose (FMC).
9. Digestion buffer: 1 mg/mL of proteinase K; 1% N-lauroylsarcosine, 4 mM dithiothreitol, 0.5 M EDTA, pH 8.0.
10. Isolation buffer: 10 mM Tris-HCl, pH 9.5; 10 mM EDTA; 100 mM KC1; 4 mM spermidine; 1 mM spermine; 0.5 M sucrose. Add 0.1% β-mercaptoethanol before use.
11. Lysis buffer: 0.5 M EDTA, pH 8.0; 1% N-lauroyl-sarcosine. Add 1 mg/mL of proteinase K before use.
12. Phenylmethylsulfonyl fluoride (PMSF) stock solution: 50 mM PMSF in isopropanol.
13. Cellulase buffer: 20 mM MES, pH 5.5; 1 mM MgCl$_2$; 0.6 M sorbitol; 2% Onozuka cellulase R10 (Gallard Schleeinger); 0.1% Macerase pectinase (Calbiochem).
14. Wash buffer: 50 mM Tris, pH 8.0; 0.6 M sorbitol; 1 mM MgCl$_2$, 100 mM β-mercaptoethanol.
15. Glycerol, Ultra Pure (Gibco-BRL).
16. SeaKem LE agarose (FMC).
17. 0.5X TBE: 45 mM Tris; 45 mM boric acid; 1 mM EDTA, pH 8.3.
18. 1X TAE: 40 mM Tris-acetate; 1 mM EDTA, pH 8.0.
19. Gene Pulser (Bio-Rad).
20. SOC: 2% Bacto-tryptone; 0.5% yeast extract; 10 mM NaCl, 2.5 mM KCl, 10 mM MgCl$_2$, 10 mM MgSO$_4$, 20 mM glucose, pH 7.0.
21. X-Gal stock: 20 mg/mL in dimethylformamide.
22. Isopropyl-β-D-thiogalactopyranoside (IPTG) stock: 200 mg/mL in ddH$_2$O.
23. LB freezing medium: LB medium supplemented with 36 mM K$_2$HPO$_4$, 13.2 mM KH$_2$PO$_4$, 1.7 mM Na citrate, 0.4 mM MgSO$_4$, 6.8 mM (NH$_4$)2SO$_4$, 4.4% (v/v) glycerol, 12.5 μg/mL of chloramphenicol.
24. GTE: 50 mM glucose; 25 mM Tris, pH 8.0; 10 mM EDTA, pH 8.0, 0.1 mg/mL of RNase A.
25. 0.2 N NaOH+1% sodium dodecyl sulfate (SDS) solution.
26. Potassium acetate solution: 60 mL of 5 M potassium acetate; 28.5 mL of glacial acetic acid, 11.5 mL of ddH$_2$O, pH 4.8–5.2.
27. AutoGen 740 DNA Isolation System (AutoGen, Japan).
28. KoAc/phenol/chloroform/ethanol (AutoGen).
29. Q-bot (Genetix, UK).
30. Biomek2000 (Beckman).
31. Hybond N+ membranes (Amersham Pharmacia Biotech).
32. Denaturing solution: 1.5 M NaCl, 0.5 N NaOH.
33. Neutralizing solution: 1 M Tris, pH 7.5; 1.5 M NaCl.
34. Proteinase solution: 50 mM Tris, pH 8.0; 50 mM EDTA, pH 8.0; 100 mM NaCl; 1% N-lauroylsarcosine, 100 mg/L of proteinase K.

3. Methods

3.1. Preparation of BAC Vector

3.1.1. Purification of BAC Vector

1. Inoculate a single *E. coli* strain DH10B colony containing the BAC vector into 5 mL of LB medium containing 30 μg/mL of chloramphenicol and grow at 37°C overnight.
2. Inoculate three culture flasks containing 1 L of LB plus chloramphenicol (30 μg/mL), prewarmed to 37°C, with 1 mL/L of culture from **step 1**. Grow at 37°C with shaking to a cell density of approx 1×10^9 cells/mL (A_{600} = 1.0–1.1).
3. Harvest the cells by centrifugation at 4°C for 15 min at 6000*g*.
4. Isolate the BAC vector using the Qiagen Plasmid Maxi Kit (five Qiagen-tip 500 columns for a 3-L preparation).
5. Use Plasmid-Safe ATP-dependent DNase to selectively digest bacterial DNA while leaving plasmid DNA intact. The efficiency of the DNase can be improved by adding two restriction enzymes that do not cut the plasmid. For 10 μg of pBeloBAC11 vector, use 150 U of DNase, 50 U each of *Cla*I and *Mlu*I *(NEB)*, and NEB buffer 2. Incubate for 2 h at 37°C.
6. Inactivate Plasmid-Safe ATP-dependent DNase by incubating at 65°C for 20 min.
7. Remove small nucleotides by using the QIAquick PCR Purification Kit *(see* **Note 1**).

3.1.2. Restriction Digestion and Dephosphorylation of BAC Vector DNA

1. Digest the BAC vector (10 μg) to completion with 100 U of *Hind*III or *Eco*RI (Gibco) in the appropriate buffer supplemented with 4 m*M* spermidine at 37°C for 2–4 h *(see* **Note 2**).
2. Clean up the digested DNA with the QIAquick PCR Purification Kit and resuspend in 100 μL of 10 m*M* Tris buffer (pH 8.0).
3. Dephosphorylate the vector DNA by adding SAP (1 U/μg of DNA) and incubating at 37°C for 2 h.
4. Clean up the dephosphorylated vector with the QIAquick PCR Purification Kit, dissolve in 100 μL of TE, and store at –20°C.

3.2. Preparation of High Molecular Weighs Genomic DNA

3.2.1. DNA Sources for BAC Cloning

3.2.1.1. PREPARATION FROM ANIMALS

1. Incubate 8–10 mL of frozen semen at 37°C for 2–3 h.
2. Suspend the semen in 30 mL of TE and centrifuge at 7000*g* for 5 min at 4°C.
3. Resuspend the sperm in 30 mL of TE and harvest by centrifugation at 5000*g* for 5 min at 4°C. Repeat the procedure two more times.
4. Embed the resuspended sperm in agarose (0.5% agarose) at a concentration of 1.5×10^8/mL using a hemocytometer for human, chimpanzee, or mouse *(see* **Note 3**).

5. Digest the agarose-embedded large DNA for 2 d with digestion buffer. Change the digestion buffer once during the digestion.
6. Rinse the sample with 0.5 M EDTA (pH 8.0) three times and store in 0.5 M EDTA at 4°C.

3.2.1.2. Preparation from Plants

There are two general methods for preparing megabase-size DNA from plants. The nuclei method is universal and works well for several divergent plants. The DNA is more concentrated and contains lower amounts of chloroplast or mitochondrial DNA. The protoplast method yields high-quality megabase-size DNA with minimal breakage, but each plant species requires a different set of conditions to generate protoplasts.

3.2.1.2.1. Nuclei Method

1. Grind 30–50 g of the fresh tissue to a fine powder in liquid nitrogen with a mortar and pestle, and transfer the powder to an ice-cold 500-mL beaker containing 200 mL of ice-cold isolation buffer.
2. Repeat **step 1** several times in order to obtain enough nuclei to embed.
3. Filter the homogenate on ice sequentially through one layer each of 140- and 80-μm nylon net or filter mesh.
4. Add 1/40 vol of isolation buffer supplemented with 20% Triton X-100 to the filtrate and mix well.
5. Pellet the nuclei by centrifugation in a fixed-angle rotor at 2000g for 15 min at 4°C.
6. Discard the supernatant fluid and resuspend the pellet in 1 to 2 mL of ice cold isolation buffer.
7. Count the nuclei with a hemocytometer and mix the nuclei with agarose in isolation buffer (without β-mercaptoethanol, 0.6% agarose) at a concentration of 2.2 × 10^8 nuclei/mL (for the diploid plants with haploid genomic sizes of 800–1000 Mb; *see* **Note 4**). The optimum number of nuclei depends on the genomic size of the plant. Usually it is difficult to count the nuclei, and, thus, when preparing nuclei for the first time, we optimize the nuclei concentration empirically. We suggest optimizing the nuclei concentration by embedding two or three different concentrations of nuclei *(see* **Note 5**). We usually pipette a 0.5 vol of 1.8% InCert agarose solution into the prewarmed nuclei suspension and mix well (1 vol of agarose solution plus 2 vol of nuclei suspension, so that the final agarose concentration is 0.6%).
8. Pour the mixture into plug molders on ice.
9. Incubate the plugs in lysis buffer for 24 h at 50°C with gentle shaking to degrade the proteins.
10. Replace this buffer with new lysis buffer for a further 24-h incubation at 50°C.
11. Wash the plugs three times (three times for a 1-h incubation at 4°C) by immersing in 0.5 M EDTA, pH 8.0, containing 0.1 mM PMSF to inactivate the proteinase K.
12. Store the plugs in 0.5 M EDTA, pH 8.0, at 4°C until use.

3.2.1.2.2. Protoplast Method. This preparation is suitable for maize and *Arabidopsis (see* **Note 6**).

1. Cross-cut 5–10 g of the young leaves into 0.5–1-mm strips.
2. Infiltrate about 80 mL of cellulase buffer through a 0.4-μm filter using a vacuum.
3. Transfer to four to six large Petri dishes and digest at room temperature for 3–5 h.
4. Remove the broken cells by sequential filtration through a 140-μm mesh and then an 80-μm mesh.
5. Pellet the protoplasts at 300*g* for 10 min and gently resuspend in 50 mL of wash buffer.
6. Pellet the protoplasts at 300*g* for 10 min and gently resuspend in 1–2 mL of wash buffer.
7. Count an aliquot under a microscope by using a hemocytometer and embed in isolation buffer (without β-mercaptoethanol). Adjust the final concentration to 8×10^7 protoplasts/mL (for the diploid plants with haploid genomic sizes of 2500–3000 Mb; *see* **Note 4**). We usually empirically optimize the protoplast concentration by embedding two or three different concentrations of protoplasts *(see* **step 7** of **Subheading 3.2.1.2.1.** and **Note 7**).
8. Make agarose plugs as described earlier *(see* **steps 8–12** of **Subheading 3.2.1.2.1.**).

3.2.1.3. PREPARATION FROM BACTERIAL CELLS

1. Grow cells in 50 mL of an appropriate medium (e.g., LB) to an OD_{600} of 0.8 to 1.0 ($4–5 \times 10^8$ cells/mL).
2. Harvest cells by centrifugation at 4000*g* for 10 min at 4°C.
3. Resuspend the cell pellet in the same volume of 10% glycerol (Ultra Pure) and spin at 4000*g* for 10 min to pellet.
4. Resuspend the cell pellet in 2.5 mL of 10% glycerol.
5. Mix cells with agarose (InCert) in water to make a final agarose concentration of 0.5%. Optimize the cell concentration empirically by embedding two or three different concentrations of cells *(see* **Notes 5** and **7**).
6. Incubate the DNA plugs in lysis buffer at 50°C with gentle shaking for 2 d and store at 4°C in 0.5 *M* EDTA (pH 8.0). Change the buffer once during the digestion.

3.2.2. Partial Digestion

Once megabase-size DNA has been prepared, it must be fragmented and DNA in the desired size range isolated. In general, DNA fragmentation utilizes two general approaches: physical shearing and partial digestion with a restriction enzyme that cuts relatively frequently within the genome. Here partial digestion with restriction enzymes is used.

1. Equilibrate 50 μg of sliced plugs with a 150-μL mixture (total reaction volume of 200 μL): corresponding reaction buffer; 0.1 mg/mL of acetylated bovine serum

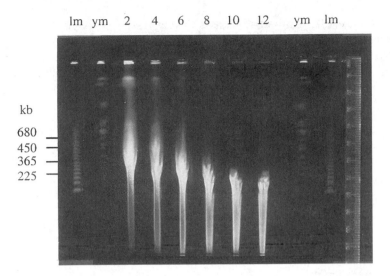

Fig. 2. Partially digested human megabase-size DNA. lm, lambda ladder; ym, *Saccharomyces cerevisiae* (Bio-Rad). Lanes 3–8, human DNA partially digested with *Eco*RI: (2) 2 U, (4) 4 U, (6) 6 U, (8) 8 U, (10) 10 U, (12) 12 U. The genomic DNA was subjected to PFGE on a 1% agarose gel in 0.5X TBE using a switch time of 90 s at 6 V/cm and 14°C for 18 h.

albumin; 4 mM spermidine; and diluted *Hind*III or *Eco*RI such as 0, 1, 2, 4, 8, 16, and 50 U/200 μL) at 4°C with appropriate shaking for 1 h (*see* **Note 8**).

2. Transfer the reaction mixture to a 37°C water bath and incubate for 1 h (*see* **Note 9**)
3. Add 1/10 vol of 0.5 M EDTA, pH 8.0, and place the tubes on ice.
4. Place the partially digested DNA plugs on an agarose gel molding plate using a comb and pour the warm (37–45°C) 1% agarose gel (SeaKem LE) in 0.5X TBE.
5. Perform pulsed-field gel electrophoresis (PFGE) using the following conditions: 6.0 V/cm, 90-s pulse, 0.5X TBE buffer, 14°C for 18 h.
6. After checking the ethidium bromide–stained gel, select the enzyme concentration giving a majority of DNA fragments ranging from about 300 to 800 kb (**Fig. 2**). It depends on the DNA concentrations of the samples, but usually the actual size of the DNA fragments from this fraction is between 50 and 400 kb in size owing to DNA trapping.

3.2.3. Size Selection of Partially Digested DNA by PFGE

1. Perform the digestion reaction on a large scale by carrying out several reactions (five to eight) under exactly the same conditions as previously determined.
2. Place the partially digested DNA plugs on an agarose gel molding plate side by side using a comb, and pour the warm (37–45°C) 1% agarose gel (SeaKem LE) in 1X TAE.

3. Perform PFGE using conditions adjusted to the DNA concentration of the plugs (high DNA concentration: 6 V/cm, between 15- and 30-s pulse, 1X TAE buffer, 12°C for 16–18 h; moderate DNA concentration: 6 V/cm, between 40- and 50-s pulse, 1X TAE buffer, 12°C for 16–18 h; low DNA concentration: 5 V/cm, between 5- and 7-s pulse, 1X TAE buffer, 12°C for 14–16 h; *see* **Note 10**).

4. Cut DNA fragments horizontally (about 5 mm each) ranging from about 200–600 kb from the gel (for the sample of low DNA concentration, excise the DNA band in the compression zone), and separately carry out a second size selection in 1% agarose (SeaKem LE) using these conditions: 4 V/cm, 7-s pulse, 1X TAE buffer, 12°C for 8 h.

5. Excise the DNA band in the compression zone and keep in 1X TAE at 4°C.

3.2.4. Recovery of High Molecular Weight DNA from Agarose Gels

1. Put the gel slice and an appropriate amount of 1X TAE in dialysis tubing (0.75 in. diameter; Gibco).
2. Elute the DNA from the gel at 3 V/cm, 10–16°C, in 1X TAE for 3 h.
3. Reverse the polarity of the current by changing the direction of the dialysis tubing and run at 3 V/cm in the same buffer for 30 s.
4. Remove the solution using a wide-bore pipet tip and use for ligation.

3.3. Ligation

Ligate the electroeluted DNA without dilution into 40–80 ng of dephosphorylated BAC vector in a total volume of 100 μL with 6 U of T4 DNA ligase (USB) plus ligase buffer at 15°C for 20 h.

3.4. Electroporation

3.4.1. Preparation of Electrocompetent Cells

1. Inoculate flasks of SOB (2% Bacto tryptone, 0.5% yeast extract, 10 mM NaCl, 2.5 mM KCl [pH 7.0] without Mg^{2+}) by diluting a fresh saturated (overnight) culture of DH10B (1:1000).
2. Grow with shaking at 37°C until the OD$_{550}$ reaches 0.7 (no higher than 0.8). This should take approx 5 h.
3. Harvest cells by spinning at 4000g for 10 min at 4°C.
4. Resuspend the pellet in 1 vol of cold, sterile 10% glycerol equal to the original culture volume.
5. Shake it vigorously several times and spin at 4000g for 10 min at 4°C.
6. Carefully pour off the supernatant (the pellet will be quite loose) and resuspend the cells in cold, sterile 10% glycerol equal to the original culture volume.
7. Shake vigorously several times and spin at 4000g for 10 min at 4°C.
8. Pour off the supernatant, resuspend the cells in the volume of glycerol remaining in the centrifuge bottle. Pool the cells in one small centrifuge tube and add a few milliliters of cold, sterile 10% glycerol.

9. Spin at 4000*g* for 10 min at 4°C.
10. Pour off the supernatant and resuspend the cells in cold, sterile 10% glycerol using 1.5–2.0 mL/L of initial culture.
11. Aliquot into microfuge tubes (100–200 µL per tube) and freeze quickly in a dry ice–ethanol bath. Store cells at –80°C.

3.4.2. Electroporation

1. Transform 1–2.5 µL of the ligation material into 20–25 µL of *E. coli* DH10B competent cells by using Gene Pulser and 0.2-cm cuvet under the conditions of 100 Ω, 12.5 kV/cm, and 25 µFa. This usually gives a time constant of approx 2.4 s (*see* **Note 11**).
2. Transfer the electroporated cells to 15-mL culture tubes with 0.5–1 mL of SOC and incubate at 37°C for 1 h with shaking.
3. Spread the SOC medium onto LB plates containing 12.5 µg/mL of chloramphenicol, 50 µg/mL of X-Gal, and 25 µg/mL of IPTG, and incubate at 37°C for 24–36 h.
4. Pick white colonies into 384-well microtiter plates containing LB freezing medium.
5. Incubate the microtiter plates at 37°C overnight and store at –80°C.

3.5. Preparation of BAC DNA

3.5.1. Manual Miniprep Method

1. Inoculate a colony into a 15-mL culture tube containing 5 mL of LB plus 12.5 µg/mL of chloramphenicol, and incubate overnight at 37°C with shaking.
2. Centrifuge the culture at 2000*g* at 4°C for 15 min using a tabletop centrifuge.
3. Pour off the supernatant and resuspend the cell pellet with the remaining solution in the tube.
4. Transfer the suspension to a 1.5-mL microfuge tube on ice, add ice-cold GTE, and mix by inversion several times.
5. Add 200 µL of freshly prepared 0.2 *N* NaOH+1% SDS solution, mix by gentle inversion several times, and incubate on ice for 5 min. At this stage the cells will lyse and the solution will grow clear and viscous.
6. Add 300 µL of the potassium acetate solution, gently invert the mixture, and return to ice. The addition of potassium acetate solution will cause the formation of a flocculent precipitate.
7. Centrifuge the mixture at full speed in a microfuge at room temperature for 15 min.
8. Transfer 750 µL of the supernatant fluid to a clean microfuge tube without disturbing the pellet.
9. Add 0.6 vol of cold isopropanol (450 µL) and centrifuge at full speed in a microfuge for 15 min to pellet the DNA.
10. Remove the supernatant, rinse the pellet with 1 mL of cold 70% ethanol, and dry upside down completely.
11. Add 40 µL of TE and digest 8–10 µL of this DNA solution with *Not*I to free the insert from the BAC vector.

lm

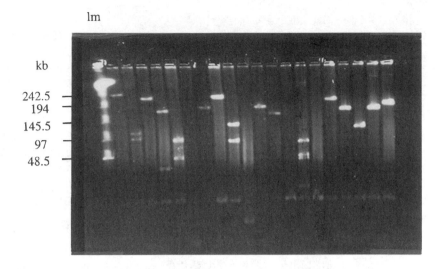

Fig. 3. Analysis of random human BAC clones by PFGE. lm, lambda ladder. Lane 1, lambda concatemer; lanes 2–21, AutoGen miniprep products of recombinant BAC clones digested with *Not*I. Note that the 6.9-kb band in each lane is the BAC vector.

12. Run 1% agarose gels in 0.5X TBE for 15 h at PFGE conditions of 6 V/cm, initial switch time of 5 s, and final switch time of 15 s (**Fig. 3**).

3.5.2. Miniprep by an Automated Robot

1. Inoculate the BAC clone into 3 mL of LB with 12.5 µg/mL of chloramphenicol within the tube specific for the AutoGen 740 DNA Isolation System and culture at 37°C with shaking overnight. Transfer the tubes into the AutoGen 740 DNA Isolation System.
2. Use the alkaline lysis method by setting up "System 1" in the panel of the AutoGen 740. Follow the user's manual provided by the manufacturer (Reagent 1: 10 mM Tris-HCl, pH 8.0, 1 mM EDTA, pH 8.0, 100 mg/L of RNase A; Reagent 2: 0.2 N NaOH, 1% N-lauroylsarcosine; Reagent 3: KoAc/phenol/chloroform/ethanol [AutoGen]; Reagent 4: isopropanol; Reagent 5: 70% ethanol).

3.5.3. Midi- and Maxipreps

Both midi- and maxipreps can be carried out by adapting the procedure given for the manual miniprep method. The volume of the added solutions (GTE, NaOH+SDS, and potassium acetate) should be adjusted proportionally to the increased culture volume. For example, if the amount of starting culture is 100 mL, 20 times more of these three solutions should be added in each step than for a 5-mL prep.

3.6. High-Density Gridding of BAC Library and Colony Hybridization

1. Grid the library out onto nylon membranes manually or using robots (Q-bot or Biomek2000), and incubate the trays on the medium plates overnight *(see* **Note 12**).
2. Transfer the membrane with bacterial colonies to a filter paper prewet with denaturing solution (colony side up).
3. Incubate at room temperature for 10 min.
4. Transfer to another filter paper prewet with neutralizing solution and let it stand for 10 min.
5. Remove the filter and dry on a clean sheet of filter paper for 5 min.
6. Invert the filter (colony side down) into a tray filled with proteinase solution and incubate at 37°C for 1 to 2 h.
7. Turn the filter colony side up and place on a clean sheet of filter paper to dry for 5 mm.
8. UV-crosslink the filter.
9. Bake the filter at 80°C for 1 to 2 h and store in a dark place at room temperature *(see* **Note 13**).

4. Notes

1. The final yield is approx 20–40 µg of DNA from 3 L of media.
2. Restriction enzyme incubation for an extended time may show exonuclease activity.
3. For other animals that have different genome sizes, you should adjust the concentration of cells.
4. For other plants that have different genomic sizes, you should adjust the concentration of nuclei, or protoplasts.
5. We suggest preparing the nuclei as described and in the final step embedding three different concentrations of nuclei (e.g., 0.5 mL of concentrated nuclei + 1.5 mL of isolation buffer, 1 mL of concentrated nuclei + 1 mL of isolation buffer, and 2 mL of concentrated nuclei + 0 mL of isolation buffer).
6. Making protoplasts is specific for every plant species and needs to be optimized.
7. We suggest preparing the protoplasts as described and in the final step embedding three different concentrations of protoplasts (e.g., 0.5 mL of concentrated protoplasts + 1.5 mL of isolation buffer, 1 mL of concentrated protoplasts + 1 mL of isolation buffer, and 2 mL of concentrated protoplasts + 0 mL isolation buffer).
8. The plugs can be sliced into fragments that are about the same size as beads without any appreciable DNA breakage and then used for partial digestion.
9. The amount of restriction enzyme and the digestion time depend on the number of restriction sites in the genome; usually 1–50 U for 5 min to 1 h.
10. When using highly concentrated DNA plugs for a partial digestion, apply a shorter pulse time (between 15–30 s) to spread out the DNA on the gel. This avoids trapping of smaller DNA segments. Conversely, for samples of low DNA

concentration, use either a very short pulse (between 5 and 7 s) or a long pulse (90 s) to avoid too much spreading of the DNA on the gel.

11. A lower field strength (9–13 kV/cm) yields a lower number of clones but a higher average insert size.

12. Using a Q-bot, 384-well microtiter plates containing BAC clones are spotted onto 22 × 22 cm Hybond N+ membranes. Bacteria from 72 plates are spotted twice onto one membrane, resulting in 27,648 unique clones on each membrane. Alternatively, smaller nylon membranes (12 × 8 cm) can be inoculated with a 384-prong High Density Replicating Tool from microtiter plates using the Biomek2000 robot.

13. The filters can be stored at room temperature for years, and each can be used for 10–20 hybridizations.

References

1. Willetts, N. and Skurray, R. (1987) Structure and function of the F factor and mechanism of conjugation. *J. Cell Mol. Biol.* **2,** 1110–1133.

2. Shizuya, H., Birren, B., Kim, U.-J., Mancino, V., Slepak, T., Tachiri, Y., and Simon, M. (1992) Cloning and stable maintenance of 300-kilobase-pair fragments of human DNA in *Escherichia coli* using F-factor-based vector. *Proc. Natl. Acad. Sci. USA* **89,** 8794–8797.

3. Kim, U.-J., Birren, B., Slepak, T., Mancino, V., Boysen, C., Kang, H. L., Simon, M., and Shizuya, H. (1996) Construction and characterization of a human bacterial artificial chromosome library. *Genomics* **34,** 213–218.

4. Cai, L., Taylor, J. F., Wing, R. A., Gallagher, D. S., Woo, S.-S., and Davis, S. K. (1995) Construction and characterization of a bovine bacterial artificial chromosome library. *Genomics* **29,** 413–425.

5. Choi, S., Creelman, R. A., Mullet, J. E., and Wing, R. A. (1995) Construction and characterization of bacterial artificial chromosome library of *Arabidopsis thaliana. Plant Mol. Biol. Rep.* **13,** 124–128.

6. Choi, S. and Wing, R. A. (2000) The construction of bacterial artificial chromosome (BAC) libraries from plants, in *Plant Molecular Biology Manual* (Gelvin, S. B. and Schilperoort, R. A., eds.), Kluwer Academic Publishers, Dordrecht, The Netherlands, pp. 45, 1–28.

7. <http://www.tree.caltech.edu/lib_status.html>.

8. Frijters, A. C. J., Zhang, Z., van Damme, M., Wang, G.-L., Ronald, P. C., and Michelmore, R. W. (1997) Construction of a bacterial artificial chromosome library containing large *Eco*RI and *Hind*III genomic fragments of lettuce. *Theor. Appl. Genet.* **94,** 390–399.

9. Choi, S., Begum, D., Koshinsky, H., Ow, D. W., and Wing, R. (2000) A new approach for the identification and cloning of genes: the pBACwich system using cre/lox site-specific recombination. *Nucleic Acid Res.* **28,** e19.

10. Hamilton, C. M., Frary, A., Lewis, C., and Tanksley, S. D. (1996) Stable transfer of intact high molecular weight DNA into plant chromosomes. *Proc. Natl. Acad. Sci. USA* **93,** 9975–9979.

11. <http:/lbacpac.med.buffalo.edu/vectorframe.html>.

7

Contiguation of Bacterial Clones

Sean J. Humphray, Susan J. Knaggs, and Ioannis Ragoussis

1. Introduction
1.1. Fingerprinting

For accurate assembly of a bacterial clone map (or contig), it is necessary to precisely detect the degree of overlap and map order of clones. One way is to generate fingerprints for all the clones in a given project. The overlap between clones is determined by the proportion of comigrating restriction fragments on either acrylamide or agarose gels, with mulitfold coverage of clones allowing rapid identification of artifacts such as rearranged or deleted clones.

There are two fingerprinting methods described here (*see* **Fig. 1**): double-digest end labeling, using either a radioactive isotope (*1*), or, as described here, fluorescent molecules (*2–4*) where fragments are resolved on a denaturing acrylamide gel and single-restriction, digestion-using agarose gels (*5*). It should be noted that the data produced by the two methods are incompatible.

The software described here for data entry and analysis are Image v3.9 and FPC v4.5. For fluorescently fingerprinted clones, the Genescan software package (Perkin-Elmer ABI, Foster City, CA) can also be used for entering gels.

Some of the main differences between the two techniques are summarized in **Table 1**. With fluorescent fingerprinting, an increased sample to gel ratio, and decrease in gel variation affects can be achieved by multiplexing finger-printed clones and a standard marker (used to assign normalized values to bands) in each well. Along with the shorter run time, this can increase the speed of data generation when using fluorescent fingerprinting.

However, once the raw data are produced it is generally quicker to enter and analyze the restriction digest agarose fingerprints. Band calling in Image is more automated, as the absorption of label and emission of signal are directly proportional to the size of the fragment (larger fragments absorb more label), a

From: *Methods in Molecular Biology, vol. 175: Genomics Protocols*
Edited by: M. P. Starkey and R. Elaswarapu © Humana Press Inc., Totowa, NJ

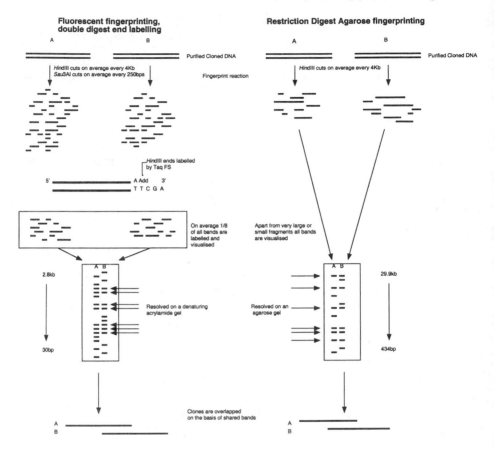

Fig. 1. A schematic of the two types of fingerprinting described here. Although the digestion, labeling, and fragment separation techniques differ significantly for both methods, and the data produced are incompatable, the same results will usually be seen after analysis of clones.

predictive decay of signal strength is seen facilitating automatic band calling. Double bands can be scored due to the additive effect of the signal. Fluorescently fingerprinted clones exhibit random signal decay as dye incorporation is determined by sequence or conformation factors at the ends of fragments *(3)* (*see* **Fig. 2**). The data produced by restriction digest agarose fingerprinting are more amenable to the automated algorithm routines used in FingerPrinting Contigs (FPC). The size information attached to the restriction digest agarose fingerprints facilitates more accurate positioning of clones within contigs, especially when picking sequence clones.

The Genome Sequencing Center (GSC) at Washington University School of Medicine (St. Louis MO) have undertaken to fingerprint the human male

Table 1
Comparison of Fluorescent End Labeling
and Restriction Digest Fingerprinting

	Fluorescent fingerprinting	Restriction digest agarose fingerprinting
Digestion	*Hin*dIII and *Sau*3AI 1 h then 1.5 h precipitation	*Hin*dIII 2 h
Labeling used	Incorporation of fluorescent dideoxy adenosine triphosphate molecule at *Hin*dIII ends	DNA stained in gel using an intercalatary dye (e.g., Vistra Green)
Resolution of fingerprints	Acrylamide gels 4.5 h run tune, mulitplexed clones and standard marker, increases throughput and accuracy	Agarose gels 16 h runtime, no multiplexing, post run stain 1.5 h
Entry of data in image	Manual, random variation of band strength	Manual, but more automation possible with decaying band strength
Raw data	Fingerprint fragments with migration values	Restriction digest fragments with size and migration values
Analysis of data in FPC	Automated with manual editing	Automated with less manual editing
Sizing overlaps	Estimated from the average size of a fingerprint band	Fragment sizes used

RPCI-11 BAC library *(6)*, using the *Hin*dIII restriction digest agarose gel method. If incorporation of data with the GSC is required, it is necessary to fingerprint novel clones using this method. The *Hin*dIII restriction digest method described here matches closely the GSC protocol *(*Marco Marra and Tammy Kucaba, personal communication, GSC, Washington University School of Medicine) especially with respect to digestion conditions and marker used and produces compatible data.

At the Sanger Centre, Carol Soderlund has written a script called *get_GSC*, which will extract chromosome specific clones from the Genome Sequencing Centre's database of fingerprints (*see* http://www.sanger.ac.uk/Users/cari/aux.shtml). These can then be imported into FPC (*see* **Subheadings 2.5.** and **3.5.**) where they are binned and ordered.

1.2. Southern Blotting and Hybridization

The aim of Southern blotting is to transfer DNA from one medium, the gel, to a stable medium which is suitable for subsequent hybridizations (*see*

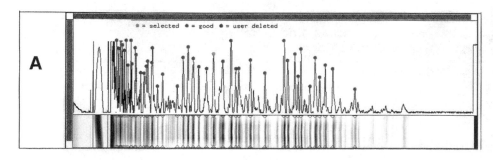

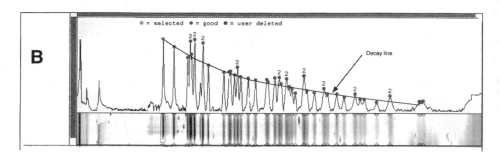

Fig. 2. Comparision from Image of the different types of band decay seen with: **(A)** *Hin*dIII, *Sau*3A-digested fluorescently labeled clone (there is random decay of the signal along the length of the gel); and **(B)** *Hin*dIII digested clone, stained with Vistra Green, displaying characteristic signal decay along the length of the gel. Bands above the decay line can be scored as doublets.

Note 1). DNA transfer is achieved by the upward movement of a reservoir of solution being drawn upward by capillary action, passing through the gel and transferring DNA onto a membrane.

This is one of the oldest techniques in molecular biology and has been modified throughout the years by the development of techniques such as downward capillary blotting and vacuum blotting *(7)*. Traditional alkaline Southern blotting *(8)* was used to transfer and fix the DNA from the gel onto a membrane for hybridization in this instance. As transfer was onto a nylon positively charged membrane, no fixation was needed after blotting. If other membrane types are used, fixation may be needed.

Once the digestion products of a bacterial clone are separated on a gel, they can be subjected to Southern blotting, and semipermanently secured on a nylon membrane. The membrane is then hybridized using a radioactively labeled probe such as an end product or the insert of a clone to determine similarities and regions of overlap between clones. Both small regions of overlap (5 kb) and large regions of overlap can be determined by this method (*see* **Figs. 3** and **4**.

dJ436H5   dJ524G21   dJ359L13
E N S NS E N   S NS E N S NS L

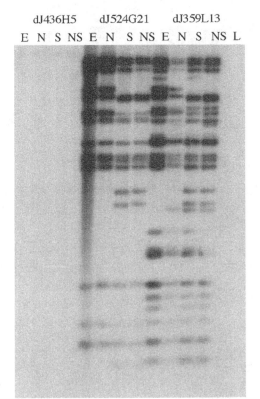

Fig. 3. Autoradiograph of Southern Blot hybridized with the insert only of dJ359L13. L = Ladder, E = *Eco*RI only digest, N = *Eco*RI and *Not*I double digest, S = *Eco*RI and *Sal*I double digest, NS = *Eco*RI, *Not*I, and *Sal*I digest. As seen from the strong hybridization signals for dJ524G21, there is an extensive overlap between this clone and dJ359L13. The absence of signal for dJ436H5 indicates no overlap between this clone and dJ359L13.

In this chapter we describe a hybridization protocol using a DNA polymerase based strand labeling, with a Rediprime labeling kit. This results in uniform labeling throughout the probe and high specific activity. Here, random oligo-nucleotide labeling was used, whereby all possible 9-mer nucleotides are present in a reaction mixture comprising of a buffered solution of dATP, dGTP, dTTP, and exonuclease-free Klenow enzyme. These random primers bind to the DNA, and the Klenow fragment of DNA polymerase I adds both labeled and unlabeled dNTPs. Uniform labeling of the probe is achieved throughout the probe due to all combinations of nonamers being present, and the random binding of these to the target DNA. In this experiment, [α-^{32}P] dCTP was used, resulting in the newly synthesized probe being radioactively labeled through-

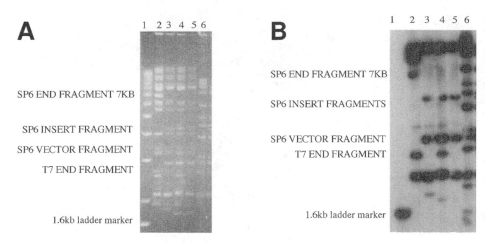

Fig. 4. **(A)** Photograph of gel prior to blotting and hybridization, and **(B)** after hybridization with dJ195C22 (whole PAC labeled, including vector). Lane 1, 1-kb ladder; Lane 2, dJ436H5 digested by *Eco*RI; Lane 3, dJ436H5 digested with *Eco*RI and *Not*I; Lane 4, dJ436H5 digested with *Eco*RI and *Sal*I; Lane 5, dJ436H5 digested with *Eco*RI, *Not*I and *Sal*I; Lane 6, dJ195C22 digested with *Eco*RI. Labeled are the SP6 end fragment of 7 kb and the two digestion products of this fragment when digested with *Not*I and *Sal*I, one the approx 3 kb vector fragment, and another approx 4 kb fragment of insert only. From the autroradiograph, it can be seen that dJ195C22 has bound strongly to the SP6 vector /insert end product, (lane 2) and equally as strongly to the insert only fragment (lanes 3–5) as to the vector fragment of approx 3 kb (lanes 3–5). Fragments other than vector only, or vector/insert fragments, have not bound the probe indicating that the region of overlap between these two clones is situated at the SP6 end of dJ436H5 and is approx 4 kb.

out *(9,10)*. Competition DNA was added to the probe as placental DNA to block out any repetitive signals that could be falsely identified as positive signals.

Relatively low stringency was used in these experiments to allow overlapping and similar clones to be easily identified. This was achieved by using a standard 65°C temperature for hybridization and posthybridization washes, and relatively high concentrations of NaCl in the posthybridization washes.

2. Materials

2.1. DNA Preparation from Bacterial Clones for Fingerprinting

1. 2X TY (per liter): Add 16 g Bacto-Tryptone, 10 g yeast extract, and 5 g NaCl. Dissolve in dH_2O, adjust pH to 7.0 with 5 N NaOH, adjust to final volume with dH_2O.
2. Combitip repeat dispenser (Eppendorf, The Netherlands).
3. 1 mL sterile deep-well microtiter plates (Beckman Instruments Inc., Fullerton, CA).

4. Deep-well microtiter plate caps (Beckman Instruments, Fullerton, CA).
5. U-bottom sterile microtiter plates and lids (Greiner Labortechnik).
6. 0.2 μm Filter bottom plates (Millipore, cat. no. MAGVN2250).
7. Multichannel pipets 5–50 μL and 50–300 μL and tips (Lab Systems, Finnpipet, Life Sciences International).
8. Sterile cocktail sticks or a 96-pin replicating tool (Denley, Labsystems Instruments).
9. RNase A (Ribonuclease A, Sigma Chemical, St. Louis, MO).
10. Orbital shaker (New Brunswick Scientific G24 environmental incubator, Edison, NJ).
11. Vortex genie fitted with a microtiter plate hold (Scientific Industries, Bohemia, NY).
12. Centrifuge with microtiter plate holding rotor (Sorvall RT7, du Pont Co., Sorvall, DE).
13. Class II microbiological safety cabinet (Walker Safety Cabinets Limited, UK).
14. Appropriate selective agents, e.g., chloramphenicol, kanamycin or ampicillin (Sigma Chemical).
15. Solution I (GTE): 4.504 g glucose (BDH Laboratory Supplies, Poole, UK), 10 mL *0.5 M* EDTA, 12.5 mL *1 M* Tris-HCl, pH 8.0. Make up to 500 mL with double-distilled H_2O and filter sterilize and store at 4°C.
16. Solution II (make fresh each time): 8.6 mL double-distilled H_2O, 1 mL 10% SDS, 400 μL *5M* sodium hydroxide (BDH Laboratory Supplies).
17. Solution III: *3 M* potassium acetate, pH 5.5. Store at room temperature.
18. Ethanol (70% with water) and isopropanol (BDH Laboratory Supplies).
19. Plate sealers (Costar, Corning, Corning, NY).

2.2. DNA Preparation from Bacterial Clones for Southern Blotting and Hybridization

1. LB broth: Yeast extract 5 g, tryptone 10 g, NaCl 10 g, made up to 1 L with deionized distilled water and autoclaved.
2. 20 μL, 200 μL, and 1000 μL pipets with tips (Gilson Medical Electronics, France).
3. 50 mL sterile falcon tubes (Greiner Labortechnik).
4. Sterile cocktail sticks.
5. Appropriate selective agent, normally kanamycin for PACs (Sigma Chemical).
6. Orbital shaker (Lh fermentation).
7. Centrifuge (Beckmann J2-21 and J-6B, Beckman Instruments).
8. Solution I: 15 m*M* Tris-HCl, pH 8, 10 m*M* ethylenediaminetetraacetic acid (EDTA), filter sterilized and stored at 4°C.
9. Solution II (make fresh each time): 0.2 M NaOH, 1% (w/v) sodium dodecyl sulfate (SDS). Stored at room temperature.
10. Solution III: *3 M* potassium acetate, pH 5.5 (chill before use).
11. Glass Corex tubes (du Pont Instruments).
12. Parafilm (American National Can).
13. Isopropanol and 70% v/v ethanol (BDH Laboratory Supplies).
14. Deionized distilled water containing 180 μg/mL RNase A (Sigma Chemical).
15. Phenol chloroform isoamyl alcohol 25:24:1 (Sigma Chemical).
16. 20, 200, and 1000 μL pipets and appropriate tips (Gilson).

17. 3 *M* Sodium acetate, pH 5.3.
18. 100% and 70% v/v ethanol (BDH).
19. 1.5 mL Eppendorfs (Eppendorf, The Netherlands).
20. –70 C freezer (Forma Scientific, Canada).
21. Microcentrifuge (MSE, Sanyo, UK).
22. Deionized distilled water.
23. Vortex (Genetic Research Instrumentation, Essex, UK).

2.3. Fluorescent Fingerprinting

1. ABI377 Sequencer (Perkin-Elmer Applied Biosystems, Foster City, CA).
2. Lambda DNA (500 ng/µL, New England Biolabs).
3. Ethanol (96% and 70% with water [BDH]).
4. 0.3 *M* sodium acetate.
5. Matrix standards for ABI; NED matrix standard (cat. no. 402996 Perkin-Elmer Applied Biosystems) and Fluorescence Amidite matrix standard kit, with tetracycline (TET), HEX, and ROX dichlororhodomide-based dyes, (cat. no. 401546 Perkin-Elmer Applied Biosystems) (*see* **Note 3**).
6. Fluorescently tagged dideoxy adenosine triphosphates, e.g., ddA-TET, -HEX and -NED Taq FS (cat. no. 4306379C, Custom Fingerprinting Kit, 1 mL each of at 10 µM NED, TET, and HEX, 3 mL Taq FS, Perkin-Elmer Applied Biosystems) (*see* **Notes 2** and **3**).
7. Fluorescently tagged dideoxy cytosine triphosphate, e.g., ddC-ROX 5.08 µM (cat. no. 402118, Dye Terminator Cycle Sequencing Core Kit, Perkin-Elmer Applied Biosystems) (*see* **Note 2**).
8. 37°C incubator (Economy Incubator Size I, Gallenkamp).
9. 80°C oven (MIND/18/CLAD, Philip Morris Ltd., UK).
10. Centrifuge with microtiter plate holding rotor (Sorvall RT7, du Pont Sorvall).
11. Benchtop centrifuge (Eppendorf 5415C, The Netherlands).
12. Blue dextran formamide dye: 9.8 mL deionized formamide, 200 µL 0.5 *M* EDTA, 0.01 g blue dextran dye.
13. 66-Well square tooth combs 0.2 mm (cat. no. 402183, Perkin-Elmer Applied Biosystems).
14. 10X (Tris-borate-EDTA) TBE buffer (cat. no. EC860, National Diagnostics, Atlanta, GA).
15. *Hin*dIII (20 U/µL, New England Biolabs), NEB2 buffer (New England Biolabs), *Sau*3AI (50 U/µL, Amersham Life Sciences), *Bsa*JI (2.5 U/µL, New England Biolabs).
16. Hamilton repeat dispenser (Hamilton, Reno, Nevada).
17. Plate sealers (Costar, Corning, Corning, NY).

2.4. Restriction Digest Agarose Fingerprinting

1. 1% agarose (SeaKem LE. FMC Bioproducts, Rockland, ME) gel, made with 1X Tris-acetate-EDTA (TAE) (*see* **Note 4**).
2. Gel tanks, Gator Wide Format System model A3-1 (Owl Scientific).

3. 121-Well comb (Marco A. Marra, personal communication, Washington University School of Medicine).
4. *Hin*dIII (40 U/ µL, Roche Molecular Biochemicals, Switzerland, formally Boehringer Mannheim, Germany).
5. Loading dye for marker (6X Buffer II for 10 mL, 1.5 g Ficoll, 0.025 g bromophenol blue, 0.025 g xylene cyanol, 10 mL sterile water). Loading dye for samples (for 10 mL: 0.1 g Orange G, 1.5 g Ficoll, 10 mL sterile water).
6. Marker mix: Analytical Marker DNA, wide band (Promega); DNA Molecular Weight Marker V (Roche Molecular Biochemicals, Switzerland, formally, Boehringer Mannheim, Germany).
7. Plate Sealers (Costar, Corning).
8. Bench top centrifuge (Eppendorf 5415C).
9. Combitip repeat dispenser (Eppendorf).
10. Hamilton repeat dispenser (Hamilton).
11. Cold room regulated to 4°C. (or recirculation system can be used).
12. Orbital platform shaker, Belly Dancer (Storvall Life Sciences, NC).
13. Vistra Green intercalating stain (Amersham Life Sciences).
14. FluorImager SI Vistra Fluorescence (Molecular Dynamics, Sunnyvale, CA).

2.5. Entry of Fingerprint Data in Image

A UNIX platform such as an, DECAlpha, solaris or linux, with 128 Mb of real memory.

2.6. Analysis of Fingerprint Data in FPC

FPC v4.5 is compatible with UNIX platforms DECAlpha and solaris, and with Silicon Graphics.

2.7. Restriction Digests of Clones
for Southern Blotting and Hybridization

1. *Eco*RI (10 U/µL), *Not*I (10 U/µL), *Sal*I (10 U/µL) and buffer D (all Promega).
2. Deionized distilled water.
3. 20, 200, and 1000 µL pipets and suitable tips (Gilson).
4. 0.5 mL Eppendorfs (Eppendorf).
5. 37°C incubator (Digi-Block, Laboratory Devices).

2.8. Electrophoresis of Digests for Southern Blotting

2.8.1. Electrophoresis for EcoRI NotI, and SalI Digest

1. 0.8% agarose (0.5% agarose for check gels), (Amresco, OH), made with 1X TAE (40 mM Tris Acetate, 2 mM Na$_2$ EDTA·2 H$_2$O).
2. Ethidium bromide 10 mg/mL (Sigma Chemical) added gel to give a final concentration of 0.1 µg/µL.
3. Gel tank, casting tray 27 × 20 cm for overnight electrophoresis, and 24-well comb (Hybaid, Hampshire).

4. One kilobase DNA ladder (Gibco-BRL Life Technologies, Paisley, UK).
5. Loading dye (15% w/v Ficoll and Orange G dye).

2.8.2. Pulsed-Field Gel Electrophoresis

1. 140 × 120 cm casting tray (Bio-Rad, Hercules, CA).
2. 100 mL 1% low melting point (LMP) gel (Gibco-BRL Life Technologies) made with 0.5X TBE (89 mM Tris base, 89 mM boric acid, 1 mM EDTA), (*see* **Note 13**).
3. Cold room at 4°C.
4. PFGE equipment (Bio-Rad, CHEF DRII, CA).
5. 24-Well comb (Hybaid).
6. Low-range PFGE marker (New England Biolabs).
7. Lambda *Hin*dIII (Promega).
8. Loading dye.

2.9. Southern Blotting

1. 3MM blotting paper (Whatmann, BDH).
2. 0.4 M NaOH.
3. 0.25 M HCl.
4. Fluorescent ruler (Promega).
5. Blotting towels (Kimberly Clark, Kleenex).
6. Hybond N+ nylon membrane (Amersham Life Sciences).
7. Saran Wrap (Dow).

2.10. Hybridization

1. Hybridization glass bottles (Hybaid).
2. Hybridization oven set at 65°C (Hybaid).
3. Nylon meshes (Hybaid).
4. Hybridization solution (10% dextran SO_4, 10X Denhardts v/v, 50 mM Tris-HCl, 6X standard saline citrate (SSC) v/v, 1% sarkosyl).
5. Rediprime labeling kit (Amersham Life Sciences).
6. [α-^{32}P] dCTP (Amersham Life Sciences).
7. Boiling water bath (Grant, Cambridge, UK).
8. Pipets and tips (Gilson).
9. 37°C incubator (Digi-Block).
10. Competition DNA, 10 µL placental DNA, 11 mg/mL (Sigma), 7.5 µL deionized distilled water, 32.5 µL 20X SSC, pH 7.
11. Shaking incubator set at 65°C (Innova 4080 Brunswick Scientific, NJ).
12. Posthybridization wash I, 0.1% w/v SDS, 1X SSC, wash II, 0.1% w/v SDS, 0.5X SSC, both preheated to 65°C (*see* **Note 7**).
13. Saran Wrap (Dow).
14. Cassette (G.R.I Hi Speed X, Essex, UK).
15. Film (Sterling Diagnostic Imaging Newark, DE).

3. Methods

3.1. DNA Preparation from Bacterial Clones for Fingerprinting

Prior to the generation of fingerprint data it is necessary to extract cloned DNA from a bacterial host. The same DNA preparation procedure is used for both methods described here. The procedure is based on an alkaline lysis method *(11)*, updated first to a 96-well format *(12)*, then improved by incorporating a filter-bottomed plate step *(5)*.

1. In a deep-well microtiter plate dispense 500 µL of 2X TY plus an appropriate selective agent.
2. Using either a 96-well inoculating tool, or sterile cocktail sticks, inoculate each well from one of the clone glycerol stocks. After sealing the wells, grow the mix for 18 h in a 37°C incubator with shaking.
3. From the overnight growth transfer 250 µL to a clean microtiter plate and centrifuge at 1550*g* for 4 min.
4. Remove the supernatant and resuspend the pellet by vortexing gently (vortex genie set to 4–5). A cocktail stick can be used for resuspending pellets still attached to the plate.
5. To the resuspended pellet add, 25 µL solution I, tap the plate gently, and add 25 µL of solution II. Mix by tapping and leave at room temperature for 5 min. The solution should clear as the bacterial clones lyse.
6. To each well add 25 µL solution III and mix by gentle tapping and leave at room temperature for 5 min. Seal the plate and vortex gently for 10 s.
7. Tape a 2-µm filter-bottomed plate to the top of a microtiter plate which contains 100 µL of isopropanol. Add the total well volume to the filter-bottomed plate and centrifuge at 1550*g* for 2 min at 20°C.
8. Remove the filter-bottomed plate and leave the microtiter plate at room temperature for 30 min. Centrifuge at 1550*g* for 20 min at 20°C.
9. Remove the supernatant and dry the DNA by inverting the plate and placing it on a clean tissue paper, being careful to avoid any disruption to the pellets.
10. Prepare RNase A: 10 µL of 1 mg/mL RNase A/1 mL of $T_{0.1}E$ (*see* **Note 5**).
11. To the dried DNA add 100 µL of 70% ethanol, mix by gentle tapping.
12. Centrifuge at 1550*g* for 10 min at 20°C.
13. For restriction digest agarose fingerprinting, repeat above wash (*see* **step 11**).
14. Remove the supernatant and dry as before, ensure that the pellet is transparent and add 5 µL of $T_{0.1}E$ with RNase A. Store samples at –20°C (*see* **Note 6**).
15. Check the preparation by separating the DNA on a small 1% agarose gel. Typical DNA yield should be between 20–30 ng/µL.

3.2. DNA Preparation from Bacterial Clones for Southern Blotting and Hybridization

In the case of PAC clones, which are used in these experiments, the DNA is inserted into a pCYPAC2 vector, which is based upon the P1 artificial chromosome (PAC) and Bacterial Artificial Chromosome (BAC) vector systems of cloning DNA *(13)*. The clones contain, on average, approximately 120 kb of insert. A rapid alkaline lysis prep is used to isolate DNA *(14)*, with average yield of 20–30 ng/μL. The protocol detailed in **Subheading 3.2.1.** can be scaled up or down depending on the yield desired. This is then followed by a standard phenol-chloroform-isoamyl alcohol cleanup of the DNA to remove protein carry over from the prep, which may interfere with subsequent digestions *(7)*.

3.2.1. DNA Preparation

1. Inoculate 20 mL LB containing 250 μg kanamycin with a single bacterial colony.
2. Incubate overnight (approx 16 h) in an orbital shaker set to 250 rpm, 37°C.
3. Centrifuge (Beckmann J2-21) for 10 min at 21,000g to pellet bacterial cells.
4. Discard supernatant and resuspend in 3 mL of Solution I.
5. Add 3 mL of Solution II and allow to stand at room temperature for 5 min. During this time, the solution should change from being fairly turbid to become clear as the bacterial cells lyse.
6. Slowly add 3 mL of Solution III and place on ice for at least 5 min. Solution III precipitates the *Escherichia coli* DNA and proteins.
7. Transfer to 30 mL Corex tubes and centrifuge (Beckmann J-6B) at 14,500g for 10 min to precipitate the *E. coli* DNA and proteins.
8. Avoiding white precipitate, remove supernatant containing PAC DNA, and add to 8 mL of ice cold isopropanol to precipitate the DNA.
9. Stand on ice for at least 5 min. At this stage, tubes may be left at –20°C overnight. Alternatively, if a lot of white precipitate is removed with the supernatant, **step 7** can be repeated.
10. Centrifuge tubes (Beckmann J-6B) for 15 min at 14,500g.
11. Without disturbing the pellet, remove the isopropanol and wash pellet with 5 mL 70% ethanol.
12. Centrifuge (Beckmann J-6B) for 5 min at 14,500g.
13. Repeat 70% ethanol wash (optional).
14. Allow pellet to air dry until translucent and resuspend in 200 μL of deionized distilled water containing RNaseA. DNA can be stored at –20°C until needed (*see* **Note 14**).
15. To determine concentration, digest 5 μL of DNA with *Eco*RI (*see* **Subheading 3.7.**), and run on a 0.8% agarose gel in 1X TBE buffer.

3.2.2. Phenol:Chloroform:Isoamyl Alcohol Cleanup of DNA

1. To DNA add an equal volume of phenol-chloroform-isoamyl alcohol. Vortex briefly to mix.
2. Centrifuge at 10,000g for 15 s and remove supernatant containing DNA into a fresh Eppendorf tube.
3. Add 1/10th volume of sodium acetate, vortex to mix, and 2X volume of cold 100% ethanol to precipitate the DNA.

4. Place at –70° C for 15 min or at –20°C for 30 min.
5. Centrifuge at 10,000*g* for 5 min.
6. Without disturbing the pellet, remove supernatant and wash pellet in 70% ethanol.
7. Centrifuge at 10,000*g* for 5 min.
8. Repeat ethanol wash (optional).
9. Resuspend pellet in 50 μL of deionized distilled water.

3.3. Fluorescent Fingerprinting

1. Prepare a 5% denaturing acrylamide gel, (20 mL acrylamide, 140 μL 10% ammonium persulphate, 28 μL *N,N,N′,N′*-tetramethylethy-lenediamine [TEMED]).
2. Set up three digest premixes, one for each fluorescent label in three 1.5 mL microfuge tubes labeled TET, HEX, and NED.
3. For one 96-well plate add to each tube, 25.5 μL $T_{0.1}E$, 24.5 μL NEB2 buffer, 5 μL *Hind*III (20 U/μL), 8 μL Taq FS (32 U/μL) and 3 μL *Sau*3AI (30 U/μL), then to the appropriate tube add 4 μL of one of the three ddA dyes .
4. Mix using a vortex, and spin in a benchtop centrifuge.
5. To the first third of the prepped DNA plate (A1-H4) add 2 μL of the TET premix using a Hamilton repeat dispenser, to the second third (A5-H8) add the HEX premix, and the to last third (A9-H12) the NED premix; cover with a plate sealer.
6. Mix the reaction by gentle agitation on a vortex, and spin the plate to 150*g* for 10 s.
7. Incubate the reaction for 1 h at 37°C.
8. Using a multichannel pipet, add 7 μL of 0.3 *M* sodium acetate and 40 μL of 96% ethanol to each well. Pool samples labeled with different dyes.
9. To column 1 add columns 5 and 9 and mix, to column 2 add columns 6 and 10 and mix, to column 3 add columns 7 and 11 and mix, and to column 4 add columns 8 and 12 and mix.
10. Incubate at room temperature for 30 min in the dark.
11. Pellet the DNA by spinning the plate at 1550*g* for 20 min at 20°C.
12. Discard the supernatant and dry the pellet by tapping the plate face down onto tissue paper.
13. Wash the pellet by adding 100 μL of 70% ethanol to each well and mix by gentle tapping.
14. Spin at 1550*g* for 10 min at 20°C.
15. Discard the supernatant and dry the pellet.
16. Resuspend the DNA in 5 μL $T_{0.1}E$.
17. To a 1.5-mL microfuge tube add 70 μL $T_{0.1}E$, 10 μL NEB2, 6 μL lambda DNA (500 ng/μL), 6 μL *BsaJ1* (2.5 U/μL), 4 μL Taq FS (32 U/μL) and 4 μL ddC-ROX.
18. Incubate for 1 h at 60°C.
19. To the reaction mix add 100 μL 0.3 *M* sodium acetate and 400 μL 96% ethanol.
20. Leave at room temperature in the dark for 15 min, then at –20°C for 20 min.
21. Spin in a benchtop centrifuge at maximum speed for 20 min.
22. Discard the supernatant and dry the pellet by tapping the plate gently onto a tissue paper.
23. Wash the pellet by adding 200 μL 70% ethanol and spin in a benchtop centrifuge at maximum speed for 5 min.

24. Discard the supernatant and dry pellet as before, this time ensuring that the DNA is clear.
25. Resuspend the pellet in 120 μL $T_{0.1}E$ and 120 μL blue dextran formamide dye.
26. Prior to loading, add 2 μL of the marker mix to each sample using a Hamilton repeat dispenser.
27. Spin the plate at 150g in a centrifuge.
28. Denature the DNA in the plate for 10 min at 80°C and load 1.25 μL of each sample on a ABI377 sequencer.
29. Use ABI Prism Collection Software v1.1.
30. After data collection, transfer the gel image to a UNIX workstation for entry into Image.

3.4. Restriction Digest Agarose Fingerprinting

1. Prepare a 1% agarose gel in 1X TAE. (for a Gator Wide format gel tank, to 4.5 g agarose add 450 mL 1X TAE) (*see* **Note 3**).
2. Set up one reaction mix to digest a 96-well plate of DNA in a 1.5-mL microfuge tube. Add 231 μL H_2O, 99 μL buffer B, and 55 μL *Hind*III.
3. Mix using a vortex, and spin in a benchtop centrifuge at maximum speed.
4. To each well add 4 μL of the reaction mix and cover with a plate sealer.
5. Mix the reaction by gentle agitation on a vortex, and spin the plate to 150g for 10 s.
6. Incubate at 37°C for 2 h.
7. Terminate the reaction by adding 2 μL of loading dye using a Hamilton repeat dispenser, and seal the plate. Either load immediately or store at 4°C.
8. Before loading the samples, make the marker in a 1.5-mL microfuge tube by adding (per gel) 19.2 μL $T_{0.1}E$, 1.5 μL analytical marker DNA wide range, 0.2 μL molecular weight marker V and 4.2 μL 6X loading dye.
9. Load 0.8 μL of the marker in the first well and then every fifth well.
10. Load 1 μL of sample between the marker lanes.
11. Run the gel at 4°C in a cold room for 15 h at 90 V.
12. Prepare a fresh stain mix for the gel by mixing 1 *M* Tris-HCl, 0.5 mL 0.1 *M* EDTA and 50 μL Vistra Green. Make up the vol to 500 mL with H_2O. Store at 4°C and use within 48 h.
13. Once run, cut the gel down so the length is 19–20 cm and stain for 30–45 min on a shaker.
14. Briefly wash with H_2O to remove excessive stain.
15. Scan the gel on a FluorImager SI. For best results, use a 530-nm emission filter.
16. For best results use the following parameters: 100 μm pixel size; normal detection sensitivity; 16-bit digital resolution; single label dye; 488 nm excitation filter; 530 nm Em filter 1, and photomultiplier tube (PMT) voltage is 800.
17. Transfer the gel image to a UNIX workstation for entry and analysis.

3.5. Entry of Fingerprint Data Using Image

Raw fingerprinting data is processed in the program Image (*see* **Fig. 5**), this was first developed in the late 1980s *(18)* and upgraded at The Sanger Centre

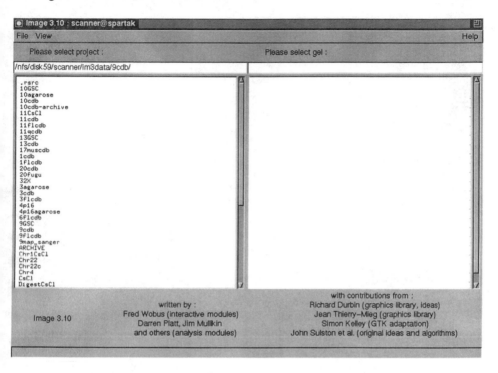

Fig. 5. Main menu in Image: list of project directories are shown.

by Darren Platt and Friedemann Wobus, current development and curation is performed by Jim Mullikin and John Attwood (*see* http://www.sanger.ac.uk/ Software/Image). Using a package of analysis algorithms, Image converts raw data to a set of normalized band values and gel images. This is achieved by interactively stepping through three main windows (*see* **Fig. 6A–D**). The first of these is lane tracking, lines matching the fingerprint lanes are traced along the length of the gel. The next step is band calling; the presence and fine position of authentic bands are edited while artifacts or nongenuine bands are removed. To analyze the clones, each fingerprint band must have a normalized integer value attached to it, this is achieved in the final step of Image, called standard marker locking. Here, the band call in the standard lane is aligned against a known standard pattern and this is used to normalize fingerprint band values.

1. Download Image via File Transfer Protocol (FTP) by selecting the appropriate file for your system.
2. Make a directory for the each project. To import a raw gel image into Image prior to data entry, use the command, imimport <project name> <gel name> <image file>.

Fluorescent Fingerprint Gel

Restriction Digest Agarose Fingerprinting Gel

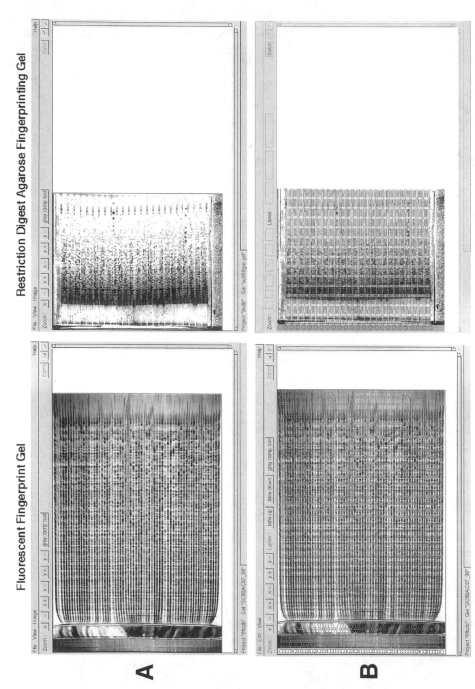

A

B

84

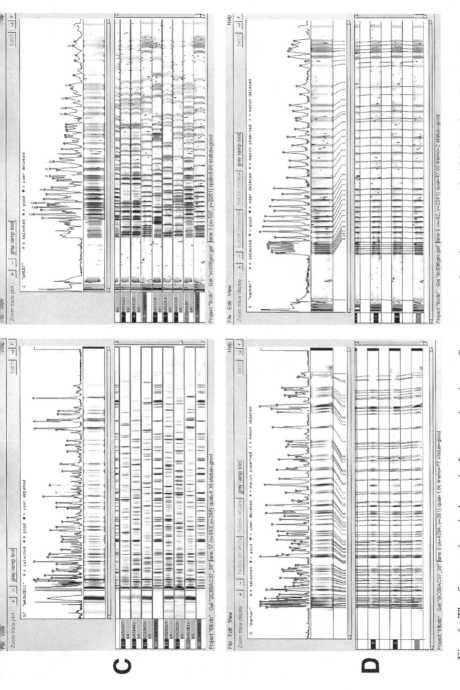

Fig. 6. The four main windows in Image, showing a fluorescent gel and agarose gel. (A) Interface for raw image manipulation, e.g., clipping down image. (B) Lanetracking. (C) Bandcalling. (D) Standard Marker locking.

85

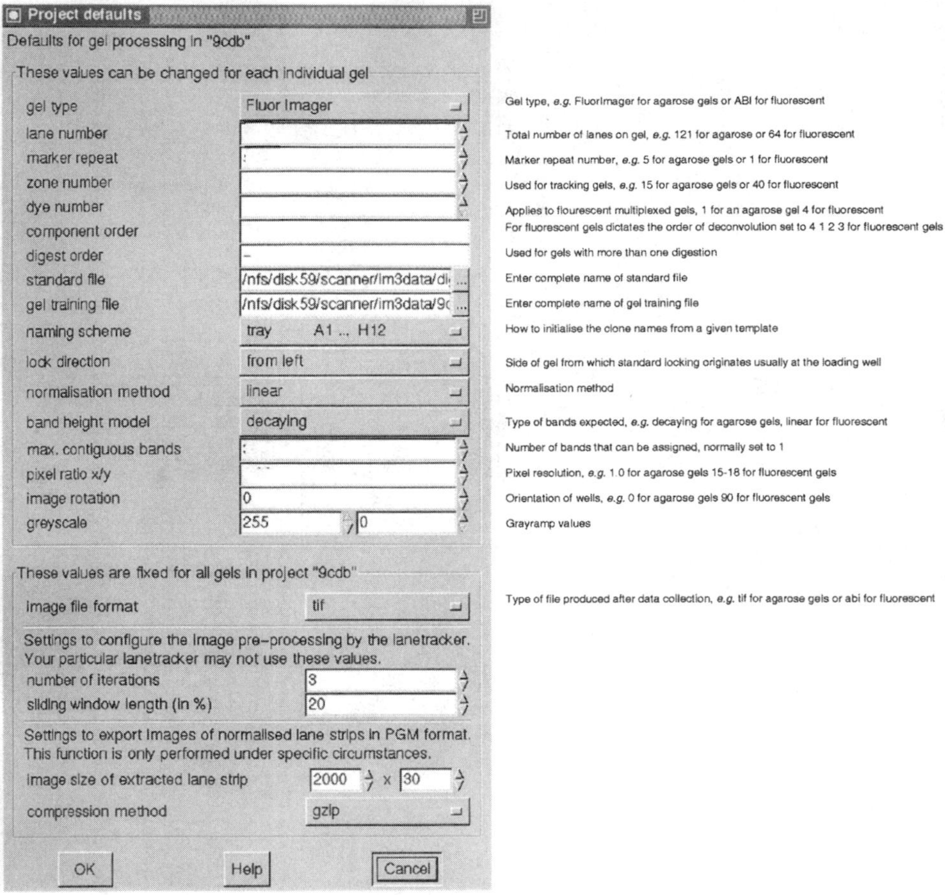

Fig. 7. Default parameters for Image. Use the up and down arrows next to the figures to alter the settings.

3. Set up default parameters need to be set for each project in Image. If all the gels in one project are to have the same characteristics, then the parameters need only be set once (*see* http://www.sanger.ac.uk/Software/Image/help/) (*see* **Fig. 7**).
4. Enter the gel number. Once the defaults are set for a project they may need to be slightly altered for individual gels, e.g., the number of sample lanes may differ between gels, however, the main defaults should remain constant for a given project.
5. Enter the FIRST CLONE NAME, and the GEL NUMBER; this can be alphanumeric. Each window has the same basic layout: scroll bars at the top and right-hand side of the image, a zoom function (400% for band calling and marker locking is appropriate), and a gray ramp tool. Use the arrows in the top right-hand corner of the window to negotiate through the different stages.

6. Clip the image and remove unwanted portions of the gel (*see* **Fig. 6A**).
7. Edit Lanetracking: The lines superimposed on the image represent the lanes on the gel, these lines must accurately delineate the lanes. On agarose-digest gels, there are two types of lines; markers (red) and samples (yellow). Moving the marker lines interpolates all sample lines in between to their regular space with regard to the neighboring marker line. For fluorescent gels, there is only one type of line, as the marker is multiplexed (*see* **Fig. 6B**) (*see* **Note 7**).

    There are two main ways to alter the position of the lines to match the lanes:
    a. Whole lines can be moved by activating (they will go black) the circular check box(es) at the left-hand end of the screen.
    b. Smaller regions can be adjusted by highlighting (they will go green) the box(es) running down the length of the line. For whole lines and groups of highlighted boxes, use the cursor keys to adjust the position, for single boxes use the mouse to drag up or down.
8. Edit Bandcalling (*see* **Fig. 6C**): Genuine, informative bands should be tagged and partials or gel artifacts removed, (*see* **Note 8**). For fluorescent gels the marker and the three clones present in a lane will be deconvoluted. On the band-calling screen, the first clone is selected and highlighted red, the top half of the screen shows an x–y plot representation of the pixel values scanned along the middle of the lane. Bands are represented by points on the plot and by triangles on the lane strip, an active band is red, nonactive ones are green. One lane is active at a time, move up or down lanes using the *cursor keys* or, **F** and **B**. Remove deleted clones (missing insert DNA few fingerprint bands) or partially cut clones (numerous fingerprint bands of equal intensity) using the *middle mouse button* on the undesirable lane. Add bands by using the *left mouse button* on the x–y plot or **M**. Move forward by using *f* or *space bar*, and back using *b*. Use *d* to delete a band and *n* or *middle mouse button* to remove one. Reposition bands by using the *left* or *right cursor keys,* if a band has been positioned on the side of a peak *r*, will roll the band to the nearest peak. At this point, clone names can be added by activating the box to the side of a lane using the *left mouse button,* then typing the name (this can be alphanumeric). All bands below a certain height can be removed by using the *left mouse button* to draw a box in the plot window and all bands within that section can be deleted.
9. Edit Standard Marker lock (*see* **Fig. 6D**), (*see* **Note 8**): The display and functions are similar to **step 3**, however, this time only the marker lanes are shown along with bands, from the standard file. To accurately interpolate the position of sample bands the standard file bands and the marker lane bands must line up. Use the x–y plot to check if the two match. To increase the match, pick a lane and move through each band checking the pattern. Once this is locked use *relock on lane*. This will apply the position of the current lane's bands onto the bands in all other marker lanes. Finally, go through each marker lane and check that each band is correctly positioned at the top of appropriate peaks. To disregard any changes made by the locking module, use *relock on whole*; the gel is then ready to finish. This will create a <gelname>.bands and a <projectname>.

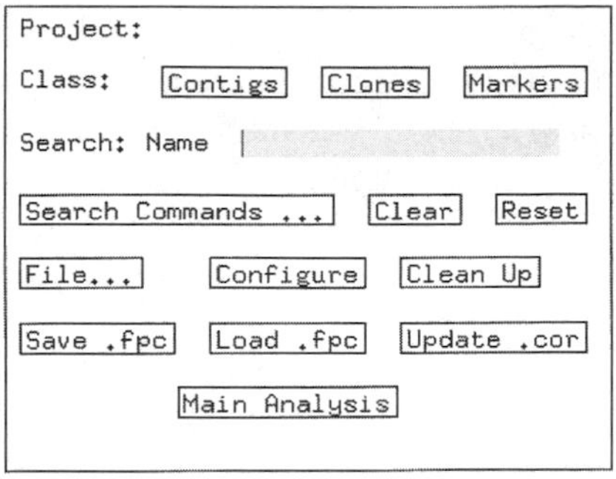

```
Project:

Class:    [Contigs]  [Clones]  [Markers]

Search: Name  |

[Search Commands ...]  [Clear]  [Reset]

[File...]    [Configure]  [Clean Up]

[Save .fpc]  [Load .fpc]  [Update .cor]

          [Main Analysis]
```

Fig. 8. The *FPC* Main Menu. Functions for different class searches are present (*Contigs*, *Clones*, and *Markers*) as well as options for more specific inquires from *Search Commands*. From *File*, new projects can be created and ACeDB-formated files can be written or read into the database. *Configure* is used to alter the display of contigs, change to variable tolerence and enter the vector file. *Save .fpc* writes the .fpc file, so after each set of edits this should be selected in order for the changes to be saved. Existing projects can be loaded with, *Load .fpc*. To read in new data from the Image directory select *Update .cor*. For details of the *Main Analysis* window *see* **Fig. 10**.

<gelname>.gel files, for restriction digest agarose gels an additional <gelname>. sizes file will be written (*see* **Note 9**).

The program "imtransfer," which comes with the Image package, will copy the finished files to the appropriate FPC directories if the name of the image project is the same as the FPC project, so, if in **step 2** the project was called 9GSC, then:

Image directory 9GSC		FPC project 9GSC
<gelname>.bands	will be copied to	/Image
<projectname>.<gelname>.gel	will be copied to	/Gels
<gelname>.sizes	if present will be copied to	/Sizes

3.6. Analysis of Fingerprirnt Data Using FPC

Once processed, the data are analyzed in another program developed at the Sanger Centre: FPC (FingerPrinting Contigs) (*19,20*; *see* **Fig. 8**). FPC is an interactive program that can operate on a selfcontained basis or interact with other programs particularly ACeDB (*21*). *It* provides rapid comparisons between fingerprinted clones using a probability-of-coincidence equation, and an interactive graphical display allowing user interface and manipulation.

Each clone is represented by a set of integer band values. Overlap between any two clones are identified by the similarity of these values, within a set tolerance. Once overlap is established, clones are organized into contigs (**Fig. 9A**),

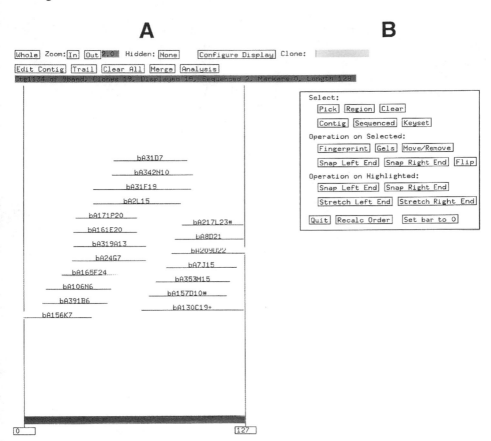

Fig. 9. (**A**) Clones are contiguated in FPC after overlaps are established. The coordinates shown on each cursor, 0–127, represent the number of bands the contig spans (each unit is equivalent to one band); the degree the clones overlap corresponds to the number of shared bands. (**B**) Selecting the *Edit Contig* function allows manual manipulation and fine positioning of clones. From this window the fingerprints or gel traces can be selected from; a single clone, *Pick*; a portion of the contig defined by the cursors, *Region*, from the whole contig, *Contig*; or from just the sequence clones, *Sequence*. Any clone's position can be refined by highlighting the clone and using the *Snap Left/Right End*. This will position the clone relative to the selected cursor.

coordinates are used to represent the clones' bands and the degree of overlap equates to the number of shared bands.

1. Download FPC along with a postscript manual, FPC.ps, by anonymous FTP from, ftp.sanger.ac.uk.pub/fpc. A User's Guide is available at http://www.sanger.ac.uk/cari/fpc_faq.shtml.

2. Create a project directory and sub-directories called Image, Bands, and Gel. When using restriction-digest agarose gels, a subdirectory called Sizes is also needed.
3. In Image (*see* **Subheading 3.5.**) the following output files and destinations can be found:

    1 Image → *.bands → /Image   fluorescent fingerprinting
    2 Image → *.bands → /Image   restriction digest fingerprinting
             *.sizes   → /Sizes   where migration values are used for analysis
    3 Image → *.sizes → /Image   restriction digest fingerprinting
             *.bands → /Bands   where size values are used for analysis

In each case;

$$\text{Image} \rightarrow *.\text{gel} \rightarrow /\text{Gel}$$

where * is the name of the gel.

    In **step 2**, the /Sizes are used only when comparing two clones and in the size calculator (written by Ken McDonald at the GSC).

    In 3, the /Bands are used with the gel data.

4. Start FPC (*see* **Fig. 8**): From *File...* drop-down menu, go to *Create new project* and name the project. This will write a <projectname>.fpc and a <projectname>.cor file.
5. To read the file(s) in the Image directory into FPC, select *Update .cor*, this will add the clones to the database and move the <gelname>.bands to the Bands directory.
6. To achieve the best results in FPC, the parameters must be set correctly, set these in the *Main Analysis* window (*see* **Fig. 10**), or *Contig Analysis* window (*see* **Fig. 11**).
   a. Tolerance: This determines the variation allowed between the position of any two bands that can be said to overlap. Set too high and spurious overlaps will be seen, too low and genuine matches will be missed. When fingerprinting human bacterial clone libraries we have found that for fluorescent gels or digest agarose gels using migration values from the <gelname>.bands set it to 7. For restriction digest agarose gels using fragment sizes from the <gelname>.sizes, use a variable tolerance (0.07% along the length of the gel). This is changed in the *Configure* menu. Migration values are generally used for both fluorescent gels and restriction digest agarose gels, this gives a more informative visual display. It is important not to change the tolerance once set as this figure is used in the overlap equation.
   b. Cutoff: This is used in the overlap equation, the higher the exponent the greater the stringency applied to the probability that two clones will overlap. The following factors are taken into account: the total number of bands in each clone, the tolerance, and number of matching bands between two clones. The number of bands in a clone is proportional to the size of the insert (given an even distribution of restriction sites), therefore it is sometimes necessary to vary the cutoff when comparing clones with different-sized inserts.
   When fingerprinting human bacterial clone libraries, we have found that for fluorescent gels a cut off of between le-06 to le-08 is appropriate, and for

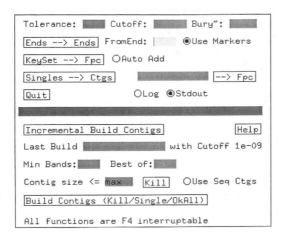

Fig. 10. The Main Analysis window of FPC. Set the *Tolerance*, *Cutoff*, and *Bury* parameters for each project here (for further details see text). Analyzing large sets of data is best done from this window.The *CB map* can be applied to all clones using *Build Contigs*, or just to new data using *Incremental Build Contigs*. A set of clones, e.g., all the clones on one gel, can be grouped together and analyzed using, *Keyset → Fpc*, or all the singletons using *Singles → Fpc*. If *Auto Add* is highlighted, overlapping clones will be automatically added to contigs.

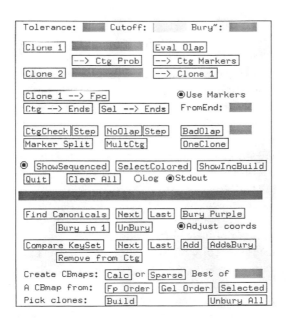

Fig. 11. The *Contig Analysis* window of FPC. From *Create CBmaps*, select *Calc* to rerun the *CB* algorithm on each contig.

restriction digest agarose gels le-10 is used. This should be set in the *Main Analysis* or *Contig Analysis* windows (*see* **Note 10**).

c. Vector file: Cloned fragments are maintained in their bacterial hosts by ligation to vector DNA, which contain resistance genes allowing selection of transformed bacterial cells. Vector DNA will normally produce at least one fingerprint band, usually present in each clone, which should be removed prior to analysis. To identify the vector bands enter at least 25 clones into FPC that do not overlap. Assemble the clones in one fingerprint (*see* **Fig. 12C**) and gel-trace window (*see* **Fig. 13**), and look for bands that are common between all of the clones. Find the migration values for these bands from the .bands file, and the sizes, if available, from the .sizes files. Take the mean value of each vector band from the 25 clones. It is these values that are added into the Vector File, e.g., for the RPCI-11 BAC library restriction digest agarose fingerprinted.

d. Migration values: bacfilter

    *

    1387
    3695
    3766

If a band lies within +/–7 it will be removed.

e. Sizes: bacfilter

    *

    6524
    510
    452

If a band lies within 7% of the value it will be removed where * is the prefix used for each clone from a library.

Only one band will be removed, so if a genuine band lies in the same position as a vector, and they were scored as a double in Image (*see* **Fig. 2**), it will remain. Enter the Vector file name in the Configure menu.

f. Bury: A facility exists to bury clones within another, this can be achieved manually using the *Edit clone* function. However FPC will automatically bury clones and the stringency for this should be set in the *Main Analysis* window. A 90% match of bands between any two clones in normally used, therefore set the *Bury* to 0.10. A clone will become buried in another if it shares 90% of its bands with the parent (or canonical) clone. As well as facilitating manual manipulation, this can also help identify potentially deleted clones and confirm the legitimacy of the canonical clone.

7. Once the parameters are correctly set the fingerprint data can be analyzed. There are two main ways large sets of data can be analyzed, (a) *CB map*, or the more interactive (b) *Keyset → FPC*.

a. The *CB map* will group together clones which share a high probability of overlap (i.e., they have a probability of coincidence score that is below the Cutoff). It uses a "greedy" algorithm, which can produce an suboptimal solution, so it generates N solutions (default is 10) and uses the best one. The

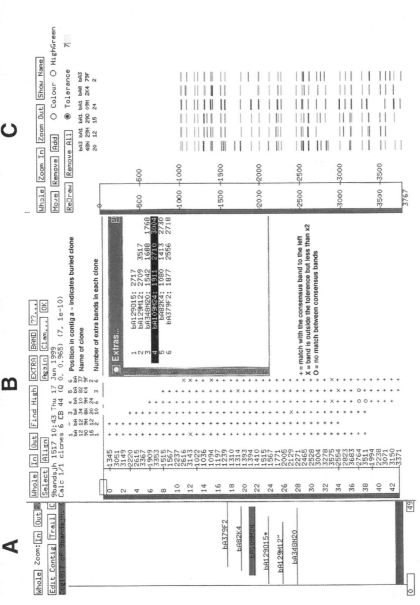

Fig. 12. The results of a consensus band map build for a new set of clones. (A) shows the contig display. The clones are represented as horizontal bars the length of which are determined by the number of bands in each clone. (B) The consensus band output. The position of the consensus bands is shown, the bars represent partially ordered groups. The precise value of each clone's extra bands can be viewed by selecting EXTRA, as shown in the figure. Other functions include zoom and clone selection facilities. The CB map can be rerun on each contig using the Contig Analysis window (Fig. 11). By selecting Again, the algorithm can be rerun on that set of clones. Once an optimal solution has been attained, minimizing the number of Os and extras, then select OK and instantiate the CB map. (C) shows an idealized electronic display of the bands identified in each clone in this contig: bA109M24 has been selected.

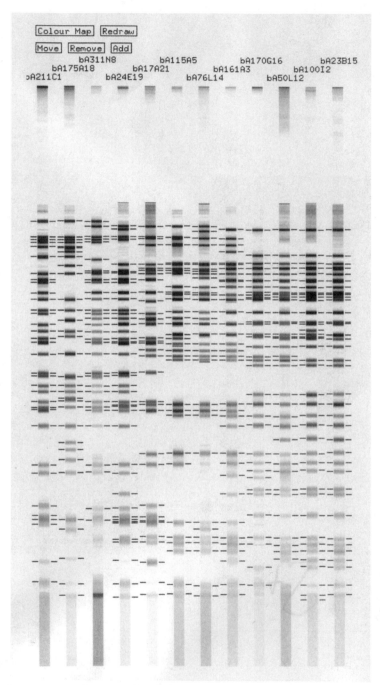

Fig. 13. Gel traces for a contig of clones from FPC. Above each clone is its name and the lines next to the trace represent bands called in *Image*.

Contig	Clones	Markers	Sequenced	Score	Qs
1549	4	2	–	1.000	0
1550	4	3	–	0.980	0
1551	4	2	–	0.966	0
1552	4	1	–	0.988	0
1553	4	4	–	0.980	0
1554	4	2	–	0.994	0
1555	5	1	–	0.945	0
1556	5	3	–	0.961	0
1557	4	5	–	0.990	0
1558	4	–	–	0.995	0
1559	7	2	–	0.869	0
1560	6	1	–	0.955	0
1561	2	–	–	1.000	0
1562	4	1	–	0.961	0
1563	5	2	–	0.977	0
1564	7	3	–	0.972	0
1565	5	1	–	0.959	0
1566	3	1	–	1.000	0
1567	3	–	–	0.985	0
1568	4	2	–	0.987	0
1569	5	2	–	0.967	0
1570	3	4	–	1.000	0
1571	6	4	–	0.927	0
1572	3	1	–	1.000	0
1573	2	–	–	1.000	0
1574	4	–	–	0.980	0
1575	4	1	–	0.966	0
1576	5	–	–	0.952	0
1577	2	–	–	1.000	0
1578	6	2	–	0.937	0
1579	3	3	–	0.994	0
1580	7	–	–	0.870	0
1581	8	2	–	0.960	0
1582	4	4	–	0.984	0
1583	3	–	–	0.980	0
1584	2	2	–	1.000	0

Fig. 14. The output from a *CB map*. Shown are the contig numbers, the number of clones in each contig, the presence of markers (e.g., Sequence Tagged Sites) in a contig and if clones have been tagged for sequencing. The *Score* is an indication as to how well the CB map solution has worked, with 1.000 being optimal. Following that are the *Q* scores; too many of these indicate a poor solution.

fingerprint bands for a contig are arranged to fit the physical order in which they lie. This is a powerful and quick tool for contig assembly. Although it can be used for fluorescent data, it is particularly useful for restriction digest agarose fingerprinting.

From the *Main Analysis* window either select *Build Contigs*, this will kill all contigs (unless a sequence clone is present and the *Use Seq Ctgs* is off) and use all the singleton data and rebuild the entire data set and construct new contigs, or *Incremental Build Contigs*, which will take only data that were added after the last build (*see* **Fig. 14**). A contig with a *Score* approaching or at 1.000 is optimal. The *Q* column indicates the number of clones that, although they overlap significantly with at least one other clone in the contig, could not be accurately aligned within the contig. This can be caused by poor fingerprints, repeat elements within clones producing similar fingerprint patterns, or sub-optimal solution as a product of the algorithm. In the latter, manual manipulation may be the only option.

For contigs with a low score it is advisable to rerun the *CB map* by selecting *Calc* on the *Contig Analysis* window (*see* **Fig. 11**). An example is shown in **Fig. 12**. Even after this point, fine manipulation of clones may be necessary to the refine the order and optimize overlap of clones especially minimum sets of sequence clones.

b. Using *Keyset → FPC* offers a less-automated approach to contig building. First, the type of keyset required should be selected as follows, using the mouse select *Clones* in the *Main Menu* (*see* **Fig. 8**), then select the *Search Commands* option. Clones can be selected on the basis of their gel, the date created or last modified, singleton status, contig number, or on the basis of a remark added to the clone (*see* **Fig. 15**). The selected clones are then compared to the database.

If there are no contigs in the database then the output will be:

>> bA88J16 ctg0 41b → Fpc (Tol 7, Cutoff le–10)

Ctg0	bA60O19 36b	25 le–12
Ctg0	bA61H8 33b	26 3e–15
Ctg0	bA215015 42b	34 le–20
Ctg0	bA317B17 37b	27 2e–14

To form a contig Edit one of these clones (*see* **Fig. 15**) so that their *Contig* does not equal 0. Select *Accept*. This number will appear in the *Clone* window. Select it with the *left mouse bottom*, to open the contig. On the *Contig Analysis* window (*see* **Fig. 11**) select *Compare Keyset* then *Next* then *Add*. The first clone (in this case, bA60O19) should appear in the contig. Highlight the new clone and define the overlap of the two clones using the *Clone1 → Ctg Prob*, in the *Contig Analysis* window and position it using the *Snap Left/Snap Right* facility in the *Edit Contig* window. Repeat the procedure for each new clone.

If there are already contigs in the database (*see* **Fig. 9**) the output window is similar to that produced after *CB map* is run (*see* **Fig. 16**). Select contigs that have clones overlapping with them and follow the same procedure of *Compare Keyset then Next then Add*. Selecting *Auto add* in the *Main Analysis* window will automatically add clones that overlap with existing contigs, so only the positioning need be done (*see* **Note 11**).

8. Once contigs have been constructed, it may be necessary to select a minimum set (*i.e.*, tiling path) of clones to sequence. The extent of sequence overlap desired depends on the sequence protocol. For full (10X) sequence clone coverage, it is critical to obtain minimally overlapping clones with as little redundancy as possible for the project to be economic. For draft (5X) sequence clone coverage, the restrictions for minimum set construction may be slightly relaxed, as two significantly overlapping FPC clones will give full coverage. The selection criteria to follow include:

a. The clone should be a true representation of the genomic DNA it contains, avoid potentially deleted clones, e.g., clones which are missing bands that

A   **B**

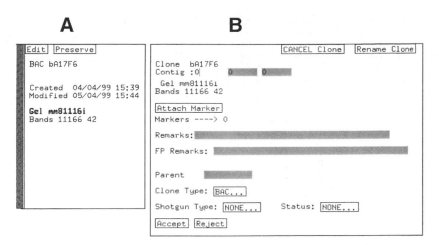

Fig. 15. (**A**) The Clone window. This indicates the name of the clone, the gel the clone's fingerprints were resolved on, the create date, and last modified date. In addition, the total number of bands in the project contained when the clone was added to the database and the number of bands in the clone are shown. By selecting *Edit*, the *Edit Clone* window is opened (**B**). The clone's name can be altered or the clone canceled all together, a contig can be selected or changed, markers attached or detached, and remarks can be entered. The clone can be buried by adding the clone's canonical name to *Parent*, and the clone's type can be changed. The sequence status of the clone can be altered and the shotgun status.

    are clearly present in overlapping clones in the contig, or clones with too many extra bands.

b. The bands in a sequence clone should be contained within at least one other clone in the contig, avoid end clones, as these may contain rearranged inserts, represent mixed library wells or even be chimeric.

c. When identifying minimally overlapping clones apply all of these criteria as well obtaining the least redundant overlap, be careful not to miss any intervening contig bands between two sequence clones.

Of invaluable use when identifying sequence clones are the gel traces of clones (*see* **Fig. 15**). Use these and the fingerprint window to identify sequence clones and minimum sets. For the latter it is often useful to use the CB map again. From the *Contig Analysis* window select, *Fp Order* (*see* **Fig. 16**).

Manual contig manipulation is often necessary when using clones of very different length or poor fingerprints as a result of chemistry or inaccurate gel entry. Using the GSC BAC data, we are currently defining the amount of automation that can be achieved in FPC (paper in progress).

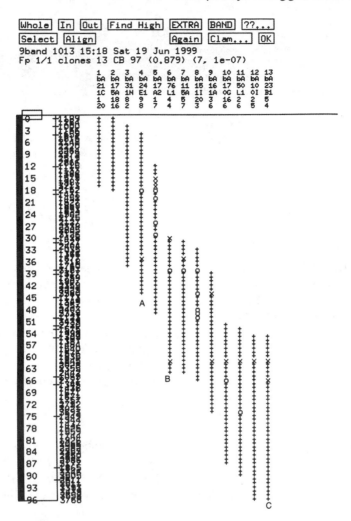

Fig. 16. CB map from the *Fp Order* on the *Contig Analysis* window. This can be used to aid in the selection of minimum sets for sequencing. A, B, and C show the tiling picked through this contig.

3.7. Restriction Digest of Clones for Southern Blotting

Following is the description for restriction digests of three enzymes, *Eco*RI, *Not*I, and *Sal*I, and their double digests. These three enzymes produce digestion fragments that are one of three different types:

1. Fragments containing a vector only.
2. Fragments containing an insert from the clone only.
3. Fragments that contain the end fragments from the clone and vector.

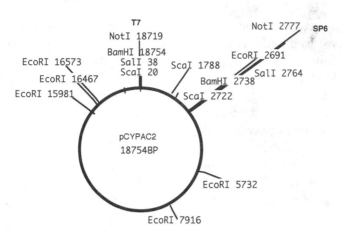

Fig. 17. Restriction sites within the pCYPAC2 vector (accession no. U09128). Restriciton sites were determined using GeneJockeyII for Macintosh. During cloning, sequential digestions of *Sca*I and *Bam*HI are used to remove the stuffer fragment. This produces four products, one the cloning vector,with *Bam*HI ends, two stuffer fragments with *Sca* 1 ends, which are incompatable with *Bam*HI and therefore will not be cloned back into the vector, and two oligonucleotide linkers with *Bam*HI/*Sca*I ends, which are removed prior to the cloning in of the insert. The *Eco*RI, *Not*I, and *Sal*I digests determine at which orientation the insert is cloned into the vector (see text for details) and identifies *Eco*RI fragments that are vector only within the digests and will be common to all clones.

Comparison between clones to detect possible overlap is based on fragments containing an insert only. Clones that have similar fingerprints for insert-only digestion fragments may be overlapping. For a precise overlap to be determined, it is necessary to determine the fragments that contain the ends of the clone and a vector end. This is possible by the digestions performed in this experiment.

The pCYPAC2 vector in which the clones are inserted contains two RNA polymerase promoters T7 and SP6. The insert, usually approximately 120 kb *(14)*, is cloned into the vector between these two promoters (*see* **Fig. 17**). *Not*I digests the PAC vector twice, at both the T7 and SP6 ends of the vector and releases the insert that can then be sized by pulse field gel electrophoresis (PFGE). *Sal*I, however, only cuts at the SP6 end of the vector (*see* **Fig. 17**). By electrophoresis of the digestion products it is possible to determine a T7 end fragment by comparison of the *Eco*RI and *Eco*RI/*Not*I and *Eco*RI/*Sal*I digests (*see* **Fig. 4**). As only *Not*I cleaves at the T7 end, there will be a fragment present in the *Eco*RI digest and the *Eco*RI/*Sal*I digest that is absent in the *Eco*RI/*Not*I digest. Likewise, it is also possible to determine the SP6 end fragment by examining the digestion fingerprint. As both *Not*I and *Sal*I *cut* at the SP6 end, there will be a fragment present in the *Eco*RI-only lane that is absent in the *Eco*RI/*Not*I and *Eco*RI/*Sal*I digests *(15)*. By studying these fragments it is also possible to determine in which orientation the insert has been cloned into the vector. *Not*I *is* a rare cutting enzyme, with a GC-rich recognition site, 5'-GC GGCC GC-3'. Such sites are not common within the genome and are indicative of potential CpG islands *(16,17)* where the dinucleotide CpG is present at higher than expected frequencies and are frequently associated with genes. Determining the length of the *Not*I fragments separated by PFGE allows us to estimate the length of the cloned insert with high accuracy. Clone size data are important for the construction of clone contigs and physical maps.

3.7.1. EcoRI Digest

1. To the appropriate volume of DNA (500 ng), add 3 μL Buffer D, 1 μL *Eco*RI enzyme and deionized distilled water to make up to 29 μL total reaction volume.
2. Incubate at 37°C for 2 h.
3. Add 1 μL of *Eco*RI and incubate a further 2 h.
4. Run a 3-μL aliquot of digest on a 0.5% agarose gel to check digestion. If digestion is not complete, add a further 1 μL of enzyme and incubate for 1 h, and recheck on a gel (*see* **Note 12**).

3.7.2. Sal*I Digests*

1. Double the amount of DNA and add 6 μL buffer, 1.5 μL *Sal*I and deionized distilled water to make up to 51 μL total reaction volume.
2. Incubate at 37°C for 2 h.
3. Add 1 μL enzyme and incubate a further 2 h.
4. Run a 2 μL aliquot of digest against undigested PAC DNA on a 0.5% agarose gel to check digestion. If digestion is not complete, add a further 1 μL enzyme and incubate for 1 h, and recheck on a check gel.
5. Remove the 10 μL digest and reserve for the PFGE. Split the remaining digest into two. To the first, add 1 μL *Eco*RI, and to the second 1 μL *Not*I.
6. Incubate at 37°C for 2 h.
7. Add a further 1 μL *Eco*RI and *Not*I, respectively, incubate for a further 2 h.
8. Run a 2-μL aliquot of digest on a 0.5% agarose gel to check digestion. If digestion is not complete, add a further 1 μL enzyme and incubate for 1 h (*see* **Note 12**).
9. To the *Not*I and *Sal*I digests add 1 μL *Eco*RI and incubate a further hour at 37°C.
10. Add 1 μL *Eco*RI and incubate at 37°C for 1 h.
11. Run a 2-μL aliquot of digest on a 0.5% agarose gel to check digestion. If digestion is not complete, add a further 1 μL enzyme and incubate for 1 h, and recheck on a check gel (*see* **Note 12**).

3.7.3. Not*I Digests*

1. To the appropriate volume of DNA, add 3 μL Buffer D, 1 μL *Not*I and deionized distilled water to make up to 37 μL total reaction volume.
2. Incubate at 37°C for 2 h.
3. Add 1 μL enzyme and incubate a further 2 h.
4. Run a 2-μL aliquot of digest against undigested PAC DNA on a 0.5% agarose gel to check digestion. If digestion is not complete, add a further 1 μL enzyme and incubate for 1 h, and recheck on a gel.
5. Remove 10 μL of digest for PFGE. To the remainder, add 1 μL *Eco*RI and incubate for a further hour.
6. Add 1 μL *Eco*RI and incubate at 37°C for 1 h.
7. Run a 2-μL aliquot of digest against undigested PAC DNA on a 0.5% agarose gel to check digestion. If digestion is not complete, add a further 1 μL enzyme and incubate for 1 h, and recheck on a gel (*see* **Note 12**).

3.8. Electrophoresis of Digest for Southern Blotting

To resolve digestion products *Eco*RI, *Eco*RI/*Not*I, *Eco*RI/*Sal*I and *Eco*RI/*Not*I/ *Sal*I, the digests should be run on a 0.8% TBE 27 × 20 cm gel. A more detailed restriction map can be produced by knowing the sizes of the clones and determining any internal *Not*I or *Sal*I sites. However fragments from these digestions will be large and need to be resolved at high resolution to accurately determine size. To produce a more detailed restriction map, *Not*I, *Sal*I and *Not*I and *Sal*I double digest should be performed, and PFGE need to be used to resolve the large DNA fragments (*see* **Fig. 18**). PFGE is suitable for electrophoresis of large fragments of DNA, as fragments are viewed with greater resolution than conventional gel electrophoresis *(7)*. This method is also used to obtain an insert for hybridization experiments as the insert and vector band of 16 kb can be seen as distinctly separate bands, lessening the chance of contamination by vector during hybridization.

3.8.1. Conventional Gel Electrophoresis

1. Prepare a 500-mL, 27 × 20 cm, 0.8% agarose, 1X TBE gel (4 g of agarose in 500 mL 1X TBE, 10 μL ethidium bromide) with a 24-well comb. Prepare 2 L 1X TBE for the running buffer.
2. Load samples onto the gel, with a marker in the first and last lanes.
3. Run the samples out of the wells and into the gel, 90 V for approximately 15 min.
4. Run gel at 45 V for 20 h.
5. Remove gel and photograph with a fluorescent ruler to facilitate band identification on the autoradiograph.

3.8.2. PFGE to Determine Sizes of Inserts and Internal Not*I and* Sal*I Sites*

1. Prepare a 1% agarose, 0.5X TBE gel (1a agarose to 100 mL 0.5X TBE) with a 24-well comb.

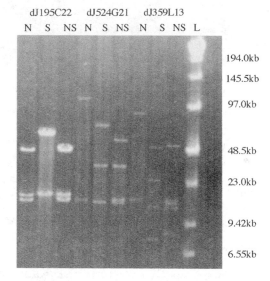

Fig. 18. A PFGE of *Not*I and *Sal*I digested clones. Digestion and electrophoresis performed as in text. Digests for each PAC are as shown for dJ195C22, N = *Not*I, S = *Sal*I, NS = *Not*I, and *Sal*I, L = ladder, sizes are given to the right. As can be seen from the gel, the vector band of 16 kb is clearly separated from the insert for all PACs. dJ195C22 contains an internal *Not*I site producing two distinct fragments of approximately 48 kb and 18 kb and also contains an internal *Sal*I site. dJ524G21 contains an insert of approx 115 kb, with apparently no internal *Not*I sites according to the *Not*I digest, yet contains two internal *Sal*I sites. When digested with both *Not*I and *Sal*I, an additional fragment is produced, suggestive of an internal *Not*I site, which is not apparent from the *Not*I only digest. dJ359L13 contains an insert of approximately 80 kb, with no internal *Not*I sites. However, three internal *Sal*I sites are present within the insert, and as for dJ524G21, an additional fragment is present when digested with *Not*I and *Sal*I, suggesting that another internal *Not*I site is present for this clone.

2. To each 10 µL digest to be loaded, add 3 µL loading dye.
3. Place PFGE marker in the first and last lanes of the gel to enable sizing of bands.
4. Carefully remove casting tray and place gel in tank. Cover with 2 L of 0.5X TBE buffer.
5. Load samples, including 500 ng of Lambda *Hind*III.
6. Running conditions: 6 V/cm, with a pulse time of 0.1–10 s, running time 14 h.
7. After 14 h running, stain gel with ethidium bromide (250 µg ethidium bromide in 500 mL of 0.5X TBE) for 50 min and photograph with fluorescent ruler to facilitate identification of bands on the autoradiograph. The gel should be handled gently, as it is fragile and will break easily.

3.9. Southern Blotting

1. Fill a large container with 0.4 M NaOH. Place a glass sheet or similar on top of the tray as a platform, and place two 3MM filters over the glass so that the ends are in the 0.4 M NaOH. This forms the wick of the blot.
2. Allow the wick to become saturated with 0.4 M NaOH; this will take approximately 30 min. This starts the capillary action, which will draw the 0.4-M NaOH upward through the gel, transferring DNA onto the membrane.
3. Cut the nylon membrane and three sheets of 3MM to the size of the gel.
4. After photographing the gel with fluorescent ruler, place in a 0.25-M HCl solution so that gel is immersed in liquid. Shake gently at room temperature for 30 min. This step causes partial depurination and strand cleavage of the DNA, resulting in shorter strands that are easier to transfer onto the membrane.
5. Discard 0.25-M HCl and rinse gel briefly in deionized distilled water.
6. Wash gel in 0.4 M NaOH for 20 min, shaking gently at room temperature. This denatures the DNA resulting in transfer of single-stranded DNA to which the single-stranded probe may bind during hybridization.
7. Invert the gel and place it on a prewetted wick. Ensure that there are no air bubbles between the wick and the gel, which could cause patchy transfer of DNA.
8. Seal the edges of the wick that are not covered by the gel using Saran Wrap to ensure that the 0.4 M NaOH is drawn up only through the gel and onto the membrane and to prevent evaporation.
9. Place membrane on top of the gel, ensuring that there are no air bubbles and full contact between the gel and the membrane to ensure even transfer. Once membrane is in place, do not move, as some DNA transfer will occur very quickly with movement of filter resulting in smeared bands on an autoradiograph.
10. Prewet three sheets of 3MM in 0.4-M NaOH and place on top of the membrane again ensure that there are no air bubbles between the membrane and the 3MM. If this occurs, remove the 3MM and replace with a fresh sheet.
11. Stack the blotting towels on top of the 3MM, ensuring that the gel is well covered by the towels. The stack should be approximately 4 in. high. The 3MM and towels will cause the capillary action.
12. Place a weight (approximately 0.4 kg) on top of the blotting towels and leave to blot overnight.
13. After blotting, dismantle the blot and mark the positions of the wells on the membrane.
14. To neutralize the membrane, wash at room temperature for 30 min in 2X SSC.
15. Blot dry with 3MM, wrap in Saran Wrap and store at room temperature until needed.

3.10. Hybridization

3.10.1. Probe Preparation

1. Digest PAC to be used with *Not*I to release the insert. To 500 ng–1 µg DNA add 3 µL of buffer D and 2 µL of *Not*I. Make up the vol to 30 µL with deionized distilled water.
2. Incubate at 37°C for 2 h and add a further 2 µL of *Not*I.

3. Electrophorese through a 0.5% 1X TBE check gel against undigested DNA to check digestion. If digestion is not complete, add a further 1 μL enzyme and incubate for 1 h, and recheck on a gel.
4. Run on a PFGE gel and develop as described in **Subheading 3.8.**
5. Excise insert band removing as little as possible agarose, and store at 4°C until needed.

3.10.2. Labeling of the Probes

These steps are common to both labeling for an insert and a whole PAC. Determine concentration of DNA. 50 ng is used per labeling.

3.10.3. Labeling Whole PAC DNA

1. When labeling a whole PAC, take 50 ng of DNA and make up to 50 μL with deionized distilled water.
2. Boil solution containing DNA for 5 min in a pierced Eppendorf tube, resulting in single-stranded DNA to which probe synthesis can occur.
3. Microcentrifuge for 15 s at 10,000g
4. Place tube on ice for 1 min.
5. Remove 45 μL and place in a Rediprime labeling tube.
6. Add 5 μL of [α-^{32}P] dCTP to the tube. Flick gently to mix until the blue pellet has dissolved.
7. Incubate at 37°C for 15 min (*see* **Note 15**).

3.10.4. Labeling of DNA within a Gel Slice

1. Weigh gel slice and add 3 mL of deionized distilled water per gram of gel.
2. Boil gel slice for 5 min in a pierced Eppendorf tube, to melt the gel and denature DNA.
3. Remove volume of DNA corresponding to 50 ng and if necessary, add deionized distilled water to give a final volume of 45 μL in the Rediprime labeling tube.
4. Add 5 μL of [α-^{32}P] dCTP radiolabel to the tube. Flick gently to mix until the blue pellet has dissolved.
5. Incubate at 37°C for 30 min.

3.10.5. Prehybridization

1. Place membranes between two nylon meshes and roll into a cylinder.
2. Place into a hybridization bottle and add 30–50 mL of hybridization solution.
3. Incubate the cylinders while rotating them in the hybridization oven at 65°C. There should be no air bubbles between the filter and the side of the bottle that may prevent the probe reaching the membrane in that region.
4. Prehybridize for a minimum of 0.5 h upward.

3.10.6. Competition of the Probe and Hybridization

1. Add competition DNA mixture to the tube and boil for 5 min. This denatures both the probe and competition DNA to single strands, allowing them to reanneal to each other.

2. Incubate tube at 65°C for 30 min (*see* **Note 16**). The competing DNA will bind to repetitive areas of the probe blocking them and preventing binding to target DNA.
3. Mix labeled probe with 5 mL hybridization mix and add to bottles containing prehybridization solution and membranes.
4. Place in rotating hybridization oven overnight (for 16–24 h) (*see* **Note 17**).

3.10.7. Posthybridization Washes

1. Preheat shaking incubator to 65°C.
2. Remove membrane from hybridization bottle and place in wash I solution.
3. Wash in shaking incubator for 30 min.
4. Pour off wash I solution and replace with wash II solution.
5. Incubate for 15 min in a shaking incubator.
6. Discard wash II solution and replace with fresh wash solution II.
7. Incubate for 15 min in the shaking incubator (*see* **Note 18**).
8. Discard wash and place membrane between two sheets of 3MM and gently blot to remove excess liquid.
9. Wrap blot in Saran Wrap to prevent filters drying out. If filters dry out while radioactive, the radiation sticks to the membrane and is very difficult to remove.
10. Place in an autoradiography cassette with film and leave at –70°C overnight or less, depending on the signal strength on the membrane.
11. Develop the film and if necessary, relay for a shorter or longer exposure.

4. Notes

1. Southern blots may be reused and probed with several different probes on different occasions as the DNA is fixed to the membrane. Between hybridizations, the membrane may be stored safely and allowed to decay naturally, or the probe can be removed by washing membrane in a boiling solution of 1% SDS, allowed to cool and monitored for signal.
2. The dichlorhodamine dyes used for fluorescent fingerprinting are extremely photolabile; they should be stored in a covered box at –20°C, any solutions containing dyes should be kept in the dark as much as possible.
3. Each new batch of fluorescent dyes should be tested before use to find the optimal amount to be added to each reaction, as batch concentrations can vary. Fingerprint a number of clones that are known to give varying strengths of signal with differing amounts of dyes. While fingerprinting human bacterial clone libraries, we have found that undiluted TET dye and 1:8 HEX and 3:4 NED give best results.
4. Care should be taken that the gel does not come into contact with TBE, ethidium bromide, or lint from tissues as these emit at the same wavelength as vistra green and will therefore affect results. It is important to use the same chemicals (especially agarose and acetic acid) as the GSC if incorporation with their data is desired. It is possible that slight variations in separation will be seen if chemicals are not duplicated.
5. RNase A can be stored for up to 4 mo at –20°C, as long as it is stored in 1 mL aliquots in 1.5 mL microfuge tubes to prevent excessive freeze-thaw cycles.

6. Prepped DNA can be stored at −20°C for up to 1 wk; after that there may be degradation in the quality of fingerprints

7. Tracking gels in Image; for 64-lane fluorescent gels put the LANE NUMBER to 70 and delete the extra tracks. With 121 lane digest gels put the MARKER RE-PEAT number to 120, then adjust the two outside marker lanes to match the ends of the gel, go back to the ENTER GEL NUMBER window and put the MARKER REPEAT number back to 5.

8. For consistent results when band calling, it is best to move through each clone one at a time, evaluating the authenticity and fine positioning of each band in the clone. Scan in to 400% and use the gray ramp tool, especially at the top and bottom of the lane. The same approach should be adopted when standard marker locking.

9. You should aim to finish a full agarose digest gel (96 clones) in about 2–3 h, and a full fluorescent gel (192 clones) in 4–5 h. The time taken to enter a gel varies with user experience, data quality, and computing power.

10. The complexity of the clone library screened can be used as a guide to establish a suitable cut off; on the *Main Analysis* window, enter a clone name and select →*FPC*, you can adjust the cut off and tolerance until the clone has an appropriate number of matches. For example, for a five-hit library;

$$>> bA202A15 \rightarrow Fpc \ (Tol \ 7, \ Cutoff \ le\text{-}10)$$

Ctg0	bA214G9 40b	35 7e-22
Ctg0	bA335N18 50b	33 Se-lS
Ctg0	bA343J19 38b	35 le-23
Ctg0	bA397112 39b	37 4e-26

11. When assembling contigs it is important to take into consideration the possible presence of mixed clones, i.e. clones containing more than one DNA insert. This can occur at library construction, through cross contamination of library wells, or mixing during prepping and fingerprinting. These clones may give misleading fingerprint overlaps. Look for large clones with up to 50% of their fingerprint bands not contained in the other clones in the contig. Supporting evidence such as, STS data, end-sequence hits, mapping information, fluorescence *in situ* hybridization data, and electronic PCR should be taken into account when merging contigs. If there is data indicating two contigs may join, it is advisable to lower the *Cutoff* to assess the fingerprint overlap.

12. It is advisable to run a check gel of all the digests together on a check gel after digestion with *Eco*RI . This allows a direct comparison of concentrations to be made, and alterations in the amount loaded per lane on the large gel to be made to ensure that each lane contains the same amount of DNA. This is also a good last-minute check for partial digestions.

13. LMP gels are more fragile than conventional agarose gels, but have the advantage that bands may be excised and used directly in hybridizations without first cleaning. If no bands are to be excised from the gel, it is better to run a conventional agarose gel that is more robust.

14. Instead of adding RNaseI to the resuspension media during the PAC preps, it can be added to the Solution I at 110 μg/mL. However, some PACs give lower yields, which can result in a pellet that is difficult to see after the precipitation in isopropanol. By not removing RNA, the size of the pellet is increased and is therefore more visible, and the RNase also has a longer period of time to act upon RNA in the sample.

15. Labeling time can be as little as 15 min at 37°C or alternatively, the labeling reaction can be left overnight at room temperature depending on the time available.

16. Depending on the repetitiveness of the region, time taken for competition to bind to the labeled DNA at 65°C can be increased to 1 h.

17. Hybridization of probe to target DNA normally occurs within this time period even for low copy numbers of target DNA However, hybridizations may be left for longer without harming.

18. Depending on the incorporation of label into the probe and the amount of target DNA, the membrane may still be very hot after these washes (200 counts or greater). It may be necessary to increase the stringency of the washes by performing another wash with 0.1X SSC and monitoring at 10 min intervals until the counts drop, or by continuing to wash at the same stringency, again with regular monitoring.

Acknowledgments

Special thanks to Drs. Carol Sunderlund, Simon Gregory, and Ian Dunham for critical review of the manuscript.

References

1. Coulson, A., Sulston, J. E., Brenner, S., and Jonathon, K. (1986) Towards a physical map of the genome of the nematode *Caenorhabditis elegans. Proc. Natl. Acad. Sci. USA* **83,** 7821–7825.

2. Carrano, A. V., Lamerdin, J., Ashworth, L. K., Watkins, B., Branscomb, E., Slezak, T., et al. (1989) A high-resolution, fluorescence-based, semisutomated method for DNA fingerprinting. *Genomics* **4,** 129–136.

3. Gregory, S. G., Howell, G. R., and Bentley, D. R. (1997) Genome mapping by fluorescent fingerprinting. *Genome Res.* **7(12),** 1162–1168.

4. Ding, Y., Johnson, M. D., Colayco, R., Chen, Y. J., Meloyk, J., Schmitt, H., and Shizuya, H. (1999) Contig assembly of bacterial artificial chromosomes clones through multiplexed fluoresence-labeled fingerprinting. *Genomics* **56,** 237–246.

5. Marra, M. A., Kucaba, T. A., Dietrich, N. L., Green, E. D., Brownstein, B., Wilson, R. K., McDonald, K. M., Hillier, L. W., McPherson, J. D., and Waterson, R. H. (1997) High throughput fingerprinting analysis of large-insert clones. *Genome Res.* **7(11),** 1072–1084.

6. Osoegawa, K., Yeong Woon, P., Zhao, B., Frengen, E., Tateno, M., Catanese, J. J., and de Jong P. J. (1998) An improved approach for construction of bacterial artificial chromosome libraries. *Genomics* **52,** 1–8.

7. Ausbel, F. M., Brent, R., Kingston, R. E., Moore, D. D., Seidman, J. G., Smith, J. A., and Struhl, K. (1995) *Current Protocols in Molecular Biology,* Greene and Wiley-Interscience, New York.
8. Southern, E.M. (1975) Detection of specific sequences amongst DNA fragments separated by gel electrophoresis. *J. Mol. Biol.* **98,** 503–517.
9. Feinberg, A. P. and Vogelstein, B. (1983) A technique for radiolabelling DNA restriction endonuclease fragments to high specific activity. *Anal. Biochem.* **132,** 16–13.
10. Feinberg, A. P. and Vogelstein, B (1984) Addenum to a technique for radiolabelling DNA restriction endonuclease fragments to high specific activity. *Anal. Biochem.* **137,** 266–267.
11. Birnboim, H. C. and Doly, J. (1979) A rapid alkaline extraction procedure for screening recombinant plasmid DNA. *Nucleic Acids Res.* **7,** 1513–1523.
12. Gibson, T. J. and Sulston, J. E. (1987) Preparation of Large numbers of plasmid DNA samples in microtiter plates by the alkaline lysis method. *Gene Anal. Technol.* **24,** 41–44.
13. Ioannou, P. A., Amemiya, C. T., Games, J., Kroised, P. M., Shizuya, H., Chen, C., Batzer, M. A., and de Jong, P. J. (1994) A new bacteriophage P1-derived vector for the propagation of large human DNA fragments. *Nature Genet.* **6,** 84–89.
14. Human Genome Mapping Project http://www.hgmp.mrc.ac.uk
15. South, A. P., Cabal, A., Ives, J. H., James, C. H., Mirza, G., Marenholz, I., Mischke, D., Bacendorf, C., Ragoussis, J., and Nizetic, D. (1999) Human epidermal differentiation complex in a single 2.5Mbp long continuum of overlapping DNA cloned in bacteria integrating physical and transcript maps. *J. Invest. Dermatol.* **112,** 910–918.
16. Brown, W. R. A. and Bird, A. P. (1986) Long-range restriction site mapping of mammalian genomic DNA. *Nature* **322,** 477–481.
17. Bird, A. P. (1986) CpG-rich islands and the function of DNA methylation. *Nature* **321,** 209–213.
18. Sulston, J. E., Mallet, F., Staden, R., Durbin, R., Horsnell, T., and Coulson, A. (1988) Software for genome mapping by fingerprinting techniques *CABIOS* **4,** 125–132.
19. Soderlund, C., Longden, I., and Mott, R (1997) FPC: a system for building contigs from restriction fingerprinted clones. *CABIOS* **13,** 523–535.
20. Soderlund, C., Gregory, S. G., and Dunham I. (1998) Sequence ready clone maps, in *Guide to Human Genome Computing* (Bishop, M. J., ed.), Academic, San Diego, CA, pp. 151–179.
21. Durbin, R. and Thierry-Mieg, J. (1994) The ACEDB genome database, in *Computation Methods in Genome Research.* (Suhai, S., ed.), Plenum, London, pp. 110–158.

8

Mapping of Genomic Clones
by Fluorescence *In Situ* Hybridization

Margaret A. Leversha

1. Introduction

Fluorescence *in situ* hybridization (FISH) provides a rapid means of placing labeled DNA segments into a wider genomic context. Mapping to banded metaphase chromosomes anchors clones for specific genes or markers in a well-recognized framework and provides a useful confirmation that clones belong to the expected region of interest.

Potential complications in physical map assembly can be eliminated by thorough characterization of resources that may not have a unique map location. Whole-genome chromosome painting using DNA from monochromosomal somatic cell hybrids or radiation hybrids onto normal human metaphases reveals the specific human chromosome content of the hybrids (*1,2*). FISH also identifies clones with sites of multiple hybridization locations, owing to clone chimerism (a significant problem with many yeast artificial chromosomes [YACs]) (*3*), regional genomic duplications, or repetitive elements.

FISH effectively spans the whole range of mapping resolution, from metaphase chromosome to DNA molecule. A wide range of nonisotopic labels is available, enabling specific identification by direct fluorescence or indirect immunochemical detection linked to fluorochromes. This means that a number of clones can be hybridized simultaneously to a single slide preparation and detected by multicolor FISH. Relative clone orders can easily be determined on metaphase chromosomes for clones separated by more than 1 to 2 Mb (*4*). A 10-fold increase in resolution is obtained using interphase nuclei, providing order for clones separated by more than 50–100 kb (*5*). The highest resolution FISH ordering is performed on linear DNA fibers with a potential resolution of 1–5 kb.

From: *Methods in Molecular Biology, vol. 175: Genomics Protocols*
Edited by: M. P. Starkey and R. Elaswarapu © Humana Press Inc., Totowa, NJ

2. Materials

2.1. DNA Preparation

1. Hycolin solution for decontaminating bacterial culture waste (William Pearson Chemicals, Coventry, UK).
2. Sterile glycerol.
3. Suspension buffer: 50 mM glucose; 10 mM EDTA; 25 mM Tris, pH 8.0.
4. Lysis buffer: 0.2 M NaOH, and 1% (v/v) sodium dodecyl sulfate (SDS), made fresh for each use from stocks of 4 M NaOH and 10% SDS.
5. 3 M Sodium acetate, pH 5.2: For 100 mL, dissolve 24.6 g of sodium acetate in 70 mL of deionized water. Adjust the pH to 5.2 with glacial acetic acid and make up to vol with deionized water. Sterilize by autoclaving.
6. 0.3 M sodium acetate, pH 7.0: Make 3 M stock to pH 7.0 as in **item 5** and dilute 1:10 with sterile deionized water.
7. Isopropanol.
8. Phenol-chloroform.
9. Ethanal, 70% (v/v).
10. TE buffer: 10 mM Tris-HCl, pH 7.4; 1 mM EDTA.
11. RNase A solution (10 mg/mL) (Sigma-Aldrich, Poole, Dorset, UK).

2.2. Nick Translation of DNA

1. 10X nick translation buffer: 0.5 M Tris-HCl, pH 7.5; 0.1 M MgSO$_4$; 1 mM dithiothreitol; 500 µg/mL of bovine serum albumin.
2. 0.5 mM dNTPs: Mix equal volumes of 0.5 mM each dATP, dCTP, and dGTP.
3. Hapten or fluorochrome-linked dUTP: 1 mM biotin-16-dUTP, digoxigenin (DIG)-11-dUTP (Roche, Lewes, East Sussex, UK), Alexa Fluor 488-5-dUTP, Alexa Fluor 594-5-dUTP (Molecular Probes, Eugene, OR).
4. DNase I: 1 µg/mL (cat. no. D4527; Sigma) diluted in 50% (v/v) 2X nick translation buffer, 50% (v/v) glycerol.
5. DNA polymerase I (10 U/µL).
6. 14°C water bath.
7. Microfuge tubes, sterile (1.5 mL).
8. Ethanol, 80% and 100%, stored at −20°C.
9. 0.5 M EDTA, pH 8.0.
10. 3 M sodium acetate, pH 7.0.
11. TE buffer: 10 mM Tris-HCl, pH 7.4; 1 mM EDTA.

2.3. Preparation of Metaphase Chromosomes from Peripheral Blood

1. Heparinized whole blood from a normal male donor.
2. Growth medium: RPMI-1640 containing 16% fetal calf serum (FCS), 100 U/mL of penicillin, 100 µg/mL of streptomycin, buffered with 20 mM HEPES.
3. Sterile centrifuge tubes, at least 30-mL vol.
4. Phytohemagglutinin (PHA) M (Life Technologies, Paisley, Scotland, UK).
5. 0.1 M Thymidine.

6. Sterile phosphate-buffered saline (PBS).
7. Colcemid, 10 μg/mL solution in PBS (Life Technologies).
8. Hypotonic solution: 0.075 *M* KCl.
9. Fixative: 3 parts methanol, 1 part glacial acetic acid, freshly prepared before use.
10. Short-form Pasteur pipets and rubber teats, or disposable pastets.
11. 37°C Incubator or water bath (*see* **Note 1**).

2.4. Preparation of Interphase Nuclei

1. Normal male fibroblast cell cultures.
2. Growth medium: minimal essential medium containing 20 m*M* HEPES, 10% FCS, 100 U/mL of penicillin, 100 μg/mL streptomycin.
3. 1X Trypsin-EDTA solution (Sigma).
4. Dulbecco's PBS, Ca^{2+}/Mg^{2+} free.
5. Hypotonic solution: 0.075 *M* KCl.
6. Fixative: 3 parts methanol, 1 part glacial acetic acid, freshly prepared before use.

2.5. Preparation of DNA Fibers

1. Normal male lymphoblastoid cell culture or isolated white blood cells.
2. PBS.
3. Hemocytometer.
4. Immunostainer Coverplate (Shandon, Runcorn, Cheshire, UK).
5. Clean microscope slides.
6. Alkaline lysis solution: 5 parts 0.07 *M* NaOH, 2 parts ethanol.
7. Methanol.
8. Slide trays.
9. Acetone.

2.6. Slide Making

1. Fixed cell suspension.
2. Glass Hellendahl jars (16-slide capacity) or Coplin jars (10 slides).
3. Fixative solution: 3 parts methanol, 1 part glacial acetic acid, freshly prepared.
4. Pasteur pipets or pastets.
5. Clean microscope slides with frosted ends: Soak in slide racks in 1% Decon 90 for several hours or overnight, rinse thoroughly with running tap water, then distilled water, followed by two changes of ethanol. Store in ethanol until required.
6. Ethanol series comprising successively 70, 70, 90, 90, and 100% ethanol.
7. Acetone.
8. Diamond pencil.

2.7. Preparation of Probe for Hybridization

1. Formamide, analytical reagent grade, deionized with mixed-bed resin beads (AG 501-X8, Bio-Rad, Hemel Hempstead, Hertfordshire, UK). Store at 4–8°C for 3 mo or –20°C for longer periods.
2. 50% (w/v) dextran sulfate, autoclaved. Store aliquots at –20°C.

3. 20X saline sodium citrate (SSC): 3 M NaCl; 0.3 M tri-sodium citrate, pH 7.0.
4. 10% (w/v) SDS, filter sterilized.
5. Hybridization buffer: 50% (v/v) deionized formamide, 10% (v/v) dextran sulfate, 1% (v/v) SDS, 2X SSC. Mix thoroughly and store aliquots at –20°C.
6. Cot-1 DNA (1 mg/mL) (Gibco-BRL) or sonicated placental DNA (10 mg/mL) (Sigma).
7. Sterile microfuge tubes (0.5 mL).
8. Water bath set at 65°C.
9. Water bath set at 37°C.

2.8. Slide Denaturation

1. Water bath set at 65°C.
2. 70% (v/v) Formamide, and 30% (v/v) 2X SSC, pH 7.0, in Hellendahl jar.
3. 70% (v/v) Ethanol in Hellendahl jar, stored at –20°C.
4. Ethanol series: jars containing 70, 70, 90, 90, and 100% ethanol.

2.9. Hybridization

1. Slide-warming bench (optional).
2. Glass cover slips, 22 × 32 mm, stored in ethanol.
3. Lint-free tissues.
4. Rubber cement obtained from bicycle or artists' suppliers.
5. 37°C Oven.

2.10. Stringency Washes

1. 42°C water bath.
2. 50% (v/v) Formamide and 50% (v/v) 2X SCC.
3. 2X SSC.
4. Coplin or Hellendahl jars.

2.11. Immunochemical Detection

1. Nonfat milk powder, any suitable brand (many appear to contain inorganic "whiteners," choose a product that dissolves to a translucent solution in 4X T).
2. Tween-20 (polyoxyethylenesorbitan monolaurate).
3. 20X SSC.
4. 4X TNFM: 4X SSC, 0.05% (v/v) Tween-20, 5% (w/v) nonfat milk. Make 500 mL or 1 L, depending on whether Coplin or Hellendahl jars are used.
5. 4X T: 4X SSC, 0.05% (v/v) Tween-20. Make 100–150 mL.
6. 37°C Water bath or incubator.
7. Moist incubation chamber: airtight box lined with moist tissues, adapted to accommodate slides.
8. Avidin-Texas Red DCS (Vector, Burlingame, CA) (2 mg/mL). Store spare aliquots of immunochemicals at –20°C.

9. Goat antiavidin, biotin-conjugated (1 mg/mL) (Vector).
10. Mouse antidigoxin, fluorescein-conjugated (2.5 mg/mL) (Sigma).
11. Goat antimouse, Alexa 488-conjugated (2 mg/mL) (Molecular Probes).
12. Temporary cover slips, 25 × 50 mm strips of Nescofilm or Parafilm.
13. 4,6-Diamidino-2-phenylindole (DAPI) stock solution (1 mg/mL) in water. Store at 4°C wrapped in foil.
14. DAPI staining solution: 0.08 µg/mL in 2X SSC. Store at 4°C wrapped in foil.
15. Antifade solution: AFl (Citifluor, London, UK) or Vectashield (Vector).
16. Clean glass cover slips, 22 × 32 mm.
17. Nail varnish.

2.12. Analysis and Interpretation of Results (see Note 2)

1. Epifluorescence microscope, equipped with a high-pressure 100 W mercury arc lamp; separate excitation filters for DAPI, fluorescein isothiocyanate (FITC) and Texas Red; a dual excitation filter for FITC and Texas Red; and a single dichroic mirror block with triple bandpass filter for all three fluorochromes.
2. Digital imaging system, including a good-quality cooled charge-coupled device black-and-white camera. This ensures quick and reliable collection of suitable images for archiving or publication.

3. Methods

3.1. Preparation of Clone DNA by Alkaline Lysis

This protocol is based on the original method of Birnboim and Doly (*6*). It usually yields 5–10 µg of bacterial clone DNA from a 10-mL overnight culture. The larger single copy clones such as bacterial artificial chromosomes (BACs) give the lowest yields (3–5 µg). The bacterial cell suspensions should be handled gently throughout to avoid bacterial genomic contamination. Provided that care is taken to avoid contaminating cell debris or protein, the final DNA quality is excellent and suitable for most purposes, including sequencing. Perform **steps 1–5** in a designated class II cabinet.

1. Make a glycerol stock: mix 850 µL from a 10-mL overnight bacterial culture with 150–200 µL of the sterile glycerol; store at –70°C.
2. Pellet the remaining 10-mL culture at 2000*g* at 4°C for 10 min, and then pour off the supernatant (the pellet may be stored at 4°C if necessary).
3. Add 200 µL of suspension buffer and resuspend the pellet gently but thoroughly.
4. Transfer the suspension to a 1.5-mL microfuge tube and stand at room temperature for 10 min.
5. Add 400 µL of fresh lysis solution and mix gently by inversion. Incubate on ice for 5 min.
6. Add 300 µL of 3 *M* sodium acetate, pH 5.2, and mix gently by inversion. Incubate on ice for 10 min (store at 4°C if necessary).

7. Microfuge at maximum speed for 5 min, and then transfer the clear supernatant to a fresh microfuge tube. If the supernatant is not clear, stand the tubes on ice for another 10–30 min.

8. Spin the original tube for another 5 min, remove the supernatant, and pool with the first supernatant.

9. Spin the pool for 5 min and transfer the clean supernatant to a fresh tube.

10. Add 600 µL of isopropanol, mix gently, and incubate at –70°C for 10 min.

11. Spin for 5 min, discard the supernatant, and allow the pellet to air-dry briefly (do not dry too long because the pellet will be difficult to resuspend).

12. Resuspend the pellet in 200 µL of 0.3 M sodium acetate, pH 7.0.

13. Add 200 µL of phenol/chloroform and vortex thoroughly.

14. Spin for 3 min and then transfer 150 µL of the aqueous phase to a fresh tube.

15. Add 50 µL of 0.3 M sodium acetate, pH 7.0, to the original tube containing the phenol/chloroform and vortex thoroughly.

16. Spin for 2 min and transfer 50 µL of the aqueous phase to pool with the other 150 µL.

17. Add 200 µL of isopropanol to the aqueous pool and mix. Incubate at –70°C for 10 min.

18. Spin for 5 min and discard the supernatant.

19. Add 500 µL of 70% ethanol, without disturbing the pellet.

20. Spin for 5 min, discard the supernatant, and air-dry the pellet.

21. Resuspend the pellet in 50 µL of TE.

22. Add 1 µL of RNaseA (10 mg/mL) and incubate at 37°C for 15 min.

23. Check the DNA quality and yield by running 1-µL aliquots in a 0.8–1% agarose gel.

24. Store the DNA at –20°C until required.

3.2. Nick translation of DNA

1. For approx 1 µg of DNA, set up a 25-µL reaction. Determine the volume of DNA required to give 1 µg and calculate the volume of sterile distilled water needed (*see* **Note 3**). Scale up as required (*see* **Note 4**).

2. Add the following in order to a 1.5-mL microfuge tube on ice: 2.5 µL of 10X nick translation buffer, x µL of sterile distilled water (to make a final volume to 25 µL), 1.9 µL of dNTPs, 0.7 µL of biotin-16-dUTP or other haptenized-dUTP, 1 µL DNase I working solution (or other volume determined by titration; *see* **Note 5**), 0.5 µL of DNA polymerase (5 U), and y µL of DNA (1 µg).

3. Mix well by lightly flicking the tube. Pulse microfuge briefly to collect the solution.

4. Incubate at 14°C for the time previously determined by titration.

5. Add 1/10 vol of 0.5 M EDTA to inactivate the enzymes.

6. Add 1/10th vol of 3 M sodium acetate, pH 7.0, and 1 mL of ice-cold absolute ethanol to precipitate the DNA. Mix well by inversion.

7. Incubate at –70°C for 30 min (or –20°C overnight).

8. Microfuge at maximum speed for 10 min. A white salt pellet should be clearly visible. Aspirate off the supernatant.

9. Add 1 mL of ice-cold 80% ethanol, without disturbing the pellet, and microfuge immediately for 10 min. Discard the supernatant immediately, leaving the pellet as dry as possible. The pellet will now be transparent and difficult to see (the pellet may be loose and the labeled probe can be accidentally lost).
10. Air-dry the pellet but do not overdry.
11. Add 10 μL of TE buffer and stand on ice for 10 min. Flick mix to resuspend the probe.
12. Check fragment sizes by running 2 μL in a 1% agarose gel (*see* **Notes 5** and **6**).
13. Store at −20°C until required.

3.3. Preparation of Metaphase Chromosomes from Peripheral Blood

1. Add 0.4–0.5 mL of whole blood to 10 mL of medium supplemented with 100–200 μL PHA solution in a 30-mL centrifuge-based universal tube. Place the tube on a sloping rack in a 37°C incubator for 48–72 h.
2. At 5 PM on the day before harvest, add 0.1 M thymidine to a final concentration of 1.2 mM (120 μL/10 mL of culture) and mix well.
3. Incubate for 16 h.
4. Centrifuge the cultures at 400g for 10 min and discard the supernatant.
5. Loosen the cell pellets by lightly flicking the tubes and resuspend in 10 mL of prewarmed PBS.
6. Centrifuge at 400g for 10 min and discard the supernatant.
7. Loosen the cell pellet and resuspend in 5–10 mL of prewarmed culture medium (without PHA).
8. Incubate at 37°C for 4 h.
9. Add 75 μL of colcemid for each 10 mL of culture.
10. Incubate for 30 min.
11. Centrifuge at 250g for 10 min.
12. Remove the supernatants, trying to leave the pellets as dry as possible. Resuspend each cell pellet thoroughly by flicking the base of the tube.
13. Add 8 mL of prewarmed 0.075 M KCl and carefully resuspend the cells by gentle swirling. Use a Pasteur pipet gently to break up any large clumps.
14. Incubate at 37°C for 8–10 min.
15. Add 1 mL of freshly prepared fixative. Mix thoroughly by swirling gently.
16. Centrifuge at 250g for 5 min.
17. Remove the supernatant and loosen the cell pellet thoroughly as before.
18. Add 5 mL of fixative and mix gently.
19. Centrifuge at 250g for 5 min.
20. Repeat **steps 17–19** twice more.
21. Resuspend the cells finally in a sufficient volume of fixative to give a very slightly milky solution (usually 0.5–1 mL of fixative/10 mL of culture).
22. Store at −20°C until required.

3.4. Preparation of Interphase Nuclei

1. Allow fibroblast cultures to reach confluency.
2. Leave undisturbed for a further 4–7 d, ensuring that mitotic activity has reached a minimum.
3. Remove the medium from the fibroblast culture, reserving 10 mL in a spare tube.
4. Rinse the flask twice with PBS prewarmed to 37°C and discard the washings.
5. Add sufficient prewarmed trypsin-EDTA to just cover the cells (1–2 mL). Monitor cell detachment by phase microscopy, tapping and shaking the flask periodically until most of the cells are loose. If necessary, incubate the flask at 37°C for 5–10 min.
6. Transfer the cells to a 20-mL centrifuge-based tube, neutralizing the trypsin-EDTA with an equal volume of the reserved culture medium.
7. Rinse the tissue culture flask with the remaining reserved medium to collect any remaining cells. Pool in the 20-mL tube.
8. Centrifuge at 250g for 5 min.
9. Remove the supernatant and loosen the cell pellet by lightly flicking the base of the tube.
10. Add 10 mL of prewarmed 0.075 M KCl and resuspend the cells.
11. Centrifuge at 250g for 5 min.
12. Repeat **steps 9** and **10**.
13. Incubate the cells at 37°C for 10 min.
14. Add 2–3 mL of methanol/glacial acetic acid fixative and mix gently.
15. Centrifuge at 250g for 5 min.
16. Remove the supernatant and loosen the cell pellet.
17. Add 5–10 mL of fixative and resuspend the cells.
18. Repeat **steps 15–17** twice more.
19. Resuspend the cells finally in 5 mL of fixative and store at –20°C.

3.5. Preparation of DNA Fibers

This method is an adaptation of the lysis methods of Parra and Windle *(7)* and Fidlerova et al. *(8)*.

1. Take 1 to 2 mL of cell suspension from a healthy culture of normal lymphoblastoid cells (isolated white blood cells can be used as an alternative).
2. Centrifuge at 250g for 5 min. Discard the supernatant and loosen the cell pellet.
3. Resuspend the cells in 5 mL of warmed PBS.
4. Spin at 250g for 5 min. Discard the supernatant and repeat PBS wash once more.
5. Resuspend the cells in 1 mL of PBS.
6. Count an aliquot of cells using the hemocytometer.
7. Dilute the cells with additional PBS to give a final concentration of approx 2×10^6/mL.
8. Spread 10 µL of cell suspension over a 1 to 2 cm area on the upper part of a clean microscope slide. Try to keep the edges of the cell spot smooth.

9. Air-dry for 30 min.
10. Fit a slide into a plastic coverplate and clamp in a nearly vertical position.
11. Apply 150 µL of lysis solution forcefully into the top of the cover plate.
12. As the level drops below the frosted edge of the slide, add 200 µL of methanol.
13. Allow to drain briefly until the level reaches the bottom of the frosted edge.
14. Holding the edges, carefully lift the slide and coverplate unit out of the clamp.
15. Pull the top of the slide back from the coverplate, allowing the meniscus to move rapidly but evenly down the slide (*see* **Note 7**).
16. Air-dry on a slide rack.
17. Monitor DNA release by examining each slide by phase microscopy before making the next slide.
18. Fix in acetone for 10 min. Slides can be stored satisfactorily at room temperature for several months.

3.6. Slide Making

1. Remove a tube of fixed cell suspension from the –20°C freezer, allowing the cells time to equilibrate to room temperature. Do not leave at room temperature for more than 30 min.
2. Prepare a jar of fresh 3:1 fixative.
3. Remove the slides from ethanol and dry with lint-free tissue.
4. Mix the cell suspension by gently flicking the tube. Take a small volume of suspension in a Pasteur pipet and place a single drop of cells onto a horizontal slide.
5. Gently apply a drop of fixative while the cell suspension is still spreading.
6. Examine the slide under a phase-contrast microscope.
   If the chromosomes are overspread, try allowing more time between the first and second drops, or position the pipet nearer the slide. It may be useful to cool the cell suspension by placing it on ice.
   If the chromosomes are not well spread, drop the cells from a slightly greater height, or add more fixative. Chromosome preparations do not spread well in cold, dry atmospheres, and it may be necessary to increase humidity around the slides by preparing them on a dampened paper towel or over a warm water bath.
7. When the required number of slides have been made, mark the edges of the slides with a diamond pencil to indicate the limits of the cell spots.
8. Fix the slides in the Coplin jar of fixative at room temperature for 30–60 min, and then air-dry.
9. Dehydrate the slides through a fresh ethanol series of 70, 70, 90, 90, and 100% ethanol, 2 min in each. Air-dry.
10. Fix in acetone at room temperature for 10 min. Air-dry.
11. Store the slides in a sealed box at room temperature for 2 to 3 wk (*see* **Note 8**).

3.7. Preparation of Probe for Hybridization

1. In a 0.5-mL microfuge tube add the following: 0.5–1 µL of labeled DNA (*see* **Note 9**), 1 µL of Cot-1 DNA (1 µg) or sonicated placental DNA (10 µg), and 14 µL of hybridization buffer.

2. Mix thoroughly and pulse microfuge.
3. Denature the probe mix at 65°C for 10 min.
4. Transfer to 37°C to preanneal for at least 15 min, up to 3 h (*see* **Note 10**).

3.8. Slide Denaturation

1. Prewarm a jar of 70% formamide to 65°C.
2. Denature the slides in 70% formamide at 65°C for 2 min (*see* **Note 11**).
3. Quench the slides in 70% ice-cold ethanol for approx 1 min.
4. Dehydrate through the ethanol series, 1 min in each.
5. Air-dry.

3.9. Hybridization

1. Place the slides on a slide-warming bench set to 37–42°C (*see* **Note 12**).
2. Pipet the first probe mix onto a labeled slide and cover with a polished 22 × 32 mm cover slip. Repeat for subsequent probe mixes (*see* **Note 13**).
3. Seal the edges of the cover slips with rubber cement.
4. Incubate the slides overnight at 37–42°C.

3.10. Stringency Washes

1. Warm three jars of 2X SSC and two jars of 50% formamide to 42°C.
2. Remove dried rubber cement from the slides.
3. Soak off the cover slips in the first jar of warmed 2X SSC (approx 5 min).
4. Transfer the slides to the first jar of 50% formamide for 5 min.
5. Transfer slides to the second jar of 50% formamide for another 5 min.
6. Wash for 5 min each in the two remaining jars of 2X SSC at 42°C.

3.11. Immunochemical Detection for Biotin and DIG-Labeled Probes

It is important that you do not allow the slides to dry out at any stage.

1. Warm a jar of 4X TNFM to 37°C.
2. Transfer the slides to the jar of 4X TNFM and incubate for 10–30 min.
3. Make the immunochemical staining solutions in 4X TNFM, allowing 100 μL per slide plus 100 μL extra:
   a. Avidin-Texas Red (1 :500 dilution) plus mouse antidigoxin (1:500).
   b. Biotinylated antiavidin (1:250) plus goat antimouse Alexa-488 (1:250).
   c. Avidin-Texas Red (1:500).
4. Mix immunochemical solutions thoroughly and allow to stand for 10 min, and then microfuge for 10 min to remove any protein precipitates. Protect from light.
5. Discard the three lots of 2X SSC from the stringency washes and replace with 4X TNFM and warm to 42°C.
6. Drain each slide and apply 100 μL of the first immunochemical solution (**a**).
7. Cover with a 25 × 50 mm strip of Nescofilm.

8. Incubate the slides in the humidified box at 37°C for 20–60 min.
9. Wash the slides in each jar of 4X TNFM at 42°C for 5 min.
10. Drain each slide and apply 100 μL of the second antibody mix.
11. Cover with a strip of Nescofilm and incubate as before.
12. Replace the wash solutions in the jars with fresh 4X TNFM and warm to 42°C.
13. Wash the slides in each jar of 4X TNFM at 42°C for 5 min.
14. Drain each slide and apply 100 μL of the third immunochemical solution (**c**).
15. Repeat **steps 11–13**.
16. Wash twice in 4X T at room temperature.
17. Stain 0.08 μg/mL of DAPI for 2 to 3 min.
18. Rinse in 2X SSC, then briefly in deionized water, and dehydrate through an ethanol series. Air-dry.
19. Apply 20-μL aliquots of antifade solution to clean 22 × 32 mm cover slips.
20. Overlay with the slides, blot, and seal with nail varnish.
21. Store the slides at 4°C, protected from light.

3.12. Analysis and Interpretation of Results

3.12.1. Chromosome Band Assignment

Chromosome band localizations are achieved using the banding pattern produced by the DAPI counterstain, similar to G-banding (**Fig. 1**). Most digital imaging systems have the facility to view the DAPI image in black and white, inverted to simulate G-banding. This should permit confident band assignments by a person with some cytogenetics experience. Automated karyotyping packages may not fully compensate for variations in chromosome morphology. If an experienced cytogeneticist is not available, it will be necessary to identify specific chromosomes by cohybridization with a known chromosome-specific probe.

Mapping of smaller DNA clones such as cDNAs can be difficult. Clones less than 1.5 kb do not always generate sufficient signal above nonspecific background levels (*9*). This may be related to the number of exons and the genomic extent of the gene, as well as accessibility of the target sequence. In these situations, it may be useful to pretreat the slides with a protease, such as 1% pepsin in 0.01 *N* HCl, at 37°C for approx 5 min before denaturation. Greater sensitivity can also be obtained using tyramide-based detection of hybridization (*10,11*).

3.12.2. Metaphase Order

Clones can be ordered by two-color hybridization on extended metaphase chromosomes when the clones are separated by 1 to 2 Mb (*4*). Even higher resolution can be obtained using chromosomes stretched by cytocentrifugation (*12*). Mapping order is achieved by analysis of sufficient numbers of chromo-

somes to give statistically significant results. In practice, this will be a`bout 15–
20 metaphases, because each chromosome has two chromatids, giving a possible set of four signals per probe in each spread (**Fig. 2**).

1. Start at one edge of the cell spot and scan systematically down the slide.
2. Locate a well-spread metaphase with long chromosomes and score the position
   of the red and green signals for each chromatid relative to the centromere,
   recording absent or uninformative signals as well: e.g., cRG/cR-; c(R/G)/cGR.
3. Analyze 15 metaphases and add the total scores for each class.
4. Perform a statistical comparison (such as the chi-squared test) on the two informative classes (cRG and cGR).
5. Analyze more cells if necessary to achieve statistical significance.

3.12.3. Interphase Order

Clones are ordered relative to known reference points, preferably not more
than 5 Mb away (*see* **Note 14**). Replicate hybridizations should be performed
with the clones to be ordered labeled with the alternative hapten. Wherever
possible, orders should be confirmed using both proximal and distal reference
clones. The two-color detection protocol can be used to compare the distribution of RRG or RGR signals, when the reference clone is biotin-labeled (**Fig. 3**).
The reference clone can be uniquely identified by including additional
DIG-labeled probe. The mixture of red and green signals for the reference clone
will be seen as orange. This allows all possible patterns to be recorded: ORG,
OGR, and ROG (*see* **Note 15**).

1. Start at one edge of the cell spot and scan systematically down the slide.
2. Choose an area of evenly distributed nuclei with uniform morphology.
3. Switch to the oil immersion lens and select the Texas Red filter combination.
4. Scan the slide under oil (a light stippling of red background signal should delineate the nuclei), and locate a nucleus with pairs of red signals. Avoid nuclei where
   it is not possible to distinguish the separate chromosomes.
5. Switch to the dual Texas Red/FITC filter and record the relative positions of the
   green signals.
6. Score at least 30–50 interphase nuclei.
7. Perform a statistical comparison on the two informative classes (ORG, OGR).

3.12.4. DNA Fiber-FISH

DNA fiber analysis is most suitable for assessing relationships such as clone
overlaps and small gaps in contigs (**Fig. 4**). Clone overlaps can usually be
confirmed with a small number of signals, but it is worth scanning more signals in case there are additional unexpected patterns. Regional duplications
can confound mapping efforts at all levels *(13)*.

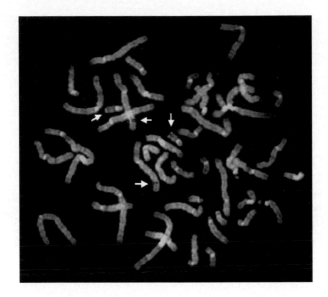

Fig. 1. FISH mapping of two P1 artificial chromosome (PAC) clones on a DAPI-banded normal male metaphase spread.

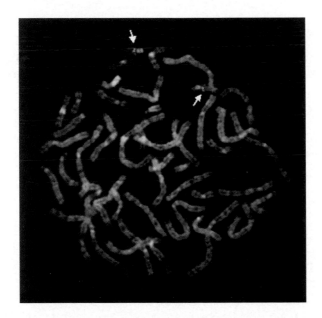

Fig. 2. Metaphase ordering of two cosmids in chromosome 22q11.

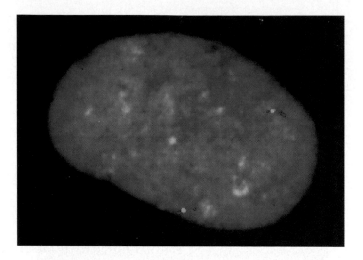

Fig. 3. Interphase ordering with three cosmids from chromosome 22.

Fig. 4. FISH on DNA fibers confirms clone overlaps of three PACs in chromosome 22. The region of overlap is seen as yellow where the red and green signals from the separate clones combine. The size of the overlap with the left biotin-labeled PAC (red) is approximately twice that of the right clone. This relationship is preserved despite the varying degrees of DNA stretching on different parts of the same slide.

In practice, assessment of contig gaps becomes more difficult with increasing separation. The farther apart two clones are, the more likely they are to be separated by random DNA breakage, and chance association of signals can occur when the fiber density is high. It is difficult to achieve uniform fiber stretching, and DNA breakage produces truncated signals, making analysis potentially confusing. It is important to avoid observer bias, preferably by analyzing coded slides. All possible combinations can be found, but the dominant pattern should be apparent after examining 20–30 signals. The precise number needed for reliable assessment depends on the size of the gap.

Estimation of the molecular size of clone signals can be derived from the average length of signals relative to signals from a known standard clone *(14)*. However, because DNA fiber stretching can be variable with this method, such estimations cannot be precise. If more accurate determination of molecular size is required, the alternative technique of molecular combing *(15,16)* may be attempted. Higher-resolution analysis can be used for placing cDNA clones or even sequence tag sites onto DNA fibers *(17)*.

As in interphase mapping, the DAPI counterstain is useful only for locating general regions of interest and the correct focal plane for screening. It is impossible to distinguish single DNA fibers. All screening is done using either the Texas Red filter or the dual Texas Red/FITC filter. When hybridizing larger clones such as PACs or BACs, signals will frequently extend over large distances, so it may be useful to scan the slides using a ×10 oil lens.

4. Notes

1. If incubating without CO_2, seal the caps of the centrifuge tubes firmly. Normal cell metabolism will restore the pH of the medium. The culture volumes should be no more than half the capacity of the tubes to allow adequate gas exchange. For further information on cytogenetic methods, *see* ref. *18*.
2. The microscope system described is for basic three-color analysis, suitable for FISH mapping. Additional FISH applications such as M-FISH may require different hardware, so the intended use of the system will influence the choice of final assemblage.
3. Successful nick translation depends on a reliable method for determining DNA concentration. If mapping clones for others, always verify their estimate of the sample concentration because this can be remarkably optimistic. A DNA fluorimeter gives the most accurate results, but any consistent method used for the initial DNase I titration should be suitable for subsequent nick translation reactions.
4. For labeling larger numbers of clones, add DNA to 1.5-mL tubes and make up the volume to 10 μL with sterile deionized water. Make up a labeling master mix (allowing excess volume for pipeting loss) and add 15 μL to each DNA sample.
5. For titration of DNase I, prepare a series of trial reactions containing 2 μg of DNA, nick translation buffer, and various volumes of DNase I working solution made up to a final volume of 50 μL with sterile deionized water. Incubate the reactions at 14°C, and transfer a 10-μL aliquot from each reaction to clean tubes after 20 min. Inactivate the DNase I by adding 1 μL of 0.5 *M* EDTA and stand on ice. Remove further aliquots at regular intervals, e.g., 30, 40, 50, and 60 min.

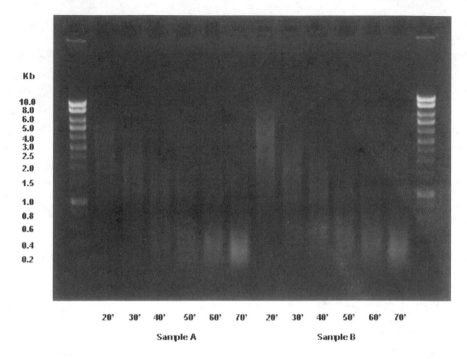

Fig. 5. DNase I titration on two DNA samples. In this example, 8 µL aliquots were sampled at intervals from 20 to 70 min incubation at 14°C. The DNA fragments were run out in a 0.8% agarose gel in 1X TAE. Sampling the reaction at different time points indicates the appropriate incubation time for nick translation to give DNA fragments of the desired length.

Run all the aliquots out on a 0.8–1% agarose gel to compare the DNA fragment sizes (**Fig. 5**). Choose a time, and DNase I concentration, that gives a smear of double-stranded fragments about 300–800 bp.

6. The conditions may vary according to the type of label used in the nick translation reaction. Fluorescein-dUTP appears to produce smaller DNA fragments than biotin-dUTP or DIG-dUTP under the same conditions. This may be owing to altered electrophoretic mobility or to additional salts in the fluorescein-dUTP solution, because divalent cations, particularly Ca^{2+}, enhance the activity of DNase I. Satisfactory fluorescein-labeled probe can be produced by reducing the incubation time by about 10 min.

7. The lysis solution needs to be injected with some force into the narrow space between the slide and cover plate to ensure that the entire cell area is covered by the lysis solution. Unevenness at the edges of the cell spot or debris on the slide can perturb the flow of solution, resulting in poor DNA release or poor fiber retention. DNA release can be affected by varying the volumes of solutions, with increased DNA loss occurring with larger volumes.

8. The storage time for slides at room temperature will vary among laboratories. Older slides will require longer denaturation. If slides are to be kept for more than a couple of weeks, they should be sealed in slide boxes containing desiccant and stored at −70°C. When removing slides from the freezer, allow the slide boxes to equilibrate to room temperature before breaking the seal, in order to prevent condensation from forming on the slides.

9. Use 1 to 2 ng for centromeric or other highly repetitive probes, 20–50 ng for single copy bacterial clones, and 80–100 ng for YACs in total yeast background. Increase the amount of Cot-1 or sonicated placental DNA when including additional complex probes in the hybridization mix. Do not use competitor DNA with simple repetitive probes.

10. Most genomic clones contain repetitive sequences such as *Alu* or *L1* that are distributed throughout the genome. Specific FISH localization of genomic clones is achieved by preannealing the probe with unlabeled competitor DNA such as Cot-1 or sonicated placental DNA *(19)*. This is known as chromosomal *in situ* suppression (CISS) hybridization *(20)*. Some clones may be particularly rich in *Alu* sequences and require extra Cot-1 DNA in the hybridization mixture to produce clean, specific signals. This competitor DNA and preannealing step is avoided when using repetitive probes such as the chromosome-specific centromeric probes. If cohybridizing a centromeric probe with another requiring CISS, make separate mixes in half the volume of hybridization buffer, denature separately, preanneal the complex probe while holding the repetitive probe on ice, and then apply together on a single slide and cover slip as usual.

11. Published slide denaturation times and temperatures vary considerably. This is partly related to variations in slide preparation and formamide quality. Overdenaturation destroys chromosome morphology, making it difficult to identify banding patterns. Chromosome morphology can also be adversely affected by steam condensation from the water bath, so minimize exposure when transferring slides to and from the formamide. It may be useful to compare denaturation times to establish the most suitable method for local conditions.

12. The slide-warming bench is not essential but it ensures that the probes are applied to warm slides, aiding the spread of the viscous probe mix under the cover slips and possibly avoiding nonspecific binding.

13. The probe mix can be placed on ice while each slide is processed but this is not essential if a small number of probes are being hybridized. Better results are obtained if the slides are prepared singly rather than applying each probe mix to its slide before placing the cover slips.

14. Clone orders can also be determined by comparing measured interphase distances between signals *(21)*. This is a more time-consuming approach, even when using an image analysis system for digital measurement, but provides useful information about the possible molecular separation between clones since interphase distance is related to molecular distances up to at least 2 Mb *(5,21)*. However, because different regions of the genome are compacted differently in the nucleus, estimations of genomic distance can only be approximate until much more is

known about interphase chromosomal structure *(22)*. Moreover, local variations in chromosomal packing can produce misleading results over larger genomic distances *(23)*.

15. A shift in image registration caused by exchanging filter blocks in the imaging pathway can complicate interphase analysis, particularly if interphase measurements are required. Using a multibandpass emission filter in the imaging pathway and separate excitation filters outside the imaging pathway minimizes this problem.

References

1. Kievits, T., Devilee, P., Wiegant, J., Wapenaar, M. C., Cornelisse, C. J., van Ommen, G. J., and Pearson, P. L. (1990) Direct nonradioactive in situ hybridization of somatic cell hybrid DNA to human lymphocyte chromosomes. *Cytometry* **11,** 105–109.
2. Boyle, A L., Lichter, P., and Ward, D. C. (1990) Rapid analysis of mouse-hamster hybrid cell lines by in situ hybridization. *Genomics* **7,** 127–130.
3. Selleri, L., Eubanks, J. H., Giovannini, M., Hermanson, G. G., Romo, A., Djabali, M., Maurer, S., McElligott, D. L., Smith, M. W., and Evans, G. A. (1992) Detection and characterization of "chimeric" yeast artificial chromosome clones by fluorescent in situ suppression hybridization. *Genomics* **14,** 536–541.
4. Lawrence, J. B., Singer, R. H., and McNeil, J. A. (1990) Interphase and metaphase resolution of different distances within the human dystrophin gene. *Science* **249,** 928–932.
5. Trask, B., Pinkel, D., and van den Engh, G. (1989) The proximity of DNA sequences in interphase cell nuclei is correlated to genomic distance and permits ordering of cosmids spanning 250 kilobase pairs. *Genomics* **5,** 710–717.
6. Birnboim, H. C. and Doly, J. (1979) A rapid alkaline extraction procedure for screening recombinant plasmid DNA. *Nucleic Acids Res.* **7,** 1513–1523.
7. Parra, I. and Windle, B. (1993) High resolution visual mapping of stretched DNA by fluorescent hybridization. *Nature Genet.* **5,** 17–21.
8. Fidlerova, H., Senger, G., Kost, M., Sanseau, P., and Sheer, D. (1994) Two simple procedures for releasing chromatin from routinely fixed cells for fluorescence in situ hybridization. *Cytogenet. Cell Genet.* **65,** 203–205.
9. Korenberg, J. R., Chen, X. N., Adams, M. D., and Venter, J. C. (1995) Toward a cDNA map of the human genome. *Genomics* **29,** 364–370.
10. Raap, A. K., van de Corput, M. P., Vervenne, R. A., van Gijlswijk, R. P., Tanke, H. J., and Wiegant. J. (1995) Ultra-sensitive FISH using peroxidase-mediated deposition of biotin- or fluorochrome tyramides. *Hum. Mol. Genet.* **4,** 529–534.
11. van Gijlswijk, R. P., Wiegant, J., Raap, A. K., and Tanke, H. J. (1996) Improved localization of fluorescent tyramides for fluorescence in situ hybridization using dextran sulfate and polyvinyl alcohol. *J. Histochem. Cytochem.* **44,** 389–392.
12. Haaf, T. and Ward, D. C. (1994) Structural analysis of alpha-satellite DNA and centromere proteins using extended chromatin and chromosomes. *Hum. Mol. Genet.* **3,** 697–709.

13. Trask, B. J., Massa, H., Brand-Arpon, V., Chan, K., Friedman, C., Nguyen, O. T., Eichler, E., van den Engh, G., Rouquier, S., Shizuya, H., and Giorgi, D. (1998) Large multi-chromosomal duplications encompass many members of the olfactory receptor gene family in the human genome. *Hum. Mol. Genet.* **7,** 2007–2020.
14. Senger, G., Jones, T. A., Fidlerova, H., Sanseau, P., Trowsdale, J., Duff, M., and Sheer, D. (1994) Released chromatin: linearized DNA for high resolution fluorescence in situ hybridization. *Hum. Mol. Genet.* **3,** 1275–1280.
15. Bensimon, A., Simon, A., Chiffaudel, A., Croquette, V., Heslot, F., and Bensimon, D. (1994) Alignment and sensitive detection of DNA by a moving interface. *Science* **265,** 2096–2098.
16. Michalet, X., Ekong, R., Fougerousse, F., Rousseaux, S., Schurra, C., Hornigold, N., van Slegtenhorst, M., Wolfe, J., Povey, S., Beckmann, J. S., and Bensimon, A. (1997) Dynamic molecular combing: stretching the whole human genome for high resolution studies. *Science* **277,** 1518–1523.
17. Horelli-Kuitunen, N., Aaltonen, J., Yaspo, M. L., Eeva, M., Wessman, M., Peltonen, L., and Palotie, A. (1999) Mapping ESTs by fiber-FISH. *Genome Res.* **9,** 62–71.
18. Rooney, D. E. and Czepulkowski, B. H. (1992) *Human Cytogenetics: A Practical Approach. Vol. I & II.* IRL, Oxford.
19. Landegent, J. E., Jansen in de Wal, N., Dirks, R. W., Baas, F., and van der Ploeg, M. (1987) Use of whole cosmid cloned genomic sequences for chromosomal localization by non-radioactive in situ hybridization. *Hum. Genet.* **77,** 366–370.
20. Lichter, P., Tang, C. J., Call, K., Hermanson, G., Evans, G. A., Housman, D., and Ward, D. C. (1990) High-resolution mapping of human chromosome 11 by in situ hybridization with cosmid clones. *Science* **247,** 64–69.
21. van den Engh, G., Sachs, R., and Trask, B. J. (1992) Estimating genomic distance from DNA sequence location in cell nuclei by a random walk model. *Science* **257,** 1410–1412.
22. Yokota, H., Singer, M. J., van den Engh, G. J., and Trask, B. J. (1997) Regional differences in the compaction of chromatin in human G0/G1 interphase nuclei. *Chromosome Res.* **5,** 157–166.
23. Yokota, H., van den Engh, G., Hearst, J. E., Sachs, R. K., and Trask, B. J. (1995) Evidence for the organization of chromatin in megabase pair-sized loops arranged along a random walk path in the human G0/G1 interphase nucleus. *J. Cell Biol.* **130,** 1239–1249.

9

Map Integration

*From a Genetic Map to a Physical Gene Map
and Ultimately to the Sequence Map*

Panagiotis Deloukas

1. Introduction

The full integration of the cytogenetic, genetic, and physical maps together with the search to identify all the genes of an organism and the effort to position them on the corresponding integrated map, has long been a key issue in genetics. In all three fields of mapping, enormous progress has been made over the past two decades through either the development of new reagents or innovations in technology. The use of sequence tag sites (STSs) as markers (*1*) however, could be singled out as the major tool toward map integration. Currently, genetic maps of complex genomes such as the human, mouse, and rat (*2–4*) are all based on microsatellite STS markers, also referred to as single sequence length polymorphisms, which in turn have been used to isolate yeast artificial chromosome, bacterial artificial chromosome (BAC), or P1 artificial chromosome (PAC) clones and build physical maps at increasing levels of resolution (*5–8*). The construction of high-resolution physical maps has also been accelerated by the use of whole genome radiation hybrid (RH) mapping (*9*). RH mapping provides a means to localize any STS to a defined map position in the genome, by the use of polymerase chain reaction (PCR). Thus, STS-based markers provide a means to integrate genetic (*2–4*), RH (*4,10–12*), and clone maps (*5–8*). EST-based STS markers have also been used to integrate the genetic, physical, and transcript maps by means of RH (*6,10–11,13*) and/or landmark contig (i.e., a set of overlapping clones) mapping. Finally, clones with a known STS content can be assigned to cytogenetic bands using tech-

From: *Methods in Molecular Biology, vol. 175: Genomics Protocols*
Edited by: M. P. Starkey and R. Elaswarapu © Humana Press Inc., Totowa, NJ

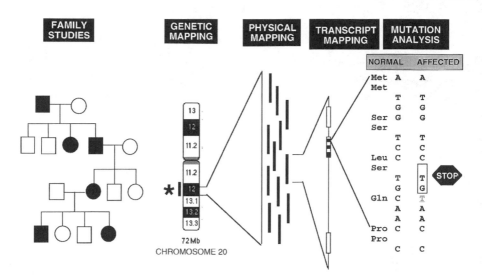

Fig. 1. The main steps involved in the positional cloning of inherited human disease genes. Genetic studies on families with affected individuals can identify an interval on the genetic map (asterisk) that most probably spans the gene causing the disease. A clone map of this region will have to be constructed and used to identify the genes within. The use of a transcript map integrated with the genetic map can accelerate this process. The genes known to map within the genetic interval associated with the disease can be evaluated early on as candidates based on their function or protein homology to other genes (also from other species). A mutation analysis will have to be conducted to identify the genetic defect causing the disease.

niques such as fluorescent *in situ* hybridization (FISH) and provide integration with the cytogenetic map *(14)*.

An integrated map that links all the different layers of information is a tool required in a wide range of projects in biomedical research, e.g., the positional cloning of inherited disease genes (**Fig. 1**)—hence the need to be accessed and comprehended by a multidisciplinary group of people including biologists, physicians, and clinicians. Although several databases in the public domain have been set up with the aim of displaying this type of information, no single site provides a complete picture so far. Furthermore, problems such as naming (i.e., several names for the same STS or gene) can complicate searches. On the other hand, the use of the World Wide Web (WWW) has allowed the different databases to build hyperlinks and cross-reference each other on-line, which has simplified searches across sites. A wealth of information is out there and what remains the task of the individual user is to assess it. To do so, it is necessary to be aware of issues such as the resolution of the method and/or reagent used in constructing each individual map, regions in the map in which distance distortions may occur owing to characteristics of the method used, problems that may arise owing to the biology of the sequence used to develop an STS marker, the conversion factors between different map units, and the confidence with which a marker has been placed on the map (applies to maps built on probabilities).

2. Materials

1. Computer (with connection to the Internet).
2. Software to browse the WWW that is compatible with the computer used, e.g., Netscape Navigator™ 3.0 for Macintosh.

3. Methods

The identification of an interval on the genetic map that is associated with, e.g., a disease phenotype (**Fig. 1**), will trigger the search for discovering and characterizing the defect that causes the disease, at the molecular level. In such a project, it is essential to use all the available resources including genetic, physical, and transcript maps as well as sequence and other biologic data; and to know the relevant databases that store this type of information. In general, there is no clear step-by-step guide to follow, and for many genomes, resources are limited or nonexistent. Many resources, however, are available for the human genome. Thus, we can follow up the example in **Fig. 1** as a hypothetical study case, with the aim of providing some insight on how to access and correctly interpret the required information.

3.1. The Use of Integrated Maps

The Genome Data Base *(15)* in collaboration with the Human Genome Organisation has created a WWW site *(16)* that lists a series of pages, one for each human chromosome.

Select a chromosome; in our example it is chromosome 20. Several links are appropriate as start points, but a typical approach is to identify and assess the genes known to map in the genetic interval of interest. Links are available for the following topics:

3.1.1. Chromosome-Specific Sites

Human Chromosome 20 Project, Sanger Centre.

3.1.2. Chromosome Resources

1. Integrated maps.
2. Genetic maps.

3. Radiation hybrid maps.
4. FISH maps.
5. Gene/transcript maps.
6. GDB chromosome 20.
7. Search by cytogenetic band.

3.1.3. DNA Sequencing

1. DNA Sequencing progress.
2. DNA Sequencing-specific sites.

3.1.4. DNA Sequence Annotation

1. The Genome Channel.
2. Gene summary tables.
3. Sanger Centre: WebACE Chromosome 20.

3.1.5. Disease Loci–Specific Sites

1. Disease loci and genes.
2. Disease and mutation databases.
3. Cancer cytogenetics.

3.1.6. Model Organism Synteny Maps

Mouse.

3.1.7. Medical Information (for Parents and Doctors)

1. Support groups.
2. Education.

3.2. An Integrated Genetic/Physical Gene Map: Search for Genes

Under "Gene/transcript maps", the following links are available:

3.2.1. Computational Biology and Informatics Laboratory

Chromosome 20 Mapped EST Query.

3.2.2. Genome Data Base

Genes on chromosome 20.

3.2.3. National Center for Biotechnology Information

1. Human gene map of chromosome 20 (96 Edition).
2. Human gene map of chromosome 20 (98 Edition).
3. Human gene map of chromosome 20 (99 Edition).
4. OMIM—Chromosome 20 Gene Map.
5. UniGene—Human Chromosome 20 Transcripts.

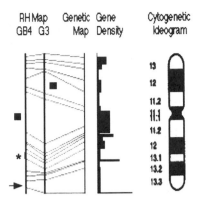

Fig. 2. Overview of the integrated human gene map of chromosome 20 on the WWW *(15)*.

3.2.4. The Wellcome Trust Centre for Human Genetics

For "Transcript map of chromosome 20," select the "Human gene map of chromosome 20 (1999 Edition)" link (*see* **Note 1**). The window shows at the top an alignment of the two RH maps, constructed using the GB4 and G3 RH panels, respectively, and the genetic map of the corresponding chromosome (**Fig. 2**). Below it, the display includes the most telomeric part of the GB4 map by default. STS markers ordered with high confidence and present on all three maps are linked with gray lines (**Fig. 2**) to define the bins of the integrated map or common reference intervals. Visibly, the order of these markers is the same on all three maps but there are regions (**Fig. 2**, solid black squares and arrow) in which a given reference interval has a significantly different size (as a fraction of the total length) on each map (*see* **Note 2**).

Click on any of the reference intervals to zoom in. Alternatively, query with a relevant genetic marker. The position of the bar (**Fig. 2**, asterisk) indicates the reference interval chosen to follow our test case (**Fig. 1**). The corresponding intervals on the GB4 map (**Fig. 3A**, only part of the map interval is shown) and the G3 map (**Fig. 3B**) are shown. All microsatellite (i.e., genetic) STS markers are highlighted and their cumulative distance on the genetic map, in centiMorgans, is reported in the first column (**Fig. 3A,B**). The cumulative distance of each marker on the RH maps is given in cR_{3000} and $cR_{10,000}$ for GB4 (**Fig. 3A**, second column) and G3 (**Fig. 3B**, second column), respectively. How do the three scales relate to physical distance? The most commonly quoted approximation in the literature of the correlation between genetic and physical distance in humans is 1 cM/Mb. Similarly, RH distances have been estimated to be 5 cR_{3000} and 40 $cR_{10,000}$ per Mb, respectively. Thus, it is possible to extrapolate distance units for all the markers using one scale and then display them in a linear order.

↑Next interval up

A

61.0	◆ **251.27**	**F**		**AFM273yh9**	**1**	**D20S119**	**Microsatellite anchor marker AFM273yh9**
	◆ 251.37	P0.00	*	SGC31967			Human putative outer mitochondrial membrane..
	◆ 251.37	"	*	SGC31967	2		Human putative outer mitochondrial membrane..
	251.37	"		U18297	3		Human stress responsive serine/threonine pr..
	251.37	"	→	stSG33865	4		Human stress responsive serine/threonine pr..
	251.37	"		U18297	5		Human stress responsive serine/threonine pr..
	251.37	P0.00		H98683	6		ESTs
	253.38	P0.00		sts-M81652	7	SEMG2	Semenogelin II
	253.69	P1.22		stSG4132	8		Homo sapiens HIV-Nef associated acyl CoA ..
	253.69	"		stSG34035	9		ELAFIN PRECURSOR
	254.62	P0.00	*	Cda1ea03	10		ESTs
	254.83	P1.33		sts-T86744	11		Human cyclin-selective ubiquitin carrier pr..
	254.93	P1.20	*	stSG10255	12		ESTs
	254.93	P1.24	*	WI-16033	13		ESTs
	254.93	P1.30	*	WI-12135	14		ESTs, Highly similar to HYPOTHETICAL ..
	254.93	P1.24	*	stSG10980	15	SDC4	Syndecan 4 (amphiglycan, ryudocan)
	255.14	P1.15		stSG4598	16		ESTs
	255.14	P1.13		stSG30061	17		EST
	255.14	P1.20		SGC30446	18		H.sapiens HE4 mRNA for extracellular prote..
	255.31	P1.09		A002A22	19		ESTs
	255.34	P1.06		sts-M33772	20		Unknown
	257.15	P0.01		A006N01	21		ESTs
	257.25	P0.01		A001X16	22		ESTs
	257.25	P0.00		stSG20113	23	PPGB	Protective protein for beta-galactosidase (..
	257.25	P0.00		AA279153	24		ESTs
	257.25	P0.00		sts-M22960	25	PPGB	Protective protein for beta-galactosidase (..
64.1	257.35	F		AFMa132xe9	26	D20S836	Microsatellite marker AFMa132xe9

B

61.0	◆ **2285**	**F**		**AFM273yh9**	**1**	**D20S119**	**Microsatellite anchor marker AFM273yh9 (SHGC-3673)**
	2289	F		SHGC-13528	2		ESTs, Highly similar to POLYADENYLATE..
	◆ 2289	F	*	SHGC-31967	3		Human putative outer mitochondrial membrane..
	2293	P1.73		SHGC-37252	4	YWHAB	Tyrosine 3-monooxygenase/tryptophan 5-monoo..
61.0	2297	F		AFM207zb10	5	D20S880	Microsatellite marker AFM207zb10 (SHGC-21..
	◆ 2305	P0	*	SHGC-31227	6		EST
	◆ 2314	F	*	SHGC-12308	7		Human mRNA for antileukoprotease (ALP) fr..
	◆ 2331	F	*	SHGC-34003	8		ESTs
64.1	◆ 2373	F		AFMb299yd1	9	D20S888	Microsatellite marker AFMb299yd1 (SHGC-21..
	◆ 2377	P0.0		SHGC-13901			ESTs
65.5	◆ 2377	F		AFMb298wb9		D20S886	Microsatellite marker AFMb298wb9 (SHGC-21..
	◆ 2399	F	*	SHGC-11751			EST
	◆ 2399	F	*	SHGC-11563			Homo sapiens protein kinase C-binding prote..
66.0	◆ **2411**	**F**		**AFM326xd5**		**D20S197**	**Microsatellite anchor marker AFM326xd5 (SHGC-1451)**

Fig. 3. An interval of the integrated human gene map of chromosome 20 (*see* **Fig. 1**). **(A)** Section of the common reference interval defined by markers AFM273yh9 and AFM326xd5 on the GB4 RH map. The markers between AFM273yh9 and AFMal32xe9 are shown. **(B)** Markers in the same reference interval on the G3 RH map. The markers used to compare the integrated map with the sequence map have been numbered 1–26 (A) and 1–9 (B).

Would it then be possible to define accurately an interval, e.g., 0.1 Mb ($\sim$0.1 cM, $\sim$0.5 cR$_{3000}$, $\sim$4 cR$_{10,000}$)? To address this question, one needs to know the resolution of each map. The resolution of the GB4 and G3 panel is on average 1 and 0.3 Mb, respectively (*see* **Note 3**), whereas the resolution of the genetic map is 1 Mb *(2)*. Thus, none of the three maps can provide this sort of resolution. For example, the correct interpretation of the GB4 map based on its resolution is that the relative order of the 25 markers between AFM273yh9 and AFMal32xe9 (**Fig. 3A**) cannot be resolved accurately using this reagent. In addition, the placement LOD score (**Fig. 2A**, third column; *see* also Chapter 11) for the markers near AFM273yh9 and AFMal 32xe9 (framework markers) is P = 0.00, which means that statistically the position of, e.g., SGC31967 can be either side of AFM273yh9. The overall resolution of the integrated map is that of the lowest resolution component. Hence, to select genes mapping between AFM273yh9 and AFMal32xe9, one needs to investigate the markers between AFM273yh9 and AFMal32xe9 on the GB4 map as well as those in the flanking framework intervals, and the markers between AFM273yh9 and AFMb298wb9 on the G3 map as well as those in the framework interval above AFM273yh9.

Does every marker represent a different gene? The map display (**Fig. 3**) reports in the last column the name of the "gene" associated with a marker. There are three STSs associated with the "Human stress responsive serine/threonine pr.." gene. For unknown genes (i.e., ESTs), this relationship is not evident by simple inspection. The map is further integrated with both sequence and biologic data through a series of links. Click on any marker. For example, stSG33865 will bring up the display shown in **Fig. 4A**. There is a link to the UniGene database (**Fig. 4B**); a list of all the STS markers on the map that represent this gene with links to the raw mapping data (**Fig. 4C**) in RHdb *(17)*; and a list of all genomic, mRNA, and EST sequences (linked to GenBank; not shown) in which the STS markers can be located by means of the electronic PCR program *(18)*.

This example also demonstrates the problem of multiple names: STK4, Krs-2, and MST1 all describe the same gene. Using MST1 to query GDB *(15)*, the user will retrieve two genes, one on chromosome 3 and one on chromosome 20. The same query in the OMIM *(19)* database will report only the gene on chromosome 3, which is the macrophage stimulating 1 factor.

3.3. The Sequence Map

It has become apparent in the past few years that sequencing entire genomes is the ultimate solution to generate fully integrated maps. A sequence map has the ability to position any STS, clone, gene, or bit of biologic information with

Cross–References		
UniGene	Hs.35140	Human stress responsive serine/threonine protein kinase Krs–2 mRNA

RH Mapping Results		
U18297 **A**	GB4 Map:	Chr.20
	Reference interval:	D20S119–D20S197 (61.0–66.0 cM)
	Physical position:	251.37 cR3000 (P0.00)
	RH details:	RHdb RH18007
	Typed by:	Genethon
U18297	GB4 Map:	Chr.20
	Reference interval:	D20S119–D20S197 (61.0–66.0 cM)
	Physical position:	251.37 cR3000 (P0.00)
	RH details:	RHdb RH70577
	Typed by:	Genethon
stSG33865	GB4 Map:	Chr.20
	Reference interval:	D20S119–D20S197 (61.0–66.0 cM)
	Physical position:	251.37 cR3000 (P0.00)
	RH details:	RHdb RH66078
	Typed by:	Sanger Centre

Electronic PCR Results

Genomic (from GenBank PRI division)

Z93016 Human DNA sequence from PAC 211D12 on chromosome 20q12–13.2. Contains Krs–2, K+ channel protein, stress responsive

STS 50135 ... 50328 bp: U18297
STS 50303 ... 50447 bp: stSG33865

mRNAs (from GenBank PRI division)

U18297 Human MST1 (MST1) mRNA, complete cds

STS 1347 ... 1491 bp: stSG33865
STS 1466 ... 1659 bp: U18297

U60207 Human stress responsive serine/threonine protein kinase Krs–2 mRNA, complete cds

STS 1370 ... 1514 bp: stSG33865
STS 1489 ... 1682 bp: U18297

ESTs (from GenBank EST division)

H56417 yq98a09.r1 Homo sapiens cDNA clone 203800 5'.

STS 132 ... 280 bp: stSG33865

R93508 yq35c11.r1 Homo sapiens cDNA clone 197780 5'.

STS 101 ... 244 bp: stSG33865

Fig. 4. Overview of the links available for each marker of the integrated human gene map. In this example, STS marker stSG33865 (**Fig. 3**) is followed. (**A**) Information on the gene represented by STS marker stSG33865; (**B**) the corresponding entry of this gene in the UniGene database; (**C**) the entry of stSG33865 in RHdb.

single base-pair accuracy. Even cytogenetic boundaries can be defined precisely on the sequence map of a chromosome based on its GC content. In contrast to recent efforts in the private domain to sequence the human-genome using whole genome shotgun *(20)*, the Human Genome Project is proceeding by building sequence-ready bacterial clone (PACs and/or BACs) maps of each

Hs.35140   *Homo sapiens*   **STK4**

Serine/threonine kinase 4

SEE ALSO   **B**

    LocusLink: 6789

SELECTED MODEL ORGANISM PROTEIN SIMILARITIES

H. sapiens:	PID:g1477791 – serine/threonine protein kinase Krs-2	**100 % / 486 aa**
M. musculus:	PID:g881958 – Mess1	**81 % / 416 aa**
R. norvegicus:	PID:g2695713 – MST2 kinase	**79 % / 477 aa**
D. melanogaster:	PID:g1335890 – serine/threonine kinase PAK homolog DPAK	**41 % / 303 aa**
C. elegans:	PID:g1255410 – Similar to serine/threonine kinase	**46 % / 358 aa**
S. cerevisiae:	PID:g508679 – Ste20p: Protein kinase	**38 % / 342 aa**

MAPPING INFORMATION

    Chromosome: 20
    Gene Map 98: Marker U18297 , Interval D20S119–D20S197
    Gene Map 98: Marker stSG33865 , Interval D20S119–D20S197

EXPRESSION INFORMATION

    cDNA sources: Brain, Germ Cell, Lung, Nose
    SAGE :   Gene to Tag mapping

mRNA/GENE SEQUENCES (3)

U60207 Human stress responsive serine/threonine protein kinase   P S
    Krs-2 mRNA, complete cds
U18297 Human MST1 (MST1) mRNA, complete cds   P S
Z93016 Human DNA sequence from PAC 211D12 on   P
    chromosome 20q12–13.2. Contains Krs-2, K+ channel
    protein, stress responsive

EST SEQUENCES (11)

N23875   cDNA clone IMAGE:255257 Nose   3′ read 1.4 kb P
AA953504 cDNA clone   3′ read 0.8 kb P C

Fig. 4B.

chromosome and sequencing a minimally overlapping set of clones (*see* **Note 4**). The Sanger Centre is currently constructing the sequence map of chromosome 20 (*see* **Note 4**), which is relevant in our study case. Follow the link "Human Chromosome 20 Project, Sanger Centre" (*see* **Subheading 3.1.**). Use the AceBrowser *(21)* to query for a relevant STS (*see* **Note 5**) such as the genetic markers defining the interval of interest. The Sanger Centre is currently using the graphic displays of ACEDB *(22)* to represent genetic, RH, and physical clone maps as well as the annotated sequence map. Information is orga-

```
AC    RH66078
XX
OS    Homo Sapiens.
XX
DT    19-AUG-1997 (Rel. 10, Created)              C
XX
RN    [1]
RA    Panagiotis Deloukas
RL    Submitted (19-AUG-1997) to EBI by: Panagiotis Deloukas, Sanger
RL    Centre, Hinxton Hall, Hinxton, Cambridge CB10 1RQ, UK
RL    Email: panos@sanger.ac.uk
XX
DR    EMBL; U60207.
DR    Sanger_STS; stSG33865.
XX
FG    FI2
XX
ST    STS46008
PS    ACCTTCAGAAGAGGCTCTTGG
PS    GGCCTTGCTCAGAAGTTTTG
PL    145 bp
PC    EI33
XX
CH    20
XX
MP    CM66; P; .1; ; RH15374; RH37523; 0; 0;
XX
SC    Genebridge4 2
      1210212001 2201111111 1001011001 1010010001 111000R000 0011001211
      0100101012 0011011102 1000011000 001
//
```

Fig. 4C.

nized per chromosome; for example, 20ace is the chromosome 20 database (*see* **Note 6**). Thus, a query with AFM273yh9 (*see* **Note 5**) will return, among other information, all the maps held in 20ace and in which this STS maps:

SANGER_chrom20_rlunap_01_12_97
Genethon_sex_average_map_March_1996
Genethon_female_map_March_1996
Genethon_male_map_March_1996
Chr_20
SANGER_rhmap_sci96
SANGER_chrom20_rhmap_09_04_97
CMG_sex_averaged_map
CMG_female_map
CMG_male_map
SANGER_chrom20_rhmap_08_04_97
SANGER_chrom20_rhmap_01_12_97
Transcript_map_98
SANGER_chrom20_rhmap_03_11_98
Chr 20ctgl25

Select "Chr_20ctgl25" to view the sequence-ready bacterial clone map. Scroll through the contig or repeat the process just described to locate the other marker defining the interval of interest. The part of this map that is relevant to

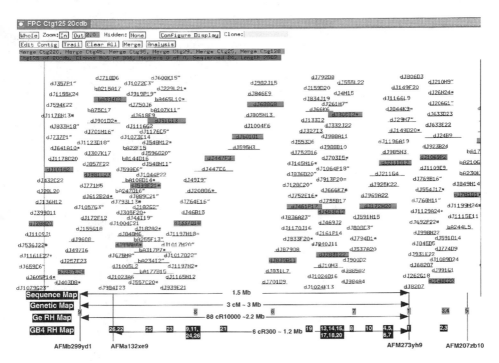

Fig. 5. Section of the sequence-ready bacterial clone map of chromosome 20. (**Top**) View in FPC (*see* Chapter 7). The clones of the sequencing tiling path are highlighted. (**Bottom**) Markers of the integrated gene map positioned according to their base-pair coordinates in the sequence map. The numbers (gray and black boxes) represent the markers shown in **Fig. 3** in the order in which they appear on the corresponding map.

our study case (**Figs. 2** and **3**) is shown (**Fig. 5**) as a view in FPC (*see* Chapter 7) that has been simplified by not displaying marker data. The clones that form the sequencing tiling path are highlighted. The sequence of these clones is now available *(23)*. This allows the calculation of the distance between AFM273yh9 and AFMb298wb9, ~1.5 Mb (*see* **Note 7**), and means that a simple sequence search by BLAST *(24)* can identify the position of any STS-based marker or sequence fragment mapping in this interval. A search using any of the sequences shown in **Fig. 4A** will return the genomic sequence of clone dJ21 lD12 (**Fig. 5**). The annotated sequence of this clone (*see* **Note 8**) can be viewed graphically through WEBACE *(25)* or as the text file submitted to the nucleotide databases (*see* **Note 9**). In either case, the exon-intron structure and complete nucleotide sequence of the stress-responsive serine/threonine protein (STK4 or Krs-2) can be obtained (*see* **Note 8**). Thus, if STK4 were a candidate gene for our study case (**Fig. 1**), this information would have been used to design assays for mutation analysis.

4. Notes

1. The construction of an integrated human gene map by RH mapping *(11)* is discussed in Chapter 11. This map is available on the WWW, and the home page *(26)* provides a link to each chromosome (except Y).

2. It is known that centromeric regions are retained in RH panels with a frequency higher than the average, which results in the overestimation of RH distances between markers flanking the centromere (**Fig. 2**, solid squares). High recombination frequency in these regions has an opposite effect on the genetic map. Genetic distances between markers near the telomere, especially in the long arm, appear to be overestimated owing to low recombination frequency (**Fig. 2**, arrow). This is not the case in RH maps which, in general, do not have the equivalent of high or low recombination spots. Thus, with the exception of centromeric regions, the correlation between RH and physical distances along the chromosome is more linear than that between genetic and physical distances.

3. Markers are ordered with odds >1000:1; *see* Chapter 11.

4. Such maps for chromosomes 1, 6, 9, 10, 13, 20, 22 (finished), and X are being constructed at the Sanger Centre. As already mentioned, genetic, RH, and gene maps can be integrated with a physical clone map using STS-based markers. Indeed, that has been an integral part of the strategy adopted at the Sanger Centre to generate sequence-ready maps *(27,28)*.

5. All markers used at the Sanger Centre have a unique identifier stSGxxxx (e.g., stSG33865). If the marker to be used in the query was developed elsewhere, try the original name prefixed with "st" (e.g., stAFM273yh9). If it fails and the accession number of the sequence used to develop this marker is known, then the query can be performed via the "Sequence" field of the query tool. Note that when you query for a contig map (e.g., Chr_20ctg125) you should use the "Map" field. GDB locus names such as D20Sxxx are stored under "Locus".

6. The chromosome-specific databases such as 20ace are available on-line through WEBACE *(29)* or can be downloaded via ftp *(30)*.

7. We can go a step back and evaluate some of the points made earlier about the use and interpretation of an integrated map by comparing the same interval on the sequence and integrated gene maps. In our example, distance is overestimated by a factor of 2 and 1.5 on the genetic and the G3 RH map, respectively, when compared with the sequence map (**Fig. 5**). The anomaly on the G3 map is owing to AFM207zb10. Placing this marker between AFM273yh9 and AFMb298wb9, although it maps outside this interval, causes an expansion of the map length. However, the distance between AFM273yh9 and AFM207zb10 is 12 $cR_{10,000}$, which is near the limit of resolution of the G3 panel. To evaluate marker order, the markers of the GB4 (**Fig. 3A**, numbered 1–26) and G3 map (**Fig. 3B**, numbered 1–9) have been placed on the sequence map (**Fig. 5**). The marker in position 12 and 2 on the GB4 and G3 map, respectively, do not map in this interval and are not shown. Hence, map distances can be distorted, and the resolution threshold of a mapping reagent determines the accuracy of map order.

8. The Sanger Centre annotates the finished sequence of every genomic clone in its pipeline *(31)*. WEBACE provides a graphic view of this information *(25)*. Scroll through the window with the clone names and select one (e.g., dJ21 lD12), select the option "Graphics" (active), and press "show object". Use the sequence coordinates to zoom into the display. For example, STK4 is between 45,000 bp and the end of the clone (at 123,933).

9. Look for the ".embl" file in the ftp directory for finished data *(25)* (e.g., dJ21 lD12.embl).

References

1. Olson, M., Hood, L., Cantor, C., and Botstein D. (1989) A common language for physical mapping of the human genome. *Science* **245,** 1434, 1435.
2. Dib, C., Faure, S., Fizames, C., et al. (1996) A comprehensive genetic map of the human genome based on 5,264 microsatellites. *Nature* **380,** 152–154.
3. Rhodes, M., Straw, R., Fernando, S., et al. (1998) A high-resolution microsatellite map of the mouse genome. *Genome Res.* **8,** 531–542.
4. Steen, R. G., Kwitek-Black, A. E., Glenn, C., et al. (1999) A high-density integrated genetic linkage and radiation hybrid map of the laboratory rat. *Genome Res.* **9,** 1–8.
5. Chumakov, I. M., Rigault, P., Le Gall, I., et al. (1995) A YAC contig map of the human genome. *Nature* **377,** 175–297.
6. Hudson, T. J. Stein, L. D., Gerety, S. S., et al. (1995) An STS-based map of the human genome. *Science* **270,** 1945–1954.
7. Nusbaum, C., Slonim, D. K., Harris, K. L., et al. (1999) A YAC-based physical map of the mouse genome. *Nature Genet.* **22,** 388–393.
8. Cai, L., Schalkwyk, L.C., Schoeberlein-Stehli, A., et al. (1997) Construction and characterization of a 10-genome equivalent yeast artificial chromosome library for the laboratory rat, *Rattus norvegicus. Genomics* **1,** 385–392.
9. Walter, M. A., Spillett, D. J., Thomas, P., Weissenbach, J., and Goodlellow, P. N. (1994) A method for constructing radiation hybrid maps of whole genomes. *Nature Genet.* **7,** 22–28.
10. Stewart, E. A., McKusick, K. B., Aggarwal, A., et al. (*1997*) An STS-based radiation hybrid map of the human genome. *Genome Res.* **7,** 422–433.
11. Deloukas, P., Schuler, G. D., Gyapay, G., et al. (1998) A Physical map of **30,000** human genes. *Science* **282,** 744–746.
12. Van Etten, W. J., Steen, R. G., Nguyen, H., et al. (1999) Radiation hybrid map of the mouse genome. *Nature Genet.* **22,** 384–387.
13. <http://ratest.uiowa.edu/> (an EST-based radiation hybrid map of the rat).
14. Bray-Ward, P., Menninger, J., Lieman, J., Desai, T., Mokady, N., Banks, A., and Ward, D. C. (1996) Integration of the cytogenetic, genetic, and physical maps of the human genome by FISH mapping of CEPH YAC clones. *Genomics* **15,** 1–14.
15. <http://www.gdb.org>.
16. <http://www.gdb.org/hugo>.
17. <http://www.ebi.ac.uk:80/RHdb/>.

18. Schuler, G. (1997) Sequence mapping by electronic PCR. *Genome Res.* **7,** 541–550.
19. <http://www.ncbi.nlm.nih.gov/Omim/>.
20. Venter, J. C., Adams, M. D., Sutton, G. G., Kerlavage, A. R., Smith, H. O., and Hunkapiller, M. (1998) Shotgun sequencing of the human genome. *Science* **5,** 1540–1542.
21. <http://webace.sanger.ac.uk/cgi-bin/ace/simple/20ace>.
22. Durbin, R. and Mieg. J.-T. (1991) A *C. elegans* database: documentation, code and data available from anonymous FTP servers at <lirmm.lirmm.fr, cele.mrc-lmb.cam.ac.uk and ncbi.nlm.nih.gov>.
23. Unfinished data: ftp://ftp.sanger.ac.uk/publhuman/sequences/Chr_20/unfinished_sequence/>; finished data: <ftp://ftp.sanger.ac.uk/pub/human/sequences/Chr_20/>.
24. <http://www.sanger.ac.uk/HGP/Chr20/Chr20_blast_server.shtml>.
25. <http://webace.sanger.ac.uk/cgi-bin/webace?db=acedb20&class=Genome_Sequence>.
26. <http://www.ncbi.nlm.nih.gov/genemap/>.
27. <http://www.sanger.ac.uk/HGP/>.
28. The Sanger Centre and the Washington University Genome Sequencing Center (1998) Toward a complete human genome sequence. *Genome Res.* **8,** 1097–1108.
29. <http://webace.sanger.ac.uk/>.
30. <ftp://ftp.sanger.ac.uk/pub/human/>.
31. <http://www.sanger.ac.uklHGP/Humana>.

10

Construction of Full-Length-Enriched cDNA Libraries

The Oligo-Capping Method

Yutaka Suzuki and Sumio Sugano

1. Introduction

The full-length cDNA, which contains the entire sequence of the mRNA, is the ultimate goal for cDNA cloning. Unfortunately, cDNA libraries constructed by many types of conventional methods have a high content of nonfull-length cDNA clones. One of the reasons for this is that reverse transcriptase (RT) tends to stop during the first strand synthesis and falls off, leaving nonfull-length cDNA. Thus, nonfull-length cDNA is an inevitable result of the use of RT for the synthesis of cDNA.

To make a full-length cDNA library, we have to devise some type of selection procedure for full-length cDNA. To select the full-length cDNA, the cDNA that contains both ends of the mRNA should be selected. For that purpose, the features that are characteristic to the 3' end and the 5' end of mRNA should be used as tags. The full-length cDNA could be selected through the selection steps for both the 3' end and the 5' end tags.

The polyA stretch is a characteristic feature of the 3' end of mRNA. Conventional methods have used the polyA as a sequence tag to select the 3' end of mRNA. According to conventional methods, the first-strand cDNA is usually synthesized from an oligo dT primer. Because dT primers mostly hybridize at the polyA tail, most of the cDNA is selectively synthesized from the 3' end of the mRNA. Thus, the conventional methods include the selection step for the 3' end tag of the mRNA. However, they include no step to select the 5' end of mRNA. As a result, the largest part of the cDNA library is occupied by cDNAs that lack the 5' end of the mRNA.

From: *Methods in Molecular Biology, vol. 175: Genomics Protocols*
Edited by: M. P. Starkey and R. Elaswarapu © Humana Press Inc., Totowa, NJ

The main reason for this lies, in our view, in the fact that mRNA does not originally have a sequence tag at the 5' end. The 5' end of mRNA also has a characteristic structure, called the cap structure, but, unfortunately, it is not a sequence tag. Unlike the polyA at the 3' end, it cannot be used for the hybridization. If the 5' end tag of the mRNA were also a sequence tag, it would be easy to use it to select the 5' end of mRNA.

To overcome this difficulty, we have developed a new method to introduce a sequence tag at the 5' end, which we call the Oligo-Capping method *(1)*. This method allows us to replace the cap structure of mRNA with a synthetic oligonucleotide enzymatically. Each mRNA product of the Oligo-Capping contains the sequence tags at the both ends—polyA at the 3' end and the cap-replaced oligo at the 5' end. With Oligo-Capped mRNA as a starting material, a new system is developed to selectively clone the cDNA that contains both of the sequence tags at the respective ends. Following the scheme shown in **Fig. 1**, a cDNA library is constructed in which the content of full-length cDNA is significantly enriched (full-length-enriched cDNA library) *(2)*.

Other groups also have presented novel methods to construct a full-length cDNA library. Kato et al. *(3)* combined the Oligo-Capping and the Okayama-Berg method, using a DNA-RNA chimeric oligo for the cap replacement. To select full-length cDNA, Edery et al. *(4)* used the cap binding protein (cap retention procedure) and Carninci et al. *(5)* chemically modified and biotinylated the cap structure (CAP trapper). All these methods make use of the cap-dependent retention of full-length cDNA on solid supports.

1.1. Principle of the Construction of a Full-Length-Enriched cDNA Library

Oligo-Capping consists of three steps of enzyme reactions. Bacterial alkaline phosphatase (BAP) hydrolyzes the phosphate from the 5' ends of truncated mRNAs, which are noncapped. The cap structure on capped full-length mRNAs remains intact during this reaction. Tobacco acid pyrophosphatase (TAP) cleaves the cap structure itself at the position indicated by in **Fig. 1A**, leaving a phosphate at the 5' ends. Finally, T_4 RNA ligase selectively ligates the synthetic oligoribonucleotide to the phosphate at the 5' end. As a result, the oligoribonucleotide is introduced only to the 5' ends of mRNAs that originally had the cap structure.

With Oligo-Capped mRNA as a starting material, first-strand cDNA is synthesized using an oligo dT adapter primer (*see* **Fig. 1**). After first-strand cDNA synthesis, the template mRNA is alkaline degraded. Polymerase chain reaction (PCR) is performed with 3'- and 5'-end primer, which have a part of the oligo dT adapter primer sequence and the cap-replaced oligonucleotide sequence,

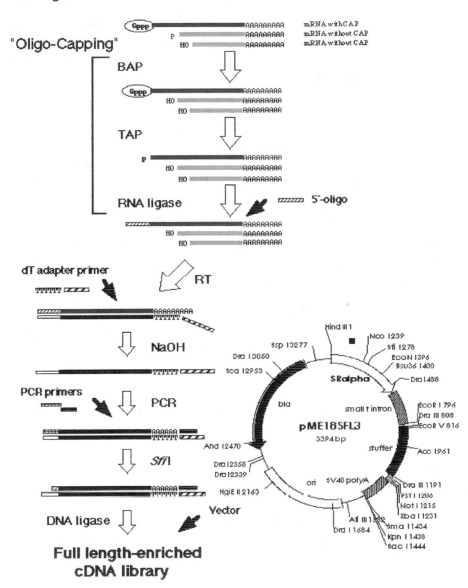

Fig. 1. Schematic representation of the construction of a full length-enriched cDNA library. Oligo-Capping replaces the cap structure of mRNA with a 5'-oligoribonucleotide by the successive functions of BAP, TAP, and T4 RNA ligase. Using Oligo-Capped mRNA as a starting material, a full-length-enriched cDNA library is constructed. As a cloning vector, we are currently using a plasmid vector, pME 18S-FL3. In this plasmid, cDNA is inserted downstream to the eukaryotic promoter, SR-α. The full-length cDNA can be directly expressed by introducing it into cultured cells.

respectively. The amplified cDNA fragments are digested with restriction enzymes, size fractionated, and cloned into a plasmid vector.

2. Materials (*see* Note 1)

1. Thermocycler.
2. Carrier for the ethanol precipitation (RNase free): Ethachinmate (cat. no. 312-01791; WAKO, Tokyo, Japan).
3. Total RNA extraction kits: RNeasy (cat. no. 75163; Qiagen, Chatsworth, CA) and Trizol (cat. no. 15596-018; Life Technologies, Rockville, MD).
4. Oligo-dT: Oligo-dT cellulose (cat. no. 20020; Collaborative, Bedford, MA) and Oligo-Tex (cat. no. W9021B; Nippon-Roche, Tokyo, Japan).
5. RNasin (40 U/μL) (cat. no. N2111; Promega, Madison, WI).
6. BAP (0.25 U/μL; cat. no. 2110; TaKaRa, Kyoto, Japan).
7. TAP (20 U/μL) purified from tobacco cells (BY-2) following the procedure described in **ref. *6***.
8. T4 RNA ligase (25 U/μL) (cat. no. 2050, TaKaRa).
9. 50% (w/v) PEG 8000 (cat. no. P2139; Sigma, St. Louis, MO; *see* **Note 2**). Add dH$_2$O to PEG 8000 so that the concentration is 50% (w/v). Dissolve the PEG 8000 at 65°C. Sterilize the solution by filtration through a 0.22-μ*M* Millex-GV membrane (cat. no. Millipore S. A., SLVG025LS; Molsheim, France).
10. DNase I (RNase free) (5.0 U/μL) (cat. no. 2215, TaKaRa).
11. Spin column: S-400HR (cat. no. 27–5140, Amersham Pharmacia Biotech, Piscataway, NJ).
12. Superscript II (200 U/μL) and 5X first-strand buffer (250 m*M* Tris-HCl, pH 8.3, 375 m*M* KCl, 15 m*M* MgCl$_2$) (cat. no. 18064-014; Life Technologies).
13. PCR kit PCGene Amp, including rTth DNA polymerase (2 U/μL) and 3.3X reaction buffer II (cat. no. N808-0192; Perkin-Elmer, Norwalk, CT).
14. *Sfi*I (20 U/μL; New England Biolabs Beverly, MA).
15. *Dra*BI (6.0 U/μL) (WAKO).
16. Gene Clean II (cat. no. GL-1131-05, Bio101, Vista, CA).
17. Agarose (cat. no. 312-01193; WAKO).
18. DNA Ligation kit (cat. no. 6021; TaKaRa).
19. 5X BAP buffer: 500 m*M* Tris-HCl, pH 7.0, 50 m*M* 2-mercaptoethanol.
20. 5X TAP buffer: 250 m*M* sodium acetate, pH 5.5, 50 m*M* 2-mercaptoethanol, 5 m*M* EDTA, pH 8.0.
21. 10X Ligation buffer: 500 m*M* Tris-HCl, pH 7.0, 100 m*M* 2-mercaptoethanol.
22. 10X STE: 100 m*M* Tris-HCl, pH 7.0, 1 *M* NaCl, 10 m*M* EDTA, pH 8.0.
23. 5'-Oligoribonucleotide A: 5'-AGCAUCGAGUCGGCCWGWGGCCUACUGGAG-3' (100 ng/μL).
24. Oligo-dT adapter primer B: 5'-GCGGCTGAAGACGGCCTATGTGGCC(T)$_{17}$-3' (5 pmol/μL).
25. 5' primer C: 5'-AGCATCGAGTCGGCCTTGTTGAG-3' (10 pmol/μL).
26. 3' primer D: 5'-GCGCTGAAGACGGCCTATGTGC-3' (10 pmol/μL).

27. 3' primer E for the EF 1-α amplification: 5'-ACGTTCACGCTCAGCmCAGAC-3' (10 pmol/μL).
28. 3' primer F for the EF1-α amplification: 5'-AACACCAGCAGCAACAATCAGAA-3' (10 pmol/μL).
29. pME18S-FL3 (Genbank acc. # AB00984).

3. Methods

3.1. Preparation of Total RNA and PolyA+ RNA

Extract total RNA from 2 to 3 g of tissue or 1 to 5×10^7 cultured cells using the acid guanidinium thiocyanate-phenol-chloroform (AGPC) method (*see* **Note 2**), and purify polyA+ RNA by binding to a commercially available oligo dT support (*see* **Subheading 2., item 4**) (*see* **Note 3**).

3.2. BAP Reaction

1. Set up a BAP reaction by combining 67.3 μL of polyA+ RNA (100–200 μg), 20.0 μL of 5X BAP buffer, 2.7 μL of RNasin, and 10.0 μL of BAP.
2. Incubate at 37°C for 60 min.
3. Add an equal volume of phenol:chloroform (1:1) to the sample and mix. Centrifuge at 13,000g for 5 min at 4°C. Transfer the upper aqueous layer to a fresh tube.
4. Repeat the phenol: chloroform extraction (1:1).
5. Ethanol precipitate the RNA by adding 2.5 vol of 100% (v/v) ethanol; $^1/_{10}$ vol of sodium acetate, pH 5.5; and 1 μL of ethachinmate. Centrifuge at 13,000g at 4°C for 10 min.
6. Remove the supernatant and rinse the pellet with 150 μL of 80% (v/v) ethanol. Drying the pellet is not necessary. Resuspend the BAP-treated polyA+ RNA in 75.3 μL of dH$_2$O.

3.3. TAP Reaction

1. Set up a TAP reaction by combining 75.3 μL of BAP-treated polyA+ RNA, 20.0 μL of 5X TAP buffer, 2.7 μL of RNasin, and 2.0 μL of TAP.
2. Incubate at 37°C for 60 min.
3. Extract the solution with phenol: chloroform (1:1) (*see* **Subheading 3.2., step 3**).
4. Ethanol precipitate the RNA (*see* **Subheading 3.2., steps 4** and **5**).
5. Resuspend the RNA in 11.0 μL of dH$_2$O.

3.4. RNA Ligation

1. Ligate the BAP/TAP-treated polyA+ RNA to the 5' oligoribonucleotide (sequence by combining with 4.0 μL of 5' oligoribonucleotide, 10.0 μL of 10X ligation buffer, 10.0 μL of 50 m*M* MgCl$_2$, 2.5 μL of 24 m*M* adenosine triphosphate, 2.5 μL of RNasin, 10.0 μL of T4 RNA ligase, and 50.0 μL of 50% [w/v] PEG 8000).
2. Incubate at 20°C for 3 h.
3. Add 200.0 μL of dH$_2$O.

4. Extract the solution with phenol:chloroform (1:1).
5. Ethanol precipitate the RNA.
6. Resuspend the RNA in 70.3 µL of dH_2O.

3.5. DNase I Treatment

1. Treat the Oligo-Capped mRNA with DNase I by combining with 16.0 µL of 50 mM $MgCl_2$; 4.0 µL of 1 M Tris-HCl, pH 7.0; 5.0 µL of 0.1 M dithiothreitol (DTT), 2.7 µL of RNasin, and 2.0 µL of DNase I.
2. Incubate at 37°C for 10 min.
3. Extract the solution with phenol: chloroform (1:1).
4. Ethanol precipitate the RNA.
5. Resuspend the Oligo-Capped mRNA in 45.0 µL of dH_2O and add 5 µL of 10X STE.

3.6. Spin-Column Purification

1. Remove excess 5' oligoribonucleotide from the RNA by spin-column chromatography (S400-HR; according to the manufacturer's instructions).
2. Ethanol precipitate the RNA.
3. Resuspend the RNA in 21.0 µL of dH_2O.

3.7. First-Strand cDNA Synthesis

1. Synthesize first-strand cDNA with RNaseH-free RT by combining the RNA with 10.0 µL of 5X first-strand buffer, 8.0 µL of 4X 5 mM dNTPs, 6.0 µL of 0.1 M DTT, 2.5 µL of oligo dT adapter primer (sequence B), 1.0 µL of RNasin, and 2.0 µL of SuperScript II.
2. Incubate at 42°C for more than 3 h (*see* **Note 4**).
3. Add 2 µL of 0.5 M EDTA, pH 8.0 to stop the reaction thoroughly.
4. Extract the solution with phenol:chloroform (1:1).

3.8. Alkaline Degradation of Template mRNA

1. Degrade the template RNA by adding 15 µL of 0.1 M NaOH and heating the solution at 65°C for 60 min.
2. Add 20 µL of 1 M Tris-HCl, pH 7.0, to neutralize the solution.
3. To remove the fragmented RNA, precipitate the first-strand cDNA by adding 2.5 vol of 100% (v/v) ethanol, $1/3$ vol of 7.5 M ammonium acetate (*see* **Note 5**), and 1 µL of ethachinmate. Centrifuge at 13,000g at 4°C for 10 min.
4. Remove the supernatant and rinse the pellet with 150 µL of 80% (v/v) ethanol. Drying the pellet is not necessary. Resuspend the first-strand cDNA in 50 µL of dH_2O.

3.9. Confirmation of First-Strand cDNA

To confirm the integrity of the first strand cDNA, PCR amplify the 5' end of the EF 1-α mRNA.

1. Combine $1/50$ of the first-strand cDNA in 52.4 µL of dH_2O with 30.0 µL of 3.3X reaction buffer II; 8.0 µL of 4X 2.5 mM dNTPs; 4.4 µL of 25 mM magnesium

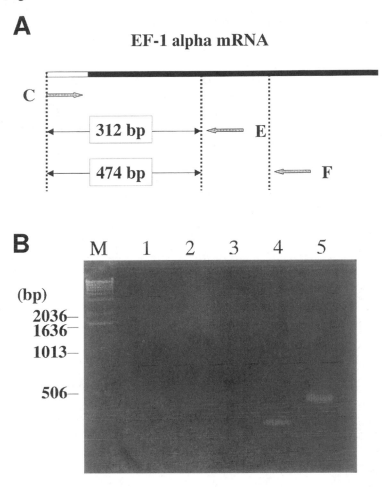

Fig. 2. PCR amplification of the 5' end of EF1-α mRNA. **(A)** Relative positions of the PCR primers against the EF1-α mRNA; **(B)** 2% (w/v) agarose gel electrophoresis of the PCR products. Lane M, molecular weight markers (the lengths of marker DNAs are indicated in base pairs on the left); lane 1, primer C; lane 2, primer E; lane 3, primer F; lane 4, primers C and E; lane 5, primers C and F.

acetate; 1.6 µL of 5' primer (sequence C), 1.6 µL of 3' primer (sequence E), or 1.6 µL of 3' primer (sequence F); and 2.0 µL of rTth DNA polymerase. Overlay with 100 µL of mineral oil.
2. Thermocycle for 30 cycles at 94°C, 1 min; 52°C, 1 min; 72°C, 1 min.
3. Analyze $^1/_{20}$–$^1/_{10}$ of the PCR products by 2% (w/v) agarose gel electrophoresis, and confirm the fragment lengths (312 and 474 bp for primer pairs C + E and C + F, respectively) (**Fig. 2**).

3.10. PCR Amplification, Size Fractionation, and Cloning of cDNA Fragments

1. Use $^1/_3$–$^1/_2$ of the of the first-strand cDNA in 52.4 µL of dH$_2$O with 30.0 µL of 3.3X reaction buffer II, 8.0 µL of 4X 2.5 mM dNTPs, 4.4 µL of 25 mM magnesium acetate, 1.6 µL of 5' primer (sequence C), 1.6 µL of 3' primer (sequence D), and 2.0 µL of rTth DNA polymerase. Overlay with 100 µL of mineral oil.
2. Thermocycle as follows: 12 cycles of 94°C, 1 min; 58°C, 1 min; 72°C, 10 min.
3. Extract the solution with phenol:chloroform (1:1).
4. Ethanol precipitate the PCR products and resuspend in 89 µL of dH$_2$O.
5. Digest the PCR products by combining with 10 µL of 10X NEB buffer 2, 1 µL of 100X bovine serum albumin (BSA) and 2 µL of *Sfi*I in a total volume of 100 µL.
6. Incubate at 50°C overnight.
7. Extract the solution with phenol:chloroform (1:1).
8. Ethanol precipitate the DNA.
9. Electrophorese the *Sfi*I-digested PCR products through a 1% (w/v) agarose gel.
10. Purify the DNA fraction longer than 2 kb (*see* **Note 6**).
11. Digest the plasmid vector pME18S-FL3 (*see* **Note 7**) with *Dra*III by combining 10 µg of pME18S-FL3 with 10 µL of 10X H buffer, 10 µL of 10X BSA, and 2 µL of *Dra*III in a total volume of 100 µL.
12. Incubate at 37°C for 6 h.
13. Extract with phenol:chloroform (1:1).
14. Ethanol precipitate.
15. Resuspend the digested pME 18S-LF3 in 100 µL of dH$_2$O and redigest the vector in order to reduce the remnants of the uncut vector.
16. Electrophorese the *Dra*III-digested DNA through a 1% (w/v) agarose gel and purify *[7]*; and *see* **Note 6**) the desired 3.0-kb vector fragment. In addition, purify the stuffer fragment (0.4 kb) to use as a mock insert.
17. In separate reactions, ligate 10–50 ng of linearized pME18S-FL3 with an equal amount of the 2-kb PCR-amplified cDNA (*see* **step 10**) and the mock insert, respectively.
18. Transform *Escherichia coli (7)* with the products of the two ligation reactions (*see* **Note 8**), and with 10–50 ng of linearized pME1 8S-FL3 cDNA (*see* **Note 9**).

4. Notes

1. Because the Oligo-Capping procedure consists of multistep enzymic reactions with long reaction times, the utmost care should be taken by ensuring that all the reagents are prepared in an RNase-free condition. The pH of each reagent should also be strictly adjusted.
2. The starting RNA material must be of the highest quality obtainable. One of the most popular methods to extract total RNA is the AGPC method. This is a convenient method that can be applicable for a wide variety of tissues. However, the total RNA isolated with the AGPC method contains a lot of fragmented RNA and

genomic DNA. RNeasy (Qiagen) contains a column to remove such unfavorable fractions. If cultured cells are used as an RNA source, the recommended method is the NP-40 method. According to this method, only the cytoplasmic RNA can be isolated *(7)*.

3. For polyA+ RNA selection, many kits are commercially available, which use latex or magnetic beads for the oligo dT support. However, it is difficult to purify high quantities of polyA+ RNA with these kits. We pack oligo-dT cellulose powder ourselves so that we can adjust the bed volume and the washing conditions more flexibly according to the quality and quantity of the total RNA.

4. To avoid the mixannealing of the oligo dT primer, do not incubate at a lower temperature. Set a long extension time so that the reverse transcription will be completed.

5. Do not use the ammonium ion for ethanol precipitation until RNA ligation is completeted because ammonium ion interferes with T_4 RNA ligase activity.

6. Employ an extended elusion time to ensure the recovery of large DNA fragments *(7)*.

7. In pME18S-FL3, cDNA is inserted downstream to the eukaryotic promoter, SR-α. The full-length cDNA can be directly expressed by introducing it into cultured cells.

8. Usually the library size is 10^5–10^6 for 20–50 µg of polyA+ RNA.

9. Include the minus insert control to estimate the background level of undigested vector. Compare the transformation efficiency for both the plus PCR products and minus insert transformation reactions. Repeat digestion and purification of the vector until the transformation efficiency of the plus PCR products reaction is 100 times that of the minus insert transformation.

10. The drawbacks for the construction of a full-length-enriched cDNA library (*see* **Fig. 3**) according to this procedure are as follows:
    a. PCR is used for the amplification of the first strand cDNA, which sometimes introduces a mutation into the cDNA.
    b. PCR can cause a strong bias in the expression profile owing to the difference in the PCR efficiency between cDNA.
    c. The restriction enzyme *Sfi*I, used for the cDNA cloning, could cleave inside cDNA, resulting in the loss of cDNA from the library.

Acknowledgments

The Oligo-Capping method was originally developed in collaboration with K. Maruyama. We thank T. Ohta and T. Isogai for helpful discussions and suggestions; H. Hata, K. Nakagawa, Y. Shirai, Y. Takahashi, and K. Mizano for their excellent sequencing work; and M. Hida, M. Sasaki, and T. Ishihara for their technical support. This work was supported by a Grant-in-Aid for Scientific Research on Priority Areas from the Ministry of Education, Science, Sports and Culture of Japan.

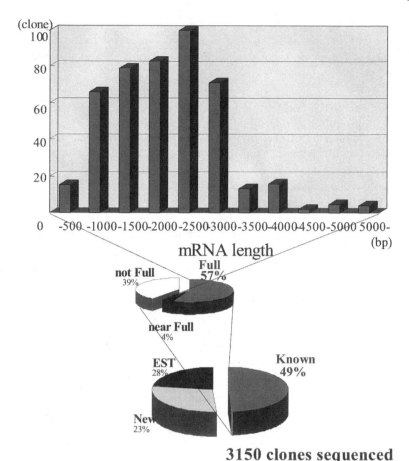

Fig. 3. Content of a full-length-enriched cDNA library. A typical example of the content of a full-length-enriched cDNA library. A full-length cDNA library was constructed from human intestine mucosal tissue. Among 3150 clones sequenced, 49% were identical to known genes, 28% were identical only to expressed sequence tags, and the remainder showed no significant homology with reported cDNA sequences. Among known clones, 57% was tentatively scored as full-length because they contained the same or longer 5' ends as compared to the matching reported cDNA sequences; four percent had shorter 5' ends but still contained the complete protein coding sequence (near Full). The others were scored not Full because they lacked the start sites of protein coding sequences. The length distribution of the mRNAs corresponding to the Full or near Full clones is shown in the top panel (*see* **Note 10**). The average mRNA size was 2.0 kb.

References

1. Marnyama, K. and Sugano, S. (1994) Oligo-capping: a simple method to replace the cap structure of eucaryotic mRNAs with oligoribonucleotides. *Gene* **138,** 171–174.
2. Suzuki, Y., Yoshitomo, K., Marnyama, K., Suyama, A., and Sugano, S. (1997) Construction and characterization of a full length-enriched and a 5'-end-enriched cDNA library. *Gene* **200,** 149–156.
3. Kato, S., Sekine, S., Oh, S. W., Kim, N. S., Umezawa, Y., Abe, N., Yokoyama-Kobayashi, M., and Aoki, T. (1994) Construction of a human full-length cDNA bank. *Gene* **150,** 243–250.
4. Edery, I., Chu, L. L., Sonenberg, N., and Pelletier, J. (1995) An efficient strategy to isolate full-length cDNAs based on an mRNA cap retention procedure (CAPture). *Mol. Cell. Biol.* **15,** 3363–3371.
5. Carninci, P., Kvam, C., Kitamura, A., Ohsumi, T., Okazaki, Y., Itoh, M., Kamiya, K., Sasaki, N., Izawa, M., Muramatsu, M., Hayashizaki, Y., and Scheider, C. (1996) High-efficiency full-length cDNA cloning by biotinylated CAP trapper. *Genomics* **37,** 327–336.
6. Shinshi, H., Miwa, M., Kato, K., Noguchi, M., Matushima, T., and Sugimura, T. (1976) A novel phosphodiesterase from cultured tobacco cells. *Biochemistry* **15,** 2185–2190.
7. Sambrook, J., Fritsch, E. F., and Maniatis, T. (1989) *Molecular Cloning: A Laboratory Manual*, 2nd ed. Cold Spring Harbor Laboratory, Cold Spring Harbor, NY.

11

Construction of Transcript Maps
by Somatic Cell/Radiation Hybrid Mapping

The Human Gene Map

Panagiotis Deloukas

1. Introduction

Systematic analysis of an organism's transcript repertoire plays a key role in molecular genetics. The complexity of this task in higher organisms such as mammals is not only owing to the large number of expected genes (70,000–100,000) in humans *(1)* but also because gene coding regions are dispersed in the genome. In addition, only a subset of all transcripts is found in a given cell type, typically in the range of 10,000, and the presence of certain transcripts is subject to the developmental stage and/or the cell's response to stimuli. The idea of a systematic approach to sequence large numbers of DNA (reverse transcribed from mRNA) clones as part of the Human Genome Project was conceived in 1990 at a time when significant advances in the field of DNA sequencing technology were in place but fewer than 2000 unique human gene sequences were available in the public databases. In 1991, Adams et al. *(2)* reported the generation of 174,172 human partial cDNA sequences and introduced the term *expressed sequence tags* (ESTs). Since then, other major sequencing efforts *(3)* have brought the number of human ESTs in databases *(4)* to more than 1,400,000.

The construction of a transcript map could be considered a first step toward the systematic study of genes in an organism. It is a tool that can accelerate the positional cloning of genes involved in genetic diseases or associated with quantitative trait loci through the candidate approach *(5)*. In addition, transcript maps of related species can be used in comparative studies and provide the basis for establishing syntenic maps. For genomes where a large pool of

From: *Methods in Molecular Biology, vol. 175: Genomics Protocols*
Edited by: M. P. Starkey and R. Elaswarapu © Humana Press Inc., Totowa, NJ

ESTs is available, the construction of a whole-genome transcript map requires two components: (1) a nonredundant set of ESTs and (2) a mapping methodology.

Sampling multiple cDNA libraries in order to achieve a high degree of representation of an organism's transcript repertoire inevitably leads to extensive redundancy. In the case of the Human Genome Project, several efforts have been made to cluster the available ESTs to nonredundant sets, with the most notable being the Genexpress Index *(6)*, the THC collection *(7)*, the Merck Gene Index *(8)*, and the UniGene *(9)*. UniGene has more recently assembled mouse and rat gene clusters. By far the most common problem in such data sets is that of multiple clusters for the same gene. Factors that make EST clustering a complex task, are the quality of the EST sequence *data per se,* the presence of genomic contaminants (i.e., nontranscribed sequences) in EST collections, and the presence of multiple ESTs for a given gene that might have been derived from different portions of a transcript or various alternatively spliced transcripts. Several research groups are currently active in developing new tools for EST clustering.

Long-range maps of complex genomes were mainly yeast artificial chromosome (YAC)-based until the advent of whole-genome radiation hybrid (RH) mapping. Although a valuable resource, YAC-based maps were shown to be either incomplete or have problems caused by chimeric or deleted clones. By contrast, RHs provide complete genome coverage (there is no evidence so far to support the opposite) and overcome the type of problems that chimerism and rearrangements often cause in mapping. Whole-genome RH cells are generated by fusing a population of donor cells irradiated with a lethal dose of X-rays to a population of recipient cells deficient in a selectable marker *(10)*. Irradiation causes the DNA of the donor cells to break randomly into pieces of an average size proportional to the dose of irradiation used. The DNA fragments either are integrated into the genome of the recipient cell or are maintained as extrachromosomal elements. Typically, recipient cells retaining 16–30% of the donor genome are suitable for mapping. A panel of 100–200 different hybrid cell lines is sufficient for the construction of whole-genome maps *(10)*. RH mapping provides a means to localize any STS to a defined map position in the genome, by use of the polymerase chain reaction (PCR). The presence or absence of an STS across the panel is scored to provide a retention pattern. The retention patterns of all assayed markers can then be subjected to two-point or multipoint analysis to evaluate statistically their similarity. The closer two STSs are in the genome, the higher the chance of being coretained and vice versa.

Detailed protocols for constructing RH panels and more in-depth coverage of the principles of RH mapping can be found in **ref. *11***. Whole genome RH panels are now available for several species such as human, mouse, rat, bovine, zebra-fish, and dog *(12–17)*. *The* RH mapping method is also amenable to automation and high throughput and has been successfully used for rapidly constructing physical and transcript maps of complex genomes *(13–18)*.

The construction of a human gene map, a project carried out at the Sanger Centre for the past 4 yr as part of an international effort, will serve as an example to discuss the experimental issues involved in this type of method.

2. Materials

1. Mapping panel 2 (Coriell Cell Repositories).
2. Control genomic DNAs: human male placental (Sigma, St. Louis, MO), Chinese hamster ovary (Lofstrand), and mouse Balb/c (Clontech).
3. $T_{0.1}E$: 10 mM Tris-HCl, 0.1 mM EDTA (pH 8.0).
4. dNTP mix: 5 mM each dATP, dCTP, dGTP, dTTP in H_2O (Pharmacia).
5. 10X PCR buffer: 450 mM Tris-HCl (pH 8.8), 15 mM MgCl$_2$, 14.53 g/L of (NH$_4$)$_2$SO$_4$, 0.43 g/L of cresol red (sodium salt; Sigma) in $T_{0.1}E$.
6. Sucrose solution: 34.6% (w/v) sucrose in H_2O.
7. Primer pair mix: 100 ng/μL each in H_2O.
8. *Taq* DNA polymerase (Amplitaq) (5 U/μL) TaqGold (5 U/μL) (Perkin-Elmer).
9. GB4 RH panel (95 samples): 93 RH DNAs plus human and hamster genomic control DNA (Research Genetics). Mix in a 2:1 ratio H_2O and $T_{0.1}E$, add 4.4 mg/L of cresol red, and adjust the pH to 8.5 using NaOH. Use this buffer to dilute the panel to 3 ng/μL and include a negative control such as H_2O or $T_{0.1}E$.
10. β-Mercaptoethanol (BDH), made up fresh as 1/10 dilution in $T_{0.1}E$.
11. Ethidium bromide (10 mg/mL) (Sigma).
12. Agarose, electrophoresis grade (Gibco-BRL).
13. 10X TBE: 108 g of Tris, 55 g of boric acid, 9.3 g of Na$_2$EDTA, made to 1 L.
14. Thermocycler (PTC-225 DNA Engine Tetrad; MJ Research).
15. 96-Well thermocycler plates (Costar Thermowell™ 6511).
16. OmniSeal TD Mats (HB-MT SRS 5; Hybaid).
17. 100-bp ladder (Pharmacia).
18. Agarose gel electrophoresis apparatus.
19. 300-nm UV-transilluminator and gel photography system.
20. UV Stratalinker 2400 (Stratagene).

3. Methods

An important issue at the start of any large-scale RH mapping project is the availability of DNA. RH cell lines are very unstable and DNA must be prepared from a single growth batch in sufficient amounts to cover the needs of the entire research community that is going to use this mapping reagent. The mapping resolution of an RH panel depends on the average size of DNA fragments of the donor cells and the frequency with which they are retained in the hybrids. As mentioned earlier, a panel of approx 100–200 hybrid lines is required for construction of whole-genome maps. Most commonly used RH panels, however, have no more than 93 hybrids, so that including controls they can be assayed in a 96-well format. Hybrids that have either too low or too high retention compared with the average retention of the panel can be excluded without loss of resolution. The selection of which resolution RH panel to use will be determined by the objectives of the mapping project. As a general rule, the higher the resolution of an RH panel, the more markers need to be assayed to obtain linkage along a whole chromosome. In other words, several hundreds of markers need to be assayed up front before assembling a map. It should also be taken into account that the distribution of gene-based markers in complex genomes is uneven. So far, only in human studies have RH panels of three different windows of resolution extensively evaluated. The Genebridge 4 (GB4) panel was constructed using 3000 rad and consists of 93 human-hamster hybrid cell lines, each retaining about 32% of the human genome in fragments with an average size of ~25 Mb *(12)*; the G3 panel was constructed using 10,000 rad and has 83 hybrid cell lines, each retaining about 18% of the human genome in random fragments of ~2.4 Mb *(13)*; and the TNG4 panel was constructed using 50,000 rad and has 90 hybrid cell lines, each retaining about 16% of the human genome in random fragments of ~0.8 Mb. Both the GB4 and G3 panel were used to construct the human gene map *(18)*. The resolution of the G3 panel is two-to-fourfold higher than the GB4 panel; that is, markers can be ordered with odds >1000:1 at an average spacing of 0.3 Mb using the G3 panel vs 1 Mb using the GB4 panel. For other species, RH panels have mainly been constructed so far using 3000 rad, and thus their characteristics resemble those of GB4.

3.1. Selection of ESTs for Mapping and Sequence-Tagged Site Primer Design

For an efficient and cost-effective mapping process, it is necessary to select a single representative sequence from each unique cluster of ESTs. A typical cluster comprises 5' and 3' reads of cDNA clones, and it may or may not include a complete mRNA sequence. It is known that genes rarely contain introns at the 3' untranslated region (UTR). In addition, when comparing at the DNA level members of a gene family in one species or orthologous genes in two species, the sequence at the 3' UTR is by far the most diverged in evolution. Thus, it is recommended to develop gene-based sequence-tagged sites (STSs) from the 3' UTRs of mRNAs. When a cluster does not include a complete mRNA sequence, an alternative is to select an EST with a putative poly-adenylation signal. In general, in my laboratory, we give a lower priority for mapping to clusters with reads of a single cDNA clone. Our main source of EST clusters is the Unigene set. In brief, Unigene was assembled as follows.

Repetitive sequences, vector contamination, and any regions that are annotated as low-quality data were removed and a sequence was considered when at least 100 bases of informative data remained. Chimeric sequences and those that do not appear to be of human origin were eliminated based on both automated and manual analysis. All remaining sequences were compared to one another and put together when they had at least 65 bases of 100% identity. From the initial set of clusters, only those believed to contain sequences of the mRNA 3' terminus were included to avoid having multiple clusters for a single gene. However, this may still occur owing to either alternative polyadenylation or alternative splicing of the 3' terminal exon.

We select the longest sequence representing the mRNA 3' terminus, based on cluster information, for mapping. The pipeline starts by screening all selected ESTs using RepeatMasker *(19)*. The output file is then used in a BLASTN search to identify duplicates (>85% identity in unmasked sequence) representing either self-matches or matches to sequences already in the database. To avoid duplication in large scale projects it is useful to have in place a central database holding all EST sequences for which primer pairs have been designed *(see* **Subheading 3.7.**). It is, however, necessary in the process of assessing map quality to have a small number of genes assayed by two or more markers *(18)*. Primer pairs are then designed for all new sequences using PRIMER version 0.5 *(19)*. A newer package, PRIMER3, is also available at the ftp address given in **ref.** *19*, but it has not been tested in our laboratory. Initially, we alter only the T_m (optimal: 60; minimum: 57; maximum: 63°C) and the product size (80–119; 120–190; 191–250 bp) compared to the default settings of PRIMER. The failures (e.g., too AT-rich sequences) are then reanalyzed using the following conditions: T_m (optimal: 60°C; minimum: 57°C; maximum: 63°C) and oligo size (optimal: 19; minimum: 17; maximum: 21 bp).

3.2. Development of Gene-Based STS Markers Suitable for RH Mapping

Gene-based STS markers, like any other marker to be used with a human-hamster RH panel such as GB4, should amplify by PCR a human genomic target of the expected length (based on the cDNA) but not coamplify a hamster-derived sequence of a similar size. In some instances, however, amplification of human genomic DNA may result in a specific product of larger size than that predicted by the EST. Although the larger product size could be attributed to the amplification of an intronic sequence, it may well be owing to a PCR artifact, and, thus, it is recommended to sequence the PCR product. The impact of pseudogenes in developing specific gene-based STS markers has not yet been fully assessed in the literature but one should expect instances in which amplification could occur preferentially from, e.g., the pseudogene rather than the expressed gene.

As already mentioned, RH mapping provides a means to localize any STS to a defined map position in the genome. Our experimental strategy includes, however, an additional mapping step prior to RH typing in which gene-based STS markers are assigned to chromosomes using Mapping panel 2, a monochromosomal somatic cell hybrid panel. Although it may seem redundant, this step allows streamlining at a later stage, the computational analysis of the raw RH mapping data, eliminating at an early point, multicopy markers and acting as an internal quality control in the mapping pipeline *(see* **Subheading 3.7.**). Mapping panel 2 includes both human-hamster and human-mouse hybrid cell lines. Thus, we determine optimal PCR conditions by testing all primer pairs against three control DNAs: human, hamster, and mouse. We perform the initial screening simultaneously at three annealing temperatures (typically 50, 55, and 60°C). All PCR reactions are carried out in 96-well plates as described in **Subheading 3.4.** *(see* **Note 1**). This approach, although it has a higher reagent cost per marker, is suitable for high throughput because only a small fraction of primer pairs needs to be rescreened. Typically, rescreening is performed at a different annealing temperature. About 75% of all primer pairs tested are successful (i.e., can be assayed against the Mapping panel 2). We have observed that markers that constantly give a low yield of PCR amplification when assayed with the human control DNA (4%) fail when typed against the RH panel. The successful fraction does not include such markers. Other failures include primer pairs that do not give a human product (5%), that show nonspecific amplification (10%), and that coamplify a hamster target of a similar size (6%).

All successful gene-based STS markers are then assayed against the Mapping panel 2 *(see* **Subheading 3.4.**; **Note 2**). About 6% of the markers assign to more than two chromosomes and are not processed further. Markers that assign to two chromosomes (about 5%) are typed against the RH panel, and we have observed that they can be successfully mapped.

3.3. Typing of Gene-Based STS Markers Against the GB4 RH Panel

Any STS marker that can amplify a specific human target in the presence of hamster DNA without interference can be typed against a human-hamster RH panel such as the GB4 panel. According to our experimental strategy *(see* **Subheading 3.2.**), we assay all the gene-based STS markers that have been assigned to no more than two chromosomes, against the GB4 panel. We perform all assays in duplicate as described in **Subheading 3.4.**, and we apply the following data quality check: markers that give discrepant results for more than three hybrids in the duplicate assay are reassayed, and if unsuccessful, they are excluded from further analysis. Note that typing all markers in duplicate safeguards against possible technical failures and/nonrobust assays and the elimination of highly discrepant results contributes to the accuracy of the map.

Most of the conventional PCR protocols described in the literature are compatible with this type of work. The one given here *(see* **Subheading 3.4.**) aims at boosting target amplification and reducing background (touchdown PCR; low Mg concentration), the number of steps involved in the assembly of the PCR reactions (oilfree), and the analysis of

PCR products (loading buffer present in the reaction mix). We have observed that the addition of sucrose in the reaction mix, although primarily serving to increase sample viscosity for direct loading onto agarose gels, clearly reduces nonspecific amplification. The PCR protocol *(see* **Subheading 3.4.**) has also been largely automated in our laboratory *(see* **Subheading 3.5.**).

3.4. PCR Protocol

1. Assemble the following master mix *(see* **Notes 1** and **3**): 2 µL of 10X PCR buffer, 0.25 µL dNTP mix, 7.0 µL of sucrose solution, 0.15 µL of β-mercaptoethanol, 0.15 µL of primer mix, and 0.1 µL of ampliTaq. These reaction volumes are given per single reaction and should be scaled up accordingly. Prepare mix with approx 10% excess when using multichannel pipets for dispensing.
2. Dispense 10 µL *(see* **Note 2**) of each of the 96 samples of the RH panel into a 96-well thermocycler plate and add 10 µL of the master mix to each well. Fit a mat *(see* **Note 4**) on top of the plate. Tap the plate gently on the bench to ensure that all the reagents are at the bottom of the well.
3. Place the plate in the thermocycler, close the heated lid, and cycle at: 94°C for 5 min followed by 10 cycles in which the temperature of the annealing step is set 5°C above the optimal annealing temperature T_{an} and is reduced by 0.5°C per cycle: 93°C for 30 s, $(T_{an} + 5°C)$ to $(T_{an} + 1°C)$ 50 s *(see* **Note 5**), and 72°C for 50 s followed by 30 cycles of 93°C for 30 s, T_{an} for 50 s, and 72°C for 50 s followed by 72°C for 5 min followed by 15°C (indefinite).
4. Remove the mat and analyze 15-µL samples on a 2.5% agarose gel in 1X TBE buffer containing 0.4 µg/mL of ethidium bromide (9 V/cm, 20 min).
5. Place the gel on a 300-nm UV-transilluminator and photograph. The experimental procedure of typing a marker against the GB4 panel is completed with the acquisition of the corresponding gel image. Depending on the scale of the project, image analysis (i.e., scoring the presence or absence of the human product) can be performed either manually or using a suitable software package *(see* **Subheading 3.5.**). The pattern of retention of each marker in the panel is encoded as a vector of values in which 1 indicates the retention of a marker in a hybrid, 0 indicates no retention, and 2 indicates an ambiguity in the duplicate typing or that the hybrid was not assayed.

3.5. Automation

In our process, all the experimental steps are PCR based, a technique amenable to automation. Automation is key to high throughput, and to achieve it we have introduced several robotic devices, commercially available or designed in-house. The first step in the process is to screen all primer pairs against three control DNAs; we have automated reaction assembly using a Genosis 100 (Tecan). We designed an adapter to hold the V-shaped reservoirs used on the Biomek 1000 (Beckman) robot in order to minimize loss of reagent. The second and third steps require the handling of DNA panels (Mapping panel 2 and GB4 panel); we use the Hydra™ 96 (Robbing Scientific), which is a 96-channel dispenser, for all dilution steps and aliquoting of the DNA into 96-well thermocycler plates. We recommend that the user perform an acid wash between operations when the same unit is used to aliquot different panels. To add the master mix (*see* **Subheading 3.4.**) to the plates carrying the Mapping panel 2, we use the Genosis 100, whereas the plates carrying the RH panel are processed on a Biomek 1000 (Beckman) equipped with an eight-channel pipeting device (MP200). Samples from the 96-well thermocycler plates are transferred on to agarose gels using a Flexys robot (Genomic Solutions PLC) equipped with an eight-channel pipeting device that was developed in-house. To ensure that the position of the wells on the gel remains constant, we designed a metal comb that hooks on one side of the gel tray but can move freely from the other side (because pouring hot agarose causes the tray first to expand and then to contract). To prevent any shrinking, gels are cast into trays without the gates (taped), which allows the agarose to set into the upper and bottom groove and thus attach to the tray. The gels are kept moistened by wrapping them with Saran™ wrap. Following electrophoresis, gel images are acquired using a high-resolution solid-state camera (Kodak MEGAPLUS, model 1.4i) attached to a Macintosh computer equipped with a Neotech IG24 image grabber card. The camera and the UV-transilluminator are accommodated in a dark cabinet, designed in-house. At the front of the cabinet, there is a metal frame that opens and closes like a drawer and allows the gel tray first to be slotted in a fixed position relative to the four circular light-emitting diodes (LEDs) of the frame and then moved above the transilluminator.

We use the Gel Gem/Gel Print software (ME Electronics) in conjunction with a Sony UP890CE thermoprinter to create image files of the gels and obtain hard copies. We then carry out image analysis using the Band Analysis software (ME Electronics). This software can call and analyze simultaneously the two image files representing a duplicate assay (i.e., an STS typed twice against the GB4 panel). For each marker, the output of the individual assays and the consensus are stored together in a report file. Report files are transferred overnight to a UNIX environment and read into our central database, rhace (**Subheading 3.7.**).

3.6. Map Construction

Construction of an RH map requires the statistical analysis of the RH vectors of the assayed markers. Two markers are considered to be linked if they have vectors of statistically significant similarity (defined by a logarithm [log10] [LOD] score) and a measure of their separation is obtained from analysis of the degree of difference between the two vectors. Thus, the estimation of both the order and the distance between markers is based on vector similarity. The unit of map distance is the centiRay and represents 1% probability of breakage between two markers for a given X-ray dosage (i.e., the one used to construct the RH panel). Therefore, the correlation between centiRay units and physical distance in base pairs will differ from one panel to the other and can only be determined by extrapolation.

The most commonly used software packages for construction of RH maps are MultiMap *(20,21)*, RHMAP version 3.0 *(23,24)*, RHMAPPER version 1.1 *(24,25)*, and SAMapper (at the time of this writing, the code was unavailable owing to updating; contact the Stanford Human Genome Center, Palo Alto, CA). We currently use Z-RHMAPPER for construction of RH maps. The Z-extensions were recently developed for RHMAPPER version 1.1 mainly to compute the totally linked markers (i.e., those that have identical vectors and therefore cannot be resolved by the RH panel used) and provide an interactive interface for querying the database and displaying maps *(26,27)*. The process of building a map using Z-RHMAPPER can be divided into four steps:

3.6.1. Setting a Project and Import of All Marker Data into the Database

Several parameters need to be specified up front. We set the two parameters that provide estimates of laboratory error—ALPHA (false negative) and BETA (false positive)—to 0.001. We recommend using higher values when analyzing pooled results generated in different laboratories. The RETENTION_ FREQUENCY is set to a value that depends on the characteristics of the RH panel used. For the GB4 panel, we set it to 0.4. Marker data should be in a tab-delimited format as shown in the following example with marker name first and RH vector last, whereas multiple fields of information can be specified in between.

```
Marker    Chr    Sequence    RH vector
10751     20     Z52150
10110010101011010011110011 0.........000110011101001010010
```

Typically, we set one project for each human chromosome and import STSs according to their chromosome assignment information. Apart from streamlining the whole process at this stage, ultimately both sets of mapping data will have to be compatible for a marker to be added on the map. Thus, a large proportion, if not all, of potential data management errors is eliminated owing to this step. In the absence of assignment information the alternative is to set a single project and then use the link_groups command at a relevant TWO_POINT_CUTOFF value (e.g., LOD 10 for the GB4 panel).

3.6.2. Creation of Groups of Totally Linked Markers

Markers with no ambiguities in the RH vector are referred to as *canonical*. The Ztl command will automatically create groups of totally linked (TL) markers. The representative of a TL group is a *canonical marker*. All other markers in a TL group are referred to as *buried*. Markers that have ambiguities in the RH vector and are not part of a TL group are termed *orphans*. If, at a later point, a marker becomes part of the framework map (*see* **Subheading 3.6.3.**), it will be preferentially used as the representative of its TL group. The canonical markers are used as input to the Zgrow and Zplace commands described next.

3.6.3. Construction of a Framework Map

Construction of a framework map is the most crucial step of the whole process. The objective is to define a set of well-ordered markers, usually with odds of 1000:1 over any other permutations of the markers, which are evenly spaced along the chromosome. Z-RHMAPPER has functions to assemble automatically a framework, but running time can increase dramatically with sets containing more than 200 markers. Canonical markers representing large groups of TL markers are the best candidates to be evaluated for framework construction using the assemble_framework command (FRAMETHRESH parameter set to LOD 3), especially in the absence of any other mapping information. Such frameworks can then be extended using the Zgrow command and all the representatives of the TL groups. Typically, we run this command by setting the FRAMETHRESH parameter to LOD 2.5. Markers added at the telomeres during this step should be carefully checked to avoid erroneous expansion of the overall map length. When independent mapping information is available, a more interactive approach can be taken. For example, a set of well-spaced markers across all human chromosomes (except Y) can be selected from the microsatellite markers ordered with high odds on the human genetic linkage map *(28)* and assayed against the RH panel up front. The order of markers on the genetic map can then be evaluated as a hypothesis in Z-RHMAPPER.

Our approach is to start with the markers at the top of the chromosome and use the Zrip command (set to 3; maximum is 5) to verify the quality of candidate orders. It works by sliding a window across an order, finding all permutations of markers within that window, and remembering the best order within that window. Once the first three most telomeric markers are defined, a framework can be assembled in a stepwise fashion by testing one marker at a time and asking that the candidate order be supported at a LOD score >2.5 over the next best order. It is recommended that the best orders also be checked using the Zevaluate command, which gives estimates of centiRay distances between markers. That was the approach we took to construct the GB4 framework of the human gene map *(18)*, which has 1079 microsatellite markers.

3.6.4. Placing of All Other Markers Relative to the Framework

A comprehensive RH map can be assembled using the Zplace command, which executes the create_placement map command to place nonburied markers on the framework. The map is automatically saved in a file called fw.map. We use the default values of LOD 5 and 15 cR for the PLACEMENT_LINKAGE and PLACEMENT_TOO_FAR parameters, respectively. Finally, the buried markers can be attached to the map using the Zprint map command. The following example given below shows a section of such a map of human chromosome 13:

RH42727	7.60	*F*			
RH24988	0.00	*P* > 3.00			
RH45841	1.14	*P* > 3.00			
RH27894	0.00	*P* > 3.00			
RH45876	1.47	*P* > 3.00			
RH48019	0.26	*P* 1.61			
RH46009	0.17	*P* > 3.00	RH17176	RH46139	RH53166
RH16918	0.00	*P* > 3.00			
RH28406	0.11	*P* 0.07			
RH39680	0.00	*P* > 3.00			
RH68572	2.40	*P* > 3.00			
RH69325	0.63	*P* 0.18			
RH44381	0.61	*P* 1.20	RH53177		
RH53404	0.10	*P* 0.98			
RH74413	2.23	*P* 0.28			
RH44442	0.10	*P* 0.01	RH53392	RH45263	RH68577
RH48999	0.00	*F*			

The first and second column in the map table report the marker name and the distance, in cR_{3000}, to the next marker, respectively. Marker names correspond to accession numbers in RHdb, a public domain repository of RH mapping data *(29)*. The third column indicates whether a marker is part of the framework, *F*, or placed relative to the framework, *P*. For the placement markers, an LOD score value is also reported. As an example, *P* > 3.00 means that the probability with which RH24988 maps into this framework interval is >1000 times higher than that of RH24988 mapping into the adjacent interval toward the telomere. The buried markers of a TL group are shown in the fourth column (e.g., RH44381 and RH53177 belong to the same TL group but only RH44381 was used to calculate the map).

The estimated distance in centiRay between two markers is influenced by certain parameters of Z-RHMAPPER such as ALPHA (false negative) and BETA (false positive). It is therefore correct to specify the running conditions of Z-RHMAPPER when giving a correlation between centiRays and physical distance. For example, we estimated that in the GB4-based human gene map, $1cR_{3000}$ corresponds on average to 250 kb under the Z-RHMAPPER conditions described in **Subheading 3.6.1.** Marker retention is not always uniform across RH panels. This has an impact on the estimated physical distance between markers. For example, the very high retention of centromeric fragments causes an overestimation of the centiRay distance between markers flanking the centromere. Very high retention frequency should also be expected for markers in the region surrounding the selectable marker used in the construction of an RH panel (e.g., in the case of GB4, the thymidine kinase gene on the q arm of human chromosome 17). As mentioned earlier, the mapping resolution of an RH panel depends on both the average size of DNA fragments of the donor cells and the frequency with which they are retained in the hybrids. Map resolution will decrease within such regions of high retention. Low retention has a similar effect on map resolution. It is therefore best to construct a chromosome X map using an RH panel made with an XX donor cell.

3.7. Data Storage

Any large-scale gene-mapping project requires a powerful and flexible type of database that allows both the storage and display of a variety of sequence and mapping data. ACeDB, A *Candida elegans* Database *(30)*, is a flexible database that allows the user to build models (configurable data files) that can be specifically tailored to the needs of different mapping projects *(31)*. Some key features of the current model used that relate to this chapter are the use of grid displays for representing individual clones of RH panels (a simple click can associate landmark data to an object in the grid); the use of graphic displays for STS-based maps; the use of a sequence display to position primers, repeats, and so on, and the ability to cross-reference a marker to the corresponding EST, cDNA clone, and EST cluster. We store all the EST sequences for which primer pairs have been designed into primace. Sequence and mapping data on markers that are successfully assayed against an RH panel are stored in rhace. A number of scripts allow the flow of information between rhace, Z-RHMAPPER, and the World Wide Web.

4. Notes

1. For testing primer pairs for optimal PCR conditions, the master mix is assembled with the appropriate control DNA template instead of the primer mix. Primer pairs to be tested are then added in **step 2**.
2. When the detection of the PCR product is obscured by the formation of primer-dimer or in cases of nonspecific amplification, we recommend the use of TaqGold. The PCR buffer needs to have a final pH of 8.1 (titrate before use).
3. Any DNA panel, such as Mapping panel 2, can be used at that point.
4. Reuse mats up to 20 times but UV-irradiate them between runs to avoid cross-contamination; use the Stratalinker with the Energy mode set at 240 mJs.
5. For T_{an} use the optimal annealing temperature of each marker.

Acknowledgments

I wish to thank all the members of the Sanger group involved in the construction of the human gene map, particularly Ele Holloway and Lisa Green for critical reading of the manuscript. This work was supported by the Wellcome Trust.

References

1. Fields, C., Adams, M. D., White, O., and Venter, C. J. (1994) How many genes in the human genome? *Nature Genet.* **7,** 345–346.
2. Adams, M. D., Kelley, J. M., Gocayne, et al. (1991) Complementary DNA sequencing: expressed sequence tags and human genome project. *Science* **252,** 1651–1656.
3. Hillier, L. D., Lennon, G., Becker, M., et al. (1996) Generation and analysis of 280,000 human expressed sequence tags. *Genome Res.* **6,** 807–828.
4. dbEST release 061199; <http://www.ncbi.nlm.nih.gov/dbEST>.
5. Collins, F. S. (1995) Positional cloning moves from perditional to traditional. *Nature Genet.* **9,** 347–350.
6. Houlgatte, R., Mariage-Samson, R., Duprat, S., Tessier, A., Bentolila, S., Lamy, B., and Auffray, C. (1995) The Genexpress Index: a resource for gene discovery and the genic map of the human genome. *Genome Res.* **5,** 272–304.
7. Adams, M. D., Kerlavage, A. R., Fleischmann, R. D., et al. (1995) Initial assessment of human gene diversity and expression patterns based upon 83 million nucleotides of cDNA sequence. *Nature* **377,** 3–17.
8. Aaronson, J. S., Eckman, B., Blevins, R. A., Borkowski, J. A., Myerson, J., Imran, S., and Elliston, K. O. (1996) Toward the development of a gene index to the human genome: an assessment of the nature of high-throughput EST sequence data. *Genome Res.* **6,** 829–845.
9. Schuler, G. D. (1997) Pieces of the puzzle: expressed sequence tags and the catalog of human genes. *J. Mol. Med.* **75,** 694–698.
10. Walter, M. A., Spillett, D. J., Thomas, P., Weissenbach, J., and Goodfellow, P. N. (1994) A method for constructing radiation hybrid maps of whole genomes. *Nature Genet.* **7,** 22–28.

11. Stewart, E. A. and Cox, D. R. (1997) Radiation hybrid mapping, in *Genome Mapping: A Practical Approach* (Dear, P. H., ed.), IRL, Oxford, pp. 73–93.

12. Gyapay, G., Schmitt, K., Fizames, C., et al. (1996) A radiation hybrid map of the human genome. *Hum. Mol. Genet.* **5,** 339–346.

13. Stewart, E. A., McKusick, K. B., Aggarwal, A., et al. (1997) An STS-based radiation hybrid map of the human genome. *Genome Res.* **7,** 422–433.

14. McCarthy, L. C., Terrett, J., Davis, M. E., et al. (1997) A first-generation whole genome-radiation hybrid map spanning the mouse genome. *Genome Res.* **7,** 1153–1161.

15. Watanabe, T. K., Bihoreau, M.-T., McCarthy, L. C., et al. (1999) A radiation hybrid map ofthe rat genome containing 5,255 markers. *Nature Genet.* **22,** 27–36.

16. Hukriede, N. A., Joly, L., Tsang, M., et al. (1999) Radiation hybrid mapping of the zebrafish genome. *Proc. Natl. Acad. Sci.* **96,** 9745_9750.

17. Priat, C., Hitte, C., Vignaux, F., et al. (1998) A whole-genome radiation hybrid map of the dog genome. *Genomics* **54,** 361–378.

18. Deloukas, P., Schuler, G. D., Gyapay, G., et al. (1998) A Physical map of 30,000 human genes. *Science* **282,** 744–746.

19. <http://www.genome.washington.edu/uwgc/analysistools/repeatmask.htm>.

20. Matise, T. C., Perlin, M., and Chakravarti, A. (1994) Automated construction of genetic linkage maps using an expert system (MultiMap): a human genome linkage map. *Nature Genet.* **6,** 384–390.

21. <http://linkage.rockefeller.edu/multimap>.

22. Lunetta, K. L., Boehnke, M., Lange, K., and Cox, D. R. (1996) Selected locus and multiple panel models for radiation hybrid mapping. *Am. J. Hum. Genet.* **59,** 717–725.

23. <http://www.sph.umich.edu/group/statgen>.

24. Slonim, D., Kruglyak, L., Stein, L., and Lander, E. (1997) Building human genome maps with radiation hybrids. *J. Comput. Biol.* **4,** 487–504.

25. <http://www.genome.wi.mit.edu/ftp/pub/software/rhmapper/>.

26. Soderlund, C., Lau, T., and Deloukas, P. (1998) Z extensions to the RHMAPPER package. *BioInformatics* **14,** 538,539.

27. <ftp.sanger.ac.uk/pub/zmapper/>; the user's manual is at <http://www.sanger.ac.uk/Users/cari/Zman.html>.

28. Dib, C., Faure, S., Fizames, C., et al. (1996) A comprehensive genetic map of the human genome based on 5,264 microsatellites. *Nature* **380,** 152–154.

29. <http://www.ebi.ac.uk:80/RHdb/>.

30. Durbin, R. and Mieg. J.-T. (1991) A *C. elegans* Database: documentation, code and data available from anonymous ftp servers at <lirmm.lirmm.fr>, <cele.mrc-lmb.cam.ac.uk>, and <ncbi.nlm.nih.gov>.

31. <http://www.sanger.ac.uk/Software/Acedb>.

12

Preparation and Screening
of High-Density cDNA Arrays with Genomic Clones

Günther Zehetner, Maria Pack, and Katja Schäfer

1. Introduction

One of the greatest improvements in the use of clone libraries in genomic research was the introduction of library arrays by storing single clones in separate wells of microtiter plates. This not only makes clones practically immortal by keeping the plates at –80°C, but it also gives each of the clones a unique reproducible identity, which allows scientists in different laboratories to be certain to use the same biological material for their various experiments, thereby enabling them to compare their results in a much more meaningful way. Equally important was the development of high-density filters, whereby thousands of these clones are transferred directly from microtiter plate wells onto nylon membranes in a regular pattern. This opened, on the one hand, a convenient way to make such libraries available to a large number of scientists, because filter membranes can be easily distributed, and, on the other hand, allowed screening of several thousand clones of a library in parallel, with a single hybridization experiment.

Using these new methods, it was possible to introduce the concept of reference libraries, which allowed many laboratories to work with identical biologic material, obtained on high-density filters, which could be used for a variety of experiments like fingerprinting, partial sequencing by oligo hybridization, high-density screening, and high-resolution mapping *(1)*. The development of robotic devices, which allowed the generation of such membranes in large quantities, soon led to the establishment of distribution centers, such as The Reference Library System at the Imperial Cancer Research Fund (ICRF), London, in 1989, which provided laboratories worldwide with high-density filters and clones from its reference libraries *(2)*.

From: *Methods in Molecular Biology, vol. 175: Genomics Protocols*
Edited by: M. P. Starkey and R. Elaswarapu © Humana Press Inc., Totowa, NJ

Whereas in earlier days mainly phage libraries were used, now a great variety of genomic cloning systems (i.e., cosmid, yeast artificial chromosome [YAC], P1 artificial chromosome, bacterial artificial chromosome, and P1 artificial chromosome [PAC]) are available, and in recent years cDNA libraries have won more and more importance, and many tissue- or development-specific libraries from human and other species can be obtained on high-density filters. Further developments in this field include DNA filters, protein expression filters *(3)*; filters from the two-hybrid system *(4)*; and the use of glass slides, instead of nylon membranes, for gridding DNA *(5)*.

The initial effort to convert a library into a reference library is quite work-intensive (**Fig. 1**), although for most of the laborious routine steps robotic devices have been developed. In particular, the picking of the original clones into microtiter plates and the generation of the high-density filter membranes can be automated to a high degree by special robots (**Fig. 2**). The following protocols describe these steps, as they are routinely used at the Resource Centre (RZPD) of the German Human Genome Project *(1,6)* for cDNA, cosmid, or other clone libraries propagated in *Escherichia coli* (YAC libraries usually require different methods), and also give examples for nonradioactive probe hybridization to high-density filters. Although many screening experiments are still done using radiolabeled probes, nonradioactive labeling techniques, with their equal sensitivity, faster detection speed, and safer experimental handling, are becoming more widely used and are very well suited for screenings by filter hybridization *(7)*.

2. Materials

2.1. Picking of Random Plated Colonies into Microtiter Plate Wells

1. 10X HMFM.
   a. Part 1: Dissolve 3.6 g of $MgSO_4 \cdot 7H_2O$ (no. 105886; Merck), 18 g of trisodium citrate·$2H_2O$ (no. 106448; Merck), 36 g of $(NH_4)_2SO_4$ (no. 101216; Merck), and 1.76 L of pure glycerol (no. 104093; Merck) in dH_2O and adjust the volume to 3.2 L. Sterilize immediately by autoclaving for 20 min.
   b. Part 2: Dissolve 72 g KH_2PO_4 (no. 104873; Merck) and 188 g of K_2HPO_4 (no. 105101; Merck), in dH_2O and adjust to 800 mL. Sterilize immediately by autoclaving for 20 min.
   c. Part 3: In a clean bench, add parts 1 and 2 together (total volume is 4 L), mix thoroughly, and dispense 400 mL in 500-mL Duran bottles to minimize future contamination.
2. LB broth: Dissolve 10 g/L of Bacto-tryptone (no. 0123-17-3; Difco), 5 g/L of yeast extract (no. 0127-17-9; Difco), and 10 g/L of NaCl (no. 106400; Merck) in dH_2O, adjust the pH to 7.0 with 5 N NaOH, and adjust to a final volume with dH_2O.

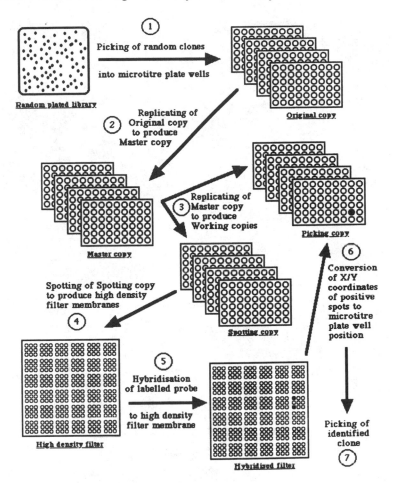

Fig. 1. Major steps in producing a reference library and screening it by filter hybridization. Starting from random plated colonies, clones are picked into an original set of microtiter plates *(1)* used only to produce the master copy *(2)* otherwise being stored permanently at −80°C. The master copy is used to produce the working copies *(3)*, from which the filters are generated (Spotting copy) *(4)*, and also those clones which have been identified in a hybridization *(5)*, converted back to the plate position *(6)*, and then isolated (Picking copy) *(7)*.

3. LB agar medium: Add 6 g of Bacto-agar (no. 0140-01; Difco) per 400 mL of LB broth (*see* **item 2**) to get 1.5% agar medium. Sterilize immediately by autoclaving for 20 min. Cool to 45°C before pouring plates.
4. 2X YT broth: Add 16 g/L of Bacto-tryptone, 10 g/L of yeast extract, and 5 g/L of NaCl. Dissolve in dH$_2$O, adjust the pH to 7.0 with 5 N NaOH, and adjust to a final volume with dH$_2$O.

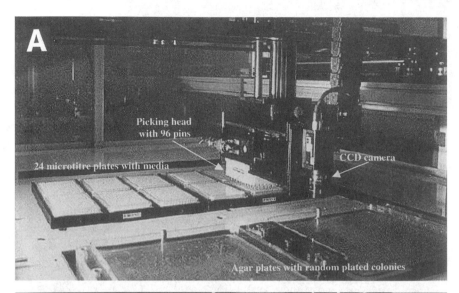

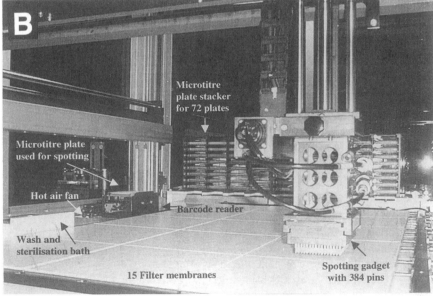

Fig. 2. (**A**) Picking robot: a charge-coupled device (CCD) camera identifies the random plated colonies on two agar plates, which are picked by a gadget with 96 individually controlled pins, and transferred into media-filled microtiter plates. (**B**) Spotting robot: One microtiter plate after the other is automatically transferred from and back to a plate stacker. A spotting gadget with 384 pins moves into each plate and transfers material onto defined positions on 15 filter membranes. Between each spotting step the needles are cleaned and sterilized.

5. 2X YT agar (1.5%) medium: Add 6 g/L of Bacto-agar (no. 0140-01; Difco) per 400 mL of 2X YT broth. Sterilize immediately by autoclaving for 20 min. Cool to 45°C before pouring plates.
6. 2X YT freezing medium: 200 mL of 2X YT broth, 22 mL of 10X HMFM, 220 μL of 30 mg/mL kanamycin (can be substituted with 220 μL of ampicillin [50 mg/mL] or tetracycline [13 mg/mL], if required).
7. Antibiotics (*see* **Note 1**).
   a. Ampicillin (50 mg/mL) (100 mL stock): Weigh out 5 g of ampicillin (sodium salt, no. A9518; Sigma, St. Louis, MO), dissolve in 50 mL of sterile dH_2O, and add 50 mL of absolute (or 95%) ethanol. Filter sterilize and aliquot 10 mL per sterile 15 mL Falcon tube. Store at –20°C.
   b. Kanamycin (30 mg/mL) (100 mL stock): Weigh out 3 g of kanamycin (kanamycin A monosulfate, no. K4000; Sigma), and dissolve in 100 mL of sterile dH_2O. Filter sterilize and store as 1-mL aliquots at –20°C.
   c. Tetracycline (13 mg/mL) (100 mL stock): Tetracycline is light sensitive; therefore, wrap with foil during preparation and storage, and wear gloves. Dissolve 1.3 g of tetracycline (hydrochloride, no. T3383; Sigma) in 50 mL of sterile dH_2O and add 50 mL absolute (or 95%) ethanol. Filter sterilize and store as 1-mL aliquots at –20°C.
8. Agar plates for picking: Melt 400 mL of agar (either LB Broth or 2X YT) per Nunc plate, and add antibiotic as required by library (i.e., 800 μL of 50 mg/mL ampicillin stock solution).
9. Microtiter plate medium: LB broth/7.5% glycerol (with appropriate antibiotic) or 2X YT freezing medium. Fill the plates with 60 μL/well (384-well plates) so that they are approximately three-fourths filled.
10. Microtiter plates: Genetix, UK (http://www.genetix.co.uk), 384-well, large volume with cover, PS material number code X7001.
11. The spotting and picking robots used at the RZPD are basically identical three-axis XYZ servo-controlled linear drive systems with 5-μ resolution from Linear Drives, UK (http://www.lineardrives.com). They have exchangeable working heads that have been especially developed for either spotting high-density filters (15 filters can be spotted in one run) or picking clones (*see* **Note 2**).

2.2. Spotting of Hybridization Filters

1. Hybond N+ membranes: article no. RPN22501, 22.2 cm², optically checked (Amersham Pharmacia Biotech Europe GmbH) (http://www.apbiotech.com).
2. Blotting paper (22.4 × 22.4 cm) GB003 (gel-blotting-paper, ref. no. 426894; Schleicher & Schuell).
3. Nunc plates (22.5 × 22.5 cm) (no. 240835; Merck).
4. Chromokult (26.5 g/L) (no. 1.10426; Merck): Dissolve in dH_2O in a microwave oven, and then cool to 45°C before pouring plates.
5. Topagar: Mix 75 μL of overnight culture (or maximum 2 d old) with 3 mL 2X YT agar (2%), and pour on agar plate.

6. 80% Ethanol: 800 mL of absolute ethanol (or 95%) + 200 mL sterile dH_2O.
7. 3% H_2O_2: 100 mL of 30% H_2O_2 + 900 mL of dH_2O.
8. Denaturation solution: 0.5 M NaOH (no. 106495; Merck), 1.5 M NaCl.
9. Neutralization solution: 1 M Tris-HCl (T3253), 1 M Tris Base (no. T1503; Sigma), 1.5 M NaCl. Adjust pH to 7.4.
10. Protein digestion with Pronase (no. 1459643; Boehringer Mannheim, now Roche Molecular Biochemicals): Prepare 50 mg/mL stock in sterile dH_2O. Make fresh each time.
11. Pronase buffer solution (per 10 L): 50 mM Tris-HCl, 1% Sarcosyl (v/v) (no. 44275; BDH). Avoid frothing by mixing gently but thoroughly.
12. Washing solution: 50 mM Na_2HPO_4 solution in dH_2O. Adjust the pH to 7.2 with phosphoric acid (H_3PO_4).
13. Stratalinker UV-crosslinker 2400 (Stratagene) (http://www.stratagene.com). It contains five 15-W 254-nm UV lightbulbs. The distance between UV lightbulbs and filter is approx 10 cm.

2.3. Hybridization Screening

1. Digoxigenin (DIG)-High Prime: (cat. no. 1585 606; Boehringer Mannheim): contains random oligonucleotides; Klenow enzyme, labeling grade; DIG-1 1-dUTP, alkali labile; dATP, dCTP, dGTP, dTTP; and an optimized reaction buffer concentrate in glycerol (50% [v/v]).
2. Polymerase chain reaction (PCR) DIG probe synthesis kit: (cat. no. 1636 090; Boehringer Mannheim): contains all reagents required for DIG labeling by PCR process.
3. DIG Quantification Teststrips (cat. no. 1 669 958; Boehringer Mannheim).
4. AmpliTaq polymerase (5 U/μL) (no. N801-0060; Perkin-Elmer).
5. *Taq* DNA polymerase (1 U/μL) (no. 1647679; Boehringer Mannheim).
6. 20X Saline solium citrate (SSC): Dissolve 175.3 g of NaCl and 88.2 g Na-citrate in 800 mL of water, adjust to pH 7.0, fill up to 1 L, and autoclave.
7. 10% Sodium dodecyl sulfate (SDS): Dissolve 100 g of SDS in 900 mL of water while heating at 68°C, cool to room temperature, adjust to pH 7.2, and fill up to 1 L.
8. 10X Maleic acid buffer: 1 M maleic acid, 1.5 M NaCl. Adjust pH to 7.5 with solid NaOH and autoclave.
9. 10X Washing buffer: Prepare like maleic acid buffer and add 3% (w/v) Tween.
10. 10X Blocking solution: Dissolve blocking reagents from Boehringer (order no. 1096176) in 1X maleic acid buffer (100 mM maleic acid, 150 mM NaCl) to an end concentration of 10% (w/v) while heating. Alternatively, dissolve 3% low-fat milk powder (1% or less fat, Nestlé) in 1X maleic acid.
11. Church buffer: 500 mM Na_2PO_4, 5% SDS, 1 mM EDTA. Adjust the pH to 7.2.
12. 1 M Tris-HCl: 121.1 g of Tris-base to 1 L of H_2O. Adjust to pH 7.5 or 9.0 with concentrated HCl and autoclave.
13. 5 M NaCl: Dissolve 292.3 g NaC1 to 1 L H_2O and autoclave to sterilize.
14. Detection buffer: 100 mL of 1 M Tris-HCl (pH 9.0), 20 mL of 5 M NaCl. Mix and make up the volume to 1 L with H_2O.
15. AttoPhos™: AttoPhos Substrate Set (cat. no. 1 681 982; Boehringer Mannheim).

3. Methods

3.1. From Random Library to Microtiter Plates: Picking of Random Plated Colonies

3.1.1. Plating the Library

It is important to plate the library at a low enough density so that colonies are well separated and not touching each other to avoid cross-contamination.

1. Determine the titer of library by plating different volumes (i.e., 1, 5, 10, 50, 100 µL) and counting the resulting colonies.
2. Plate the optimal volume onto 22 × 22 cm agar plates to attain approx 2500 colonies/plate (*see* **Note 3**).
3. Grow at 37°C until colonies have desired size (usually overnight).

3.1.2. Choosing the Clones to Pick

To avoid any contamination within a microtiter plate well, either with a second clone or with another microorganism, it is important to pick only those clones from the random plated library that show the desired appearance (check size, shape, color and surface) and that grow well separated from any other colony. If a robotic device is used, a camera takes digital images of the plate and then an image analysis program is employed to identify colonies on the plate that satisfy the predefined quality criteria. If all suitable colonies within the analyzed region are detected, the position of each colony is transmitted to the picking robot.

3.1.3. Picking of the Colonies

1. Prepare enough microtiter plates by filling the wells with the appropriate medium. This can be done using either a multichannel pipet or an automatic plate-filling robot (i.e., IGEL from Opal-Jena (*8*) or QFill2 [Genetix]). Fill each well of a 384-well plate with approx 60 µL or each well of a 96-well plate with approx 90 µL. Always fill an extra plate with media and incubate at 37°C to check for contamination.
2. Transfer the colonies from the agar plate to a microtiter plate well. This can be done by two methods:
   a. By hand: although it is very inefficient to pick a large library by hand, it is possible to pick clones from a few plates this way. Use sterile wooden toothpicks to pick a single chosen colony (*see* **Note 4**). Transfer a toothpick into the medium in the microtiter plate well. Rotate the toothpick several times to ensure optimal transfer and discard.
   b. Using a robot (**Fig. 2A**): place two 22 × 22 cm agar plates (with growing colonies) of the random plated library and 24 filled microtiter plates on the working surface of the picking robot. After starting the program most of the work is done automatically. A CCD camera takes successive slightly

overlapping images of 1/48 of an agar plate and each image is immediately analyzed, whereby first the contour of each potential colony is traced, and then, using parameters specifying the area size, roundness, and diameter, those colonies that should be picked are selected. The picking head consists of 96 independently controlled metal pins, which are positioned one after the other over a selected colony and then moved down into the colony by air pressure. After all the pins are loaded with transfer material, the head moves over a microtiter plate, lowers into the medium-filled wells, and moves slightly up and down to ensure adequate transfer. The pins are then cleaned and sterilized, and the cycle continues until either all colonies of all areas of the plate are picked or all wells are filled. Our robot (**Fig. 2A**) picks approx 2000 clones/h.

3. Transfer the inoculated microtiter plates into a warm room or incubator. Cosmids, cDNAs, PACs, and Pls are best grown for approx 16 h at 37°C.
4. If necessary, edit the plates to remove those plates with too little growth and then label each plate with the appropriate library name/identification and consecutive plate numbers (*see* **Note 5**).
5. Freeze the microtiter plates:
   a. Keep the microtiter plates at 4°C for a few hours before freezing, to prevent heavy condensation inside the lids.
   b. Blot the inside lids with sterile 3MM Whatman paper to remove condensation.
   c. Freeze either as single plates on dry ice or as a brick of 24 plates (three stacks of eight, all oriented the same way) in a –80°C freezer (*see* **Note 6**).

3.2. From Microtiter Plates to High-Density Membranes: Spotting Hybridization Filters

3.2.1. Defrosting Microtiter Plates

1. Cosmids, cDNAs, P1 s and PACs should be defrosted as quickly as possible. Best results are obtained by immediately unwrapping the plates and laying them on the bench in a single layer at room temperature for approx 60 min (*see* **Note 7**). If a defrosted library copy does not give satisfactory results, a new spotting copy must be replicated from the master copy.
2. After defrosting, if there is condensation on the lids, remove by blotting with sterile 3MM Whatman paper (*see* **Note 8**).

3.2.2. Filter Spotting

1. To avoid contamination and growth problems on a large number of filters generated during a production run, make a test spotting first. Spot three filters, laying one down on a 2X YT agar/LB agar plate (to check growth), one on a Chromokult plate (to check for contamination with microorganisms, producing white, yellow, or purple colonies, in contrast to *E. coli*, which gives blue colonies), and one on a Topagar plate (to check for plaques owing to phage contamination). Remove any contaminants by cleaning the wells with 80% ethanol and leaving them empty.

Remove phage contaminations by treating the wells with 0.8 *M* HCl for 15 min, cleaning with dH$_2$O, and leaving them empty.

2. Moisten one GB003 Whatman paper with medium (2X YT or LB broth containing appropriate antibiotics) and place in the center of a Plexiglas plate.
3. Carefully lay a positively charged nylon membrane on top of the Whatman paper and roll out any air bubbles with a sterile pipet. Roll firmly enough to dispel the excess liquid medium. It is important to keep the filters in a fixed position, so that they are firmly held using a table lock system.
4. Place the microtiter plates into the stacker system in the correct order and orientation (from there each plate is automatically moved to a plate holder while the plate is spotted, and afterward it is returned to its original position in the stacker). To avoid contaminating the filters, treat the spotting gadget and empty bath with UV light before spotting. Also treat the ethanol bath with 3% H$_2$O$_2$. Clean the 384-pin gadget before each new microtiter plate by dipping into an 80% ethanol bath and subsequently drying with a hot-air fan. Use a 250-μm (pin diameter) gadget if 72 plates of a library are to be spotted in 5 × 5 duplicate spotting pattern (*see* **Subheading 3.2.3.**). For other less dense patterns, a 400-μm gadget may be used. Start the spotting program on the robot (**Fig. 2B**).
5. After spotting, place the filters on predried 2X YT/LB agar plates for 60–90 min and incubate at 37°C for 12–15 h. Slowly lay the filters down on the agar, if necessary, lifting again to dispel air bubbles. If the same microtiter plates are being spotted again the following day, store them at 4°C (wrapped in Saran Wrap to prevent evaporation); otherwise freeze store the plates.

3.2.3. Spotting Patterns

The spotting pattern determines the number of clones transferred onto the filter and therefore the density of the clones on the filter. It is also very important for the later analysis of the screening results because it ensures that the correct position of each positive spot can be determined on the image of the hybridized filter.

To improve the readability of high-density filters, the following aids may be used: blocks, guide dots, and internal duplicates. Blocks are 3 × 3, 4 × 4, 5 × 5, or 6 × 6 grids of spotted colonies, in which each such block has a slightly farther distance to its neighboring blocks than the distance between the colonies within the block. This gives a visible pattern that allows determination of the approximate position of a positive spot by simply counting the blocks. Guide dots are spotted instead of colonies in the center of an odd-numbered size block. If a guide dot is spotted on an even-numbered size block, one additional spot position is also left empty owing to the spotting of internal duplicates. Guide dots consist of either ink alone or ink mixed with a DNA solution. In the latter case, the hybridization probe also contains labeled DNA, which

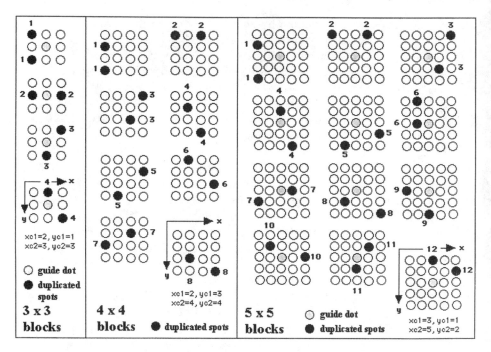

Fig. 3. All possible positions of internal duplicates within one block of a 3×3, 4×4, and 5×5 spotting pattern are shown. The centers of the 3×3 and 5×5 blocks contain the guide dots. In each block, the black marked positions indicate identical clones (for clarity each doublet is shown separately and is labeled by numbers). For each pattern, one example of calculating the block internal coordinates is given.

binds to the DNA in the guide dots. They allow, in case of a very weak background on the hybridization image, identification of the otherwise nonvisible blocks. To help to define the exact position within a block, each clone is spotted twice, so that the position to its duplicate is unique within a block. Therefore, it is possible, by simply viewing the relative position of a doublet, to determine its exact position within the block (**Fig. 3**). The following block sizes are spotted for the indicated number of microtiter plates: 3×3 without duplicates for 54 plates (20,736 clones/filter), 3×3 with duplicates for 24 plates (9216 clones/filter), 4×4 with duplicates for 48 plates (18,432 clones/filter), 5×5 with duplicates for 72 plates (27,648 clones/filter), and 6×6 with duplicates for 108 plates (41,472 clones/filter).

3.2.4. Processing

1. Prewet precut blotting paper (23×23 cm; Whatman GB002 [ref. no. 426691]) in denaturing solution by pouring approx 100 mL of denaturing solution into a clean

Nunc plate lid. Submerge the paper, roll out air bubbles using a test tube, and then pour off the excess liquid to avoid contact with the colony surface.

2. Handle the filter with forceps, holding it by diagonal corners. Transfer the membrane from the agar to prewetted blotting paper in denaturing solution and leave for 4 min (avoid air bubbles).

3. Lay the filter on fresh prewetted blotting paper in denaturing solution and transfer the filter with the paper onto a glass plate sitting above water level in a steaming water bath. Leave it for 4 min.

4. Take out the filter (without the paper), place on prewet blotting paper in neutralizing solution, and leave for at least 4 min.

5. Add 0.5 mL of pronase to 100 mL of prewarmed buffer (100 mL of buffer/filter in a Nunc plate), and, holding by two adjacent corners, slowly submerge the filter. Be sure that the filter is completely submerged and not floating on the surface. Leave in the buffer at 37°C for 30 min.

6. Wash the filter in $NaPO_4$ buffer (250 mL for four filters) for 10 min.

7. Dry the filter on blotting paper at room temperature for 1 to 2 d. Cover the filter with a the Nunc plate and be careful not to place the Nunc plate on any area of drying colonies.

8. UV crosslink the filters for 2 min or use the auto crosslink program on the Stratagene crosslinker (exposure of 120,000 $\mu J/cm^2$ for approx 25–50 s).

3.3. Hybridization Screening
Using Nonradioactive DIG Labeled Probes

3.3.1. Preparation of Probes

Probes can be DIG labeled (*see* **Note 9**) by random priming or PCR (**Fig. 4**).

3.3.1.1. RANDOM PRIMED DNA LABELING

1. Dissolve 0.1–1 μg of template DNA (*see* **Note 10**) in 1X TE buffer (e.g., 300 ng of DNA in a 16-μL final volume in 1.5 mL tube).
2. Denature by heating to 95°C for 2–10 min.
3. Transfer immediately to ice/NaCl or ice/ethanol bath.
4. Add 4 μL of DIG-High-Prime, mix, and centrifuge briefly.
5. Incubate for 1–20 h at 37°C (best overnight).
6. Stop the reaction by adding 2 μL of 0.2 *M* EDTA (pH 8.0) and/or heat to 65°C for 10 min.
7. Quantify the amount of labeled probe to check the efficiency of the labeling reaction using DIG Quantification Teststrips.

3.3.1.2. DIG LABELING WITH PCR

1. Set up PCR mix on ice (500 μL, divide as 10 × 50 μL): 375 μL of H_2O, 50 μL of 10X PCR buffer (Perkin-Elmer, including $MgCl_2$), 50 μL of DIG mix (vial 2 of PCR DIG Probe Synthesis Kit; *see* **Note 11**), 5 μL of AmpliTaq (or 25 μL of *Taq* DNA polymerase from Boehringer Mannheim), 10 μL (20 μ*M*) of primer 1, 10 μL (20 μ*M*) of primer 2, and 10 μL of template DNA (*see* **Note 12**).

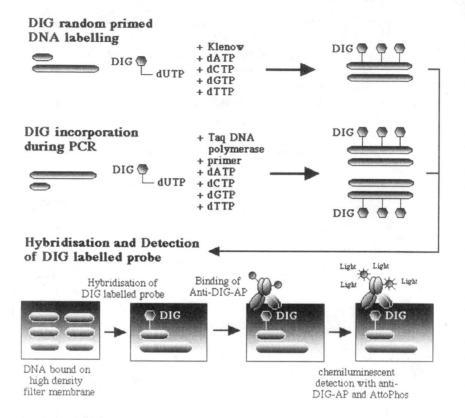

Fig. 4. Two possible DIG labeling methods (random priming and PCR incorporation) are shown, as well as the schematic steps in using such probes for hybridization screening and signal detection.

2. PCR cycles; 10 cycles of 95°C for 10 s, 65°C for 30 s, and 72°C for 2 min; 20 cycles of 95°C for 10 s, 60°C for 30 s, and 72°C for 2 min; plus an additional 20-s elongation per cycle (cycle 11, additional 20 s; cycle 12, additional 40 s; cycle 13, additional 60 s; and so on); and, 7 min at 72°C (last elongation).
3. Analyze the labeled probe by agarose gel electrophoresis. A single band should be visible after ethidium bromide staining. Because of the multiple incorporation of DIG-dNTPs during the PCR process, the molecular weight of the labeled PCR product is increased compared with that of a nonlabeled product.

3.3.2. Hybridization

Hybridization can be performed in flasks, plastic bags, or Nunc plates. If two filters are hybridized in a bag, they should be placed back-to-back with the DNA side exposed. If Nunc plates are used, transfer to a plastic bag before anti-DIG-AP is added, to reduce the volume, and finish the procedure in the bag. Hybridizations in Nunc plates give the best quality hybridizations, followed by plastic bags, and finally flasks.

3.3.2.1. PREHYBRIDIZATION

1. Roll up the moist, UV-treated filter (the surface with the spots facing inside) slightly and transfer into a hybridization flask with 20 mL of Church buffer (*see* **Note 13**).
2. Unroll the filter by slowly turning the flask until the filter lies straight against the flask wall.
3. Leave for at least 60 min at 65°C in a hybridization oven.

3.3.2.2. HYBRIDIZATION

1. Remove the prehybridization solution and leave the flask upside down on a paper towel to drain.
2. Mix denatured probe with 20 mL of Church buffer and fill slowly into the flask to avoid any bubbles.
3. Hang flask in a hybridization oven and leave to rotate overnight at 65°C.

3.3.2.3. STRINGENCY WASH

1. Pour probe from the flask into a 15-mL Falcon tube and freeze at –20°C for reuse (*see* **Note 14**).
2. Wash the lid of the hybridization flask with clear water.
3. Wash the filter sequentially with each of the following solutions for 15 min each: 2X SSC, 0.1% SDS at room temperature; 2X SSC, 0.1% SDS at room temperature; 0.1X SSC, 0.1% SDS at 65°C; 0.1X SSC, 0.1% SDS at 65°C.
4. Discard the solutions, put the flask upside down on a paper towel, and leave to drain.
5. Wash the lid of the hybridization flask with clear water.

3.3.3. DIG Detection

1. Wash the filter with 20 mL of each 1X solution at room temperature for the indicated times. Leave the flask upside down on a paper towel to drain between each wash (take care not to rub the filters after the washing steps are finished; otherwise, the signals might get smeared):
   a. Washing solution for 5 min.
   b. Blocking solution (dilute fresh from 10X stock solution) for 30 min.
   c. Anti-DIG-AP in blocking solution (mix fresh 1.25 μL of anti-Dig AP [750 U/mL] per filter with 25 mL of blocking solution) for 20 min.
   d. Washing solution for 15 min.
   e. Washing solution for 15 min.
   f. Detection buffer for 10 min.
2. Add 20 mL of detection buffer plus 1 mL of AttoPhos (*see* **Note 15**) stock solution for 5 min (remove immediately).

3. Remove the filter from the flask.
4. Put the filter between two sheets of plastic and remove air bubbles.
5. Incubate for 2–24 h in the dark (signals will diffuse if the membranes are left longer at room temperature, but they can be stored at –20°C to keep the signal intact for longer periods).

3.3.4. Scanning

1. Clean the glass plate of the STORM 860 Phosphor Imager (*see* **Note 16**) and place the filter with the spots facing downward on the glass; use forceps to gently lower the membrane onto the glass, starting with one edge, carefully avoiding trapping any air bubbles or scratching the glass. Treat the filter very carefully to avoid smearing owing to mechanical force. Do not touch the filter or glass because oil from fingerprints and powder from gloves may leave a print that can be detected.
2. Scan in blue light and save the image for later analysis (*see* **Note 17**).

3.3.5. Detection of Positive Clones

Positive hybridization signals can usually be easily distinguished from low nonspecific background hybridization (**Fig. 5**).

3.3.6. Calculation of Well Positions

It is usually easy to determine the X/Y coordinate of a positive spot on a filter grid using the aid of the blocks, guide dots, and internal duplicates. Using the X/Y values on the filter grid (preferably from both positions of a doublet, because this can be used as the internal control to ensure that both sets of coordinates result in the same well position), the microtiter plate well that contains the positive clone can be calculated. Methods can vary depending on the source of the filter (*see* **Note 18**). The conversion from coordinates to well positions can be done by employing a formula that depends only on the spotting program used for a filter. Alternatively, as is done in case of the RZPD, the microtiter plate well is determined dynamically, whereby the X/Y coordinates and identity numbers of the used filters are entered into a form on the World Wide Web *(6)*, and a program retrieves the actual spotting information for these filters from a database, taking into account any specific variation or errors in the spotting procedure of a particular filter. It also provides links to any additional information that is known about identified clones (such as sequence or mapping information, genes or markers contained in the clone) in either the RZPD database or an external database (e.g., Genbank, GeneCards, GDB). A simple formula that can be used to determine the X/Y coordinates of a positive spot, assuming an RZPD filter is used, in which the $X = 1, Y = 1$ position is located at the top left corner, is as follows:

$$X = s(xb-1) + xc$$

$$Y = s(yb-1) + yc$$

where X and Y are the final X and Y coordinates; s is the block pattern (three for 3×3 blocks, four for 4×4 blocks, five for 5×5 blocks); xb and yb are the coordinates of the block containing the spot on the filter; and xc and yc are the coordinates of the spot within the block.

3.3.7. Retrieving Clones for Further Analysis

Because the well positions are the unique identifier of clones from an arrayed (reference) library, there is a direct correlation between this well position and the clone name/identifier, which can be used to order an identified clone for further analysis or retrieve additional information about the clone. In some special cases, as with the clones from the IMAGE clone collection, clones have an external unique identification number, which can be used to identify a clone, and to which a well position has to be converted (*see* **Note 19**).

It is always important to check the identity of a clone received after identifying it in a screening experiment, because usually the clone spotted on a filter comes from a different copy of microtiter plates than the clone picked for distribution, and neither internal deletions, or rearrangements nor erroneous X/Y coordinate determination can ever be completely ruled out. Therefore, before any further analysis is performed on a clone, it should be rehybridized with the original probe to ensure that the hybridizing insert DNA is still present.

1. Use sterile loops to streak out a clone to single colonies on an agar plate containing the appropriate antibiotics from the stab in which the clone was received.
2. Grow for several hours or overnight at 37°C.
3. Lie the filter membrane onto colonies and carefully remove the filter again.
4. Process the filter with the same procedure as described for spotted filters.

3.3.8. Stripping of Hybridized Filters

Wash the filters in: ethanol for 10 min, H_2O for 10 min, 0.4 M NaOH for 10 min, neutralizing solution for 10 min, and 1X TE for 10 min.

3.3.9. Drying of Hybridized Filters

1. Place the filters in 96% ethanol for 10 min.
2. Wash in deionized H_2O for 10 min.
3. Air-dry.

4. Notes

1. Antibiotics may be weighed directly into water to prevent provocation of any allergies caused by the powder.

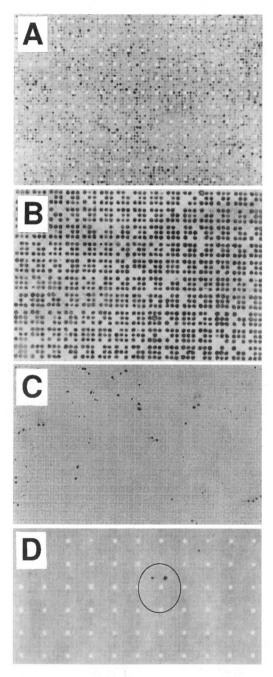

Fig. 5. Sections of different DIG hybridizations to high-density filters scanned with STORM phosphor imager with blue light. (**A**) Total genomic DNA of *Callithrix jacchus* labeled by random priming after partial digestion with *Mbo*I and hybridized to

2. These type of robots were originally developed at the ICRF in London to produce high-density filters for The Reference Library System and have been further improved over the years. They are available from several companies, e.g., Linear Drives, KayBee Systems *(9)*, and Genetix. Smaller laboratory benchtop robots, such as the BioGrid from BioRobotics *(10)*, can also be used to produce high-density filters on a smaller scale.
3. The optimal number of colonies depends on their size and the method by which they are picked. Working with our robotic picking device (**Fig. 2A**) and image analysis system, 2500 colonies give the optimal yield. Glass beads can be used to obtain a very even plating distribution. Apply the desired volume of your library titration on the surface of the agar plate, add 20–30 sterile glass beads (about 0.5 cm diameter), cover the plate with lid, and shake the plate to allow the beads to roll over the whole surface. Remove the beads by dropping them into an alcohol solution.
4. Alternatively, a metal disc with a central handle and 12 protruding needles, equally distributed around the outer rim, can be used. The needles are sterilized using ethanol and heat, and then 12 individual clones are picked by turning the wheel between each picking event, so that a new needle faces the agar plate. After all the pins are loaded with material, one needle is lowered into the first well of a row of a microtiter plate and quickly rolled along the row of wells so that each needle inoculates a new well. Rolling the disc forward and backward ensures that the material transfer is complete.
5. Depending on the number of libraries and plates used in a laboratory, the labeling of the plates can be done either manually or, as in our case, by using a barcode sprayer made by Domino Amjet GmbH *(11)*, which prints not only the required information on each microtiter plate, but also a bar code that is read during the filter-spotting process, to identify each used plate automatically, with the help of a bar-code reader (**Fig. 2B**).
6. If plates are frozen in a –80°C freezer, put a note on the outside door to prevent others from accidentally moving freshly freezing plates, which could lead to cross-contamination. Each single plate or brick should be wrapped airtight with shrink-wrap or Saran wrap to prevent evaporation at –80°C.

---

filter (5 × 5 spotting pattern with duplicates, white spots indicate guide dots) containing *Callithrix* cosmid clones. Strong signals indicate repetitive sequences. (**B**) Amp fragment probe labeled by PCR (as described in text) and hybridized to mouse adult brain cDNA filter (3 × 3 spotting pattern, no duplicates, no guide dots). Note that some spotted clones did not grow on the filter. (**C**) Human-actin probe labelled by PCR and hybridized to human keratinocyte cDNA filter (3 × 3 spotting pattern with duplicates, center dot within blocks empty but no guide dots spotted). (**D**) Single-copy RNA polymerase I specific transcription factor gene (approx 600 bp) labeled by PCR as probe and hybridized to mouse testis cDNA filter (5 × 5 spotting pattern with duplicates, white spots indicate guide dots). Positive signal (circled) at position 2 within 5 × 5 block (*see* **Fig. 3**) corresponds to clone in microtiter plate 8, row F, column 21.

7. Always handle defrosted plates gently because well-to-well cross-contamination can be a very serious problem. If a set of microtiter plates is used a second time for spotting, it is better to vortex the plates after defrosting by using a sterile replicator to resuspend the cells. This will lead to more even and complete growth of colonies on the filters.

8. Plates should not be left at room temperature or at 4°C for longer than necessary (keep frozen as long as possible). When plates are left at 4°C or in an incubator for any length of time, extra care should be taken to wrap all the plates properly to prevent evaporation of liquid from the wells.

9. Direct DIG-labeled probes can be used for hybridization screening, as well as for other hybridization techniques and are detected by an antibody conjugated to the enzyme alkaline phosphatase, which catalyzes a color or a chemiluminescent reaction. Other possible methods of DIG labeling include DIG RNA labeling, DIG labeling by nick translation, DIG oligonucleotide tailing, and DIG oligonucleotide 3'-end or 5'-end labeling.

10. DNA of different lengths, from 200 bp to linearized plasmid, cosmid, and λ DNA, can be labeled. If the DNA fragment to be labeled is isolated from low-melting-point agarose, excise the fragment cleanly and transfer to a 1.5-mL centrifuge tube. Add sterile dH$_2$O to 3 mL/g of gel and heat the tube to 100°C for 7 min to melt gel and denature the DNA. Cool to 37°C and use in a standard labeling procedure.

11. Vial 2 contains 125 µL of a mixture containing dATP, dCTP, dGTP (2 m*M* Bach), dTTP (1.3 m*M*), and DIG–11-dUTP (0.7 m*M*) (alkali labile, pH 7.0); DIG-11-dUTP will, in contrast to normal PCR, label approximately every twentieth nucleotide with DIG. This mix contains a DIG-dUTP:dTTP ratio of 1:2, which is recommended for producing probes with the highest sensitivity. If the target gene exists in high copy numbers, a labeling ratio of 1: 19 might be sufficient for probe synthesis.

12. Genomic or cDNA clones can be used as template DNA and specific oligos, designed to amplify the desired piece of DNA from the clone, as primers. The final concentration of the template DNA can vary. For single-copy genes, 1–100 ng of human genomic DNA and 10–100 pg of plasmid DNA could be used. As an example, DNA from the cosmid vector scos-1 (SuperCos 1; Genbank access. no. M99566 M27232) is used as template DNA (a miniprep solution was diluted 1:20, 10 µL of dilution was mixed with 90 µL of TE and denatured at 94°C for 10 min, and 10 µL of denatured mix was used in PCR reactions) to label a fragment of the ampicillin gene. The primers which are used (primer 1: 5'-TTCGTTCATCCATAGTTGCC-3', primer 2: 5'-GCCTGTAGCAATGG-CAACAACG-3') amplify a sequence from this gene and produce a probe suitable to light up all clones on a filter from a library made with a vector also containing the ampicillin gene. Such images (**Fig. 5B**) can be used for quality control or to normalize images from hybridizations with more specific probes.

13. When hybridization is carried out in a plastic bag, add at least 15 mL of Church buffer per filter. Add 5–10 mL for each additional filter. Up to eight filters can be prehybridized in one bag. In Nunc plates use a buffer volume of 50 mL. Instead

of Church buffer other hybridization buffers can be used (i.e., Easy Hyb [Boehringer] or Quick Hyb [Stratagene]), but in these cases the hybridization temperatures and times have to be adjusted according to the recommended protocols from the buffer producer.

14. DIG-labeled probes are stable for about 1 yr. Hybridization solutions with DIG-labeled probes can be reused several times.

15. AttoPhos is a highly sensitive fluorimetric substrate for the detection of alkaline phosphatase with an optimal excitation wavelength of 430–440 nm and the emission maximum at 560 nm.

16. We use a STORM 860 Phosphor Imager from Molecular Dynamics *(12)* to analyze hybridizations. The instrument scans and processes samples by illuminating the scan area one pixel at a time with a beam that is red (635 nm) for red-excited fluorescence scan, or blue (450 nm) for a chemofluorescence/blue-excited fluorescence scan. When blue or red light hits an area of the sample containing an appropriate fluorochrome (i.e., AttoPhos), the fluorochrome emits light with a characteristic spectrum. The optical system collects the emitted light and passes it through an optical filter to the photomultiplier tube, converting it to an electric current, which varies with the intensity of this light. The analog signal is then converted into digital information and stored as an image on the hard disk.

17. Filters can be scanned in red light *before* AttoPhos is applied, in order to detect background signals.

18. Several noncommercial and commercial organizations distribute high-density screening filters, i.e., RZPD *(6)*, UK-HGMP-RC *(13)*, BACPAC Resource Center *(14)*, Research Genetics *(15)* Genome Systems *(16)*.

19. Clone names based on microtiter plate positions are usually made up from the following components: library ID/name, plate number, row character, and column number. For example, the clone with the official name AC1OA3 *(17)* is from chromosome 3–specific cosmic library from Lawrence Livermore National Laboratory (LLNL). *AC* is the short name of the LL03NCO1 *AC* library, *10* is the microtiter plate number, *A* is the row character, and *3* is the column number. However, the order of these essential parts of a clone name can vary and also be supplemented (i.e., by information about the originating laboratory or the exact plate copy). The same clone would have, at the RZPD, the more detailed and automatically parsable identifier LLNLc129A0310Q2 (*LLNL* is the originating laboratory, *c* indicates a cosmic clone, 129 is the internal library ID, *A* is the row character, *03* the two-digit column number, *10* is the plate number and *Q2* is the plate copy identifier) to satisfy the more demanding needs of a distribution service that must deal with different copies of several hundred libraries from many different origins. However, all nomenclature schemes based on the microtiter plate well position where the clone is stored allow unambiguous identification of the frozen clone and hence retrieve the colonies from the specific clone. (Note, however, that the same clone from different plate copies might not necessarily be exactly the same biologic entity owing to possible deletions or other rearrangements that are most likely to be specific to a given copy only.)

Acknowledgments

The described protocols and methods were developed and improved over several years by the staff of the Resource Centre (RZPD) of the German Human Genome Project (http://www.rzpd.de or info@rzpd.de), mainly by Andreas Vente (lab manager); Barbara Koller (nonradioactive hybridizations, quality control); Katrin Welzel, Carolin Anthon-Hoeft, Annette Poch-Hasneck, and Effi Rees (library production and picking); Anja Kellermann (PCR), Lisa Gellen (chief technician); and Susan Kirby, Marika Peters, and Silvia Brandt (library management). Robot hardware and software are maintained by Klaus Bienert and Heiko Kraack. We thank Lisa Gellen for help in preparing the manuscript. The Resource Centre is funded by the German Federal Ministry for Science, Education, Research and Technology (BMBF) and jointly conducted by the Max-Planck-Institute for Molecular Genetics, Berlin (Prof. Hans Lehrach), and the Deutsches Krebsforschungszentrum, Heidelberg (Prof. Annemarie Poustka). On July 1, 2000, the RZPD changed its status from a branch of the Max-Planck Society to a nonprofit private limited company registered as "RZPD Deutsches Resourcenzentrum für Genomforschung GmbH."

References

1. Vente, A., Korn, B., Zehetner, G., Poustka, A., and Lehrach, H. (1999) Distribution and early development of microarray technology in Europe. *Nature Genet.* **22,** 22.
2. Zehetner, G. and Lehrach, H. (1994) The Reference Library System—sharing biological material and experimental data. *Nature* **367,** 489–491.
3. Bussow, K., Cahill, D., Nietfield, W., Bancroft, D., Scherzinger, E., Lehrach, H., and Walter, G. (1998) A method for global protein expression and antibody screening on high density filters of an arrayed cDNA library. *Nucleic Acids Res.* **26,** 5007, 5008.
4. Wanker, E. E., Rovira, C., Scherzinger, E., Hasenbank, R., Walter, S., Tait, D., Colicelli, J., and Lehrach, H. (1997) HIP-I: a huntingtin interacting protein isolated by the yeast two hybrid system. Hum. *Mol. Genet.* **6,** 487–495.
5. The chipping forecast (1999) *Nature Genet.* **21(Suppl.),** *(entire issue).*
6. <http://www.rzpd.de>.
7. Maier, E., Roest-Crollius, H., and Lehrach, H. (1994) Hybridisation techniques on "gridded high density DNA and *in situ* colony filters based on fluorescence detection. *Nucleic Acids Res.* **22,** 3423, 3424.
8. <http://www.bioinstrumente-jena.de>.
9. <http://www.kaybee.co.uk>.
10. <http://www.biorobotics.co.uk>.
11. <http://www.domino-printing.com>.
12. <http://www.moleculardynamics.com>.
13. <http://genomics.roswellpark.org>.
14. <http://bacpac.med.buffalo.edu>.
15. <http://www.resgen.com>.
16. <http://www.genomesystems.com>.
17. McNinch, J. S., Games, J. A., Wong, B. S., Alleman, J., Gingrich, J., and de Jong, P. J. (1993) Chromosome 3 Cosmid Library LL03NCO1 "AC" Library Information Sheet, Lawrence Livermore National Laboratory, Berkeley, CA.

13

Direct Selection of cDNAs by Genomic Clones

Daniela Toniolo

1. Introduction

During the last decade, major advances in genomic research have resulted in the development of a variety of tools and technologies for gene identification that were successfully applied to the construction of transcriptional maps and to the identification of genes responsible for genetic disorders. Once genomic DNA sequences become available, *in silico* gene identification will be the most widely used method. However, established techniques for gene identification will still be relevant, especially to identify specific genes, mapped to defined regions of the genome.

Depending on the type and amount of information available, different techniques can be used to identify genes of interest. One of the most commonly used is direct selection of cDNAs, a technique that takes advantage of the specificity of DNA-DNA hybridization to extract from complex mixtures of cDNAs transcribed sequences of interest. In cDNA selection, cloned double-stranded genomic DNA and a mixture of cDNAs are combined, denatured, and allowed to anneal. Most of the cloned genomic DNA molecules reanneal to each other but some will hybridize to cDNAs. The hybrid molecules can be separated from the cDNA mixture by polymerase chain reaction (PCR) amplification and can be cloned for further analysis.

Several variations of the aforementioned procedure have now been reported. Main differences in various procedures lie in the hybridization conditions to capture the cDNAs, which are based on either labeling or filter immobilization of genomic DNA *(1–3)*. In both cases, the selection has been shown to work efficiently and not to be highly dependent on the level of gene expression. Moreover, direct cDNA selection has a normalizing effect on the distribution of the end products. High- and low-abundance mRNAs are eventually represented at levels

From: *Methods in Molecular Biology, vol. 175: Genomics Protocols*
Edited by: M. P. Starkey and R. Elaswarapu © Humana Press Inc., Totowa, NJ

much more similar to each other than they were originally. In addition, sequences expressed at very low levels can also be efficiently captured from complex mixtures such as highly heterogeneous tissues and a mixture of mRNAs from different tissues. In general, cDNAs present at levels as low as 1 in 10^6 can be isolated. The only relevant technical limitation to the method is that the genes of interest must be expressed in the tissue or cell types used for cDNA preparation and the pattern and the level of expression must be known or predictable.

This chapter is aimed at providing a stepwise protocol for direct cDNA selection, the use of different sources of genomic DNA and cDNAs, and some of the possible procedures for analysis of the recovered cDNAs. **Figure 1** presents a scheme of the general strategy for cDNA selection.

2. Materials

1. Cloned genomic DNA of choice.
2. Nick translation kit (Amersham or other manufacturers).
3. Biotin-dUTP (Roche).
4. 3 *M* Ammonium acetate, pH 5.
5. 96% Ethanol.
6. Salmon sperm DNA (100 mg/mL) (Sigma, St. Louis, MO).
7. cDNA synthesis kit (Life Technologies or other manufacturers).
8. Thermal cycler.
9. *Taq* polymerase and buffer (Promega, Madison, WI).
10. 1.5 m*M* MgCl$_2$.
11. 1.25 μ*M* dNTP.
12. RoRi(dN)$_{11}$ primer (25 μ*M* stock): 5'-AAGGATCCGTCGACATCGATAAT-ACGACTCACTATAGGGANNNNNNNNNNN-3'
13. RoRint primer (25 μ*M* stock): 5'-ATCCGTCGACATCGATAATACGACTC-3'
14. Agarose (normal and low melting).
15. 10X TBE buffer.
16. Total genomic DNA sheared to 400 to 500-bp fragments or Cot 1 DNA (Promega).
17. Competitor DNAs.
18. 2X Hybridization buffer: 10X SSPE, 0.2% Denhardt's solution, 1% sodium dodecyl sulfate (SDS).
19. Hybridization oven.
20. Streptavidin-coated magnetic beads (Dynabeads 280; Dynal).
21. Magnet for 1.5-mL tubes (Dynal or Promega).
22. 10X saline sodium citrate (SSC).
23. Ligation kit (TaKaRa).
24. Competent XL1Blue or DH5α cells.
25. LB medium and LB agar plates.
26. TE buffer: 1 m*M* Tris-HCl, pH 8.0, 1 m*M* EDTA.

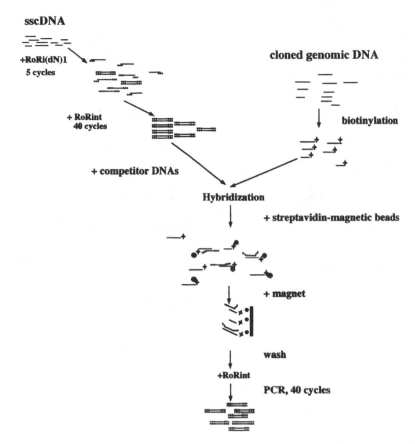

Fig. 1. Schematic representation of the cDNA selection procedure described in the text. RoRi(dN)11: 51 nt primer containing 11 random nt at the 3' end. RoRint: primer containing a 28-nt sequence, internal to RoRi, stars: biotin; dots: streptavidin; thick vertical line: magnet.

27. Diethylpyrocarbonate (DEPC)-treated water.
28. 37°C Incubator.
29. 96-Well plates, flat bottomed.
30. 96-Pin replicating tool.
31. 30% Glycerol in LB medium.
32. Nylon membranes (Hybond, Amersham).
33. Microcentrifuge.

3. Method

3.1. Choice and Preparation of Genomic DNA

Direct cDNA selection depends on the use of cloned DNA fragments derived from genomic DNA. Genomic DNA cloned in yeast artificial chromosomes (YAC), cosmids, bacterial artificial chromosomes (BAC), and P1 artificial chromosomes (PAC) clones that are suitable for cDNA selection methodologies. However, there are advantages and disadvantages of using each of the cloning systems. The two most relevant parameters are the size of the genomic DNA inserts and the purity of the cloned genomic DNA obtainable with any particular vector.

The size of the genomic DNA insert is significant for the complexity of the cDNA that will be isolated, but it does not seem to interfere with the efficiency of selection. Large genomic inserts may carry multiple transcripts. This may be a disadvantage considering that the different transcripts have to be subsequently distinguished, but it is an advantage in the analysis of large genomic regions, because fewer clones will have to be used to cover a given region and fewer hybridizations and PCR amplifications will be required.

The second point to consider is the purity of the cloned genomic DNA. There is no need to use highly purified genomic DNA, but host cell DNA contaminating a genomic DNA clone can result in the isolation of cDNAs not corresponding to the cloned insert, but to the contaminant DNA. The best example of this kind of problem comes from the use of YAC clones. The purification of a YAC clone by pulsed-field gel electrophoresis (PFGE) is feasible *(4)* but is a very inefficient procedure. Although total DNA from yeast (*Saccharomyces cerevisiae)* can also be used in general circumstances *(5)*, the presence of yeast mitochondrial DNA (mtDNA) and rRNA genes (rDNA) contaminating either the purified YAC or the yeast DNA preparation may sometimes lead to enrichment of cDNAs with homology to contaminating yeast DNA molecules.

DNA from bacterial and yeast clones can be prepared using standard procedure *(6)*. Bacterial DNA can be easily purified and will not need further treatments thereafter (*see* **Note 1**).

3.2. Labeling of Genomic DNA

In direct cDNA selection, genomic DNA and the hybridized cDNA molecules must be separated from the mixture of cDNAs. To achieve this, the DNA can be bound to a nylon membrane *(1)* or labeled with biotin in solution *(2,7)*. Biotin-labeled DNA can be extracted from the solution by mixing with streptavidin-coated magnetic beads. The very high affinity of biotin for streptavidin allows tight binding of the labeled DNA to the beads, which may then be separated from unlabeled DNA using a magnet. DNA is biotinylated by incorporation of biotinylated-dNTPs into genomic DNA.

1. Label up to 1 μg of cloned DNA with biotin-dUTP using commercial nick translation kits and following the manufacturer's instructions.
2. Add 5 μL of carrier salmon sperm DNA (100 mg/mL) and precipitate with 0.1 vol of 3 M NH$_4$-acetate (pH 5.0) and 2.5 vol of 96% ethanol.
3. Centrifuge at 10,000g for 15 min at 4°C.

4. Wash the pellet with 250 μL of 70% ethanol by centrifuging as in **step 3**.
5. Air-dry and resuspend the pellet in TE buffer at a concentration of 100 ng/μL (*see* **Note 2**).

3.3. Choice and Preparation of cDNAs

The cDNAs can be obtained from two sources: from a cDNA library or as double-stranded uncloned cDNA. The use of a cDNA library can be convenient, and vector primers can be used in the subsequent steps of PCR amplification, but some major disadvantages must be taken into account. The first is the reduction of the complexity of the cDNA owing to the cloning step and reamplification of the library for distribution to multiple users. The second relates to the size of the inserts of cDNA libraries. If the cloned inserts are larger than 1 kb, PCR amplifications from vector primers during various steps of cDNA selection are strongly biased toward amplifying smaller fragments, thus further reducing the complexity of the cDNA. Hence, a better source for cDNA is uncloned double-stranded cDNA made from one or more tissue sources. The complexity of such cDNA is much higher, and the amount of RNA and cDNA required is quite low and less than what is needed to construct a cDNA library.

Another important parameter is the source of the mRNA, which depends on the pattern of expression of the gene of interest. When the tissue or the RNA of choice is not available, it may be useful to use RNA prepared from tissues with a complex pattern of expression, such as fetal brain or embryo, in the case of mammals.

Once the source of the mRNA is chosen, care should be taken in the preparation of mRNA (*6*), which has to be free of unspliced and immature RNA that could very efficiently hybridize to genomic DNA and, on being selected, complicate the analysis of the results. To this aim, it may be useful to prepare cytoplasmic mRNA, when possible. It is always important to treat the mRNA with RNase-free DNase to remove contaminating DNA (*6*). In some instances, it may be important to purify the mRNA from rRNA as much as possible either by multiply passing through an oligo-dT column or by passing the DNA through rDNA bound to activated cellulose (*8*). This last step is necessary when total yeast DNA containing YAC is used.

cDNA synthesis can be performed according to the manufacturer's instructions using reverse transcriptase (RT) enzyme. The method described next is used in my laboratory, but other methods can also be used, because they are all compatible with cDNA selection.

3.3.1. First-Strand Synthesis

For cDNA synthesis we have used M-MLV RT. However, several other RTs are also available in the market and they all may work equally efficiently.

1. Resuspend 2 μg of PolyA⁺ RNA (treated with RNase-free DNase) in 30 μL of DEPC-H_2O.
2. Add 10 μL of SX RT buffer (supplied by the manufacturer).
3. Add 2.5 μL of 10 mM dNTP, 3 μL of 250 mM oligo·dT and 2 μL of random primers.
4. Add 2.5 μL of M-MLV and incubate at 37°C for 60 min (*see* **Note 3**).
5. Stop the reaction by incubating at 95°C for 5 min.

3.3.2. Second-Strand Synthesis

The second strand of the cDNA can be synthesized using different methods. The following method is based on PCR *(8)*. The second strand of the cDNA can be primed and linkers added in a two-step PCR reaction using a 51-nt primer, RoRi(dN)$_{11}$, with a degenerated tail of 11 nt at the 3' end and a known sequence of 40 nt at the 5' end (*see* **Subheading 2.**). The single-stranded cDNA is copied for five cycles of synthesis at low annealing temperature (40°C) to allow priming from the 11-nt tail. Thereafter, another primer (RoRint) is used for the subsequent steps of amplification at high temperature. Using this set of primers, a 26-nt tail is directly added to the cDNA, after second-strand synthesis. cDNAs from 3 to 0.3 kb can be synthesized this way *(8)*.

1. Dilute the product of the first-strand synthesis to 200 μL with TE buffer and use 2 μL in the reaction (corresponding to 1 to 2 ng of cDNA).
2. Add 1 μL of 25 μM RoRi(dN)$_{11}$ oligo, 5 μL of *Taq* polymerase 10X buffer, 3 μL of 1.5 mM $MgCl_2$, and 8 μL of 1.25 μM dNTPs.
3. Denature at 94°C for 5 min (hot start).
4. Add 1 U of *Taq* polymerase and continue the PCR for five cycles at 94°C for 1 min, 40°C for 2 min, and 72°C for 4 min.
5. Prepare a mix containing 1.4 μL of 25 μM RoRint oligo, 2 μL of *Taq* polymerase 10X buffer, 1.2 μL of 1.5 mM $MgCl_2$, 3.2 μL of 1.25 μM dNTPs, 1 U of *Taq* polyrnerase, and H_2O to 20 μL.
6. Add this 20-μL mix to the PCR reaction at the end of **step 4** (five cycles) and continue for another 40 cycles at 94°C for 1 min, 65°C for 1 min, and 72°C for 3 min plus a 2-s increment every cycle.
7. Analyze 1 μL and 5 μL of the PCR products on a 2% agarose gel in 1X TBE buffer. The largest products should be approx 2 kb.
8. Run the PCR products on 2% low melting agarose gel to remove the primers, unincorporated dNTPs, and products below 400–500 bp size (*see* **Note 4**).
9. Determine the amount of cDNA by agarose gel method with comparison to DNA of known concentration and similar size.

3.4. Hybridization and Selection

Direct cDNA selection is based on hybridization between cloned genomic DNA and a mixture of cDNAs. The hybridization occurs in two steps. In the first step, the cDNA is hybridized to unlabeled total genomic DNA to block repetitive sequences in the cDNA. Because random priming is used for cDNA synthesis to obtain better representation of the full length cDNAs, this also leads to synthesis of cDNA copies of the rRNA contaminating the mRNA preparation. It is therefore advisable to add cloned rDNA and mtDNA to compete for rRNA and mitDNA contaminating the cDNA preparation.

In the second step, the prehybridized cDNAs are hybridized to the biotinylated cloned genomic DNA. This reaction will end with the labeling of the selected cDNA with biotin and its capture by the streptavidin-coated magnetic beads.

3.4.1. Prehybridization of the cDNA

1. In a 1.5-mL Eppendorf tube, mix 2 µg of PCR-amplified cDNA with 25 µg of Cot1 DNA or the same amount of total genomic DNA (sheared to 500-bp fragments).
2. Add 2–5 µg of cloned rDNA and/or mtDNA, if required.
3. Precipitate with 0.1 vol of 3 *M* Na acetate (pH 5.2) and 2.5 vol of 96% EtOH.
4. Centrifuge at 10,000*g* for 15 min at 4°C.
5. Wash with 70% EtOH by centrifuging as in **step 4**.
6. Remove the EtOH and air-dry the pellet at room temperature.
7. Resuspend the pellet in 25 µL of H_2O by mixing.
8. Add 25 µL of 2X hybridization buffer.
9. Overlay with one drop of mineral oil, heat at 95°C for 5 min, and incubate for 24 h at 65°C.

3.4.2. Hybridization

1. Add 150 ng of cloned genomic DNA to 50 µL of hybridization buffer.
2. Heat at 95°C for 5 min.
3. Mix quickly with prehybridized cDNA and further incubate at 65°C for 48 h.

3.4.3. Selection

1. Resuspend the streptavidin-coated magnetic beads by vortexing.
2. Transfer 100 µL of beads into a 1.5-mL tube.
3. Add 1 mL of bead washing buffer (0.1 mg/mL of bovine serum albumin in phosphate-buffered saline).
4. Place the tube on a magnet for 30 s to allow the beads to settle on the magnet and the supernatant to become clear.
5. While on the magnet, remove the supernatant.
6. Perform two more washes (**steps 3–5**).
7. Transfer the hybridization mix to the tube with the beads and incubate at room temperature for 40 min. Keep the contents mixed by inverting the tube throughout the incubation. At the end of the incubation repeat **step 5**.
8. Add 1 mL of the first hybridization washing buffer (2X SSC, 0.1% SDS) and incubate for 5 min at 65°C. Repeat **steps 3–5** using hybridization washing buffer.

9. Perform two more washes as in **steps 3–5**, but using: 2x in 2X SSC, 0.1% SDS; 2x in 0.2X SSC, 0.1% SDS; and 1x in 0.2X SSC.
10. Resuspend the beads in 100 μL of H$_2$O. Store at 4°C until required.

3.4.4. PCR Amplification of Selected cDNA

1. Mix the beads very thoroughly and use 1, 5 and 10 μL (per 100 μL PCR reaction) from the 100 μL suspension. Use RoRint oligo at a final concentration of 0.5 μ*M* as described earlier (*see* **Subheading 3.3.2.**) for cDNA amplification (*see* **Note 5**).
2. Analyze 1–5 μL of the PCR reaction on a 2% agarose gel, determine the concentration, purify, and repeat the selection once more as described in **Subheading 3.4.3.**

3.4.5. Cloning Selected cDNAs

1. After two selections, clone the PCR amplification products using any of the commercially available cloning kits.
2. After ligation and transformation in *Escherichia coli* **(6)**, plate an aliquot of the transformation to determine the number of colonies obtained. Store the remaining stock of transformed bacteria at 4°C (up to 1 wk).
3. Based on test plating, determine the volume of aliquot to be plated using the remaining transformation mix.
4. Plate the remaining transformation mix as per the calculated volume and incubate overnight at 37°C (*see* **Note 6**).

3.4.6. Picking of Recombinant Clones

1. Fill 100 μL of LB medium, plus the appropriate antibiotic, into the wells of 96-well microtiter plates.
2. Inoculate each well with a colony, cover, wrap with plastic, and incubate in a humidified chamber at 37°C overnight.
3. Check for growth, and make two replicas of each microtiter plate using a 96-pin replicating tool.
4. To the original plate, add 100 μL of 30% glycerol in LB, and store at –80°C wrapped in Saran wrap.
5. Incubate the replicated plates at 37°C overnight, and after checking for growth, freeze them at –80°C as well. They can be kept frozen until needed (*see* **Note 7**).

3.5. Analysis of the Selected cDNAs

The method of gene identification by direct cDNA selection described in this chapter produces many cDNAs highly enriched in transcribed sequences from the genomic region of interest. The cDNAs obtained will have to be analyzed to demonstrate that they correspond to genomic sequences used in the experiment and that they are expressed in mature mRNA. It will also have to be excluded that they correspond to the most common artifacts in cDNA selection, rRNA, mitDNA, and repetitive sequences. The presence of the artifacts was discussed in the previous sections and their detection is rather easy: they can be identified by hybridization of the cDNA clones on filters to specific probes and the corresponding clones can be discarded. More difficult is the identification of artifactual clones derived from low copy number repeats or host cell-derived DNA sequences. Eventually, identity of the genomic DNA can be demonstrated by hybridization of inserts from single colonies to Southern blots of the corresponding genomic clones or by sequencing and comparison of partial sequences to available genomic sequence. Specific experiments are required to definitely demonstrate which of the selected clones correspond to the gene of interest.

3.5.1. PCR Amplification of the Inserts of the Clones

1. Grow a copy of each microtiter plate on an agar plate, plus antibiotic at 37°C, overnight.
2. Touch each colony with a sterile toothpick and inoculate into 100 μL of H_2O.
3. Use 1–5 μL of the bacterial colony as a template in a 25-μL PCR reaction. Primers and PCR conditions depend on the vector used for cloning.
4. After amplification under optimal conditions, analyze 5–10 μL of each PCR product on a 1.5–2% agarose gel stained with EtBr.
5. Determine the size of the inserts by comparing with molecular weight standards.

3.5.2. Hybridization Analysis

1. Place a rectangular or round nylon filter on a plate of the appropriate size containing LB agar medium plus antibiotic.
2. Using a 96-pin replicating device, stamp each plate twice on the same nylon membrane.
3. Grow the colonies on the membrane by incubating overnight at 30°C. Do not overgrow.
4. When the colonies are still very small, fix their DNA to the filter by standard colony hybridization technique *(6)*.
5. Hybridize the filters to mitDNA and rDNA probes, total genomic DNA, PCR product of isolated colonies and any other probe of interest (*see* **Note 8**).

4. Notes

1. Care should be taken in subsequent steps to compete and handle contaminating sequences in genomic DNA prepared from yeast.
2. Biotinylated DNA can be stored at –20°C for long periods.
3. Ten microliter of the mix can be transferred to a second tube containing 1 μCi of [α-^{32}P] dCTP. After incubation at 37°C for 60 min, the second tube can be used to count the efficiency of incorporation and to determine the size of the cDNA by agarose gel electrophoresis in denaturing conditions *(6)*.

4. Electrophoresis must be long enough to distinguish the lower size bands. Cut the agarose from the wells to the 400 to 5000-bp bands in the marker DNA. Melt the agarose at 65°C until it is dissolved. Extract once with 1 vol of phenol (without chloroform). EtOH precipitate and resuspend in an approximate volume (assume approx 30% recovery).

5. The PCR reaction conditions are extremely critical to maintain the complexity of the cDNA. The same final volume of 100 μL, needed for preparative PCR, is used throughout the experiment because conditions may vary considerably if the final volume of the PCR reaction is changed.

6. The number of colonies to analyze depends greatly on the size of the genomic clones used in the selection. Considering the average size of a gene to be 30 kb, one could expect 1 exon/kb of genomic DNA. The variability is, however, very great and it is hard to know what to expect. It is therefore very useful to pick a few hundred colonies, array them in microtiter plates, and use them for multiple analyses.

7. Frozen microtiter plates can be thawed only four to five times. Repeated freeze-thaw results in the gradual loss of cell viability. The master copy should always be kept frozen (at –80°C), and all clone analyses should be done using the replica plates.

8. DNA filters can be used several times after stripping them following manufacturer's instructions.

Acknowledgment

I thank all the people in my laboratory who have contributed to the development of the methods described in this chapter. M. Mancini, S. Rivella, S. Bione, and S. Papadimitriou, at different times, have used and tested the methods of cDNA selection.

References

1. Lovett, M., Kere, J., and Hinton, L. M. (1991) Direct selection: a method for the isolation of cDNAs encoded by large genomic regions. *Proc. Natl. Acad. Sci. USA* **88,** 9628–9632.
2. Parimoo, S., Patanjali, S. R., Shukla, H., Chaplin, D. D., and Weissman, S. M. (1991) cDNA selection: efficient PCR approach for the selection of cDNAs encoded in large chromosomal DNA fragments. *Proc. Natl. Acad. Sci. USA* **88,** 9623–9627.
3. Peterson A. S. (1998) Direct cDNA selection, in *Genome Analysis: A Laboratory Manual* (Birren, B., Green, E. D., Klapholz, S., Myers, R. M., and Roskams J., eds.), Cold Spring Harbor Laboratory, Cold Spring Harbor, NY, pp. 159–171.
4. Parimoo, S., Kolluri, R., and Weissman, S. M. (1993) cDNA selection from total yeast DNA containing YACs. *Nucleic Acids Res.* **21,** 4422–4423.
5. Sambrook, J., Fritsch, E. F., and Maniatis, T. (1989) *Molecular Cloning: A Laboratory Manual,* 2nd ed., Cold Spring Harbor Laboratory, Plainview, NY.

6. Sedlacek, Z., Korn, B., Koneki, D. S., Siebenhaar, R., Coy, J. F., Kioschis, P., and Poustka, A. (1993) Construction of a transcription map of a 300 kb region around the human G6PD locus by direct cDNA selection. *Hum. Mol. Genet.* **2,** 1865–1869.
7. Goldberg, M. L., Lifton, R. P., Stark, G. R., and Williams, J. G. (1979) Isolation of specific RNAs using DNA covalently linked to diazobenzyloxyrnethyl cellulose or paper. *Methods Enzymol.* **68,** 206–220.
8. Mancini, M., Sala, C., Rivella, S., and Toniolo, D. (1996) Selection and fine mapping of chromosome specific cDNAs: application to chromosome 1. *Genomics* **38,** 149–154.

14

Exon Trapping

Application of a Large-Insert Multiple-Exon-Trapping System

Martin C. Wapenaar and Johan T. Den Dunnen

1. Introduction

Exon trapping (**Fig. 1**) is a technique that has been developed to identify genes in cloned eukaryotic DNA (*1–7*). Compared with other techniques for gene identification, exon trapping has two main characteristic features. First, it is independent of the availability of an RNA sample in which the gene to identify is expressed. Second, the sequences isolated directly derive from the input DNA. Some 10–20% of all genes might be expressed at very low levels or only during very short stages of development, making it difficult to isolate them based on their expression using cDNA hybridization or cDNA selection protocols. Exon trapping uses an assay isolating sequences based on the presence of functional splice sites. Consequently, sequences are isolated directly from the clone under analysis without knowledge or availability of tissues expressing the gene to be identified. Furthermore, because isolation is not based on hybridization, it is not possible to isolate highly similar sequences that derive from other parts of the genome, not under analysis.

Through the efforts of the Human Genome Project, the number of mammalian genes that are currently being identified is increasing at an incredible rate. Most of these sequences derive from large-scale sequencing efforts in combination with comparisons against databases containing known genes and large collections of cDNA sequences (expressed sequence tags) and using software tools to identify genes. It is unclear, however, which proportion of the genes will be missed by such efforts. Therefore, to complete the human gene catalog, alternative methods such as exon trapping will be required to identify genes independent of expression.

From: *Methods in Molecular Biology, vol. 175: Genomics Protocols*
Edited by: M. P. Starkey and R. Elaswarapu © Humana Press Inc., Totowa, NJ

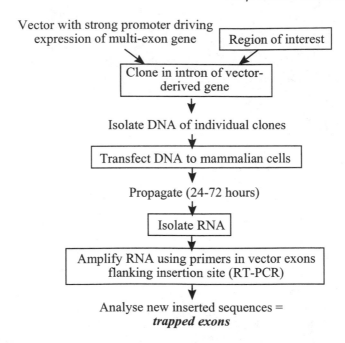

Fig. 1. Principle of exon trapping.

Initial exon-trapping systems were plasmid-based *(3,5)*, that is, they scanned 1 to 2-kb inserts. We have established a large-insert, cosmid-based multiple-exon-trapping system *(4)*, which is described herein. This system was developed to bypass the inherent problems related to small-insert systems: including: (i) the small chance to clone multiple exons together, and, consequently the isolation of single often small exons; (ii) the loss of the intrinsic information of "order" and the eradication of the genomic context, i.e., the overall structural exon/intron information, which increases the background of false positive clones (mainly trapped purely intronic sequences) considerably; and (iii) because the single trapped exons are usually used as probes (because they are small and yield weak signals) for cDNA library screening, the initial advantage of working with a system that is independent of expression will be lost.

1.1. Principle of Cosmid-Based Exon Trapping

The basic element of all exon-trapping vectors is a strong promoter that drives expression of a gene containing a cloning site in one of its introns (**Fig. 1**). The cosmid-based vectors (4) use a mouse metallothein promoter (mMT) to drive expression of the human growth hormone (hGH) gene with a multiple

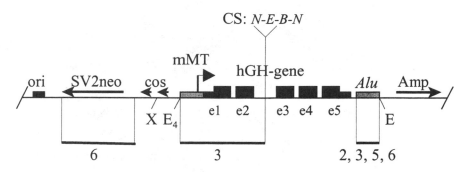

Fig. 2. The sCOGH-exon-trapping vectors. The basic figure shows sCOGH1, with the heavy bars below highlighting the segments that have been removed in the derived vectors, indicated by their number (e.g., 2 for the part missing in sCOGH2, i.e., the Alu-repeat [*Alu*] directly downstream of the hGH-gene). Amp, ampicillin resistance gene; cos, bacteriophage lambda derived cos sites; CS, *Bam*HI cloning site flanked by *Not*I sites; E, *Eco*RI site, e1 e5, exons 1–5 of the hGH gene; mMT, mouse metallothein promoter; ori, origin of replication for propagation in Escherichia coli; SV2neo, eukaryotic neomycin resistance marker; and X, *Xba*I site (used for linearization of the vector).

cloning site in intron two (**Fig. 2**). On transfer of the cloned DNA to mammalian cells, the hGH gene with insert is transiently transcribed from the mMT promoter. After propagation of the cells, RNA is isolated and hGH-derived transcripts are amplified using reverse transcriptase polymerase chain reaction (RT-PCR). If exonic sequences are present in the insert DNA, they will be trapped between the insert-flanking hGH exons 2 and 3. On agarose gel electrophoresis, the presence of trapped sequences becomes visible because PCR-products increase in size compared with the products derived from only the vector (**Fig. 1**).

Two consequences of large-insert exon trapping deserve special attention. First, when (part of) a gene is cloned, it can be expected that all exons are trapped in one product (**Fig. 2**). Consequently, RT-PCR amplification of the trapped products requires great care to ensure amplification of large products (>4 kb). Especially when 3'-terminal exons are present, the products may span several kilobases. Second, inserts may contain one or more 5'-first and/or 3'-terminal exons, and it is unclear whether the splicing machinery recognizes all these elements and how it will cope with them. 5'-First exons are probably not recognized since the promoter will be inactive in the cell line used for transformation and transcription probably runs over these exons. 3'-Terminal exons, however, will probably be recognized and produce a transcriptional stop although the formation of a fusion-gene-transcript, splice skipping an internal

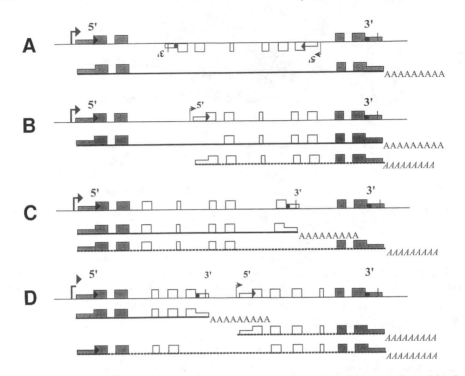

Fig. 3. Exon trapping with large-insert vectors: examples of inserts cloned in the vector-derived gene and the possible effects on RNA transcription and processing. Inserts (in white) are flanked by the vector-derived gene (gray). The transcripts that are most likely produced are represented by thick lines, transcripts that are probably not made, either because the promoter-driving transcription of the 5'-first exon is likely to be inactive in the cell type used for transfection or because transcription terminates at a 3'-terminal exon, are represented by broken lines. (**A**) Exons cloned in the wrong transcriptional orientation; no exons will be trapped. (**B**) Cloned 5'-first and internal exons; even when the promoter in the insert would be active, transcripts will run over the 5'-first exon and sequences can be trapped using vector-derived exon primers. When the promoter is active, a 5'-RACE protocol can be used to trap it (including downstream exons). (**C**) cloned several internal and one 3'-terminal exon; since the 3'-terminal exon will probably be recognized, the transcript will terminate there and a 3'-RACE-protocol will be required to trap the exons. (**D**) internal, a 5'-first and a 3'-ter-minal exon; the RT-PCR protocol to be used depends on the transcript(s) produced and the exons to be trapped. Large boxes represent internal exons and small boxes the 5' or 3'-untranslated regions of the 5'-first and 3'-terminal exons, respectively. The prominent arrow represents a promoter, the A-stretch, a transcript's poly A-tail.

3'-terminal exon, might also occur (**Fig. 3**). A 3'-RACE protocol (*6,7*) will be required to trap exons between a 5' vector–derived and a 3'-terminal insert-derived exon. Gene segments downstream will most probably be missed unless the cloned gene's promoter is active and a 5'-RACE protocol is used for amplification.

2. Materials

1. Qiagen Plasmid Midi and Maxi Kit (Qiagen, Santa Clarita, CA).
2. *Xba*I (10 U/µL); *Bam*HI (10 U/µL), *Sau*3AI (5 U/µL), SuRE/Cut™ buffers A, B, and H (Boehringer Mannheim, Germany).
3. 1X TBE buffer: 90 m*M* Tris; 90 m*M* boric acid; 1 m*M* EDTA, pH 8.3.
4. Agarose SeaKem LE and Seakem Gold (FMC, Rockland).
5. Phenol:chloroform (1:1).
6. 3 *M* NaAc, pH 5.6.
7. Ethanol.
8. TE buffer: 10 m*M* Tris-HCl; 1 m*M* EDTA, pH 7.4.
9. Shrimp alkaline phosphatase (SAP) (1 U/µL) and 10X SAP buffer (Amersham Life Science, Cleveland, OH).
10. T4 DNA ligase and 10X ligase buffer (Boehringer Mannheim).
11. Bovine serum albumin (BSA) (100 µg/mL) (Boehringer Mannheim, Germany).
12. H$_2$O and Milli-Q H$_2$O diethylpyrocarbonate (DEPC). DEPC treatment: Add 0.05–0.1% (v/v) of DEPC (Sigma, St. Louis, MO), leave overnight, and autoclave.
13. CHEF electrophoresis system, including cooling and programmable power supply (*see* **Note 1**).
14. Ethidium bromide solution (stock 10 mg/mL), used at a final concentration of 5 µg/mL.
15. Gigapack III Plus packaging extract and SM buffer (Stratagene, La Jolla, CA).
16. 10 m*M* MgSO$_4$.
17. LB broth: 10 g/L of Bacto@-tryptone; 5 g/L of Bacto@-yeast extract, 5 g/L of NaCl; pH 7.0, including 0.2% maltose and 10 m*M* MgSO$_4$.
18. Ampicillin (10 mg/mL stock).
19. LB plate with ampicillin; LB medium with 1.5% agar and 100 µg/mL of ampicillin
20. *Escherichia coli* strain XL1-Blue (Stratagene).
21. Glycerol.
22. Dulbecco's modified Eagle's medium (DMEM) with GlutaMAX I™, 4500 mg/L of D-glucose, 25 m*M* HEPES, without sodium pyruvate (Gibco-BRL, Life Technologies, Paisley, UK).
23. Fetal calf serum (FCS), mycoplasma and virus screened (Gibco-BRL).
24. Dulbecco's Phosphate Buffered Saline (DPBS), without Calcium and Magnesium (Gibco-BRL).
25. 10X Trypsin-EDTA, liquid (Gibco-BRL).
26. FuGENE™-6 Transfection Reagent (Boehringer Mannheim.
27. Reporter vector pcDNA3.1 (–)/Myc-His/*lacZ* (Invitrogen, Carlsbad, CA).
28. β-Gal Staining Set (Boehringer Mannheim).
29. hGH enzyme-linked immunosorbent assay (ELISA) Kit (Boehringer Mannheim).
30. RNAzol™ B (Biotecx, Houston, TX).
31. Magnetic mRNA Isolation Kit (HT Biotechnology, Cambridge, UK).

32. PBS: 8 mM Na$_2$HPO$_4$·2H$_2$O, 1.5 mM KH$_2$PO$_4$, 2.7 mM KCl, 0.137 mM NaCl.
33. Binding/elution buffer (BE buffer): PBS with 1 M NaCl, RNase free.
34. Tween-20.
35. BE2 buffer: BE buffer, 0.1% Tween-20 (RNase free).
36. Gene Amp® XL RNA PCR Kit (Perkin-Elmer, Norwalk, CT).
37. Expand™ Long Template PCR System (Boehringer Mannheim).
38. Primers (all listed 5' to 3'):
    a. hGHex 1/2: ATGGCTACAGGCTCCCGGA.
    b. hGHex4/5: TTCCAGCCTCCCCCATCAGCG.
    c. PolyT-REP: GGATCCGTCGACATCGATGAATTC(T)$_{25}$.
    d. hGHa: cgggatccTAATACGACTCACTATAGGCGTCTGCACCAGCTG-
       GCCTTTGAC (with *Bam*HI site facilitating cloning and a T7 RNA poly-
       merase promoter).
    e. hGHb: cgggatccCGTCTAGAGGGTTCTGCAGGAATGAATACTT (with
       *Bam*HI site facilitating cloning).
    f. REP: GGATCCGTCGACATCGATGAATTC.
    g. hGHaORF1: [TT]-CAGCTGGCCTTTGACACCTACCAGGAG.
    h. hGHaORF2: [TT]-GCAGCTGGCC TTT*C* ACACCTACCAGGAG (note *C*.
       differs from hGH sequence to provide an open reading frame [ORF]).
    i. hGHaORF3: [TT]-GGCAGCTGGCCTTTGACACCTACCAGGAG.
    j. [TT]-tail: cgggatccTAATACGACTCACTATAGGACAGACCACCATG
       (containing a *Bam*HI site for cloning, a T7 RNA polymerase promoter, and a
       Kozak translation initiation sequence).

3. Methods

3.1. Subcloning of PAC or BAC DNA in sCOGH2

The sCOGH system facilitates the scanning of large genomic regions, in one instance, for the presence of exons. Therefore, it would be advantageous to use the sCOGH vector already at the stage of contig construction in positional cloning projects since this facilitates a direct transition to the stage of gene identification. Cosmids can be generated, e.g., by subcloning a yeast artificial chromosome (YAC), PAC, or bacterial artificial chromosome (BAC) contig or by constructing a total genomic library and subsequent isolation of the clones spanning the region of interest.

The sCOGH system consists of several different vectors *(4)*. sCOGH2 is used for standard exon trapping. sCOGH5, missing the 3' end of the hGH gene (exons 3–5), was designed to trap 3'-terminal exons although such exons can probably also be isolated using sCOGH2 applying a 3'-RACE protocol (*see* **Subheading 3.4.1.**). sCOGH3 misses the mMT promoter and hGH exons 1 and 2 and can be used to trap 5'-first exons (isolated only when the clones are transformed to cells that can activate the gene's natural promoter). sCOGH3 should facilitate the targeted isolation of tissue-specific genes.

3.1.1. Preparation of Vector DNA

1. Digest 100 μg of purified sCOGH2 DNA (e.g., isolated with Qiagen Plasmid Maxi Kit) in 300 μL with 300 U of *XbaI* and 30 μL SuRE/Cut buffer H for 1 to 2 h at 37°C.
2. Check for complete linearization of the vector by running a 200-ng sample on a 0.8% agarose gel in 1X TBE.
3. Add an equal volume of phenol:chloroform (1:1) and vortex.
4. Centrifuge in an Eppendorf centrifuge for 5 min at maximum speed.
5. Collect the upper phase and precipitate the DNA by adding 1/10 vol of 3 *M* NaAc (pH 5.6) and 2 vol of ethanol. Keep on ice for 5 min and spin down for 10 min at maximum speed.
6. Resuspend the DNA pellet in 200 μL of TE (final concentration of 0.5 μg/μL). Set aside a 5-μL sample for a test ligation (*see* **step 8**).
7. Add 5.6 U of SAP and 23 μl, of 10X SAP buffer. Incubate for 90 min at 37°C followed by a deactivation of the enzyme at 65°C for 15 min.
8. Check for a proper SAP reaction by self-ligating the SAP-treated and nontreated *XbaI* digested vector. Add to 1 μL of each DNA sample 0.5 U of T4 DNA ligase, 1 μL of 10X ligase buffer, and 7.5 μL of H_2O. Incubate overnight at 15°C.
9. Run the samples side-by-side with the linearized vector without ligation on a 0.8% agarose gel in 1X TBE. Only the ligated vector without SAP treatment should give larger fragments owing to concatemerization of the vector.
10. Purify the *XbaI*/SAP-treated vector by phenol:chloroform (1:1) extraction and ethanol precipitation as described in **steps 3–5**. Dissolve the DNA pellet in 250 μL of H_2O.
11. Add 300 U *of BamHI*, 30 μL of SuRE/Cut buffer B, and H_2O to 300 μL and incubate for 1 to 2 h at 37°C. Check for complete digestion by running a 200-ng sample on a 0.8% agarose gel.
12. Extract with phenol:chloroform (1:1), ethanol precipitate as before, and redissolve the DNA in 100 μL (final concentration of 1 μg/μL).
13. Test self-ligation with 0.5 μL of the treated vector (**step 8**) and check on the gel (**step 9**). The intensity of the new (larger) bands appearing in the ligated sample gives an impression of the proficiency of the vector for cloning.

3.1.2. Partial Digestion of Insert DNA

Start with DNA of good quality, e.g., isolated with the Qiagen Plasmid Midi Kit.

1. Set up four parallel digestions of 2.5 μg of PAC or BAC DNA in a 12.5-μL vol including 1X SuRE/Cut buffer A and 100 μg/mL of BSA. Keep on ice (*see* **Note 2**).
2. Dilute the *Sau*3AI stock solution to 0.05 U/μL in 1X SuRE/Cut buffer A and 100 μg/mL of BSA (always prepare fresh and keep on ice).
3. Add 0.5, 1.0, 1.5, and 2.0 μL of the enzyme dilution to the respective DNA solutions, mix gently, and set immediately at 37°C for 1 h.
4. Stop the digestions by incubation at 65°C for 15 min and store the samples at 4°C.

5. Load 5 μL (1 μg) of each sample (including 1 μg of PAC/BAC DNA without digestion as control) on a 1% SeaKem Gold agarose gel in 0.5X TBE. The gel is placed
   in a CHEF electrophoresis tray and run at 5.5 V/cm for 12 h at 18°C (*see* **Note 1**).
6. After the run, stain the gel in an ethidium bromide solution and inspect on a
   UV-transilluminator. The ideal sample should have most of its DNA in the 30 to
   50-kb size range. Useful size markers are (concatenated) lambda DNA and
   *Hind*III digested lambda DNA.

3.1.3. Ligation and Packaging

1. Ligate 5 μL (1 μg) of the optimal partially digested DNA by adding 1 μL (1 μg)
   of *Xba*I/SAP/*Bam*HI-treated sCOGH2, 0.5 U of T4 DNA ligase, 0.8 μL of 10X
   ligase buffer, and H_2O to a final volume of 8 μL. Incubate overnight at 15°C.
2. Add 4 μL of the ligation to 25 μL of Gigapack III Plus packaging extract and
   incubate at 22°C for 2 h.
3. Add 500 μL of SM buffer and 20 μL of chloroform, mix, and spin briefly to
   sediment the debris. The phage solution is ready for titration (store at 4°C).
4. Grow an overnight culture of XLl-Blue (Stratagene) at 37°C in 2 mL of LB
   including 0.2% maltose and 10 mM $MgSO_4$. The next day inoculate 5 μL of this
   culture in 5 mL of the same medium and grow for another 4–6 h (keep OD_{600}
   below 1.0). Pellet the bacteria at 500g for 10 min and resuspend in 2.5 mL of 10
   mM $MgSO_4$.
5. Prepare a 1:10 and 1:50 dilution of the phage stock in SM buffer.
6. Mix 25 μL of the bacterial suspension with 25 μL of phage dilutions and incubate
   at 22°C for 30 min.
7. Add 200 μL of LB and incubate at 37°C for 1 h with intermittent shaking of the tube.
8. Plate the bacteria on an LB plate with ampicillin, incubate overnight at 37°C, and
   calculate the number of clones appearing from the titer of the phage stock (we
   usually obtain a cloning efficiency of about 1×10^6 clones/μg of insert DNA).
9. Isolate sufficient clones to cover the complexity of subcloned PAC or BAC. We
   grow the clones in microtiter plates with selection medium and 7.5% glycerol for
   efficient storage (at –80°C) and retrieval.

3.2. Transfection of Mammalian Cells

Transfection can be performed using many protocols, such as, lipofection,
electroporation, and calcium phosphate precipitation. In general, the standard
laboratory protocol is most effective. However, a test is recommended to
determine the transfection efficiency of the cosmid-sized DNA in combination
with the cell line used (*see* **Note 3**).

3.2.1. Lipofection

3.2.1.1. PREPARATION OF THE CELLS

1. Start with a 250-mL tissue culture flask of healthy, well-spread, Chinese hamster
   ovary (CHO) cells, growing in log phase in DMEM medium supplemented with
   10% FCS (*see* **Notes 4** and **5**).

2. Remove the culture medium, rinse the cells with 5 mL of DPBS, add 2 mL of 1X trypsin solution, and incubate at 37°C until the cells detach from the flask.
3. Stop the trypsin reaction by adding of 8 mL of DMEM. If the cells appear to clump together, carefully pipet the cells up and down until a single-cell solution is obtained.
4. Count the cells (e.g., with a Fuchs-Rosenthal counting chamber) and make a dilution of 1.5×10^5 cells/mL in DMEM with 10% FCS.
5. Plate 2 mL (3×10^5 cells) in a 35-mm dish (or 6-well plate) and incubate overnight at 37°C. The next day the cells are ready for transfection.

3.2.1.2. TRANSFECTION

1. Add 3 μL of FuGENE-6 Transfection Reagent directly into 97 μL of serum-free DMEM in a sterile tube, and incubate for 5 min at room temperature.
2. Add 1 μg (0.5–10 μL) of clone DNA (*see* **Notes 3** and **6**).
3. Dropwise, add the diluted FuGENE-6 solution to the DNA, mix gently, and incubate for 15 min at room temperature to allow for formation of complex.
4. Taking care to evenly distribute over the plate, add the FuGENE-6/DNA complex dropwise to the cells, swirl gently, and place back in the incubator (*see* **Note 7**).
5. After 24–48 h of propagation, RNA can be isolated for subsequent RT-PCR analysis, i.e., the actual exon trap experiment, or the expression of a reporter gene can be determined (*see* **Notes 8–10**).

3.3. RNA Isolation and Poly(A)⁺ Selection

The quality of the RNA preparation is one of the most critical elements of the entire procedure, especially for the reverse transcription reaction. RT-PCR analysis can be performed using total RNA, but, especially when long products need to be generated, we have obtained better results using polyA⁺ RNA. For polyA⁺ RNA isolation, several excellent techniques and kits are available. We have most successfully applied the Magnetic mRNA Isolation Kit (HT Biotechnology), using the manufacturer's protocol.

3.3.1. Isolation of Total RNA

1. Wash the tissue culture dishes twice with 2 mL of ice-cold DPBS.
2. Remove all the DPBS and add 2.5 mL RNAzol™ B. Allow the cells to lyse. This may take some time. If necessary, check lysis under a microscope.
3. Divide the solution over two vials (i.e., 1.25 mL each).
4. Add 125 μL of chloroform, shake vigorously for 15 s, and leave on ice for 15 min.
5. Pellet the suspension by centrifugation at 10,000*g* for 15 min at 4°C.
6. Transfer the upper aqueous phase to a fresh tube and add an equal volume of isopropanol.
7. Incubate for 5 min on ice.
8. Centrifuge at 10,000*g* for 15 min at 4°C.
9. Wash the pellet once with 1 mL of 75% ethanol by vortexing.

10. Centrifuge at 10,000g for 10 min at 4°C.
11. Remove all the supernatant, dissolve the pellet in 50 μL of Milli-Q H$_2$O/DEPC, and incubate for 10 min at 65°C.
12. Take 1 μL and analyze the RNA on a 2% TBE agarose gel. Use autoclaved RNase-free solutions and a clean electrophoresis tank.

3.3.2. Selection of Poly(A)+ RNA

1. Add an additional 50 μL of Milli-Q H$_2$O/DEPC. Heat the samples for 2 min at 65°C to disrupt secondary RNA structures and place directly on ice.
2. Wash the magnetic beads two to three times with BE buffer.
3. Resuspend the beads in BE2 buffer.
4. Add 100 μL of magnetic bead solution to the tubes containing the RNA samples. Incubate at 18–25°C for at least 10 min. Gently mix the beads during incubation.
5. Capture the beads with the magnetic stand, remove the supernatant, and wash twice with BE buffer.
6. Wash the beads once or twice with a twice-diluted BE buffer.
7. Resuspend the beads in 20 μL of Milli-Q H$_2$O/DEPC.
8. Elute the mRNA by heating to 65°C for 10 min.
9. RNA quality and quantity can be checked on the gel (optional). In general, 2 μL of the final RNA sample is sufficient for one RT-PCR analysis.

3.4. RT-PCR Amplification

The RT reaction is the most critical step of the entire procedure. Its efficiency largely determines the ultimate success of the approach. Generally, we perform two separate amplification reactions for each transfected cosmid (*see* **Note 11**): one to trap internal exons and another to trap 3'-terminal exons (with coamplified upstream internal exons). Reverse transcription and first- and second-round PCR can be performed according to standard laboratory protocols or following the directions of the suppliers of the various RT, PCR, and integrated RT-PCR systems. In large-insert exon trapping, it is absolutely essential to amplify large fragments. Especially when 3'-terminal exons are present, it can be expected that exon-containing fragments in excess of 4 kb need to be amplified, requiring special care during amplification. Therefore, these steps are performed using so-called long-range amplification systems such as the Gene Amp-XL RNA PCR kit (Perkin-Elmer) and the Expand Long Template PCR System (Boehringer Mannheim).

3.4.1. cDNA Synthesis (RT) and First-Round PCR Amplification

1. Set up two parallel reactions per transfected cosmid, to trap internal (a) and 3'-terminal exons (b). Use 2 μL of RNA sample per reaction.
2. Prime the RT reaction with primer hGHex4/5 (a) or primer PolyT-REP (b) (*see* **Note 11**).

3. Perform first-round PCR by adding primer hGHexl/2 (a) or primer hGHex1/2 (b). Use the following conditions for PCR cycling: one cycle of 5 min at 94°C; 30 cycles of 1 min at 94°C, 1 min at 60°C, and 2 min at 72°C; and a final extension of 10 min at 72°C. Amplification products should be stored at 4°C (*see* **Note 12**).

3.4.2. Second-Round PCR Amplification

Although the exon-trapping vector contains a strong promoter, expression is generally too low to yield visible amplification products after one round of PCR; a second PCR-round is thus required.

1. Use 1 µL of product of the RT-PCR reaction in the second-round PCR.
2. The nested PCR reaction is performed with primers hGHa and hGHb (trapping internal exons) or with primers hGHa and REP (trapping 3'-terminal exons) (*see* **Note 13**). Use the temperature cycling conditions as mentioned before (*see* **Subheading 3.4.1., step 3**).
3. Analyze the size and yield of the PCR products by loading 1/10 of the reaction on a 0.8% agarose gel run in 1X TBE (*see* **Notes 14** and **15**).

3.5. Characterization of Exon-Trapping Products

Depending on the size and number of exon-trapping products obtained, several of subsequent experiments can be envisaged. Sequencing in combination with database searches provides the most direct way to obtain detailed information of the trapped sequences. Trapped products are putative cDNAs and can also be used as such, e.g., to probe cDNA libraries, Northern blots, or tissue sections. However, no database hits or positive signals indicate that expression is below detection or that the correct tissue or developmental stage was not analyzed yet. Because an expression-independent gene identification system was used and expression of 10–20% of the genes may be very low (*see* **Subheading 1.**), this phenomenon might not be rare.

Because they provide an excellent marker to identify genuine coding gene sequences, we have designed an in vitro transcription/translation protocol to scan the trapped products for the presence of large ORFs (*4*). For this purpose, three second-round PCR reactions must be performed using three alternative forward primers, one for each ORF to test (*see* **Note 13**).

As soon as sequences are available from the ends of the trapped products, primers can be designed for further analysis. Two analyses are most obvious: amplification on genomic DNA to determine whether the amplified segment is interrupted by introns and a nested RT-PCR reaction on RNA (able to detect extremely low expression levels) to verify expression and to determine the expression profile. If in these analyses patient-derived material is used, one can directly proceed into the stage of mutation detection although neither the gene sequence nor the gene structure has been determined yet. Especially a combination with in vitro transcription/translation protocols (i.e., a protein truncation test *[8]*) is very attractive as a possibility to quickly scan a large set of patients for truncating mutations *(9)*.

4. Notes

1. Electrophoresis conditions should be chosen such that a good separation is obtained between 20 and 100 kb. Although very low percentage agarose gels can be used, we prefer pulsed-field gel electrophoresis. The CHEF electrophoresis equipment we use is homemade *(10)*. To obtain the separation mentioned, this system requires running conditions of 5.5 V/cm for 12 h at 18°C, using four identical cycles with a linear switch time increase from 1 to 7 s.

2. Although we have obtained partials in the proper size range in a reproducible fashion at enzyme concentrations of 1 to 4×10^{-2} U *Sau*3AI/µg of DNA, local laboratory conditions often vary, and it is recommended to start with testing a wider range of enzyme dilutions (for each enzyme dilution 2.5 µg of PAC- or BACBAG-DNA will be required).

3. The hGH-gene facilitates testing of the transfection efficiency by assaying the cell culture medium for hGH concentration *(4)*. Note, however, that using an empty sCOGH vector (measuring ~10 kb) to determine the optimal transfection protocol is probably not fully conclusive for the transfection efficiency obtained with a ~50-kb insert-containing cosmid clone. Most protocols that yield DNA that can be digested with restriction enzymes, without recognizable degradation (e.g., isolated with the Qiagen Plasmid Midi Kit), can be used for transfection. Note, however, that transfection efficiency depends on the quality of the DNA and it may vary from batch to batch.

4. Cell culturing should start about 1 wk before the transfection will be performed, depending on the growth rate of the cells and the number of cells required. Always start with a fresh inoculate derived from a batch of cells stored in liquid nitrogen. Do not culture cells for longer than 3 wk before transfection. During growth, take care that the cells are nicely spread and that the flasks are not too full.

5. Because the mMT promoter of the sCOGH vector is active in most cells, exon trapping can be performed using any rapidly growing mammalian cell line that can be transfected with high efficiency using cosmid-sized DNA. To facilitate low-background RT-PCR amplification of sCOGH-derived exon-trapping products, rodent cell lines are used since these enable the design of human-specific GH primers that do not amplify endogenous transcripts *(4)*. We have worked most successfully with CHO cells, but other Chinese hamster (V79 *[4]*), rat, and murine cells also gave good results.

6. Theoretically, 50% of the clones will contain the genomic insert in the wrong transcriptional orientation (*see* also **Note 14**). Because the splicing machinery will not recognize exons in the cloned segment, this exon-trapping procedure will generate an "empty" (0.2-kb) hGH exon 2 to 3 splice product. Different large-insert clones should thus not be mixed in an exon-trapping experiment since

this will favor isolation of the smallest (i.e., the least interesting) empty exon-trapping products.

7. Because the reagent/DNA complex does not appear to have a cytotoxic effect, it is not necessary to replace the medium during lipofection.

8. The transfection efficiency can be determined using a LacZ reporter vector (e.g., pcDNA3.1[–]/Myc-His/*lacZ*); the number of blue cells appearing after X-Gal staining is a simple measure for the transfection efficiency. Using the lipofection protocol provided, we usually obtain a frequency of 5–10% blue-staining CHO cells. The level of expression of the hGH gene after lipofection with an empty sCOGH2 vector can also be used to measure the transfection efficiency. Excreted hGH protein in the culture medium can be sampled at different time intervals and determined in an hGH ELISA assay. Using this latter protocol, it is also possible to determine the optimal time for harvesting of the cells prior to RNA isolation (i.e., the point when the expression of the transfected DNA is at its peak). We usually measure about 40 ng/mL of excreted hGH protein in the medium 24–48 h posttransfection.

9. Expression from the mMT promoter can be boosted by culturing the cells in the presence of heavy metal ions such as Zn^{2+} and Cd^{2+} *(11)*. However, owing to the death of a large fraction of cells, the total RNA yield will not increase the concentration of the desired transcript. This may be advantageous to decrease the background of undesired RT-PCR products and thus the chance to amplify large regions (*see* **Note 11**). For clones constructed in sCOGHl-5, successfully transfected cells can be selected using neomycin *(4)*.

10. Nonsense-mediated mRNA decay is a well-known process that destroys mRNAs containing internal stop codons *(12)*. Incubation of the cells with cycloheximide (100 µg/mL for 4–8 h prior to harvesting) can be used to specifically increase the yield of these RNAs *(13)*. Because most RNAs generated by the exon-trapping procedure will not be in-frame with that of the hGH-gene, the cycloheximide treatment may be advantageous.

11 The RT reaction is the most critical step of the entire procedure. The primers used during amplification determine whether internal, 5'-first, or 3'-terminal exons are isolated (**Fig. 3**). In general, two RT-PCR amplifications are performed on each cosmid: one to trap internal and one to trap 3'-terminal exons, the latter using a 3'-RACE protocol. Amplification of long RT-PCR products critically depends on the absence of small target sequences, since these will be highly favored during the two-step amplification procedure (*see* also **Note 6**). Consequently, no endogenous growth hormone transcripts should be amplified, because these yield RT-PCR products of 0.2 kb. We achieve this by using rodent cell lines (*see* also **Note 5**). Background is further reduced by the use of primers that are not able to amplify genomic or vector DNA; primers such as hGHex1/2 and hGHex4/5 span two flanking exons and anneal exclusively on correctly spliced RNA.

12. After reverse transcription, RNA can be degraded by performing an RNaseA treatment, which may significantly increase the yield of the RT-PCR products obtained.

13. To facilitate a scan of the trapped products for the presence of large ORFs, perform three independent second-round PCR reactions, replacing primer hGHa with primers hGHaORF1, hGHaORF2, and hGHaORF3, respectively. The PCR products can be tested for the presence of large ORFs using an in vitro transcription/translation assay *(4)*.

14. Theoretically, each clone should yield a product. Clones containing the insert in the wrong transcriptional orientation (50% of the clones) or containing an insert from "exonless" (i.e., intragenic or purely intronic, regions produce the 0.2-kb "empty" hGH exon 2 to 3 spliced vector product (*see* **Note 6**). Clones containing exons should yield products of >0.2 kb up to a size determined by the technical limitation of the RT-PCR protocol applied, usually 2–4.5 kb. Each RT-PCR reaction should include a positive control to determine the actual size limit obtained experimentally. When no product is obtained and all controls (transformation efficiency, RNA isolation, and RT-PCR) indicate that there were no technical failures, the most attractive conclusion is that the trapped sequences were too large to amplify. A positive control for this conclusion can be a clone containing the same region in the opposite transcriptional orientation, yielding the 0.2-kb empty trap product (*see* **Note 11**).

15. The sCOGH vectors contain *Not*I sites flanking the cloning site, facilitating the isolation of the insert and the construction of clones in which the orientation of the insert is reversed (by *Not*I digestion and ligation, i.e., recircularization). To avoid the isolation of clones that contain only circularized cosmid vector, a packaging step is essential in this procedure (*see* **Subheading 3.1.3.**). Another possibility is to perform the exon trapping using a clone contig of high redundancy, thereby increasing the chance that every segment is covered by more than one clone and thus in both transcriptional orientations.

Acknowledgments

We acknowledge Hans Dauwerse, Nicole Datson, Esther van de Vosse, Paola van de Bent-Klootwijk, and Gert-Jan van Ommen for technical assistance and scientific input during the development of the sCOGH exon-trapping system. The exon trap system was developed with financial support from the Dutch Scientific Organization for Pure Research (NWO) and the European Union (BIOMED-2 grant PL962674).

References

1. Auch, D. and Reth, M. (1990) Exon trap cloning: using PCR to rapidly detect and clone exons from genomic DNA fragments. *Nucleic Acids Res.* **18,** 6743, 6744.
2. Duyk, G. M., Kim, S., Myers, R. M., and Cox, D. R. (1990) Exon trapping: a genetic screen to identify candidate transcribed sequences in cloned mammalian genomic DNA. *Proc. Natl. Acad. Sci. USA* **87,** 8995–8999.
3. Church, D. M., Stotler, C. J., Rutter, J. L., Murrell, J. R., Trofatter, J. A., and Buckler, A.J. (1994) Isolation of genes from complex sources of mammalian genomic DNA using exon amplification. *Nature Genet.* **6,** 98–105.

4. Datson, N. A., Van De Vosse, E., Dauwerse, J. G., Bout, M., Van Ommen, G. J. B., and Den Dunnen, J. T. (1996) Scanning for genes in large genomic regions: cosmid-based exon trapping of multiple exons in a single product. *Nucleic Acids Res.* **24,** 1105–1111.

5. Burn, T. C., Connors, T. D., Klinger, K. W., and Landes, G. M. (1995) Increased axon-trapping efficiency through modifications to the pSPL3 splicing vector. *Gene* **161,** 83–87.

6. Datson, N. A., Duyk, G. M., Van Ommen, G. J. B., and Den Dunnen, J. T. (1994) Specific isolation of 3'-terminal exons of human genes by exon trapping. *Nucleic Acids Res.* **22,** 4148–4153.

7. Krizman, D. B. and Berget, S. M. (1993) Efficient selection of 3'-terminal exons from vertebrate DNA. *Nucleic Acids Res.* **21,** 5198–5202.

8. Roest, P. A. M., Roberts, R. G., Sugino, S., Van Ommen, G. J. B., and Den Dunnen, J. T. (1993) Protein truncation test (PTT) for rapid detection of translation-terminating mutations. *Hum. Mol Genet* **2,** 1719- 1721.

9. Petrij, F., Giles, R. H., Danwerse, J. G., Saris, J. J., Hennekam, R. C. M., Masuno, M., Tommerup, N., Van Ommen, G. J. B., Goodman, R. H., Peters, D. J. M., and Breuning, M. H. (1995) Rubinstein-Taybi syndrome caused by mutations in the transcriptional co-activator CBP. *Nature* **376,** 348–351.

10. Den Dunnen, J. T., Grootscholten, P. M. and Van Ommen, G. J. B. (1993) Pulsed-field gel electrophoresis in the analysis of genomic DNA and YAC clones, in *Human Genetic Disease Analysis: A Practical Approach* (Davies, K. E., ed.), Oxford University Press, Oxford, pp. 35–58.

11. Searle, P. F., Stuart, G. W., and Palmiter, R. D. (1985) Building a metal-responsive promoter with synthetic regulatory elements. *Mol. Cell. Biol.* **5,** 1480 1488.

12. Hentze, M. W. and Kulozik, A. E. (1999) A perfect message: RNA surveillance and nonsense-mediated decay. *Cell* **96,** 307–310.

13. Carter, M. S., Doskow, J., Morris, P., Li, S., Nhim, R. P., Sandstedt, S., and Wilkinson, M. F. (1995) A regulatory mechanism that detects premature nonsense codons in T-cell receptor transcripts in vivo is reversed by protein synthesis inhibitors in vitro. *J. Biol. Chem.* **270,** 28,995–29,003.

15

Sequencing Bacterial Artificial Chromosomes

David E. Harris and Lee Murphy

1. Introduction

Over the last 7 years, there have been enormous changes to the methods being used to sequence DNA. These changes include the increased use of fluorescent dyes to label DNA in the sequencing reaction, improvements to automated sequencers, and the use of high-throughput methods for preparing and sequencing DNA samples. The results of these developments have been to improve sequence accuracy, greatly increase the rate of sequence output, and, most important, reduce the cost. While further developments are to be expected, note that the basic sequencing chemistries are direct developments of the dideoxy chain-termination method of Sanger et al. *(1)*.

Many sequencing projects involve mapped bacterial clones, and although at one time cosmids were the most widely used vector system, bacterial artificial chromosomes (BACs) are now preferred owing to their large insert size and stability. This chapter describes methods for sequencing BACs that have been used successfully in several sequencing projects to produce large amounts of data.

The methods have been written with the assumption that the objective of the sequencing project is to produce contiguous, high-quality sequence (i.e., sequence better than 99.99% accurate). The approach involves two stages. An initial random (shotgun) phase involves fragmentation of the BAC DNA and ligation of the 1.4 to 2.0-kb fragments into a suitable sequencing vector. Preparation and sequencing of a large number of these subclones generates many sequences derived at random from the target DNA. Assembly of these sequences (reads) and correction of disagreements by editing provides most of the BAC sequence, much of which will be highly accurate (i.e., finished). At the end of this shotgun stage it is likely that the sequence will contain a number

From: *Methods in Molecular Biology, vol. 175: Genomics Protocols*
Edited by: M. P. Starkey and R. Elaswarapu © Humana Press Inc., Totowa, NJ

of gaps and also some regions of poor quality. To bring the sequence to the desired accuracy, a second stage of directed sequencing (finishing) is performed.

There is clearly a balance between the shotgun and finishing stages, that is, projects containing a large number of randomly generated reads from the shotgun are likely to need less finishing than those containing fewer shotgun reads. On the other hand, it is wasteful to put an unnecessarily large number of shotgun reads into a project. The sequencing strategy should be planned so as to produce the finished sequence in an efficient manner, performing as few sequencing reactions as possible in order to achieve the required sequence quality.

The result of much experience suggests that if a sequence meets the following criteria it is likely to be better than 99.99% accurate:

1. The consensus must be produced from a minimum of two high-quality sequences that agree and that have been obtained from different subclones (i.e., the entire sequence should be covered with sequence from at least two subclones).
2. These high-quality sequences must be obtained from reads from the two opposite DNA strands (i.e., the sequence must be double stranded) or high-quality sequences from several subclones (all from the same DNA strand) must be obtained using at least two different sequencing chemistries. This can be either a combination of dye-primer and dye terminator reads or a combination of two different dye-terminator chemistries (e.g., AmpliTaqFS/dye terminator and BigDye terminator).

Before starting, it is necessary to decide how many shotgun reads should be produced. For efficient sequencing, the shotgun should give double-stranded coverage of most of the target sequence, and although a small number of gaps are likely to be present when the shotgun reads are first assembled, these should be sequence gaps (not clone gaps). The shotgun should give complete clone coverage even if it has not produced complete sequence coverage. The experience from many sequencing projects shows the optimum shotgun stage is reached when the average coverage of the target sequence is six- to eightfold. Thus, for a BAC containing a 150-kb insert, the shotgun should produce 90,0000 to 1,200,000-bp of sequences from the insert. The number of sequences needed to provide this coverage depends on the average read length, and, therefore, a project yielding an average of 450 bp per read will need 2000–2700 good-quality reads from the insert to achieve the desired coverage.

The shotgun will actually need more reads because there will be losses owing to the fact that the shotgun is performed on the complete BAC (assume that 5–10% of the sequences will be from the BAC vector) and also losses because of poor-quality sequence (assume 10–15% loss).

A further decision needs to be made as to which sequencing vector to use. Two widely used systems are the single-stranded vector M13mp18 (M13) and the double-stranded plasmid pUC 18. There are useful features of both systems. Libraries produced with M13 as the sequencing template can give more random representation of the target sequence than those produced in pUC18. M13s are particularly useful in giving representation of "difficult" sequences (i.e., DNA showing extreme compositional bias), and sequences obtained from M13 templates are typically longer and "cleaner" than those obtained from double-stranded templates. pUC18 templates are useful because they provide two reads for each template prepared. In addition, the two reads obtained from a pUC template will be in a known orientation and will be a known distance apart. The paired reads from pUCs provide information that is very useful in confirming assemblies and in helping to identify misassemblies owing to the presence of sequence repeats, and they often help connect contigs (e.g., if the two reads from a pUC template assemble into different contigs, then the orientation of the two contigs and the size of the sequence gap between them will be known).

In summary, the shotgun stage to sequence a BAC with a 150-kb insert (in which the composition of the DNA is 35–55% G+C) should consist of 14 × 96-well plates of pUC18 templates (this will produce 2688 reads) and 6 × 96-well plates of M13 templates (giving 576 reads). Starting with a total of 2964 reads, the assembled shotgun should contain >2200 reads (allowing for vector and quality losses), which should give between six- and eightfold coverage.

If the DNA sequence is known to be of extreme composition (particularly if it is high G+C), then the proportion of reads produced from M13 templates should be increased.

2. Materials

2.1. Preparation of BAC DNA

1. 2X TY: 16 g of tryptone, 10 g of yeast extract, 5 g of NaCl, and double-distilled water (ddH$_2$O) to a final volume of 1 L. Adjust to pH 7.4 with NaOH, dispense into required portions, and autoclave.
2. Chloramphenicol (Sigma-Aldrich, Poole, Dorset, UK).
3. 10 m*M* EDTA, pH 8.0.
4. Sodium dodecyl sulfate (SDS)/NaOH: Combine 25 mL of 20% (w/v) SDS, 25 mL of 4 *M* NaOH, and 450 mL of ddH$_2$O.
5. 3 *M* Potassium acetate (KOAc): Mix 100 mL of 7.5 *M* KOAc (*see* **item 8**) and 46 mL of glacial acetic acid with 254 mL of ddH$_2$O.
6. Isopropanol (propan-2-ol).
7. 10 m*M* Tris-HCl, pH 8.0, 50 m*M* EDTA.
8. 7.5M KOAc: Dissolve 368.03 g of KOAc in ddH$_2$O to a final volume of 500 mL (do not adjust the pH of the solution).
9. 96% (v/v) Ethanol.

10. 50 m*M* Tris-HCl, pH 8.0, 50 m*M* EDTA.
11. RNase (DNase-free) solution (10 mg/mL).
12. Phenol-chloroform.
13. Chloroform.
14. 70% (v/v) Ethanol.
15. TE (10:0.1): 10 m*M* Tris-HCl, pH 8.0, 0.1 m*M* EDTA.

2.2. Preparation of Subclone Libraries

2.2.1. Preparation of DNA Fragments

1. 10X mb buffer: 300 m*M* sodium acetate (NaOAc), pH 5.0; 500 m*M* NaCl; 10 m*M* ZnCl$_2$, 50% (v/v) glycerol.
2. Mung bean nuclease (100 U/μL) (Promega UK, Southampton, UK).
3. 1 *M* NaCl.
4. 96% (v/v) ethanol.
5. TE (10:0.1): 10 m*M* Tris-HCl, pH 8.0, 0.1 m*M* EDTA.
6. Ficoll loading dye solution: 0.5 mL of 10X TBE, 0.5 g of Ficoll 400 (Amersham Pharmacia Biotech, Amersham, UK), 5 mg of bromophenol blue, 4.5 mL of ddH$_2$O.
7. Dye mix: 625 μL of TE, 75 μL of 10X TAE, 200 μL of Ficoll loading dye solution.
8. Low melting point agarose.
9. AgarACE (Promega, UK).
10. Pellet paint (Cambridge Bioscience, Cambridge, UK).
11. TE-equilibrated phenol.

2.2.2. Preparation of M13 Library

1. M13mp18 *Sma*I-CIP: M13mp18 digested with *Sma*I and treated with calf intestinal phosphatase; prepared in-house or obtained from Appligene Oncor (Illkirch, France).
2. T4 DNA ligase (5 U/μL) and 10X ligase buffer (Roche, Lewes, East Sussex, UK).
3. Premix for each ligation: 3.8 μL of ddH$_2$O, 0.2 μL of M13mp18 *Sma*I-CIP, and 1 μL of 10X ligase buffer.
4. Ficoll 400 (Amersham Pharmacia Biotech).
5. Prep-A-Gene DNA purification kit (Bio-Rad, Hemel Hempstead, Hertfordshire, UK).

2.2.3. Preparation of pUC18 Library

1. pUC18 *Sma*I-CIP: pUC18 digested with *Sma*I and treated with calf intestinal phosphatase; prepared in-house or obtained from Appligene Oncor.
2. 5 DNA ligase (U/μL T4) and 10X ligase buffer (Roche).

2.2.4. Transformation by Electroporation

1. 10% (v/v) Glycerol solution.
2. H-top agar: 8 g of bacto agar, 10 g of bacto tryptone, 8 g of NaCl and ddH$_2$O to 1 L. Heat to dissolve the agar, autoclave, and dispense into portions.

3. SOB medium: 20 g of tryptone, 5 g of yeast extract, 10 mL of 1 M NaCl, 0.15 g of KCl and ddH$_2$O to 1 L. Autoclave, add MgCl$_2$ to 20 mM, and dispense in 10-mL portions.
4. SOC medium: Heat 10 mL of SOB to 45°C and add 200 μL of 20% (w/v) glucose.
5. Isopropyl β-D-thiogalactopyranoside (IPTG) (40 mg/mL) in ddH$_2$O.
6. 5-Bromo-4-chloro-3-indolyl-β-D-galactopyranosie (X-gal) (50 mg/mL) in dimethylformamide.
7. TYE plates for M13s: 15 g of agar, 8 g of NaCl, 10 g of bacto tryptone, 5 g of yeast extract, and ddH$_2$O to 1 L. Autoclave and pour plates.
8. Ampicillin (Sigma-Aldrich).
9. TYE-amp plates for pUCs: 15 g of agar, 8 g of NaCl, 10 g of bacto tryptone, 5 g of yeast extract, and ddH$_2$O to 1 L. Autoclave and allow to cool. Add ampicillin to 100 μg/mL, IPTG to 208 μg/mL, and X-gal to 167 μg/mL.
10. Gene Pulser (Bio-Rad).

2.3. Preparation of DNA Sequencing Templates

2.3.1. Preparation of Single-Stranded M13 DNA by Triton-Based Method (Triton Preparation)

1. Circlegrow (Anachem, Luton, Bedfordshire, UK).
2. 20% (w/v) Polyethylene glycol (PEG) 8000/2.5 M NaCl: Dissolve 200 g of PEG 8000 and 146.1 g of NaCl in ddH$_2$O to a final volume of 1 L.
3. Triton-TE extraction buffer: 10 mM Tris-HCl, pH 8.0, 1 mM EDTA, 0.5% (v/v) Triton X-100 (Sigma-Aldrich).
4. 3 M NaOAc, pH 4.8: Dissolve 408.2 g of NaOAc·3H$_2$O in approx 700 mL of ddH$_2$O. Adjust the pH of the solution to 4.8 with glacial acetic acid and make up to 1 L with ddH$_2$O. Filter through a Costar bottle-top filter (0.2-μm) and autoclave.
5. 96% (v/v) Ethanol.
6. 70% (v/v) Ethanol: Store at –20°C in a sparkproof freezer. Use cold.
7. Deep-well 96-well microtiter plates (cat. no. 140504; Beckman, Fullerton, CA).
8. Plate Sealer (cat. no. 5701; Dynex, Chantilly, VA).
9. Falcon Pro-Bind U-Bottom Plate (cat. no. 35-3910; Becton Dickinson, Cowley, Oxford, UK).
10. Metal foil tape (cat. no. ZSF-A-100; Warth International, East Grinstead, Sussex, UK).

2.3.2. Preparation of Double-Stranded pUC18 DNA

1. Circlegrow (Anachem).
2. Ampicillin (Sigma-Aldrich).
3. GTE: 2.3 mL of 20% (w/v) glucose, 5.0 mL of 0.1 M EDTA, 1.3 mL of 1 M Tris-HCl, pH 7.4, and 42 mL of ddH$_2$O.
4. Lysis solution: 2.5 mL of 4 M NaOH, 2.5 mL of 20% (w/v) SDS, and 45 mL of ddH$_2$O. Store at room temperature and use within 2 d.

5. 3 *M* KOAc: 147.2 g of KOAc, 7.5 mL of glacial acetic acid, and ddH$_2$O to 500 mL. Store at 4°C.
6. RNase A solution (20 mg/mL): 200 mg of RNase A, 100 µL of 1 *M* Tris-HCl, pH 7.4, 150 µL of 1 *M* NaCl, and ddH$_2$O to 10 mL. The solution should be dispensed into small portions and stored frozen at –20°C.
7. Deep-well 96-well microtiter plates (cat. no. 140504; Beckman).
8. Plate Sealer (cat. no. 5701; Dynex).
9. Falcon Pro-Bind U-Bottom Plate (cat. no. 35-3910; Becton Dickinson).
10. 3M Scotch Pad sealer (UPC part no. 021200-61618; 3M Center, St. Paul, MN).
11. Multiscreen filter plate (MAGVN2250; Millipore [UK], Watford, UK).
12. Falcon 3910 96-well plate (Becton Dickinson).

2.4. Sequencing Single or Double-Stranded Templates with AmpliTaq FS/Dye Terminators

1. Dye Terminator Ready Reaction Kit (PE Applied Biosystems, Warrington, Cheshire, UK). Dispense into 1.6-mL portions in 2-mL Eppendorf tubes and store at –20°C.
2. Primer (*see* **Note 1**): 1 pmol/µL in TE (10:0. 1) dispensed in 500-µL portions in 1.5-mL Eppendorf tubes and stored at –20°C.
3. Ethanol/acetate: Mix 16 mL of 96% (v/v) ethanol with 0.5 mL of 3 *M* NaOAc, pH 4.8.
4. 70% (v/v) Ethanol.
5. Costar Thermowell 96-well plate (Model C) (cat. no. 6510; Corning Costar, Acton, MA).
6. Rubber mat (cat. no. HB-TD-MT-SRS-5; Hybaid, Teddington, Middlesex, UK).
7. Thermal cycler, e.g., Omnigene (Hybaid), or PTC-225 (MJ Research, Braintree, Essex, UK).
8. Rubber cushion (used to support a thin-walled microtiter plate during centrifugation) (cat. no. 11174207; Jouan S.A., Saint-Herblain, France).

2.4.1. Directed Sequencing Using BigDye Terminator

1. BigDye Terminator Cycle Sequencing Ready Reaction Kit (PE Applied Biosystems).
2. Primer (*see* **Note 2**).
3. 96% (v/v) Ethanol/3 *M* sodium acetate, pH 4.8, mixed at 16:1 ratio. Store at room temperature.
4. 70% (v/v) Ethanol. Store at –20°C.
5. Costar Thermowell 96-well plate (Model C) (cat. no. 6510; Corning Costar).
6. Rubber mat (cat. no. HB-TD-MT-SRS-5; Hybaid).
7. Thermal cycler, e.g., Omnigene (Hybaid), or PTC-225 (MJ Research).
8. Rubber cushion (cat. no. 1114207; Jouan).

2.4.2. Directed Sequencing Using BigDye Primer

1. BigDye Primer Cycle Sequencing Ready Reaction Kit (PE Applied Biosystems).
2. 96% (v/v) ethanol. Store at 4°C.

3. Costar Thermowell 96-well plate (Model C) (cat. no. 6510; Corning Costar).
4. Rubber mat (cat. no. HB-TD-MT-SRS-5; Hybaid).
5. Thermal cycler, e.g., Omnigene (Hybaid) or PTC-225 (MJ Research).
6. Rubber cushion (cat. no. 1114207; Jouan).

2.4.3. Preparation of Sequencing Template by PCR

1. 4X 1.25 mM dNTPs (dNTP mix) (Amersham Pharmacia Biotech).
2. 10X *Taq* buffer: 1.0 mL of 1 M Tris-HCl, pH 8.5, 2.5 mL of 2M KCl, 75 µL of 2 M MgCl$_2$, and 6.4 mL of ddH$_2$O.
3. AmpliTaq polymerase (5 U/µL) (PE Applied Biosystems).
4. Primer (*see* **Note 3**).
5. 20% (w/v) PEG 8000/2.5 M NaCl: Dissolve 200 g of PEG 8000 and 146.1 g of NaCl in ddH$_2$O to a final volume of 1 L.
6. Costar Thermowell 96-well plate (Model C) (cat. no. 6510; Corning Costar).
7. Rubber mat (cat. no. HB-TD-MT-SRS-5; Hybaid).
8. Thermal cycler, e.g., Omnigene (Hybaid) or PTC-225 (MJ Research).
9. Rubber cushion (cat. no. 1114207; Jouan).

3. Methods

3.1. Preparation of BAC DNA

1. Pick a single colony into 200 mL of 2X TY containing the appropriate antibiotic (e.g., chloramphenicol at 25 µg/mL for vector pBACe3.6) in a 500-mL conical flask and shake at 300 rpm at 37°C for 18 h.
2. Transfer the culture to a 250-mL centrifuge tube and centrifuge at 3500g at room temperature for 5 min.
3. Pour off the supernatant and allow the pellet to drain for a few minutes.
4. Resuspend the pellet in 20 mL of 10 mM EDTA, pH 8.0, and leave to cool in ice for 5 mm.
5. Pour 40 mL of fresh SDS/NaOH into the centrifuge tube, but do not mix the solutions by agitation (the solutions will mix sufficiently as the SDS/NaOH is added). Leave to cool in ice for 5–10 min.
6. Add 30 mL of ice-cold 3 M KOAc, but do not mix. Leave to cool in ice for 15 min.
7. Centrifuge at 9600g at room temperature for 15 min.
8. Pour the supernatant into a fresh 250-mL centrifuge tube and centrifuge at 9600g at room temperature for 15 min.
9. Pour the supernatant into a fresh 250-mL centrifuge tube, add 45 mL of isopropanol and mix.
10. Centrifuge at 2400g at room temperature for 15 min.
11. Pour off and discard the supernatant and resuspend the pellet in 8 mL of 10 mM Tris-HCl, pH 8.0, and 50 mM EDTA.
12. Transfer the solution to a 50-mL centrifuge tube and add 4 mL of 7.5 M KOAc. Leave the tube at –70°C for 30 min.
13. Thaw the solution and centrifuge at 2400g at room temperature for 30 min.

14. Place 24 mL of 96% (v/v) ethanol in a fresh 50-mL centrifuge tube and add the supernatant from **step 13**. Mix gently.

15. Centrifuge at 1200*g* at room temperature for 10 min.

16. Pour off and discard the supernatant and resuspend the pellet in 700 µL of 50 m*M* Tris-HCl, 50 m*M* EDTA.

17. Transfer the solution to a 1.5-mL Eppendorf tube and add 10 µL of RNase solution (DNase free).

18. Incubate at 37°C for 1 h.

19. Extract the solution twice with 800 µL of phenol:chloroform and once with 800 µL of chloroform. After each extraction remove and discard the non-aqueous layer.

20. Add 700 µL of isopropanol to the aqueous solution.

21. Centrifuge at 13,000*g* at room temperature for 5 min.

22. Remove and discard the supernatant and wash the pellet with 500 µL of 70% (v/v) ethanol.

23. Centrifuge at 13,000*g* at room temperature for 5 min.

24. Remove and discard the supernatant and dry the pellet.

25. Resuspend the supernatant in 40 µL of TE.

26. Make a 10-fold dilution (10XD) by mixing 0.5 µL of BAC DNA and 4.5 µL of TE in a 0.5 mL Eppendorf tube.

27. Estimate the concentration of BAC DNA by gel electrophoresis of 1 µL of a 10XD in 0.5% (w/v) agarose with markers containing known amounts of DNA (*see* **Note 4**).

28. Estimate the volume of undiluted BAC stock solution that contains 10 µg of DNA.

3.2. Preparation of Subclone Libraries (2)

3.2.1. Preparation of DNA Fragments

1. Transfer a measured volume of BAC stock solution equal to 10 µg of DNA into a fresh 1.5-mL tube. Add 6 µL of 10X mb buffer, followed by ddH$_2$O to a final volume of 60 µL.

2. Fragment the BAC DNA by sonication (*see* **Note 5**).

3. Add 0.3 µL of mung bean nuclease, mix gently, briefly centrifuge to settle contents, and incubate for 10 min in a water bath at 30°C.

4. Add 14 µL of ddH$_2$O, 20 µL of 1 *M* NaCl, and 560 µL of ice-cold 100% (v/v) ethanol. Leave at –20°C overnight (or at –70°C for 30 min). Pellet the DNA by centrifugation at 13,000*g* at 4°C for 30 min. Wash with 500 µL of ice-cold 70% (v/v) ethanol and dry.

5. Resuspend the DNA pellet in 9 µL of dye mix.

6. Separate the DNA fragments by electrophoresis through a 0.8% (w/v) low melting point agarose gel with a range of molecular weight markers (*see* **Note 6**).

7. On a long-wave UV-transilluminator, cut out the agarose blocks containing 0.6 to 1 kb, 1 to 1.4, 1.4 to 2, and 2 to 4-kb DNA fragments. Place each block in a labeled 1.5-mL Eppendorf tube (*see* **Note 7**).

8. Melt each gel slice to be extracted at 65°C for 5 min. Transfer each tube to 42°C, and after 5 min, add 5 μL of AgarACE per 200-μL volume and incubate at 42°C for at least 20 min.

9. Add an equal volume of TE-equilibrated phenol, mix thoroughly, and centrifuge briefly at 13,000*g* to separate the two liquid phases. Transfer the upper (aqueous) layer to another 1.5-mL tube.

10. Ethanol precipitate by adding 1/10 vol of 1 *M* NaCl, 2.5 volumes of 100% (v/v) ethanol, and 1 μL of pellet paint.

11. Centrifuge at 13,000*g*, 4°C for 30 min, wash with 500 μL of ice-cold 70% (v/v) ethanol and air dry.

12. Resuspend in 8 μL of TE (10:0.1).

13. Store the DNA fragments at –20°C.

3.2.2. Preparation of M13 Library

1. Add to a 0.5-mL Eppendorf tube, 21 μL of the 1.4 to 2-kb DNA solution from **step 7** in **Subheading 3.2.1.**, 5 μL of premix, 3 μL of 50% (w/v) Ficoll, and 0.5 μL of T$_4$ DNA ligase.

2. Pipet to mix. Centrifuge briefly to settle the tube contents and then incubate overnight at 12–14°C.

3. Purify the ligated DNA using Prep-A-Gene kit (following the manufacturer's instructions) eluting twice with 10 μL of ddH$_2$O.

4. Store the library cold at all times and frozen when not in use.

3.2.3. Preparation of pUC18 Library

1. Add to a 0.5-mL Eppendorf tube 3 μL of 1.4 to 2-kb DNA solution from **step 7** in **Subheading 3.2.1.**, 0.3 μL of pUC18 *Sma*I-CIP, 0.4 μL of 10X ligase buffer, and 0.3 μL of T4 DNA ligase.

2. Pipet to mix. Centrifuge briefly to settle contents and then incubate overnight at 12–14°C.

3. Incubate the ligation at 65°C for 10 min (to denature the ligase).

4. Add 46 μL of ddH$_2$O to give a total volume of 50 μL.

5. Store the pUC18 library in the cold at all times and frozen when not in use.

3.2.4. Transformation by Electroporation

1. Chill a 0.5-mL Eppendorf tube on ice.

2. Add 10 μL of 10% (v/v) glycerol and 0.2 μL of a ligation reaction (either M13 or pUC18).

3. Add 40 μL of electrocompetent cells (*see* **Note 8**), and then transfer the mixture into the bottom of a prechilled 0.1-cm gap electroporation cuvet.

4. Transfer the cuvet to an electroporator and apply a voltage at 1.7 kV, 2000 Ω, and 25 μF.

5. Immediately add 0.5 mL of warm SOC medium.

6. After electroporation do the following:

a. For M13 libraries, add 3 mL of molten H-top agar to a sterile tube at 45°C. Add 50 μL of 40 mg/mL IPTG and 50 μL of 25 mg/mL X-gal, and mix. Add the contents of the cuvet, mix gently, and pour over a prewarmed TYE plate. Allow to set and incubate overnight at 37°C.

b. For pUC libraries, add the contents of the cuvet to a sterile tube and incubate at 37°C for 1 h, then add 50 μL each of 40 mg/mL IPTG and 50 mg/mL X-gal, and spread the contents over two TYE-amp plates. Incubate overnight at 37°C. For the expected results, *see* **Note 9**.

3.3. Preparation of DNA Sequencing Templates

3.3.1. Preparation of Single-Stranded M13 DNA by Triton-Based Method (Triton Preparation)

The method that involves PEG precipitation of the phage followed by solubilization of the M13 DNA in a Triton buffer was developed by Elaine Mardis, GSC, St. Louis (**3**).

1. Fill each well of a deep-well microtiter plate with 1.0 mL of Circlegrow.
2. Using a sterile cocktail stick, pick a plaque into each well. Leave the sticks in the wells as markers until the entire box has been picked. Remove the sticks carefully a few at a time and try to prevent cross-contamination between the wells.
3. Seal the box with a Dynex plate sealer and pierce a hole in the sealer over each well with a large syringe needle. Place the box in a shaker at 37°C for 16 h at 360 rpm.
4. Centrifuge the box at 4000g at room temperature for 20 min.
5. Add 150 μL of 20% PEG 8000/2.5 M NaCl into each well of a new deep-well microtiter plate.
6. Transfer 600 μL of each supernatant to a separate aliquot of PEG/NaCl and mix by pipetting.
7. Make a glycerol archive (*see* **Note 10**) of each M13 clone by resuspending each pellet in the remaining supernatant. Transfer 75 μL of each clone into a separate well of a Falcon Pro-Bind U-Bottom Plate containing 50 μL of 50% (v/v) glycerol. Mix and freeze immediately at –70°C.
8. Turn on a water bath and warm to 80°C.
9. Incubate the deep-well microtiter plate at room temperature for 20 min, and centrifuge at 4000g at room temperature for 20 min.
10. Decant the supernatants by inverting the box and leaving to drain on a piece of tissue for 1 min.
11. Place a piece of tissue into a centrifuge bucket, invert the deep-well microtiter plate and centrifuge at approx 8g for 2 min to remove residual PEG.
12. Add 20 μL of Triton-TE extraction buffer to each well and cover with metal foil tape.
13. Centrifuge briefly to collect the sample in the bottom of each well and move quickly to the next step.
14. Vortex for 2 min moving the deep-well microtiter plate about the vortex mat to resuspend the phage, centrifuge briefly to collect the sample in the bottom of each well, and then repeat once more. Move quickly to the next step.

15. Place the deep-well microtiter plate in an 80°C water bath for 10 min to lyse the phage, and centrifuge rapidly to bring down condensation. Move quickly to the next step.
16. Remove the metal foil tape, add 40 µL of ddH$_2$O to each well, and pipet to mix.
17. Centrifuge briefly to collect the sample in the bottom of each well.
18. Transfer the contents of each well to a well of a Falcon Pro-Bind U-Bottom Plate containing 10 µL of 3 M NaOAc, pH 4.8, and pipet to mix.
19. Add 160 µL of 96% (v/v) ethanol to each well and pipet to mix.
20. Precipitate at –70°C for 20 min or –20°C overnight.
21. Centrifuge at 4000g at 4°C for 1 h and pour off the ethanol as soon as the centrifuge has stopped. Otherwise, repeat the centrifugation.
22. Invert the plate to empty.
23. Add 200 µL of 70% (v/v) ethanol (*see* **Note 11**) Do not mix the ethanol and precipitate.
24. Centrifuge at 4000g at 4°C for 10 min and pour off the ethanol as soon as the centrifuge has stopped. Otherwise, repeat the centrifugation.
25. Invert the plate to empty.
26. Dry immediately and resuspend each pellet in 100 µL of ddH$_2$O (*see* **Note 12**).
27. Store template DNA frozen at –20°C.

3.3.2. Preparation of Double-Stranded pUC18 DNA

The high throughput alkaline-lysis (microprep) method which is described below was developed by the Development Group at The Sanger Centre *(4)*.

1. Fill each well of a deep-well microtiter plate with 1 mL of Circlegrow containing ampicillin at 100 µg/mL.
2. Pick colonies with a sterile cocktail stick into the media. Seal the box with a Dynex plate sealer and pierce each well with a needle to allow aeration during growth.
3. Place the deep-well microtiter plate in a shaker at 37°C at 320 rpm for 22 h (*see* **Note 13**).
4. Make a glycerol archive (*see* **Note 10**) by transferring 75 µL of each clone into a separate well of a Falcon Pro-Bind U-Bottom Plate containing 50 µL of 50% (v/v) glycerol. Mix and freeze immediately at –70°C.
5. Centrifuge the microtiter plates at 3000g at room temperature for 5 min to pellet the cells.
6. Discard the supernatants and leave the microtiter plate to drain on a tissue for 1 min.
7. Add 250 µL of GTE solution to each well and vortex the cells until each pellet has been completely resuspended.
8. Centrifuge the microtiter plate at 3000g at room temperature for 5 min to pellet the cells.
9. Discard the supernatant and leave to drain.
10. Add 250 µL of GTE solution to each well and vortex the cells for 2 min to resuspend.
11. Add 4 µL of RNase A solution to each well of a Falcon Pro-Bind U-Bottom Plate.
12. Transfer 60-µL aliquots of resuspended cells to a separate well in the plate containing RNase A.

13. Add 60 µL of NaOH/SDS solution to each well. Seal the plate with a 3M Scotch Pad sealer and mix by inversion 10 times.
14. Leave on the bench for 10 min.
15. Remove the plate sealer and add 60 µL of 3 *M* KOAc to each well. Seal the plate with a new 3M Scotch Pad sealer and mix by inversion 10 times.
16. Leave on the bench for 10 min.
17. Remove the plate sealer and place the microtiter plate in oven at 90°C for 30 min.
18. Cool the plate by placing it on ice for 5 min.
19. Tape a Multiscreen filter plate to the top of a Falcon 3910 96-well plate ensuring that the filters and the receiving wells line up.
20. Transfer the full volume of each well of the Falcon Pro-Bind U-Bottom Plate to a separate well in the filter plate and centrifuge at 2000*g* at 20°C for 2 min.
21. Remove and discard the filter plate and add 110 µL of isopropanol to each filtrate.
22. Seal with a new 3M Scotch Pad sealer and mix by inversion twice.
23. Centrifuge at 2500*g* at 20°C for 30 min.
24. Discard each supernatant and add 200 µL of 70% (v/v) ethanol (*see* **Note 11**) to each well.
25. Centrifuge for 5 min. Discard each supernatant and leave the plate to dry.
26. When the plate is completely dry, resuspend each DNA sample (typical yield is approx 5 µg) overnight in 100 µL of ddH$_2$O.

3.4. Sequencing Single- or Double-Stranded Templates with AmpliTaq FS/Dye Terminators

1. For 4 × 96-well microtiter plate's worth of templates, mix 2160 µL of ABI Prism Dye Terminator Ready Reaction with 432 µL primer solution (*see* **Note 1**). This is the reaction mix.
2. Using a 12-channel pipet, dispense 9 µL of template DNA solution from each well of a stock plate into the corresponding well of a Thermowell plate.
3. Add 6 µL of reaction mix to each well (*see* **Note 14**).
4. Centrifuge the plates briefly to make sure all the liquid is at the bottom of the wells.
5. Seal each plate with a rubber mat and put the plates on a cycler.
6. Cycle the reactions with the following program: 96°C for 20 s, 50°C for 20 s, and 60°C for 180 s, for 25 cycles.
7. Remove the plates from the thermal cycler and centrifuge briefly.
8. Remove the rubber seals and add 100 µL of ethanol/NaOAc to each well and mix well by pipetting.
9. Place the Thermowell plate in a rubber cushion and centrifuge at 3000*g* at 4°C for 1 h (*see* **Note 15**).
10. Remove the plates and discard the supernatant.
11. Add 100 µL of ice-cold 70% (v/v) ethanol (*see* **Note 11**) (do not mix the precipitate and the ethanol), and centrifuge at 3000*g* at 4°C for 10 min (*see* **Note 15**).
12. Remove the plates from the centrifuge and remove the supernatant.
13. Briefly centrifuge the plates inverted (at ~8*g*) on a piece of tissue to remove any remaining supernatant.

14. Dry the samples either by leaving the plates inverted on a tissue or in a vacuum desiccator.
15. Store the samples dry at –20°C.

3.5. Running Automated Fluorescent DNA Sequencers and Completing the Shotgun Phase

The samples of sequenced DNA produced in **Subheading 3.4.** are analyzed on ABI 373 or ABI Prism 377 sequencers operated according to the manufacturer's instructions *(5)*. The gel file collected by each sequencer run is analyzed to create individual sample files. These are then processed further to complete the shotgun phase. The selection of software for data processing depends on the available computing resources. At The Sanger Centre, the software *(6)* used currently includes a Unix-based system (gelminder) for retracking and data extraction, phred for base-calling *(7,8)*, and a series of modules (asp) for processing individual sample files *(9)*. When all the sample files for a BAC project have been processed, the good-quality reads are assembled using phrap *(10)* and a gap4 database *(11)* is created for project viewing and sequence editing.

3.6. Directed Sequencing Reactions

When the shotgun is complete, the assembled project is manually edited by an experienced operator but is likely to consist of a number of contigs and regions of low-quality data. Further directed sequencing is required to close all gaps, to add high-quality sequence to regions of low quality, and to include other sequencing chemistries into single-stranded regions so that the entire sequence meets the required finishing criteria. Subclones from low-quality and single-stranded regions can be resequenced using BigDye terminator or primer chemistry to produce better-quality data and to add a second chemistry. Contigs can be joined by choosing a custom primer adjacent to the gap and sequencing, using BigDye terminator chemistry, on subclones near the end of the contig and in the correct orientation (primer walking).

3.6.1. Directed Sequencing Using BigDye Terminator

1. In a Thermowell 96-well plate, combine 4 μL of BigDye mix (*see* **Note 16**), 1 μL of primer (*see* **Note 2**), and 4 μL of template DNA.
2. Centrifuge the plate briefly to make sure all liquid is at the bottom of the wells.
3. Seal the plate with a rubber mat and place on a thermal cycler.
4. Cycle the reactions with the following program: 96°C for 30 s, 50°C for 15 s, and 60°C for 4 min for 25 cycles.
5. Remove the plates from the thermal cycler and centrifuge briefly to make sure all liquid is at the bottom of the wells.
6. Add 50 μL of ethanol/NaOAc to each well and mix well by pipetting (*see* **Note 17**).

7. Place the plate in a rubber cushion and centrifuge at 3000g at 4°C for 30 min (*see* **Note 15**).
8. Remove the plates and the supernatant.
9. Add 100 μL of ice-cold 70% (v/v) ethanol (*see* **Note 11**) and centrifuge at 3000g at 4°C for 2 min (*see* **Note 15**).
10. Remove the plates from the centrifuge and discard the supernatant.
11. Centrifuge the plates inverted for 20 s (at approx 8g) on a piece of tissue to remove any remaining supernatant.
12. Dry the samples either by leaving the plates inverted on a tissue or in a vacuum desiccator.
13. Store the samples dry at –20°C.

3.6.2. Directed Sequencing Using BigDye Primer

1. Primer sequencing requires each nucleotide reaction, i.e., A, T, C, and G, to be carried out in a separate well. Dispense 2 μL of template DNA into each of four wells of a Thermowell 96-well plate. Add 4 μL of mix A to the first well, 4 μL of mix C to the second, 4 μL of mix T to the third, and 4 μL of mix G to the fourth well (*see* **Note 18**).
2. Centrifuge the plate briefly to make sure all liquid is at the bottom of the wells.
3. Seal the plate with a rubber mat and place on a thermal cycler.
4. Cycle the reactions with the following program: 95°C for 30 s, 55°C for 30 s, and 70°C for 1 min for 15 cycles; and 95°C for 30 s and 70°C for 1 min for 15 cycles.
5. Remove the plate from the thermal cycler and centrifuge briefly to make sure all the liquid is at the bottom of the wells.
6. Add 50 μL of 96% (v/v) ethanol (stored at 4°C) to one well and then pool the four reactions that contain the same template. Leave at room temperature for 10 min.
7. Place the plate in a rubber cushion and centrifuge at 3000g at 4°C for 20 min (*see* **Note 15**).
8. Remove the plates from the centrifuge and discard the supernatant.
9. Centrifuge the plates inverted for 20 s (at approx 8g) on a piece of tissue to remove any remaining supernatant.
10. Dry the samples either by leaving the plates inverted on a tissue or in a vacuum desiccator.
11. Store the samples dry at –20°C.

3.6.3. Preparation of Sequencing Templates by Polymerase Chain Reaction

Polymerase chain reaction (PCR) is used in the finishing stage to close any physical gaps (regions of the BAC that are not covered by subclones) and to double strand M13 subclones, to produce the sequence from the 3' end of the insert. For this purpose, the following simple PCR method is suitable. However, for difficult regions, such as those with extreme base bias of high G+C, and for PCR from genomic DNA, this method may not work well and optimization may be required or an alternative PCR kit used. The primers used in the PCR are utilized in the sequencing reaction (*see* **Note 19**).

1. In a Thermowell 96-well plate, combine for each template 2 µL of DNA, 2 µL of each primer (*see* **Note 3**), 8 µL of dNTP mix, 5 µL of 10X *Taq* buffer, 0.5 µL of AmpliTaq polymerase, and 32.5 µL of ddH$_2$O.
2. Centrifuge the plate briefly to make sure all the liquid is at the bottom of the wells.
3. Seal the plate with a rubber mat and place on a thermal cycler.
4. Cycle the reactions with the following program: **Step 1**—95°C for 1 min, 65°C for 1 min, and 72°C for 3 min for 10 cycles, reducing the annealing temperature from 65 to 56°C by 1°C each cycle; **step 2**—95°C for 1 min, 55°C for 1 min, and 72°C for 3 min for 12 cycles, reducing the annealing temperature from 55°C to 50 by 1°C every second cycle.
5. Remove the plate from the thermal cycler and centrifuge briefly to make sure all liquid is at the bottom of the wells.
6. Add 30 µL of PEG/NaCl to each well, mix with a pipet, and centrifuge briefly to place all the samples at the bottom of the wells. Leave for 25 min at room temperature.
7. Place the plate in a rubber cushion and centrifuge at 3000*g* at 4°C for 60 min (*see* **Note 15**).
8. Remove the plate from the centrifuge and discard the supernatant.
9. Centrifuge the plate inverted for 3 min (at approx 8*g*) on a piece of tissue to remove any remaining supernatant.
10. Resuspend each pellet in 50 µL of ddH$_2$O and store at 4°C.
11. Check that each PCR reaction has been successful by assessing the products on a 0.8% (w/v) agarose gel, and sequence all the products.

4. Notes

1. The primers used in the reactions are at follows: for M13 and pUC18 forward sequence (M13-21f), TGTAAAACGACGGCCAGT; for M13 reverse sequence (after PCR to double strand the M13 template, *see* **Subheading 3.6.3.**), CAGGAAACAGCTATGACC; and for pUC18 reverse (pUCr), GCGGATAAC-AATTTCACACAGGA.
2. The primer can be universal forward or reverse (1 pmol/µL) (*see* **Note 1**). Alternatively, a custom primer can be used to produce sequence from farther along the subclone (primer walking).
3. To double strand M13 subclones, add M13 forward and reverse primer (6 pmol/µL) to the reaction mix (*see* **Note 1**). Again, custom primers can be used.
4. A suitable marker is lambda DNA digested with *Hind*III (New England Biolabs, Hitchin, Hertforshire, UK). One microliter of a 1 in 10 dilution of this marker contains 25 ng of the largest DNA fragment (23,130 bp).
5. The exact conditions for efficient fragmentation will depend on several factors, including the type of sonicator used. At The Sanger Centre (using an XL2020 Sonicator manufactured by Heat Systems, Farmingdale, NY; for more details,

see http://www.sanger.ac.uk/Teams/Team53/sonication.shtml), samples are sonicated two times for 15 s each and then a 1-μL aliquot is analyzed by 0.8% (w/v)
agarose gel electrophoresis to determine the extent of sonication. There are three
possible outcomes: (1) complete sonication (no sign of high molecular weight
DNA, with a smear between 4 kb and 500 bp), (2) near complete sonication
(smear and faint high molecular weight DNA), and (3) unsonicated (faint smear
and substantial high molecular weight DNA). In the second case of (ii), the
sample is resonicated for 5 s and the extent of sonication is rechecked. In the
case, the sample is resonicated two times for 10 s each and rechecked.

6. Suitable markers include lambda DNA digested with *Hin*dIII and pBR322
    digested with *Bst*NI (available from New England Biolabs).
7. It is usual to make libraries from only the 1.4 to 2.0-kb fraction. The unused
    agarose blocks can be stored at –20°C.
8. Many *Escherichia coli* stains are suitable hosts for the production of sequencing
    templates. We have the most experience using TG1 (a moderately fast-growing
    strain) for M13 preparations and either TG1 or SURE cells (Promega UK) for
    pUC preparations.
9. For each ligation, it is usual to perform a single test transformation to determine
    the quality of the library (i.e., the vector + insert content) and the transformation
    efficiency. The expected result for the test electroporation is a plate covered with
    >50 (and usually 100–200) plaques or colonies. The blue plaques (or colonies)
    should be <10% of the total transformants. For each series of electroporations,
    it is usual to include a positive control (e.g., use 1 μL of ϕX174 digested with
    *Hae*III, available from New England Biolabs, as the DNA library) and a nega-
    tive control (containing no DNA). When the quality of the ligation has been
    determined, the number of plates needed to provide the required plaques (or
    colonies) can be decided. For example, if 0.2 μL of an M13 ligation gave 200
    plaques, then five electroporations should produce enough plaques for a typical
    BAC project.
10. Glycerol archive cultures are useful for generating additional DNA for sequence
    finishing when the original DNA template is exhausted. DNA templates are pre-
    pared from glycerol stocks by the appropriate method (*see* **Subheading 3.3.1.** or
    3.3.2.). If only a small number of templates are being prepared, phenol extraction
    is incorporated into the DNA preparation procedure to give high-quality DNA.
11. Store 70% (v/v) ethanol in a –20°C freezer so that it is cold when used.
12. The volume used to resuspend template DNA (100 μL) should be reduced if the
    yield of template DNA is low (as indicated by agarose gel electrophoresis or a
    weak fluorescence signal when the template is sequenced).
13. If the yield of plasmid is low (as indicated by weak fluorescence sequence sig-
    nal), the growth time can be extended up to 48 h.
14. For sequencing plasmids, the following reaction mix has also been used to
    increase the fluorescent signal: 5 μL of plasmid DNA, 8 μL of terminator
    mix, 1 μL of primer, and 6 μL of ddH$_2$O. The primer for this suggested mixture
    is either M13-21f (forward) (6 pmol/μL) or pUCr (reverse) primer (10 pmol/μL).

15. Precool the centrifuge to 4°C before use.
16. Using only 4 μL of BigDye terminator for each reaction is classed as a 0.5X reaction and has always been a sufficient amount for all our sequencing needs. If greater sensitivity is required, use 8 μL.
17. Unincorporated BigDye terminator can sometimes be carried through the precipitation step leading to "dye blobs" in the sequence. This is usually seen at the start of a run and can mask the true sequence peaks below, causing problems for base-calling software. If this phenomenon is seen regularly, try adding 2.5 μL of 5% propan-2-ol (isopropanol) to each reaction along with 50 μL of the ethanol/ NaOAc mix.
18. Primer chemistry suffers from compressions caused by small GC hairpins in the sequence that do not occur in BigDye terminators, and, therefore, primer sequencing is of limited use in the sequencing of high G+C DNA. However, BigDye terminators cannot sequence through larger hairpins, >20 bp, so primer chemis try has to be used. Adding 5% (v/v) dimethylsulfonide to the sequencing mix helps break down the secondary structure, and running an automated DNA sequencer at an elevated temperature of 52°C also helps limit compressions.
19. The PCR product can be sequenced, using BigDye terminator chemistry, with either of the two primers used in the PCR reaction. If BigDye primer chemistry is required for sequencing the PCR product, then the initial PCR will need to be carried out using tailed custom primers. By adding a universal forward primer to the 5' end of one of the oligonucleotides, primer chemistry can be used.

Acknowledgments

We wish to thank everyone at The Sanger Centre and at The Genome Sequencing Centre, St. Louis, MO, who were involved in developing the methods described herein. In particular, we thank Karen Oliver, Michael Quail, and Sarah White for helpful comments.

References

1. Sanger, F., Nicklen, S., and Coulson A. R. (1977) DNA sequencing with chain-terminating inhibitors. *Proc. Natl. Acad. Sci. USA* **74,** 5463–5467.
2. Jones, M. and Quail, M. <http://www.sanger.ac.uklTeams/Team53/methods.shtml>.
3. Mardis, E. (1994) High-throughput detergent extraction of M13 subclones for fluorescent DNA sequencing. *Nucleic Acids Res.* **22,** 2173–2175.
4. Baron, L. and Smith, A. <http://www.sanger.ac.uk/Teams/Team51/MicroPrep. shtm>.
5. PE Applied Biosystems (1998) *Automated DNA Sequencing: Chemistry Guide* (P/N 4305080 Rev. A).
6. <http://www.sanger.ac.uk/Software/>.
7. Hillier, L., Wendl, M. C., and Green, P. (1998) Base-calling of automated sequencer traces using phred. I. Accuracy assessment. *Genome Res.* **8,** 175–185.

8. Ewing, B. and Green, P. (1998) Base-calling of automated sequencer traces using phred. II. Error probabilities. *Genome Res.* **8,** 186–194. Also *see* <http://bozeman. genome.washington.edu/phrap.docs/phred.html>.

9. <http://www.sanger.ac.uk/Software/sequencing/docs/asp/>.

10. <http://bozeman.genome.washington.edu/ phrap.docs/phrap.html>.

11. Dear, S. and Staden, R. (1991) A sequence assembly and editing program for efficient management of large projects. Nucleic Acids Res. **19,** 3907–3911. Also *see* <http://www.mrc-lmb.cam.ac.uk/pubseq>.

16

Finding Genes in Genomic Nucleotide Sequences by Using Bioinformatics

Yvonne J. K. Edwards and Simon M. Brocklehurst

1. Introduction

You have, we hope, come to this chapter wishing to know how to use bioinformatics to locate genes in genomic sequences. You probably want to know which are the easiest and best tools to use, to treat them largely as black boxes, and to know how to assess the likely accuracy of the results you obtain. If so, you have come to the right place. In the absence of knowing which genome(s) you are interested in, we have chosen to take our examples from a variety of human, plant, pathogenic bacterial, and fungal genomes (*see* **Table 1**). Because access to computational resources varies greatly, we have chosen to restrict ourselves to describing methods that make use of computational resources (software and databases) that are publicly available on the Internet via the World Wide Web (*see* **Table 2**). We assume that you have access to the Internet, and that you know how to use a graphical Web browser such as Netscape Navigator or Microsoft Internet Explorer. We also assume that this is not your first acquaintance with using bioinformatics tools. Before attempting to work through this chapter, you should have run BLAST and be familiar with techniques for retrieving gene or protein sequences from data banks such as Swissprot or EMBL.

Genomes possess significant diversity in many aspects of their structure. Their sizes vary enormously from just a few thousand bases for small viral genomes, to more than a hundred million bases for some plant genomes. Whereas cellular genomes are always DNA based, viral genomes may be either DNA or RNA based. Some genomes are single stranded; in this case, information may be read in the 5'-to-3' direction, the 3'-to-5' direction, or even in both directions (the last kind are termed *ambisense genomes*). Other genomes are

From: *Methods in Molecular Biology, vol. 175: Genomics Protocols*
Edited by: M. P. Starkey and R. Elaswarapu © Humana Press Inc., Totowa, NJ

Table 1
Genomic DNA Fragments Used to Demonstrate Gene Prediction Methods by Using Bioinformatics

Organism	Division	Description	EMBL entry name	Accession no.	Sequence length (bp)
Homo sapiens	Human	Interleukin-2 receptor γ-chain	HSIL2RGA	L19546	4038
Mycobacterium tuberculosis	Prokaryote	Erdman sigma factor rpoV	MT21134	U21134	2745
Oryza sativa	Plant	Receptor kinase-like protein (Xa21)	OS37133	U37133	3921
Saccaromyces pombe[a]	Fungi	Data not submitted to EMBL at time of writing	Not applicable	Not applicable	4250

[a]The last fragment (c1592) was obtained from the *S. pombe* sequencing project based at the Sanger Center (http://www.sanger.ac.uk/Projects/S_pombe/). Fragment c1592 is from chromosome III.

Table 2
List of URLs for Tools Used to Predict Protein-Coding Regions in Genomic Sequences

Name	Home page URL for gene prediction programs	Refs
BCM Gene Finder	http://dot.imgen.bcm.tmc.edu:9331/gene-finder/gf.html http://genomic.sanger.ac.uk/gf/gf.shtml	*1*
WebGeneMarkHmm WebGeneMark	http://dixie.biology.gatech.edu/GeneMark/eukhmm.cgi http://dixie.biology.gatech.edu/GeneMark/hmmchoice.html	*2,3*
GeneID3	http://www1.lmmes/software/geneid/geneid.html	*4*
Genie	http://www.fruitfly.org/seq_tools/genie.html	*5*
Genscan	http://bioweb.pasteur.fr/seqanal/interfaces/genscan.html	*6*
Grail	http://compbio.ornl.gov/Grail-1.3/	*7,8*
HMMgene	http://www.cbs.dtu.dk/services/HMMgene/	*9*
BLASTX 2.0.10	http://www.ncbi.nim.nih.gov/BLAST/	*10*

double stranded, in which case information is read only in the 5' to 3' direction on either strand. Genomes may be constructed from a single molecule or from multiple component chromosomes. Such is the diversity of genome structure that even genomes of organisms that belong to the same taxonomic class often exhibit enormous diversity. For example, genome sizes of species belonging to the same class often vary by several orders of magnitude. Given the often strong sequence similarities between related *genes* from even the most diverse of organisms, it is perhaps surprising that *genomes* are so dissimilar.

From the gene-finding perspective of this chapter, one of the most important aspects of genome diversity is gene density, i.e., the amount of the genome that codes for genes. This varies widely from a minimum of 1 to 2% up to a maximum of about 90%. Genomes with low gene density can cause some of the biggest problems in accurately identifying genes.

During the last 5 years, computational methods for analysis of nucleotide sequences have increased in sophistication. Herein, we show how to use some current approaches for tackling problems relating to finding proteincoding genes in genomic sequence for a variety of types of genome. We give a flavor of the diversity of gene-finding approaches that are available and introduce methods based on both homology-based searching and machine-learning approaches (*see* **Notes 1** and **2**). If you follow the approach given, you should be able to undertake gene-finding projects using not only the tools we recommend, but be able to start using new tools as they become available.

As you read the subsequent sections, keep in mind that they are intended to form a "beginner's guide" to gene finding. There are many pitfalls in genome analysis that can trap the unwary gene hunter. We tell you how to watch out for some of these. Some problems, however, can be difficult or impossible to deal with using bioinformatics techniques alone. For example, pseudo-genes (conventional and processed), overlapping genes, genes within genes, and alternative splicing can lead you down spurious paths. These are not covered in the text. Computational approaches do not work with 100% success, and, thus, you should not necessarily expect to come away from digesting this chapter being able to take a piece of genomic sequence and identify the genes precisely and accurately. Rather, our aim is to provide the knowledge you will need to take sections of genomic sequence and identify regions that potentially code for expressed functional protein products.

2. Materials

2.1. Hardware Computers

Computers with access to the Internet, e.g., Intel PC running Microsoft Windows NT 4.0, Intel PC running Red Hat Linux 6.1, Apple Macintosh, Silicon Graphics O2 workstation running IRIX 6.3, Sun Microsystems Ultra 10 workstation running Solaris 7.

2.2. Software Access to Internet

Web browser Netscape Navigator version 4 or Microsoft Internet Explorer version 5.

2.3. Programs

Particular bioinformatics software applications (*see* **Table 2**) accessible via Internet front ends.

3. Methods

3.1. Overall Strategy and Recommended Software Tools

We recommend that you follow these three rules for successful gene finding:

1. Do not rely on a single piece of software. In appropriate cases (*see* **Subheading 3.3.**), you will gain more confidence in a gene prediction by using a variety of tools and gathering together a consensus of the results.
2. Do use software that can be tailored to the particular genome(s) you are working on. If the software does not let you select the genome you are interested in, try to choose the most closely related genome available. Remember that if the software does not explicitly model the genome you are interested in, then the results are frequently less accurate than if it does. If only one of the available prediction programs models your genome, you should use that program to the exclusion of others. In that case, you are likely to find it important to make use of the BLASTX results (*see* **Subheading 3.2.**) to give some confidence to your results.
3. Do remember that if your genome has low gene density (i.e., introns are many and exons are frequently short), then the predictions will often be less accurate than those for genomes with high gene density.

At the time of writing, of the many gene-finding sites on the Web, we recommend that you use those detailed in **Table 2**. Note that Web sites often cease to exist or change address without notice. Do not be surprised if one or more of these sites does not exist when you try to access them. The three rules just given will hold for the foreseeable future—do not be afraid to try new sites as they become available.

3.2. Using Gene-Finding Software

Next we provide information on the recommended software tools (**Table 2**). The programs fall into two categories: pure gene-prediction programs and sequence similarity searches using programs such as BLAST. For the most part, the gene-prediction programs work using so-called machine-learning algorithms (*see* **Notes 1** and **2**). These tools can be regarded as black boxes; however, considerable benefits can be reaped from understanding how the programs work (*[1–10]* and references therein). Additionally, it is important to set applicable parameters in order for the programs to work optimally and for you to derive the most from your analysis.

3.2.1. BCM Programs; Fgenes, Fgenesh, Fgenes-M, BestORF, Fgene, FgeneP, Fex, CDSB

This suite of programs models the following organisms: *Homo sapiens, Drosophila melanogaster, Caenorhabditis elegans, Saccharomyces cerevisiae,* plant, and *Escherichia coli.* The software predicts the number of genes and exons, the positions of predicted genes and exons, and predicted amino acid sequences of coding regions.

3.2.2. WebGeneMarkHmm, WebGeneMark

There are 60 species modeled, including, *H. sapiens, D. melanogaster, C. elegans, S. cerevisiae, E. coli, Oryza sativa, Mycobacterium tuberculosis,* and *Saccharomyces pombe.* Setting the window size, step size, and threshold frame-shift indicator parameters can affect the prediction. You may wish to experiment with these. GeneMark provides a list of open reading frames (ORFs) and regions of interest. The list of ORFs is defined here as coding sequences with alternate starts (regions from start to stop codon with a coding function >0.50; *see* **Note 3**). The list of regions of interest, defined by GeneMark, comprises fragments with a coding signal enclosed within two stop codons.

3.2.3. GeneID3

Vertebrates and plants are modeled. The GeneID3 program is based on a statistical model of codon usage and nucleotide frequency in genes in DNA sequences. The program also translates putative exons and performs a database search and rescores exons showing sequence similarity to known sequences.

3.2.4. Genie

D. melanogaster and H. sapiens are modeled. Genes are predicted on both forward and reverse strands. The maximum length of input sequence here is restricted to 90,000 bases. Multiple sequences can be added if each is in Fasta format (i.e., the first line is not sequence, and starts with a ">" character).

3.2.5. Genscan

Arabidopsis thaliana, H. sapiens (or vertebrates), and *Zea mays* are modeled. Options can be chosen to display suboptimal exons and choose an exon cutoff parameter. The software predicts number and position of genes and exons. Predicted exon sequence and predicted amino acid sequence can also be output.

3.2.6. Grail (Graill, Grailla, and Grail2)

H. sapiens, Mus musculus, A. thaliana, D. melanogaster, and *E. coli* are modeled. Features that can be predicted by the software include exons, CpG islands, and frameshift errors. There are eight features that can be predicted. Associated with each feature, a variety of parameters can be altered. You may wish to experiment with these.

3.2.7. HMMgene

H. sapiens (other vertebrates); and *C. elegans* are modeled. The output is a "best" predicted sequence.

3.2.8. BLAST

For gene finding, you should use the program BLASTX (at least version 2.0.10). When using BLASTX, we recommend that you set the various parameters to the following values. Set the number of descriptions to 500 and the number of alignments to 500. Leave the Expect value cutoff at the default value of 10. **Figure 1** presents an example of the results of such a search. The aim of this search is to predict protein-coding regions. For such predictions, it is important that the computations be performed at the level of protein-protein sequence comparisons. The most computationally efficient way of doing this is to use amino acid sequence databases and translate the query sequence (your sequence) automatically into the six frames. This functionality is provided by BLASTX.

By comparison, BLASTN performs searches at the level of nucleotide sequence and is a much less sensitive search. Thus, BLASTN is significantly less useful for the present purpose. Possibly the best option would be to use TBLASTX, which translates both query and database sequences "on the fly" and makes comparisons at the protein level. Because of its computational expense, many Web sites do not allow the use of TBLASTX over the Internet for searching large databases.

Most BLAST servers filter query sequence for low compositional complexity regions by default. Low-complexity regions commonly give spuriously high scores that reflect compositional bias rather than significant position-by-position alignment. Filtering can eliminate these matches (e.g., hits against proline-rich regions) from the BLAST reports, leaving regions whose BLAST statistics reflect the specificity of pairwise alignment. Query searches at the protein level use the program SEG to filter low-complexity sequences found. The residues are substituted using the letter X in the query protein sequences.

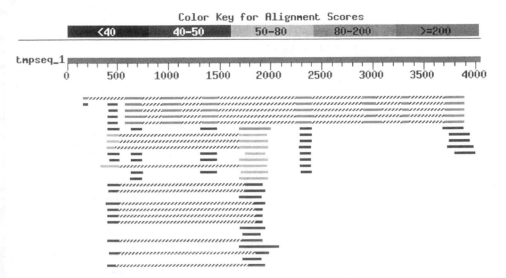

Fig. 1. A summary of BLASTX report of genomic sequence hsil2rga against a nonredundant protein sequence database. The BLASTX searches are carried out at the protein level by translating the query genomic sequence into all six reading frames. This provides a sensitive search relative to searching at the nucleotide level using BLASTN. Ignoring the BLASTX matches to the human interlcukin 2 (IL-2) receptor common γ-chain precursor, the BLASTX matches defined in **Table 3** are those made with the *Canis familiaris* IL-2 receptor common γ-chain precursor gene. The first exon of the gene is not detected because it is proline and leucine rich. An Alu sequence is interspersed between exon 1 (D1) and exon 2 (D2) and also exon 4 (D4) and exon 5 (D5).

3.3. Deriving a Consensus Gene Prediction

There are several ways to go about making use of results from multiple gene predictions. The approach we suggest is to construct a "winner takes all" consensus prediction. The steps to take are as follows:

1. Assemble the results of exon predictions from the various programs such that you can determine where equivalent regions are located. For example, *see* **Table 3**.
2. Initially discard any sets of results from programs in which your species of interest is not modeled. If this leaves you with some data, use these results as your main guide as to where the genes are likely to be located. If this leaves you with no data, use the results from programs in which available species are closely related to your chosen genome. The latter should be a last resort, because relative synonymous codon usage in even closely related species can be quite different.
3. Using the remaining results, total the number of times a particular position in the sequence appears as a boundary for an exon. Take the position in the sequence

Table 3
The Gene Prediction Results for hsil2rga DNA Fragment (from the human genome) Using a Variety of Programs[a]

	CDS	BCM Fgenes (H.sapiens)	WebGene MarkHmm (H.sapiens)	GeneID3 (H.sapiens)	Genie (H.sapiens)	Genscan (H.sapiens)	Grail 2 (H.sapiens)	HMMgene (H. sapiens)	Consensus Gene Prediction	BLASTX matches
D1	88-202	179-230	133-202	179-230	-	88-202	133-230	88-202	88*-202* 88*-230* 133*-202* 133*-230* 179*-202* 179*-230*	-
D2	581-734	581-734	641-771	641-771	737-771	641-771	581-771	581-734	581*-771 641*-771	580-741
D3	943-1127	943-1127	-	1022-1127	943-1127	943-1127	943-1165	943-1127	**943-1127**	944-1126
D4	1336-1475	1588-1645	-	1354-1475	-	1299-1475	1308-1475	1354-1475	1354*-**1475**	1335-1475
D5	2239-2401	2205-2401	2239-2401	2239-2401	-	2239-2401	2239-2356	2239-2356	**2239-2401**	2239-2400
D6	2934-3030	2934-3030	2934-3030	2934-3030	2934-3030	2934-3030	-	2934-3030	**2934-3030**	2900-3031
D7	3283-3352	3283-3352	3283-3352	3283-3370	3283-3370	3283-3352	3283-3370	3283-3352	**3283-3352**	3281-3352
D8	3708-3893	3708-3893	-	-	-	3708-3780	3708-3893	3708-3893	**3708-3893**	3708-3890
R1	-	-	-	-	1968-1909	-	-	-	-	-
R2	-	-	-	-	1813-1634	-	-	-	-	-

[a]Each program is named in the column headings, along with the model of species selected. The consensus gene prediction column represents a prediction collated from the individual program results. In the consensus gene prediction column, correct predictions are highlighted in bold (by comparison with the data shown in the CDS column). Note the difficulty in predicting the position of the first exon. This is a common problem in gene prediction. The legend to **Fig. 1** explains why the BLASTX searches missed out on finding exon 1. An asterisk indicates low certainty for a start or end position of an exon. A summary of the BLASTX search using a data bank comprising nonredundant translated DNA sequences is shown in the BLASTX matches column. The coding sequence (CDS) is annotation in EMBL files. The letter *D* followed by a number depicts (likely) protein coding regions, and the letter *R* followed by a number designates (likely) coding regions in the reverse complement direction.

that is most frequently predicted to be a consensus boundary position. For example consider an exon that is predicted, using three different programs, in regions defined as 67–102, 55–102, and 55–117. The winner takes all consensus for the predicted exon would be 55–102. In **Table 3** you will see that the results for row D1 are not clear, whereas the prediction for row D6 has high confidence.

4. The fewer the sets of results you have, the more you should focus on the results from the BLASTX predictions that will show with high confidence where poten-

Table 4
Gene Prediction Results for *M. tuberculosis* Fragment
each program is named in the column heading)[a]

	CDS	BCM CDSB (E. coli)	WebGene Mark (M. tuberculosis)	GeneID3 (plants)	Genie (H. sapiens)	Genscan (A. thaliana)	Grail 1 (E. coli)	HMMgene (C. elegans)	Gene prediction	BLASTX matches
D1	-	-	2-661	-	-	62-623	51-621	553-685	**2-661**	2-658
D2	-	-	-	-	-	699-815	-	-	-	699-808
D3	841-2427	841-2424	835-2427	-	-	848-2403	841-2391	-	**835-2427**	826-2424
D4				1148-1438	-			-		
D5				1543-2427	1627-2248			1460-2262		
D6	-	-	-	-	2404-2474	-	-	-	-	-
D7	-	-	2551-2745	-	-	2503-2709	2491-2691	2553-2745	**2551-2745**	2470-2742
R1	-	-	-	-	2388-2286	-	-	-	-	-
R2	-	-	-	-	1448-790	-	-	-	-	-

[a]WebGeneMark is the only program that models the genome of interest. The results from this program are highlighted in boldface in the Gene prediction column. A summary of the BLASTX search using a data bank comprising nonredundant translated DNA sequences is shown in the BLASTX matches column. The coding sequence (CDS) is annotation in EMBL files. The letter *D* followed by a number depicts (likely) protein coding region, and the letter *R* followed by a number designates likely coding regions in the reverse complement direction. The D1 BLASTX match is to a hypothetical protein in *Mycobacterium leprae*. The D3, D4, D5 BLASTX matches are to the DNA-directed RNA polymerase sigma factor from *M. leprae*. The D7 match is a hypothetical 17.5-kDa protein in chromosome 1 in *Schizosaccharomyces pombe*. Some of these matches (e.g., D7) could form the basis of further analysis and lead to further annotation.

tial exons are located. Note that the exon boundaries are not expected to be precise from the BLASTX results (*see* **Note 4**).

3.4. Worked Examples

So that you can see that you are using the tools correctly, we provide four examples. From the human genome, we use a region of genomic sequence that includes the γ-chain of the interleukin-2 receptor. From the *Mycobacterium tuberculosis* genome, a region of sequence coding for Erdman sigma factor (rpoV) is selected. From *O. sativa,* we chose a fragment of genomic sequence that codes for a receptor kinase-like protein (Xa21). Finally, from the *S. pombe* genome, we chose a region of the genome that was not submitted to the EMBL database at the time of writing and has no existing annotation. Information relating to database accession for these regions of sequence is provided in **Table 1**. The output from the gene-finding programs (**Table 2**) is summarized in **Tables 3–6**. Note that for the BLASTX homology searches, we exclude hits

Table 5
The Gene Prediction Results for *O. sativa* Fragment[a]

	CDS	BCM Fgenesh (Plant)	WebGene MarkHmm (O. sativa)	GeneID3 (Plant)	Genie (H. sapiens)	Genscan (A. thaliana)	Grail 2 (A. thaliana)	HMMgene (C. elegans)	**Gene prediction**	BLASTX matches
D1	1-2677	1-956	1-2677	-	1-493	1-2677	139-410	-	**1-2677**	115-2676
D2				-			447-493	-		
D3				557-559	-		569-956			
D4				-	753-781					
D5		-		910-1603	-			838-956		
D6		-			-		1137-1468	-		
D7		1680-2712		1988-2677	-		1501-2712	1812-2677		
D8	-	-	-	2748-2768	-	-	-	-	-	-
D9	-	-	-	3391-3416	-	-	-	-	-	-
D10	3521-3921	3664-3921	-	-	-	3521-3901	3521-3921	3494-3921	-	3499-3879
R1	-	-	-	-	1930-1901	-	-	-	-	-
R2	-	-	-	-	1292-1215	-	-	-	-	-
R3	-	-	-	-	-	-	-	858-820	-	-
R4	-	-	-	-	-	-	-	399-136	-	-

[a]Each program used is named in the column heading, along with the model of species selected. Only the WebGeneMarkHmm program modeled the genome of interest. Thus, the gene prediction column is not a consensus; rather, it uses the results from the single program (shown in boldface). The results from WebGeneMarkHmm are in the Gene prediction column. A summary of the BLASTX search using a data bank comprising nonredundant translated DNA sequences is shown in the BLASTX matches column. The coding sequence (CDS) is annotation in EMBL files. The letter *D* followed by a number depicts (likely) protein coding region, and the letter *R* followed by a number designates (likely) coding regions in the reverse complement direction. The detectable sequence similarity that exists with known proteins in the regions covered by the predicted exons gives added confidence to the predictions. All the BLASTX matches came from receptor kinase-like protein from *Oryza longistaminata* or long-staminate rice. Note that in this case, the BLASTX match did not identify the start of the gene. At the amino acid level, this protein is leucine rich. A leucine-rich region is typically masked by a low-complexity filters, and this is an example in which masking low-complexity repeats may reduce the accuracy of identifying coding regions using sequence similarity searches.

to the genes themselves to give you an impression of what the results might look like from a blind prediction.

4. Notes

1. Sequence similarity searches are based on the idea that proteins fall into families that are related by evolution. Homologous sequences are derived from a common ancestry. Such relationships are apparent in the similarities in sequences of related proteins. Some of these similarities can be found in rapid database-searching

Table 6
Gene Prediction Results for *S. pombe* DNA Fragment
Using a Variety of Programs[a]

	CDS	BCM Fgene (yeast)	WebGene Mark (S. pombe)	GeneID3 (Plant)	Genie (H. sapiens)	Genscan (A. thaliana)	Grail 2 (A. thaliana)	HMMgene (C. elegans)	**Gene prediction**	BLASTX matches
D1	npa	-	-	-	-	-	-	-	-	(w)266-532
D2	npa	-	-	-	-	621-677	-	-	-	-
D3	npa	-	-	716-755	-	-	-	-	-	-
D4	npa	2702-3071	2702-3109	2922-3071	2702-3071	2639-3071	2702-3075	-	**2702-3109**	2723-3262
D5	npa	3123-3228	-	3199-3228	-	3106-3228	3131-3228	3131-3228	-	-
D6	npa	3287-3681	-	3481-3689	3481-3685	3481-3681	3287-3685	3287-3681	-	3312-4235
D7	npa	-	-	-	3736-3793	3736-3900	3695-3941	-	-	
D8	npa	-	3918-4250	-	-	3973-4218	3973-4077	-	**3918-4250**	
D9	npa	-	-	-	-	-	4120-4218	4120-4218	-	
R1	npa	-	-	-	-	-	3777-3517	-	-	-
R2	npa	-	-	-	3436-3411	-	-	-	-	-
R3	npa	-	-	-	2707-2641	-	-	-	-	-
R4	npa	-	-	-	-	-	-	-	-	(w)1524-1246

[a]Each program is named in the column heading, along with the model of species selected. In this case, only one program (WebGeneMark) modeled the genome of interest. The gene prediction column here is not a consensus; rather, it uses the results from the single program (shown in boldface). A summary of the BLASTX search using a data bank comprising nonredundant translated DNA sequences is shown in the BLASTX matches column. The letter *D* depicts likely protein coding region, and the letter *R* followed by a number designates (likely) coding regions in the reverse complement direction. The BLASTX matches with known proteins in the regions covered by the predicted exons give added confidence to the predictions. npa signifies that the coding sequence (CDS) has not previously been annotated. The D1 region makes a weak sequence similarity match (w) to the DNA-directed DNA polymerase involved in DNA binding, DNA biosynthesis, and nucleotidyltransferase. At the protein level, the D4–D9 regions share sequence similarity with a membrane transporter protein responsible for antibiotic resistance. These genes are present in low copy numbers in the genome of various fungal species such as *Candida albicans*, *S. cerevisiae*, and *S. pombe*. The sequence identity between the query and subject is typically about 30% covering 500 amino acids. The R4 region makes a weak sequence similarity match (w) to a C-terminal section of a transcription factor involved in transactivation and repression in the mouse brachyury protein. This is not likely to be biologically significant because this region is rich in histidines, prolines, serines, leucines, and glycines. Additionally, the expectation values are positive and scores are low. A match with a positive expectation value may be statistically insignificant but could be biologically meaningful; for example, many members of a superfamily have diverged sufficiently that they do not make significant sequence similarities in BLASTX searches.

software such as the widely used program BLAST. BLAST comes in several versions: BLASTN, BLASTP, BLASTX, TBLASTN, and TBLASTX. It is important that you use the versions of the program that are best suited to particular tasks. Additionally, it is important to use the correct databases for your particular searches.

2. Machine-learning computational approaches allow a computer to learn how to solve particular problems by training it. Rather than programmers writing code to solve a problem directly, they write computer software that can modify itself in various ways according to how successfully it finds patterns in a well-understood set of data. If the software can accurately find patterns or features in this training set of data, it is hoped that it can find patterns accurately in new data. Examples of machine-learning approaches to problems that you might have encountered include neural networks and hidden Markov models.

3. GeneMark uses Markov models to parameterize the differences between coding and noncoding sequences based on the correlations in adjacent nucleotides such as in-phase-hexamer statistics in data-training sets *(2,3)*. The coding function is a probability calculated for query sequences by GeneMark using a phased Markov chain model quantifying the likelihood of the region coding for protein.

4. Additional information provided by the prediction programs, such as donor and acceptor splice sites located close in sequence to the boundaries of exons, can provide clues to exon boundary positions. Such signals can be species specific, and their characteristic sequence motifs may be provided from the scientific literature.

Acknowledgments

Y.J.K.E. thanks Peter Keller for constructive discussions while this chapter was being written.

References

1. Solovyev, V. V. and Salamov A. A. (1997) The Gene finder computer tools for analysis of human and model organisms genome sequences, in *Proceedings of the Fifth International Conference on Intelligent Systems for Molecular Biology* (Rawling, C., Clark, D., Altman, R., Hunter, L., Lengauer, T., and Wodak, S., eds.), AAAI Press, Halkidiki, Greece, pp. 294–302.
2. Lukashin, A. V. and Borodovsky, M. (1998) GeneMarkHmm: new solutions for gene finding. *Nucleic Acids Res.* **26,** 1107–1115.
3. Borodovsky, M. and McIninch, J. (1993) Genmark—parallel gene recognition for both DNA strands. *Comput. Chem.* **17,** 123–133.
4. Guigo, R., Knudsen, S., Drake, N., and Smith, T. (1992) Prediction of gene structure. *J. Mol. Biol.* **226,** 141–157.
5. Reese, M. G., Eeckman, F. H., Kulp, D., and Haussler, D. J. (1997) Improved splice site detection in Genie. *J. Comput. Biol.* **4,** 311–323.
6. Burge, C. and Karlin, S. (1997) Prediction of complete gene structures in human genomic DNA. *J. Mol. Biol.* **268,** 78–94.
7. Uberbacher, E. C. and Mural, R. J. (1991) Locating protein-coding regions in human DNA sequences by a multiple sensor-neural network approach. *Proc. Natl. Acad. Sci. USA* **88,** 11,261–11,265.

8. Uberbacher, E. C., Xu, Y., and Mural, R. J. (1996) Discovering and understanding genes in human DNA sequence using GRAIL. *Methods Enzymol.* **266,** 259–281.

9. Krogh, A. (1997) Two methods for improving performance of an HMM and their application for gene finding, in *Proceedings of the Fifth International Conference on Intelligent Systems for Molecular Biology* (Gaasterland, T., Karp, P., Karplus, K., et al., eds.), AAAI Press, Menlo Park, CA, pp. 179–186.

10. Altschul, S. F., Madden, T. L., Schaffer, A. A., Zhang, J. H., Zhang, Z., Miller, W., and Lipman, D. J. (1997) Gapped BLAST and PSI-BLAST: a new generation of protein database search programs. *Nucleic Acids Res.* **25,** 3389–3402.

17

Gene Identification Using the Pufferfish, *Fugu rubripes*, by Sequence Scanning

Greg Elgar

1. Introduction

The major goal of the Human Genome Project must be to identify, sequence, characterize and assign specific function to all the genes spread through our 3000 Mb of haploid DNA. Owing to the uniformity and simplicity of the DNA code, it is not an easy task to identify genes even after the region in which they lie has been fully sequenced. The average length of a human coding sequence in the DNA databases is approx 1.2 kb, and sensible estimates of the total number of genes in the human genome lie between 50 and 100,000. A gene number of 70,000 would give a total coding sequence of 85 Mb, <3% of our genome. Herein lies one of the major problems. A 3% return on investment, even when genes are identifiable, is rather poor, especially when sequencing is an expensive business. As if that is not enough, a large percentage of highly reiterated dispersed repeats serves to exacerbate the problem.

Consequently, other more direct approaches are being used, mostly to identify coding sequences within large genomic regions of DNA, and it is only by using a combination of these more elegant strategies that "gene hunters" are able to operate economically. Some of these methods compare human sequences with sequences from other organisms, using the premise that conserved sequences have some function. An extension of this, particularly among mammals but also with chicken, is to identify conserved linkage groups, and this may have particular value in positional cloning projects and the identification of new human genes. Conserved linkage, or conserved synteny, can in fact be used to great advantage in comparative genomics, particularly if a genome is smaller and easier to work with than the human genome.

From: *Methods in Molecular Biology, vol. 175: Genomics Protocols*
Edited by: M. P. Starkey and R. Elaswarapu © Humana Press Inc., Totowa, NJ

In the early 1990s, a group of researchers in Cambridge, England *(1)*, defined a simple genomic approach to gene identification and characterization. They reasoned that all vertebrates would have a similar repertoire of genes, owing to the way in which genomes have evolved. Thus, a vertebrate with a small genome should be the starting point for investigation. The pufferfish *(Fugu rubripes)* was known to have the smallest recorded vertebrate genome of just 400 Mb and, therefore, was presented as the choice of model vertebrate genome.

Why is the genome of the pufferfish so much smaller than mammalian genomes? First, the genes are smaller. Although the coding sequence is the same size, intron sizes are greatly reduced. Second, the intergenic distances are much smaller, and third, there is very little repetitive DNA and virtually none of that is dispersed. Critically, however, the pufferfish has a very similar gene repertoire to other mammals, including humans. The structure of genes is also conserved, with splice sites falling in positions identical to those found in humans. Finally, and critically, homology between fugu and mammalian genes is high enough to facilitate easy identification through both hybridization and database comparison. This forms the basis of the suitability of using fugu in comparative genomics *(1–4)*.

With such a small genome, the proportion of coding sequence is high—in the region of 20%, as opposed to about 3% for mammals. This makes fugu an attractive model for the analysis of large regions, because it is far more economical to use its compact genome than the genomes of mammals, cluttered with "junk" DNA. However, to be of real value to gene hunters, the extent of regions showing conserved synteny with mammalian genomes had to be evaluated. Different studies from both the zebrafish *(5,6)* and fugu *(7–13)* genomes suggest that large regions of conserved synteny do exist, but with variable degrees of intrachromosomal rearrangement. A more genomewide assessment suggests that over some regions at least, the fugu genome provides a useful resource for gene hunters *(4)*.

The sequence scanning methodology used in **ref.** *4* may also be applied specifically to a region or gene of interest and is the topic of this chapter. It may be applied to any organism and region, provided the necessary resources (usually a genomic library of some sort) are available but is particularly efficient in gene-dense organisms such as fugu *(see* **Note 1***)*. Several short, single-pass sequences are randomly generated from a genomic clone and are then compared against known sequence data in the public databases. In this way the gene content of a given genomic clone may be analyzed. In particular, sequences may be identified as homologous to expressed sequence tag (EST) database entries, as well as *Caenorhabditis elegans* genomic DNA indicating the presence of an unknown gene. The high gene density in the fugu genome

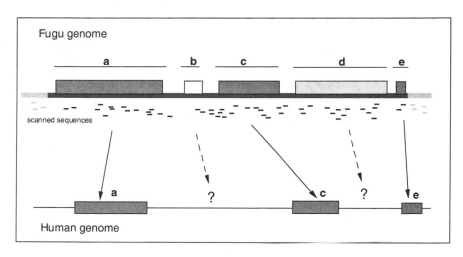

Fig. 1. Schematic of the sequence scanning procedure and how data from the fugu genome may help in locating and identifying genes in the human genome. The top half represents a fugu cosmid clone that contains genes a, b, c, d, and e. Note that the cosmid vector arms, which represent about one-eighth of the clone, are included in the scanning procedure and hence will be represented in the sequence scans. Underneath the cosmid, and to scale, are representations of some random sequence reads that are of sufficient coverage to "hit" all the genes on the cosmid. Fifty sequences are represented here, which is a good starting figure for cosmid clones (about 200 are usually sufficient for a BAC clone). Homology searches of these clones against DNA and protein databases allow identification of three known genes, a, c, and e, all of which map to the same region of the human genome. Gene b shows homology only to an EST and therefore allows the gene to be sequenced and identified in fugu. Gene d has already been identified in the human genome but is only partially characterized and unmapped. The sequence scanning information provided by the fugu clone therefore allows identification and characterization of genes as well as giving an indication of possible mapping positions in the human genome, provided synteny is conserved.

(one gene every 6 to 7 kb) allows a number of genes to be identified from a single cosmid or bacterial artificial chromosome (BAC) clone. Because some of these may have been identified and mapped to a specific location in the human genome, any newly identified genes on that clone may also map to that region of the human genome (**Fig. 1**).

This chapter describes the laboratory work involved in generating the sequence reads and a gives basic outline of how to carry out the homology searches against DNA and protein databases. More extensive interpretation of genomic data using bioinformatic approaches is covered in Chapter 16.

2. Materials

1. TB: 12 g of Bacto tryptone, *24* g yeast extract and *4* mL of glycerol in 900 mL of ddH$_2$O. After autoclaving add 100 mL of filter-sterilized 0.1*7 M* KH$_2$PO$_4$, and 0.72 *M* K$_2$HPO$_4$·3H$_2$O.
2. 50% (v/v) Glycerol.
3. GTE: 50 m*M* glucose, 25 m*M* Tris-HCl (pH 8.0), 10 m*M* EDTA.
4. RNase A (10 mg/mL). Boil and allow to cool slowly to room temperature. This will ensure that it is DNase free.
5. 3 *M* Potassium acetate (KAc): To 60 mL of 5 *M* potassium acetate add 11.5 mL of glacial acetic acid and make up to 100 mL with dH$_2$O.
6. 10 *M* NaOH.
7. 10% SDS.
8. 100% Ethanol.
9. 70% Ethanol.
10. TE buffer: 10 m*M* Tris-HCl (pH 7.4), 1 m*M* EDTA (always disodium salt).
11. Restriction enzymes: *Eco*RV with 10X buffer (New England Biolabs).
12. Loading dye: 20% Ficoll 400, 0.4% bromophenol blue, and 0.1 *M* EDTA.
13. Agarose (Bioline, http://www.bioline.com/).
14. DNA molecular weight marker Hyperladder I (Bioline).
15. 10X TBE: 108 g of Tris base, 55 g of boric acid, and 9.3 g of EDTA made to 1 L with dH$_2$O.
16. 2 m*M* dNTPs: 2 m*M* each of dATP, dCTP, dGTP, and TTP (Bioline).
17. T4 DNA polymerase and 10X buffer (New England Biolabs, http://www. neb.com/).
18. Polyethylene glycol (PEG) solution: 26.2% PEG 8000, 6.6 m*M* MgCl$_2$, and 20 mL of 3 *M* potassium acetate made up to 100 mL with dH$_2$O
19. Calf intestinal alkaline phosphatase (CIAP) and 10X buffer (Boehringer).
20. 100 m*M* Trinitrilo-acetic acid (Sigma, Poole, Dorset).
21. T4 DNA ligase and 10X buffer (New England Biolabs).
22. XL-2 Blue MRF' ultracompetent cells (cat. no. 200150; Stratagene, http://www.stratagene.com).
23. Sterile pop-top tubes 12 mL (Becton Dickinson, Franklin Lakes, NJ).
24. SOC: 20 g of tryptone, 5 g of yeast extract, 10 mL of 1 *M* NaCl, and 0.15 g of KCl made up to 1 L with dH$_2$O. After autoclaving add MgSO$_4$ and MgCl$_2$ to 10 m*M* each and 0.2% glucose.
25. TYE+amp plates: Dissolve 15 g of Bacto agar, 8 g of NaCl, 10 g of Bacto tryptone, and 5 g of yeast extract in dH$_2$O and make up the volume to 1 L. Sterilize by autoclaving. Add ampicillin (stock of 100 mg/mL in ddH$_2$O) to a final concentration of 100 µg/mL once the medium has cooled to 50°C and then pour into large agar plates.
26. 200 m*M* Isopropyl-β-D-thiogalactopyranoside (Melford, Chelsworth, Ipswich, UK).
27. 8% X-Gal: Dissolve 8 g of X-Gal in dimethyl formamide (Melford).
28. Sterile toothpicks or cocktail sticks.
29. 96-Well sterile culture plates.

30. 96-Pin replicator (plastic disposable preferred; *see* **Note 2**) (cat. no. X5051/L; http://www.genetix.co.uk; Genetix UK).
31. T7 short primer: 5' AATACGACTCACTATAG 3' primer.
32. T3 short primer: 5' ATTAACCCTCACTAAAG 3' primer.
33. 96-Well polymerase chain reaction (PCR) plates (Costar; Corning Costar, Acton, MA).
34. BioTaq and 10X buffer (Bioline).
35. Long KS: 5' CTCGAGGTCGACGGTATCG 3' primer diluted to 6 μM.
36. Big Dye™ terminator sequencing kit (cat. no. 4303154; PE Applied Biosystems).
37. Round-bottomed 96-well PCR plates (Costar "T" Thermowell™ plates).
38. Formamide loading dye: For PE ABI 377 sequencers, this is a 5:1 mix of deionized formamide and 25 m*M* EDTA + 50 mg/mL of blue dextran.
39. 37°C Incubator.
40. Sonicator suitable for sonicating small volumes with a cup probe (Misonix Ultrasonic Processor XL; http://www.misonix.com/).
41. 96-Well plate thermocycler (MJ Research, http://www.gri.co.uk).
42. Microtiter plate centrifuge capable of spinning to 3200*g* (Jouan, http://wwwjouan.com/).
43. ABI 377 Sequencer (http://www.pebio.com/ab/).
44. Gene-PAGE plus acrylamide (Amresco, Solon OH).

3. Methods

3.1. Isolation of Cosmid/BAC DNA

This basic alkaline lysis miniprep method results in relatively clean DNA, with minimal *Escherichia coli* contamination if carried out carefully and is perfectly adequate for restriction digests and sonication. It is therefore appropriate for sequence scanning protocols and allows the preparation of many different clones at one time.

1. Grow a 5-mL culture in TB overnight at 37°C *(see* **Note 3**). Make a glycerol stock with 1 mL of the culture by adding 0.5 mL of 50% glycerol. Transfer 2 mL to an Eppendorf tube. Centrifuge for 2 min at 9500*g*. Discard the supernatant, add a further 2 mL of culture, and repeat spin. Pour off the supernatant and resuspend the pellet in 200 μL of GTE, add 5 μL of RNase A stock solution, vortex for 2 min ensuring that the pellet has completely dispersed, and incubate at room temperature for 10 min.
2. Add 400 μL of 0.2 *M* NaOH/1% SDS (freshly made). Mix gently by inversion. Place on ice for 10 min.
3. Add 300 μL 3 *M* KAc. Invert gently to mix *(see* **Note 4**). Place on ice for 45 min.
4. Microfuge for 10 min at 9500*g*. Decant the supernatant into a fresh Eppendorf tube containing 1 mL of cold ethanol, vortex briefly, and allow to stand for 1 min. Centrifuge for 10 min (9500*g*), remove the ethanol, wash the pellet in 70% ethanol, and dry the pellet.

5. Add 50 µL of TE buffer to pellet and leave to resuspend at 4°C overnight. Check 1 µL on a 0.8% agarose gel by digestion.

3.2. Restriction Digest Check of Cosmid/BAC Miniprep

Restriction digestion is the most useful way of determining the yield of miniprep DNA. Trying to determine concentration by absorbance at OD_{260} will give an artificially high reading, as any RNA or degraded DNA, as well as proteins, will increase the absorbance. It is also useful for determining the order and extent of overlap between clones selected for a particular region.

1. Set up a 20-µL reaction to include 2 µL of 10X buffer, 5 µL of miniprep DNA, 1 µL of appropriate restriction enzyme, and 12 µL of dH_2O.
2. Incubate at 37°C for 1 h.
3. Add 5 µL of loading dye to the reaction mix and run on a 0.8% agarose gel. Use lambda *Hind*III marker.

3.3. Cosmid/BAC Shotgun Protocol: Preparation of Sheared DNA

Random breaks are introduced into the clone DNA using sonication. This procedure produces uneven ends that need "tidying" with T4 DNA polymerase. DNA over about 500 bp is then selectively precipitated using a PEG mix ready for ligation into blunt-end cut vector *(see* **Note 5**).

1. Mix the following in a 1.5-mL Eppendorf tube: 20 µL of cosmid DNA (approx 1 µg), 5 µL of 2 m*M* dNTPs, 5 µL of 10X T4 DNA polymerase buffer, and 20 µL of sterile dH_2O.
2. Sonicate for 25 s at a power setting of 4 to 5. Check 5 µL on a 1.5% gel before adding polymerase to ascertain the effectiveness of the sonication.
3. Add 0.5 µL of T4 DNA polymerase. Incubate at 16°C overnight.
4. Add an equal volume of 20% PEG solution. Vortex and incubate at room temperature for 5–10 min. Spin for 30 min (9500*g*).
5. Remove the supernatant and rinse the pellet with 100 µL of 70% ethanol. Dry the pellet and resuspend in 12 µL of sterile dH_2O.
6. Run 2 µL on a 1.5% agarose gel to check recovery *(see* **Note 6**). Use an appropriate DNA ladder to get a good idea of the size range of the DNA fragments produced.

3.4. Preparation and Ligation of Vector

The vector of choice here is Stratagene's pBluescript II KS (pBS), but any vector with a unique blunt-ended restriction site in the multiple cloning site will suffice. As will be clear, it is also useful if there are good primer sites (in the case of pBS, T3, T7, KS, and SK) flanking the restriction site. Uncut vector can either be purchased from a company or made using the miniprep method described in **Subheading 3.1.** The vector is dephosphorylated to reduce background nonrecombinants.

1. Set up the following restriction digest: 10 µg of plasmid vector DNA, 10 µL of 10X reaction buffer, and 5 µL of *Eco*RV enzyme *(see* **Note 7**). Make up to a final volume of 100 µL with dH$_2$O.
2. Incubate at 37°C for 2 h. Check 5 µL on a 0.8% agarose gel to determine whether it has digested properly.
3. Add 1/10 vol of 10X CIAP reaction buffer and 1 µL of CIAP. Incubate at 37°C for 30 min.
4. Add TNA to a final concentration of 15 m*M*. Incubate at 68°C for 20 min.
5. PEG precipitate and resuspend in TE buffer.
6. Check a small sample on a 0.8% agarose gel and then dilute the DNA to approx 50 ng/µL ready for use directly in ligation reactions.
7. Set up a 10-µL ligation containing 0.5 µL of dephosphorylated vector *(Eco*RV cut pBS), 1 µL of sheared DNA (alternatively, set up a number of ligations, using different amounts of insert), 1 µL of 10X ligation buffer, 6.5 µL of dH$_2$O, and 1 µL of T4 DNA ligase *(see* **Note 8**).
8. Incubate overnight at any temperature between 4°C and ambient. Store at –20°C until required for transformation.

3.5. Plasmid Transformation Protocol

Transformations are notoriously variable in their success rate, because they are dependent on several parameters, all of which need to be correct in order to achieve success. One of the most critical of these is, of course, the transformation efficiency of the competent cells. Despite everyone having their own favorite recipes and distant memories of that batch of competent cells that gave 1×10^9 colonies per microgram, the cold truth is that commercial sources are better and more reliable. They can also be more economical *(see* **Note 9**) than taking 3 mo and 12 batches of homemade competent cells in order to produce a decent transformation. The following protocol relates to Stratagene XL-2 cells and may vary for other cells and suppliers. Reference should be made to the individual supplier's instructions.

1. Add 1 µL of ligated DNA to 15–20 µL of competent cells *(see* **Note 9**) in a 12-mL pop-top tube. Leave on ice for 10 min.
2. Heat-shock the cells at 42°C for 47 s.
3. Add 500 µL of SOC (prewarmed to 37°C) to each tube and incubate with shaking at 37°C for 45 min.
4. While the cells are incubating, dry TYE+amp plates by briefly incubating at 37°C.
5. After 1 h, add 75 µL of IPTG/X-Gal mix (25 µL of 200 m*M* IPTG and 50 µL of 8% X-Gal) to the cell/SOC culture. Add this mix to the plates, spread over the surface, and leave to soak in.

6. Incubate the plates overnight at 37°C. Transformed colonies containing vector and insert are white, and religated vector colonies are blue (*see* **Notes 10** and **11**).

3.6. Storage and Growth of Recombinant Clones

Once the cultures have been transformed and white colonies obtained, they have a limited storage life on the plates (1-mo maximum). It is therefore best to pick them immediately using sterile toothpicks (or cocktail sticks) into 96-well culture plates.

1. Prepare the appropriate number of 96-well plates by filling each well with 100 μL of TB plus ampicillin (100 μg/mL) medium.
2. Using a sterile toothpick or cocktail stick, gently pick white colonies and place into the wells of the 96-well plates.
3. Grow overnight at 37°C. The following morning, add 40 μL of 50% glycerol to each well of the microtiter plates. Store at –20°C (short term) or –80°C (long term).
4. To regrow these stored cultures, scrape the frozen cultures with either a wire inoculating loop or sterile toothpick and inoculate either an agar plate or liquid culture containing the appropriate antibiotics. Grow overnight at 37°C.
5. It is advisable to duplicate the plates using a 96-pin replicator to transfer culture over to another 96-well plate containing 100 μL of media + antibiotic. Grow overnight at 37°C. Add glycerol and store at either –20 or –80°C.

3.7. Preparation of PCR Template for Sequencing

There are many ways to sequence DNA templates, but the choice of method here is designed for speed and economy and can be tailored to any throughput rate. It can be performed by any reasonably equipped molecular biology laboratory. The methodology uses PCR products as templates that give highly reproducible results. Furthermore, the procedure is rapid, because it requires no additional prepping of templates (i.e., the PCR product is derived directly from the bacterial cultures) and no purification of template, because the PCR uses limiting concentrations of dNTPs and primers, and the sequencing reaction uses a primer with a much higher annealing temperature than the PCR primers, thereby ensuring that only the sequencing primer takes any part in the sequencing reaction. The following protocol relates to PCR amplification of templates from a full 96-well culture plate.

1. Make up a PCR master mix of 2 mL (*see* **Note 12**): 200 μL of 10X buffer, $MgCl_2$ to a final concentration of 1.5 mM, T3 and T7 primers to a final concentration of 125 nM, dNTPs to a final concentration of 30 μM (30 μL of 2 mM stock), and 50 U of *Taq* polymerase (usually 10 μL).
2. Dispense 20 μL of the mix into each well of a 96-well PCR plate (make sure that the appropriate plate is used for the type of machine being used).
3. Transfer approx 1 μL of each culture across to the PCR plate using a 96-well replicator (*see* **Note 13**). Seal appropriately.

4. Incubate the plate initially at 96°C for 2 min and then cycle 33 times as follows: 96°C for 20 s, 49°C for 20 s, and 72°C for 45 s (*see* **Note 14**). There is no need for a final additional extension time.
5. Once finished, bring the final volume up to 50 μL by adding 30 μL of dH_2O to each sample (*see* **Note 15**).
6. Check 5 μL of each PCR product on a 1.5% agarose gel using a suitable DNA marker to estimate sizes (*see* **Note 16**).

3.8. Sequencing PCR Products Using Dye Terminators

This protocol describes sequencing with dye terminator chemistry, which gives more flexibility as to which primer can be used. The reactions are also straightforward to set up and precipitate. The particular reactions detailed below are for running on a PE Applied Biosystems 377 automated sequencer, but it should be possible to adapt to any particular machine or, indeed, use manual sequencing techniques. Because of the way in which the PCR products are generated, there is no need for any purification. The key to the sequencing primer is that it has an annealing temperature of at least 60°C, thereby allowing the cycle sequencing to be carried out at temperatures at which any residual T3 and T7 primers (annealing temperatures of just 49°C) cannot take any part in the reaction.

1. Set up the sequencing reaction in round-bottomed 96-well PCR plates (regardless of thermocycler; *see* **Note 17**) as follows: 6 μL of PCR template, 4 μL of dye terminator mix, and 0.5 μL of KS primer (6 μ*M* stock solution).
2. Cycle sequence for 25 cycles using the following parameters: 95°C for 20 s and 60°C for 140 s.
3. When the reactions are complete, add 30 μL of a 25:1 100% ethanol/3 *M* KAc mix. Spin at 3200*g* for 30 min at 4°C in a plate centrifuge (*see* **Note 18**). Tip the ethanol down the sink by inverting the plate (the pellets will not disappear down the sink).
4. Add 50 μL of 70% ethanol to each well. Pour down the sink. Add a further 50 μL of 70% ethanol to each well. Pour down the sink. Tap the inverted plate on a paper towel. Put the plate upside down on the towel and spin until the centrifuge reaches 150*g*, and then press the stop button.
5. The reactions are now dry and can be stored dried down at –20°C until required.
6. Add formamide loading dye when ready to load the gel (the amount added will depend on the number of lanes in the gel).
7. Heat denature the samples at 95°C for 2 min.
8. Prepare and load acrylamide gel as per the supplier's instructions.

3.9. Preparation of Sequence Data for Database Searching

Once the sequencing gel has completed its run, the data generated will need to be analyzed. In the case of ABI 377 sequence machines (and other automated sequencers), analysis software is provided making this a straightforward task. However, particular care should be taken in tracking samples all the way through the procedure, so that bacterial clones may be indexed correctly and referred back to in light of the results of the sequence scans. For instance, a clone may be required for further sequencing or probing that can be performed from some of the remaining PCR product from that clone or its glycerol stock.

A variety of DNA and protein databases can be accessed freely or purchased. The most complete collections of publicly accessible databases are found at the National Center for Biotechnology Information, US *(14)*, and at the UK Human Genome Mapping Project Resource Centre *(15)*. These databases are essentially copies of each other, so it is not necessary to search both. To search these databases, sequence data generated from the scans must be edited to remove any unwanted vector contamination. Leaving vector attached to the sequences will result in a long list of similarity matches to vector sequences in the databases, thus effectively masking any good matches made by the insert sequence itself. **Figure 2** presents a schematic of the kinds of sequence that need to be removed.

This removal of contaminating sequences can be done manually, involving an initial database search with unedited sequences that serves to highlight which bases of any clone match vector (or *Escherichia coli*). These bases can then be removed from the clone sequence and a second database search carried out with the edited sequence. Alternatively, and preferably if large batches of sequences are to be generated, a vector-clipping program, such as the PreGap module of the Staden Package (available free), should be used *(16)*. Full documentation for the use of these programs is also available from this Web site.

Once sequences have been efficiently clipped, database searches should reveal what is contained within the cosmid/BAC. When looking for matches across species, amino acid similarities are more informative than DNA matches. This is primarily because there are 20 amino acids compared with only four bases; the chances, therefore, of having the same residue in the same position is much lower when aligning protein sequences.

Map locations of human genes are available primarily (but not exclusively) through Genemap'99 *(17)*, the online Mendelian Inheritance in Man database *(18)*, and Unigene *(19)*.

4. Notes

1. The fugu cosmid library (as well as many others) is available as gridded filters from the HGMP Resource Centre (http://www.hgmp.mrc.ac.uk/), and any data arising from the use of these can also be integrated into the fugu database (http://fugu.hgmp.mrc.ac.uk/).

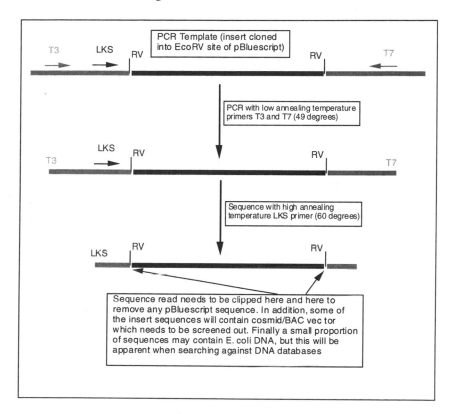

Fig. 2. Sequence scanning process. Subclones containing insert (white colonies) are PCR amplified from bacterial stocks using T3 and T7 primers. The resulting PCR products require no purification and are sequenced using the universal LKS primer from one end. After sequencing, any vector needs to be removed from the clone before searching against DNA and protein databases.

2. Sterile, disposable 96-pin replicators are available from Genetix and are preferred to metal replicators because they avoid any cross-contamination of samples. With metal replicators, even when thoroughly flamed, there is some carryover of material from earlier replications, and this is particularly problematic when using them to set up PCR reactions.

3. With some BAC clones in particular, yields are low and it may be necessary to grow several 5-mL cultures overnight and pool more than one miniprep together. This always appears to give better yields than setting up one large culture. If yields are still low with BAC clones, try growing from a seed culture for 6–8 h during the day rather than overnight.

4. It is critical that the 3 *M* Kac be mixed in gently by inversion. This allows large protein aggregates to form, which will precipitate readily and will be efficiently

removed before ethanol precipitation. If the mixture is vortexed or shaken, it will form very small aggregates and these will not precipitate effectively, leaving protein in the DNA pellet after ethanol precipitation.

5. PEG precipitation provides a rapid way of size selecting DNA fragments >500 bp. In this way, any very small DNA fragments, that would not make very good templates for sequencing yet would be efficiently cloned, are removed.

6. A clearly visible smear should be apparent on the gel, with the smear tailing off below 500 bp. The upper size limit varies but there should not be any unsonicated DNA left at the top of the gel, which appears as a band. If a band is present, or a smear is not visible, a fresh aliquot of the clone should be sonicated again.

7. The usual blunt-end restriction sites in multiple cloning regions of vectors are *Eco*RV or *Sma*I. *Eco*RV *is* much more stable and cuts DNA much more cleanly than *Sma*I. Because *Sma*I *is* unstable, it should be used at 25–30°C rather than 37°C, and for short incubation times.

8. T4 DNA ligase buffer contains dATP, which can deteriorate rapidly if continually frozen and thawed. When new stock arrives, aliquot buffer into tubes in 10-µL vol and store at –20°C. Use each tube once and throw away the rest.

9. Stratagene supplies individual vials of 100–150 µL of cells, and this is supposed to be for one transformation. However, I have found that just 15–20 µL of cells is sufficient as long as only small (1-µL) volumes of ligation are used. Therefore, it is useful to save up half a dozen ligations ready for transformation and then split up a single tube of competent cells.

10. If the blue color is not well developed, leave the plates in the refrigerator overnight; this will darken the color. This step can be important because false positives can be produced, and picking colonies while the color is faint will increase the chance of this happening.

11. If the transformation fails (i.e., there are no white colonies or hardly any colonies at all), there are many possible reasons. It is therefore particularly important to include appropriate controls among the transformations carried out. This includes transforming a calibrated amount of uncut vector (usually supplied) to check the efficiency of the cells and the transformation itself, transforming unligated and self-ligated (i.e., no insert) vector and, if necessary, transforming SOC alone to check that there is no source of contaminating colonies. If all these controls look good, it may be necessary to go back and perform more ligations with different concentrations of insert, or even reprep the original genomic clone and start again (it is not a very long protocol).

12. If a large number of culture plates are to be screened by PCR, then a larger master mix may be made (e.g., aliquots of 50 mL) without the addition of the *Taq* polymerase. This mix can then be stored at 4°C ready for use.

13. Plastic 96-well replicators transfer approx 1 µL of culture across if dipped and stirred around in culture plates that have not yet had glycerol added. If glycerol has already been added, the culture becomes much more viscous and care must be taken to just dip the very tip of the replicator into the culture. This will transfer sufficient cells for the PCR reaction.

14. An extension time of 45 s will allow PCR products of up to 2–2.5 kb to be amplified efficiently. Above this size, the limiting concentrations of dNTPs mean that products are faint and not particularly good for sequencing. Most inserts will be <2 kb anyway, if sonication is good.

15. Adding water to the PCR products means that any remaining dNTPs and primers are diluted still further. It also means there is a greater volume of template for subsequent sequencing reactions.

16. If a number of gels are to be run over a period of time, it may be worth considering using multichannel pipets in wells that are arranged accordingly. Some gel apparatuses have multichannel combs available (alternatively, they may be cut very cheaply from Perspex by a workshop).

17. It is important to use round-bottomed 96-well PCR plates in this protocol, because these allow the resulting sequenced DNA to be precipitated and washed efficiently in the plates. Conically shaped bottoms do not allow efficient precipitation or washing. Alternatively, the sequencing can be carried out in individual tubes, but the setting up and precipitation stages become much longer and more tedious. 18. If a plate centrifuge is not available, reactions will have to be carried out in or transferred to tubes in order to be precipitated in a microfuge (at 9500g).

References

1. Brenner, S., Elgar, G., Sandford, R., Macrae, A., Venkatesh, B., and Aparicio, S. (1993) Characterization of the pufferfish *(Fugu)* genome as a compact model vertebrate genome. *Nature* **366,** 265–268.

2. Elgar, G., Sandford, R., Aparicio, S., Macrae, A., Venkatesh, B., and Brenner, S. (1996) Small is beautiful: comparative genomics with the pufferfish *(Fugu rubripes)*. *Trends Genet.* **12,** 145–150.

3. Elgar, G. (1996) Quality not quantity: the pufferfish genome. *Hum. Mol. Genet.* **5,** 1437–1442.

4. Elgar, G., Clark, M. S., Meek, S., Smith, S., Warner, S., Edwards, Y. J., Bouchireb, N., Cottage, A., Yeo, G. S., Umrania, Y., Williams, G., and Brenner, S. (1999) Generation and analysis of 25 Mb of genomic DNA from the pufferfish *Fugu rubripes* by sequence scanning. *Genome Res.* **9,** 960–971.

5. Postelthwait, J. H., Yan, Y. L., Gates, M. A., et al. (1998) Vertebrate genome evolution and the zebrafish gene map. *Nature Genet.* **18,** 345–349.

6. Gates, M. A., Kim, L., Egan, E. S., Cardozo, T., Sirotkin, H. I., Dougan, S. T., Lashkari, D., Abagyan, R., Schier, A. F., and Talbot, W. S. (1999) A genetic linkage map for zebrafish: comparative analysis and localization of genes and expressed sequences. *Genome Res.* **9,** 334–347.

7. Aparicio, S., Hawker, K., Cottage, A., Mikawa, Y., Zuo, L., Venkatesh, B., Chen, E., Krumlauf, R., and Brenner, S. (1997) Organization of the *Fugu rubripes* Hox clusters: evidence for continuing evolution of vertebrate Hox complexes. *Nature Genet.* **16,** 79–83.

8. Brunner, B., Todt, T., Lenzuer, S., Stout, K., Schulz, U., Ropers, H. H., and Kalscheuer, V. M. (1999) Genomic structure and comparative analysis of nine

Fugu genes: conservation of synteny with human chromosome Xp22.2-p22.1. *Genome Res.* **9,** 437–448.

9. Gellner, K. and Brenner, S. (1999) Analysis of 148 kb of genomic DNA around the wntl locus of *Fugu rubripes. Genome Res.* **9,** 251 –258.

10. Gilley, J. and Fried, M. (1999) Extensive gene order differences within regions of conserved synteny between the *Fugu* and human genomes: implications for chromosomal evolution and the cloning of disease genes. *Hum. Mol. Genet.* **8,** 1313–1320.

11. Miles, C., Elgar, G., Coles, E., Kleinjan, D. J., van Heyningen, V., and Hastie, N. (1998) Complete sequencing ofthe *Fugu* WAGR region from WT1 to PAX6: dramatic compaction and conservation of synteny with human chromosome 11p13. *Proc. Natl. Acad. Sci. USA* **95,** 13,068–13,072.

12. Schofield, J. P., Elgar, G., Greystrong, J., Lie, G., Deadman, R. Micklem, G., King, A., Brenner, S., and Vaudin, M. (1997) Regions of human chromosome 2 (2q32-q35) and mouse chromosome 1 show synteny with the pufferfish genome *(Fugu rubripes). Genomics* **45,** 158–167.

13. Trower, M. K., Orton, S. M., Purvis, I. J., et al. (1996) Conservation of synteny between the genome of the pufferfish *(Fugu rubripes)* and the region on human chromosome 14 (14q24.3) associated with familial Alzheimer disease. *Proc. Natl. Acad. Sci. USA* **93,** 1366–1369.

14. <http://www.ncbi.nlm.nih.gov/BLAST>.

15. <http://www.hgmp.mrc.ac.uk>.

16. <http://www.mrc-lmb.cam.ac.uk/pubseq/staden home.html>.

17. <http://www.ncbi.nlm.nih.gov/genemap99>.

18. <http://www.ncbi.nlm.nih.gov/Omim>.

19. <http://www.ncbi.nlm.nih.gov/UniGene>.

18

Isolation of Differentially Expressed Genes Through Subtractive Suppression Hybridization

Oliver Dorian von Stein

1. Introduction

Despite the fact that the genetic blueprint in every cell is identical, an organism is composed of a multitude of different cell types. This cell type complexity or phenotypic differences are the result of differential expression of identical genes. For example, a normal cell expresses a different repertoire of genes than a tumor cell derived from the same cell type. Moreover, to identify those genes would provide an entry point for understanding the biologic processes responsible for these phenotypic differences. This in turn could lead to the development of novel therapeutic strategies against cancer.

Isolation of such differentially expressed genes would require methods capable of rapid and efficient comparisons of the transcriptional status between two cell types (e.g., a normal cell vs a tumorigenic cell). The recent description of a novel equalizing cDNA subtraction method called suppression subtractive hybridization (SSH) *(1)* provides the technical basis for such comparisons. SSH is particularly efficient in isolating both rare and abundantly differentially expressed genes. In addition, this method is not biased for genes that differ largely in their initial abundance, and is also able to isolate genes that demonstrate a three- to fourfold change in expression level. SSH can be adapted to any cellular system in which expression profiling is required. It relies on the efficient polymerase chain reaction (PCR)-based suppression of genes that are common to both populations with the concomitant exponential amplification of genes that are differentially expressed. Throughout this chapter the term *tester* refers to that mRNA population containing differentially expressed genes of interest (i.e., the treated sample), and the term *driver* indicates that mRNA population obtained from the same cells without treatment. **Figure 1** outlines the general strategy.

From: *Methods in Molecular Biology, vol. 175: Genomics Protocols*
Edited by: M. P. Starkey and R. Elaswarapu © Humana Press Inc., Totowa, NJ

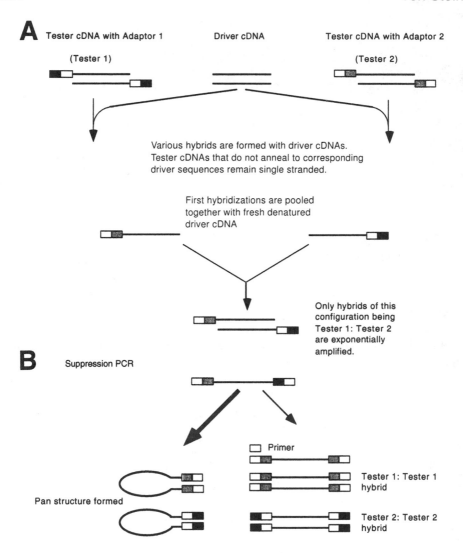

Fig. 1. **(A)** Schematic of the method employed. **(B)** A primer anneals to one of the complementary sequences (adapter) present on each end of the single-stranded cDNA molecule. It is extended through the action of the *Taq* polymerase, such that the resulting double-stranded cDNA molecule also now has inverted terminal repeats, as in the case of the original template. During the denaturing cycle of a PCR thermocycle, the two strands dissociate and during the annealing step form a panlike structure thereby

2. Materials

2.1. Primers

1. Oligo d(T) primer: 5'-TTTTGTACAAGCTTTTTTTTTTTTTTTTTTTTTTTT-TTTTTT-3'.
2. AD1a: 5'-CTAATACGACTCACTATAGGGCTCGACCGGGCAGGCGGCC-GCGT-3'.
3. AD 1b: 5'-ACGCGGCCGCCT-3'.
4. AD2a: 5'-TGTAGCGTGAAGACGACAGAAAGGGCGGGAGGCCGTCG-ACCGT-3'.
5. AD2b: 5'-ACGGTCGACGG-3'.
6. P1: 5'-CTAATACGACTCACTATAGGGC-3'.
7. P2: 5'-TGTAGCGTGAAGACGACAGAAA-3'.
8. PN1: 5'-TCGACCGGGCAGGCGGCCGCGT-3'.
9. PN2: 5'-AGGGCGGGAGGCCGTCGACCGT-3'.

2.2. RNA Isolation

1. Ultra-Turrax T25 (IKA®-Labortechnik, Staufen, Germany).
2. Drethylpyrocarbonate (DEPC)-treated water.
3. peqGOLD RNA Pure™(peqlab GmbH, D-91058 Erlangen-Tennenlohe, Germany).
4. Phosphate-buffered saline (PBS): 0.14 M NaCl, 2 mM KCl, 8 mM Na$_2$HPO$_4$, 1 mM KH$_2$PO$_4$.
5. Oligo-dT cellulose (type VII; Amersham Pharmacia Biotech, Amersham, UK).
6. STE-sodium dodecyl sulfate (SDS): 20 mM Tris-HCl, pH 7.4, 100 mM NaCl, 10 mM EDTA, 0.5% (w/v) SDS.
7. Proteinase K (Sigma-Aldrich, Poole, Dorset, UK).
8. Econo-Pac columns (20 mL) (Bio-Rad, Hemel Hempstead, Hertfordshire, UK)
9. mRNA washing solution: 100 mM NaCl, 20 mM Tris-HCl, pH 7.4, 10 mM EDTA, 0.2% (w/v) SDS.
10. mRNA Elusion solution: 1 mM Tris-IICl, pII 7.4, 1 mM EDTA, 0.2% (w/v) SDS.
11. TAE: 40 mM Tris-acetate, 1 mM EDTA.

2.3. cDNA Synthesis

1. T$_4$ DNA polymerase (1 U/μL), *Escherichia coli* DNA ligase (7.5 U/μL), *E. coli* DNA polymerase I (10 U/μL), and *E. coli* RNase H (2 U/μL) (Roche, Lewes, East Sussex, UK).
2. SuperScript II RT, dithiothreitol (DTT), and 5X first-strand buffer: 250 mM Tris-HCl, pH 8.3; 375 mM KCl; 15 mM MgCl$_2$ (Gibco-BRL, Paisley, UK).

---

preventing the successful annealing of a much shorter primer sequence. In this fashion, such template amplification is suppressed. Consequently, only the amplification of single-stranded DNA templates, having two different adapters on their ends, is possible because no inverted repeats are present to form the pan structure. In the SSH protocol, these can only originate from the tester population.

3. dNTPs, 10 mM each.
4. 5X Second-strand buffer: 94 mM Tris-HCl, pH 6.9, 453 mM KCl, 23 mM MgCl$_2$, 750 μM β-NAD, 50 mM (NH$_4$)$_2$SO$_4$.
5. PCR purification kit (Qiagen, Crawley, West Sussex, UK).
6. T buffer: 10 mM Tris-HCl, pH 8.0.
7. *Rsa*I (10 U/μL) and 10X buffer: 0.1 M Tris propane-HCl, pH 7.0, 0.1 M MgCl$_2$, 10 mM DTT (New England Biolabs, Hitchin, Herts, UK).
8. T4 DNA ligase (10 U/μL) and 10X buffer: 0.5 M Tris-HCl, pH 7.5, 0.1 M MgCl$_2$, 0.1 M DTT, 10 mM adenosine triphosphate; 250 μg/μL of bovine serum albumin (BSA) (New England Biolabs).

2.4 Hybridization Buffers

1. 4X subtractive hybridization buffer: 50 mM HEPES, pH 8.2; 0.5 M NaCl; 20 mM EDTA; 10% (w/v) PEG 8000.
2. Church hybridization buffer: 0.5 M Na$_2$PO$_4$, pH 7.2; 7% (w/v) SDS.
3. QuickHyb (Stratagene, Cambridge, UK).

2.5. Reagents for Bacterial Transformation

1. ELECTROMAX *E. coli* bacteria strain DH10B (Gibco-BRL Life Technologies).
2. Electroporation cuvet (0.1-cm gap) and *E. coli* purser (Bio-Rad).
3. Disposable polypropylene tubes (14 mL) (Greiner, Stonehouse, Gloucestershire, UK).
4. 1 M Isopropyl β-D-thiogalactopyranoside in water (IPTG). Store in 1-mL aliquots at −20°C.
5. 5-Bromo-4-chloro-3-indolyl-β-D-galactopyranoside in dimethylformamide (X-Gal) (20 mg/mL). Store in the dark at −20°C).
6. Ampicillin (Sigma-Aldrich) (50 mg/mL) in water. Store in small aliquots at −20°C.
7. SOC broth: 2% (w/v) Bacto-tryptone; 0.5% (w/v) Bacto-yeast extract; 10 mM NaCl, 2.5 mM KCl, pH 7.5. Sterilize by autoclaving, and supplement with Mg^{2+} (MgCl$_2$ and MgSO$_4$) to 10 mM, and glucose to 20 mM, prior to use.
8. LB broth: 1% (w/v) Bacto-tryptone; 0.5% (w/v) Bacto-yeast extract, 1% (w/v) NaCl.
9. LB agar: LB broth + 1.5% (w/v) agar.

2.6. Sundry Reagents

1. Amicon Microcon concentrators (Millipore, Watford, Herts, UK).
2. 50X Advantage DNA polymerase mix and 10X buffer: 400 mM Tricine-KOH, pH 9.2; 150 mM potassium acetate; 35 mM magnesium acetate, 37.5 μg/mL BSA (Clontech, Basingstoke, Hants, UK).
3. Random primer labeling kit *(redi* Prime kit; Amersham Pharmacia Biotech).
4. [α-^{32}P]dCTP (370 MBq/mL, 10 mCi/mL) (Amersham Pharmacia Biotech).
5. Elutips (Schleicher & Schuell, Dassel, Germany).
6. High-density TAE agarose gels (Centipede gel electrophoresis chambers; Owl Scientific, Woburn, MA).
7. Nylon membrane (Hybond N+; Amersham Pharmacia Biotech).
8. Saline sodium citrate (SSC) 20X: 2.99 M NaCl, 0.34 M trisodium citrate.

9. Plasmid vector containing *Not*I and *Sal*I restriction sites flanked by T7 and T3 RNA polymerase promoter sites (e.g., pBluescript II; Gibco-BRL Life Technologies).
10. *Not*I *(*10 U/μL) and 10X buffer: 1 M NaCl; 0.5 M Tris-HCl, pH 7.9, 0.1 M MgCl$_2$, 10 mM DTT (New England Biolabs).
11. *Sal*I (10 U/μL) and 10X buffer: 1.5 M NaCl, 0.1 M Tris-HCl, pH 7.6, 0.1 M MgCl$_2$, 10 mM DTT (New England Biolabs).
12. *Taq* polymerase (3 U/μL) and 10X standard PCR reaction buffer: 200 mM Tris-HCl, pH 8.4, 500 mM KCl, 15 mM MgCl$_2$ (Amersham Pharmacia Biotech).

3. Methods

3.1. Generation of Adapters

Adapters used for the subtraction protocol can be generated by simply annealing two complementary oligonucleotides together in the following manner:

1. Mix equimolar amounts of AD1a with AD1b in 150 mM NaCl; 10 mM Tris-HCl, pH 8.0; and 1 mM EDTA.
2. Add to a beaker of preheated water (94°C) and allow to cool slowly to room temperature.
3. Repeat **steps 1** and **2** for AD2a with AD2b.
4. Remove contaminating salts from each adapter using an Amicon microcon concentrator, according to the manufacturer's instructions. Adjust the adapters to a concentration of 100 pmol/μL. Adapters AD1 and AD2 contain internal *Not*I and *Sal*I restriction sites, respectively, thereby allowing selective cloning into a suitably digested vector.

3.2. Isolation of Total RNA and Poly(A)+ RNA from Tissue or Cell Culture

3.2.1. Isolation of Total RNA

If the intended mRNA source is tissue, one should first extract total RNA from the tissue using the following protocol. If, however, total RNA is to be extracted from cell culture, refer to **Subheading 3.2.2.**

1. Ground approx 200–500 mg of frozen tissue (in a prechilled stone pestor) to a fine powder under liquid nitrogen. Immediately pour the powder with the nitrogen into a 50-mL tube and allowed to stand briefly until all the nitrogen has dissipated.
2. Add 5 mL of peqGOLD RNA Pure. For fresh wet tissue, omit **step 1** and homogenize the tissue directly in 5 mL of peqGOLD RNA Pure.
3. Homogenize using an Ultra-Turrax T25 at 20,000 rpm for 5–10 min, and incubate for 3–10 min at room temperature to allow the nucleic acids to dissolve into the solution.
4. Add 1 mL of pure chloroform (0.2 mL of chloroform per 1 mL of peqGOLD RNA Pure used), and vortex vigorously until the solution takes on a milky white appearance.

5. After brief incubation at room temperature, transfer the mixture to a 14-mL polypropylene tube and centrifuge for 15 min at 10,000g in a 4°C-cooled swing-out rotor.
6. Transfer the top aqueous RNA-containing phase to a clean polypropylene tube containing 3 mL of pure chloroform, and vortex the contents.
7. Centrifuge (as in **step 5**) and remove the top phase for a further round of chloroform extraction. After the last extraction, add an equal volume of isopropanol and place at –20°C for 30 min.
8. Centrifuge the tubes at 12,000g for 30 min in a 4°C-cooled swing-out rotor. The total RNA should be visible as a whiteish pellet.
9. Decant the liquid and wash the pellet twice with 75% (v/v) ethanol before resuspending in 150 µL of bidistilled water. Store at –80°C for further use. To isolate poly(A)$^+$ RNA, follow the protocol described in **Subheading 3.2.2. (step 4)**.

3.2.2. Isolation of Poly(A)$^+$ RNA

When isolating poly(A)$^+$ RNA from cell cultures, it is not necessary to isolate the total RNA first; one can proceed directly as outlined next:

1. Grow cells to a confluency of approx 70–80%, remove the medium, and wash the cells briefly in PBS.
2. Lyse the cells immediately in 20 mL of STE-SDS containing 300 mg/mL of proteinase K.
3. Homogenize the lysed cell mixture using an Ultra-Turax (this shears high molecular weight DNA and breaks up the cellular membrane), and incubate at 50°C for 30 min in order to degrade cellular proteins.
4. To total the RNA isolated from the tissue, add 10 mL of STE-SDS and incubate at 50°C for 30 min (since total RNA preparations are never free of cellular proteins).
5. To the incubated RNA samples add NaCl to a final concentration of 0.5 M, and mix well before adding 100–200 mg of oligo-dT cellulose. Rotate the resulting mixture overnight to allow binding of the poly(A)$^+$ RNA to the oligo-dT cellulose.
6. Wash the oligo-dT cellulose by pouring the contents into a 20-mL Econo-Pac column, allowing the liquid to drain out while retaining the oligo-dT cellulose.
7. Apply 20 mL of mRNA washing solution to the column and allow to drain through.
8. Elute the poly(A)$^+$ RNA from the oligo-dT cellulose by adding 4 mL of elusion solution, and collect the contents in a 14-mL polypropylene tube on an ice bed.
9. Determine the RNA concentration from 400 µL of the eluate by spectroscopic measurement of the extinction coefficient at 260 and 280 nm. An optical density (OD) of 1 at 260 nm is equivalent to 40 mg/mL of RNA. The OD_{280nm} is used as an indication of purity and should be approx 50% of the OD_{260} value. Pure RNA should have an OD_{260}/OD_{280} ratio of 1.8–2.0 in bidistilled water.
10. Precipitate the remaining 3.6 mL of RNA by adding 350 µL of 3 M sodium acetate, pH 5.2, and 0.8–1 vol of isopropanol, followed by centrifugation at 12,000g for 30 min at 4°C.

11. Decant the aqueous phase and wash the poly(A)$^+$ RNA pellet twice with 70% (v/v) ethanol, before air-drying the pellet for 10 min (take great care not to allow the RNA pellet to dry completely because it is often very difficult to redissolve). Resuspend the pellet in bidistilled H$_2$O at a concentration of 0.5–2.0 mg/mL, before storing at –80°C.

12. Monitor the integrity of the poly(A)$^+$ RNA by visualizing on a 1.4% (w/v) TAE agarose gel. A smear of equal intensity should be seen that runs from approx 500 bp up to 10 kb. It is extremely important that the quality of the poly(A)$^+$ RNA is high (*see* **Note 1**).

3.3. Double-Stranded cDNA Synthesis

3.3.1. First-Strand cDNA Synthesis

1. Heat approx 1 µg of poly(A)$^+$ RNA with 500 ng of oligo dT$_{30}$ primer in a volume of 11 µL to 70°C for 5 min in a thermal cycler, before rapidly chilling on ice.

2. Adjust the reaction mixture to 20 µL by adding 4 µL of 5X first-strand reaction buffer, 2 µL of 0.1 *M* DTT, and 1 µL of dNTPs. Initiate reverse transcription by adding 1 µL of Superscript II RT, and incubate the reaction mixture at 42°C for 1 h in an air incubator. Place the reaction on ice.

3.3.2. Second-Strand cDNA Synthesis

1. Add 91.8 µL of sterile bidistilled water, 32 µL of 5X second-strand buffer, 3 µL of dNTPs, 6 µL of 0.1 *M* DTT, 2 µL of *E. coli* DNA ligase, 4 µL of *E. coli* DNA polymerase I, and 0.7 µL of *E. coli* RNase H.

2. Incubate at 16°C for 2.5 h and blunt-end the double-stranded cDNA by adding T$_4$ polymerase (10 U/µg of mRNA used), followed by further incubation at 16°C for 20 min.

3. Remove the salts and proteins by using a PCR purification kit according to the manufacturer's instructions. Elute the cDNA in 35 µL of T buffer. Retain a 5-µL aliquot of the double-stranded cDNA with which to monitor the subsequent restriction digest.

3.4. Restriction Digestion of Double-Stranded cDNA

1. Digest the remaining 30 µL of double-stranded cDNA with 30 U of *Rsa*I in a 50-µL reaction containing 5 µL of 10X *Rsa*I restriction buffer. Allow the digestion to proceed overnight in a bacterial incubator set at 37°C (*see* **Note 2**).

2. Remove unwanted salts using a PCR purification kit (Qiagen) and elute the restricted double-stranded cDNA with 30 µL of T buffer.

3. Analyze 5 µL of the digested double-stranded cDNA alongside 5 µL of the undigested double-stranded cDNA on a 1% (w/v) TAE agarose gel. In the undigested double-stranded cDNA, you should see a smear of DNA from 500 bp to 9 to 10 kb to of roughly equal intensity, whereas the restricted sample should have a clear size shift such that the middle of the smear runs at approx 1 to 2 kb. At this point you have restricted cDNA populations from both the tester and driver. For the

driver cDNA, no further preparation is required and the sample should be stored at −20°C for later use.

3.5. Adaptor Ligation to Restricted Tester cDNA

There are two types of adapters AD1 and AD2 (*see* **Subheading 2.**) used in the subtraction protocol. Use the adapters made in **Subheading 3.1.** and perform all the steps in 0.2-mL PCR tubes. For each subtraction, a small aliquot (*see* **Note 3**) of the digested tester double-stranded cDNA is taken and divided into two equal portions. Each portion is ligated to a different adapter.

1. Mix 3 μL of restricted tester double-stranded cDNA with 2 μL of 100 pmol/μL AD1 or AD2, 1 μL of 10X T_4 DNA ligase buffer, 3 μL of bidistilled water, and 1 μL of T_4 DNA ligase. Store the remainder of the digested double-stranded cDNA for later use (e.g., screening).
2. Remove 2 μL from each tester ligation reaction and combine in a separate tube. This reaction is only used to verify adapter ligation and is, in addition, a negative control for subtraction.
3. Ligate overnight at 16°C (PCR machine). Remove 1 μL from the control reaction, add to 0.5 mL of bidistilled water, and store at −20°C for later use. Remove the salts and excess adapters from the other two ligation reactions (Qiagen PCR purification column), eluting in a volume of 10 m*M* Tris-HCl, pH 8.5, no greater than 30 μL.

3.6. Subtractive Hybridizations

3.6.1. Primary Hybridization (normalization step)

For each subtraction, set up two hybridizations, as follows:

1. Take 2 μL from each of the two ligation reactions and place into clean tubes.
2. Add to the tubes 4 μL of the corresponding restricted driver double-stranded cDNA from **Subheading 3.4.** (*see* **Note 4**). Dry down (Speed-vac) the two samples to near dryness (watch this carefully because it is sometimes difficult to resuspend the totally dried DNA pellet).
3. Resuspend each pellet in 3 μL of bidistilled water, and when completely dissolved, add 1 μL of 4X subtractive hybridization buffer. Transfer each solution to a separate 0.2-mL PCR tube and overlay each with 10 μL of PCR-grade mineral oil. Incubate (PCR machine) as follows: 98°C for 1.5 min, 68°C for 8 h.

3.6.2. Second Hybridization

Following the first hybridization step, there will exist cDNA molecules that have remained single stranded, simply because they have not found a complementary sequence in the driver cDNA population. The second round of hybridization targets these single-stranded cDNA molecules. With both tester fractions pooled, like genes anneal such that double-stranded cDNA molecules flanked by two different adapters (i.e., AD1 and AD2) are generated. Only these heterohybrids are consequently exponentially amplified and enriched.

1. Place 3 µL of the driver double-stranded cDNA into a clean PCR tube and add 1 µL of 4X subtractive hybridization buffer. Overlay with oil and denature at 98°C for 2 min, and then place on ice.
2. Remove 1 µL of the denatured driver double-stranded cDNA, add carefully to one of the primary tester hybridizations (e.g., tester with AD1), and mix. Finally, add the second primary tester hybridization (e.g., tester with AD2) to this tube and mix carefully (*see* **Note 4**). Overlay with oil and incubate overnight (PCR machine) at 68°C.
3. Add 200 µL of T buffer and heat in a PCR machine at 72°C for 7 min. Store the sample at –20°C.

3.7. PCR Amplification

3.7.1. Outer (primary) PCR Amplification

This section describes the PCR amplification of the hybridized cDNAs. The amplification is performed in two steps using primers that are complementary to the adapter sequences that have been previously ligated. The first step of PCR amplification utilizes two primers that anneal to the outer half of the linker sequence. The first primer pair gives rise to the so-called suppression effect (*see* **Note 5**), whereas the second PCR uses nested primers that exponentially amplify only those templates that are differentially expressed.

1. To 1 µL from the diluted hybridization (from **Subheading 3.6.2., step 3**) and 1 µL from the control ligation reaction (**Subheading 3.5., step 3**) add in the following order: 23.5 µL of bidistilled water, 3 µL of 10X PCR reaction buffer, 1 µL of 4X 10 m*M* dNTP mix, 1 µL of 10 µL PCR primer P1, 1 µL of 10 µ*M* PCR primer P2 and 0.51 µL of 50X Advantage cDNA Polymerase Mix.
2. Thermocycle as follows: 75°C for 5 min (this extends the adapters), 94°C for 25 s, (94°C for 20 s, 66°C for 30s, and 72°C for 2 min for 28 cycles (*see* **Note 6**).
3. Remove 3 µL from the PCR reaction and add to 27 µL of bidistilled water. This diluted template is the starting material for the second PCR step using the nested primers.

3.7.2. Nested PCR Amplification

After the primary PCR step, the subtracted cDNAs are further enriched by performing a second round of PCR with primers that are in juxtaposition to the cDNA ends.

1. Remove 1 µL of the diluted templates from **Subheading 3.7.1. (step 3)** and add the following components in order: 23.5 µL of bidistilled water, 3 µL of 10X PCR reaction buffer, 1 µL of 4X 10 m*M* dNTP mix, 1 µL of 10 µ*M* PCR primer

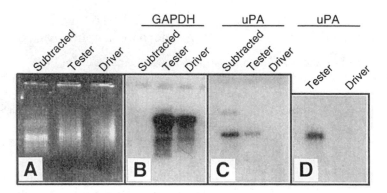

Fig. 2. Equal amounts of PCR-amplified driver, tester, and subtracted cDNA were fractionated on a 1.4% (v/v) agarose gel (**A**), blotted, and hybridized with ^{32}P-dCTP labeled GAPDH (**B**), and urokinase plasminogen activator (uPA) (**C**). (**D**) Differential expression of the uPA gene as shown by Northern analysis.

PN1, 1 µL of 10 µ*M* PCR primer PN2 and 0.5 µL of 50X Advantage cDNA Polymerase Mix.
2. Thermocycle as follows: 94°C for 25 s, 94°C for 20 s, 66°C for 30s, and 72°C for 2 min for 18 cycles.
3. Perform the minimum number of cycles that gives a product as visualized by agarose gel electrophoresis. Remove 5-µL aliquots after cycles 12, 14, 16, and 18, respectively, and visualize on a 1.4% (w/v) TAE gel. One should see a 200 to 2-kb smear in the unsubtracted control. In the case of the subtracted sample, there could be a distinct banding pattern with a light background smear, although bands are not always seen.

3.8. Evaluation of Subtraction Efficiency

Evaluation is best performed by monitoring the expression status of a number of genes that are either known to be of differential status in one mRNA population or known to show no differential expression (e.g., housekeeping genes such as glyceraldehyde-3-phosphate dehydrogenase GAPDH or actin). **Figure 2** gives an example of evaluation of subtraction efficiency.

1. Resolve equal amounts of amplified cDNA from the unsubtracted and the subtracted cDNAs by electrophoresis through a 1.5% (w/v) TAE agarose gel.
2. Prepare a Southern blot of the agarose gel on a nylon membrane.
3. Radiolabel a gene probe (*see* **Subheading 3.10.1.**) and screen the Southern blot in Church hybridization buffer *(1)* at 62–65°C.
4. Wash the blot twice in 2X SSC, 0.5% (w/) SDS at 68°C, then once in 0.1X SSC, 0.1% (w/v) SDS at 68°C, and expose the blot to X-ray film.

3.9. Cloning into a Vector

After evaluation of the subtraction efficiency, the subtracted library cDNA is cloned directly into a suitable cloning vector (*see* **Note 7**).

1. Digest approx 400 ng of PCR-amplified cDNA using 10 U of *Not*I and 10 U of *Sal*I, and purify the digested cDNA using a PCR purification column (Qiagen).
2. Ligate 100 ng of digested cDNA to 30 ng of *Not*I and *Sal*I-linearized vector using 1–3 U of T_4 DNA ligase, in a total volume of 10 μL, at 16°C overnight.
3. Remove 1 μL of the ligation reaction and add to 33 μL of ELECTROMAX bacteria strain DH10B in a 1.5-mL Eppendorf tube on ice.
4. Pipet the contents into a prechilled electroporation cuvet and electroporate at 1.8 kV.
5. Immediately add 700 μL of SOC medium to the cuvet, transfer to a 14 mL Greiner tube, and incubate for 40 min at 37°C with shaking.
6. Plate serial dilutions of the library on LB agar + 50 μg/mL of ampicillin plates in order to determine the titer. Once established, plate out on larger 22 × 22 cm LB agar plates containing 100 μg/mL of ampicillin, 100 μM IPTG, and 50 μg/mL of X-Gal.
7. Incubate at 37°C until small colonies are visible, and incubate further at 4°C until blue/white coloration can be clearly distinguished.

3.10. Reverse-Northern High-Density Blot Screening

3.10.1. Radioactive Labeling of Probes

Individually radiolabel tester and driver double-stranded cDNA probes as follows:

1. Denature approx 25 ng of tester or driver double-stranded cDNA (from **Subheading 3.4., step 3**), in a volume of 45 μL, by heating to 100°C for 1 to 2 min and cool rapidly on ice.
2. Add to a ReadyPrime reaction vial, and add 5 μL of $[\alpha\text{-}^{32}P]$dCTP.
3. Incubate for 15–30 min at 37°C (or for 1 h at room temperature), and remove unincorporated nucleotides from the labeled DNA using Elutips, according to the manufacture's guidelines.
4. Elute the labeled DNA in 600 μL of 1.0 *M* NaCl, 20 m*M* Tris-HCl, 1.0 m*M* EDTA, pH 7.4, and denature at 100°C for 2 -to 3 min immediately before use.

3.10.2. Screening of the Subtracted Library

This section describes one method of screening the library, but others are possible (*see* **Note 8**). **Figure 3** gives a typical result seen when screening subtracted libraries by reverse Northern analysis.

1. Pick recombinant bacterial clones into sterile 96-well microtiter plates containing LB broth plus 100 μg/mL of ampicillin.

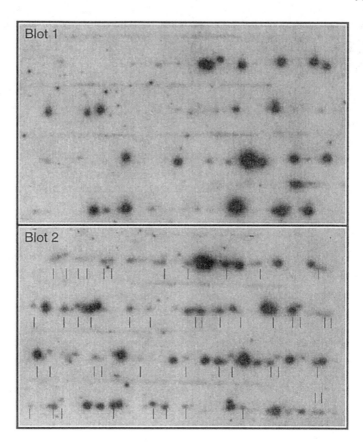

Fig. 3. Colony PCR was performed as described (*see* **Subheading 3.10.2.**) and the products were resolved on 1% (w/v) agarose gels in parallel. The gels were stained with ethidium bromide and photographed to ensure equal loading, and then were blotted onto nylon membrane under alkaline conditions. Duplicate filters were hybridized with double-stranded ^{32}P-labeled driver (blot 1) and tester (blot 2) cDNA of equal specific activity under stringent conditions. After washing, the filters were exposed to X-ray film at –80°C for 10–12 d. Bars indicate those clones that show differential hybridization and therefore represent clones harboring cDNA fragments that originate from only the tester cDNA population. Additionally, clones that show only very weak differential expression are detected.

2. Incubate on a gyratory shaker for 4 h at room temperature, and transfer 5 µL of each culture into 100 µL of sterile bidistilled water in a 96-well microtiter format PCR tube plate.
3. Lyse the bacterial suspensions by heating to 100°C for 2 min, and transfer 5 µL of each bacterial lysate into a fresh well of a 96-well microtiter format PCR tube plate.

4. To each clone lysate, add 5 μL of 10X standard PCR reaction buffer, 1 μL of 4X 10 mM dNTP mix, 1 μL of each of a pair of suitable vector PCR primers and 0.5 U of *Taq* polymerase, in a final volume of 50 μL.
5. Thermocycle as follows: 94°C for 20 s, 46°C for 20 s, and 72°C for 45 s for 30 cycles (the annealing temperature noted here is intended for T3 and T7 primers).
6. Electrophorese 12 μL of each PCR reaction through a high-density TAE agarose gel.
7. Using 0.4 M NaOH as the blotting buffer, transfer the DNAs onto nylon membranes. Wash the membranes briefly in 4X SSC.
8. Hybridize membranes in Church hybridization buffer at 62–65°C with equivalent amounts of *Rsa*I-restricted ^{32}P-labeled double-stranded cDNA of approximately equal specific activity, derived from driver and tester mRNA, respectively.
9. Wash the membranes twice in 2X SSC, 0.5% and (w/v) SDS at 68°C, and then once in 0.1X SSC, and 0.1% (w/v) SDS at 68°C, and expose the blot to X-ray film for up to 12 d at –80°C. Compare the signals derived from each clone with the alternative probes.

3.11. Confirmation of Differential Expression by Northern Analysis

1. Size fractionate 2-μg aliquots of driver and tester poly(A)$^+$ RNA on a 1.4% (v/v) formaldehyde agarose gel and blot in 10X SSC overnight onto a nylon membrane.
2. Radiolabel individual cloned DNAs (*see* **Subheading 3.10.1.**), representing putatively differentially expressed mRNAs, and screen the Northern blot in QuickHyb at 65°C.
3. Wash the northern blot twice in 2X SSC and 0.5% (w/v) SDS at 68°C, then once in 0.1X SSC and 0.1% (w/v) SDS at 68 °C, and expose the blot to X-ray film until a clear signal is seen (*see* **Note 9**).

4. Notes

1. It is of great importance that the quality of the mRNA be very high, because the quality of the generated cDNA is dependent on the integrity of the mRNA. This ultimately affects the success of the overall subtraction efficiency. Therefore, all necessary precautions should be taken when working with RNA. This includes making all buffers with DEPC-treated water. DEPC is a powerful protein denaturant and denatures ribonucleases irreversibly. DEPC is added to water at 0.2% (v/v) and left to stand for 30 min before being autoclaved. At high temperatures, DEPC decomposes to water and carbon dioxide. Kits are also available that allow the rapid isolation of high-quality poly(A)$^+$ RNA from either tissue of isolated cells. (Note that one can also perform cDNA synthesis for the subtration analysis directly from total RNA. The advantage here is that low abundant mRNAs are not lost as can happen during standard mRNA isolation.)
2. We have noticed that a digest time of 1– to 2 h is often not sufficient to digest completely all double-stranded cDNA (as monitored by agarose gel electrophoresis). It is also important for the subtraction procedure that all cDNAs used be

completely digested, so that like genes generate like cDNA fragments. Therefore, overnight cDNA digestion is recommended.

3. The volume of double-stranded cDNA added depends on its concentration but
   usually about 3 μL of the restricted double-stranded cDNA stock is sufficient
   (provided one started with at least 1 μg of mRNA).

4. One should exercise a little care to ensure correct and accurate pipetting, as well
   as thorough mixing, when working with small volumes. A pipet with a total handling volume of 10 μL is preferred, because it tends to be more accurate than a
   pipet with a total handling volume of 20 μL.

5. The suppression effect takes place only on those cDNA molecules that have,
   after the hybridization steps, the same linker sequence on either end, i.e., cDNA
   molecules that have adapter AD 1 on either end. The adapter functions as internal
   tandem repeats such that the cDNA is flanked with complementary regions of
   sequence. These complementary regions anneal together forming a so-called pan
   structure (see **Fig. 1**), thereby preventing the less competitive annealing of a PCR
   primer. In this manner, these cDNAs are largely inactive during the PCR cycle.
   By contrast, those cDNA molecules that are flanked by two different adapter
   sequences undergo normal exponential amplifications, because their ends are not
   complementary and the PCR primer pair is free to anneal.

6. It is important to optimize the number of cycles in both PCR steps (outer and
   nested PCR), such that the least number of cycles is employed. This in turn will
   help reduce unwanted background. To monitor the best number of amplification
   cycles employed for both outer and nested PCR steps, the following should be
   done. For the outer PCR step, remove from the unsubtracted and subtracted controls 1 μL of the PCR reaction after cycles 22, 24, 26, and 28, respectively.
   Amplify these aliquots using the nested primers, and for each of the four reactions, remove 5-μL aliquots after cycles 12, 14, 16, and 18, respectively. Run all
   samples on an agarose gel, blot, and hybridize with either a housekeeping gene or
   a gene known to be differentially expressed. The result will indicate which cycle
   number combination provides the best signal.

7. Any suitable plasmid vector can be utilized. However, recommended are those
   (containing, e.g., T7 and T3 RNA polymerase promoter sequences) that allow
   one to generate *in vitro* riboprobes for subsequent *in situ* hybridization studies.
   The adapters used here contain *Not*I and *Sal*I sites that allow directional cloning
   into a likewise restricted vector. This greatly reduces unwanted background
   because only those cDNA molecules that are exponentially amplified harbor the
   two restriction sites mentioned. One can modify the restriction sites in the adapters to suit the vector in which the library will be constructed.

8. This type of library screening is more laborious than others, but it is extremely
   sensitive. The inserts can be amplified from the vector using primers that flank
   the insert. For example, if the subtracted library has been cloned into pBluescript,
   T3 and T7 primers can be used. The annealing temperature is dependent on the
   primer sequence. Alternatively, one can screen the membranes with subtracted
   cDNA probes; that is, one labels the subtracted PCR product. In this case, it will

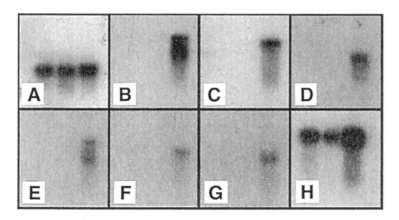

Fig. 4. Northern blot analysis of seven clones **(B–H)** demonstrating differential expression with respect to the tester cell line. GAPDH is used as a loading control **(A)**. Clones B–D represent highly abundant differentially expressed cDNAs, whereas clones E–G display low-level differential expression. Clone H demonstrates a three- to fourfold induction.

be necessary to perform a "reverse subtraction" in which the original tester becomes the driver and vice versa *(2)*. If one has access to a DNA arrayer robot capable of generating DNA microarrays and a scanner, one could screen the subtracted library in this manner *(3)*. One can also perform a direct colony lift of the library and hybridize the filter to Cy3 and Cy5 fluorescently labeled cDNAs from the tester and driver, respectively. These membranes can be scanned with a suitable imaging system (e.g., fluorimager Alpha, Vallac).

9. **Figure 4** shows a selection of differentially expressed clones that were identified through reverse northern screening *(4)*. These clones were then monitored for differential expression at the mRNA level. As is evident, all clones demonstrated strong differential expression with respect to the tester (i.e., a signal is only seen in the right-most lane of all the blots).

10. In contrast to display techniques, the method described here allows the identification of hundreds of differentially expressed genes in one hybridization experiment. The differentially expressed clones can be collectively screened against other suitable cell lines, thereby increasing the likelihood of narrowing down the number of real target genes. Using SSH in conjunction with a high-throughput differential screening method such as colony PCR (or microarrays) allows the rapid and easy identification of rarely and frequently transcribed, differentially expressed genes. Additionally, with careful handling one can achieve true positive rates of >90%.

Acknowledgment

This work was supported by a grant from the Dr. Mildred Scheel Stiftung fur Krebsforschung (grant W53/94/Hol).

References

1. Church, G. M. and Gilbert, W. (1984) Genomic sequencing. *Proc. Natl. Acad. Sci. USA 81,* 1991–1995.
2. Diatchenko, L., Lau, Y.-F. C., Campbell, A. P., Chenchik, A., Moqadam, F., Huang, B., Lukyanov, S., Lukyanov, K., Gurskaya, N., Sverdlov, E. D., and Siebert, P. D. (1996) Suppression subtractive hybridization: a method for generating differentially regulated or tissue-specific cDNA probes and libraries. *Proc. Natl. Acad. Sci. USA* **93,** 6025–6030.
3. Yang, G. P., Ross, D. T., Kuang, W. W., Brown, P. O., and Weigel, R. J. (1999) Combining SSH and cDNA microarrays for rapid identification of differentially expressed genes. *Nucleic Acids Res.* **15,** 1517–1523.
4. von Stein, O. D., Thies, W. G., and Hofmann, M. (1997) A high throughput screening for rarely transcribed differentially expressed genes. *Nucleic Acids Res.* **25,** 2598–2602.

19

Isolation of Differentially Expressed Genes by Representational Difference Analysis

Christine Wallrapp and Thomas M. Gress

1. Introduction
1.1. Overview

Representational difference analysis of cDNA (cDNA RDA) is designed to compare two different mRNA populations resulting in the isolation of differentially expressed genes. RDA was originally developed for genomic DNA as a method to isolate the differences between two complex genomes (*1*) and later was adapted for cDNA to examine differential gene expression (*2*).

Basically, RDA is a subtractive DNA enrichment technique. Common to such methodologies is that one DNA population (the driver) is hybridized in excess against a second population (the tester) to remove sequences present in both populations, thereby enriching target sequences unique to the tester. The general strategy, therefore, is to combine subtractive hybridization and subsequent, selective polymerase chain reaction (PCR) amplification of the differentially expressed sequences (**Fig. 1**). The procedure is performed in two stages: the generation of amplicons and the enrichment of differences.

1.1.1. Generation of Representations

The procedure starts with poly(A)⁺ RNA from two different populations, e.g., two cell lines or tissues. cDNA is synthesized and restricted with a four-base cutting enzyme (*Dpn*II). The ligation of an oligonucleotide adapter to the end of all DNA fragments allows the PCR amplification of 150- to 1500-bp fragments, resulting in a considerable quantity of the so-called representations or amplicons. The cDNA pool in which the differentially expressed genes can be found yields a representation called tester, and the cDNA pool in which the target genes are absent yields a representation called driver. Next, the adapter

From: *Methods in Molecular Biology, vol. 175: Genomics Protocols*
Edited by: M. P. Starkey and R. Elaswarapu © Humana Press Inc., Totowa, NJ

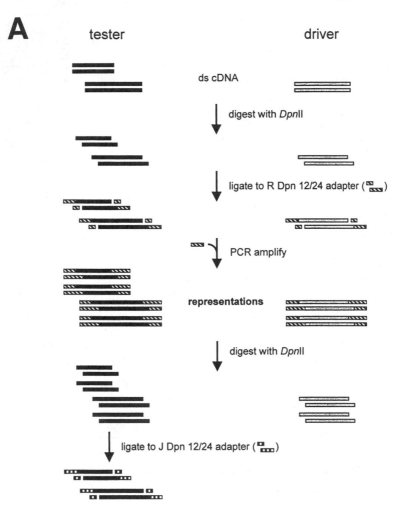

Fig. 1. Schematic diagram of cDNA RDA based on the protocol of Hubank and Schatz *(2)*. (**A**) Outline of the generation of tester and driver amplicons. Starting material is double-stranded cDNA obtained from two different mRNA populations. Genes present in both tester and driver populations are represented as long bars, and differentially expressed genes of the tester population represented as short bars. cDNA is digested with the restriction endonuclease *Dpn*II and ligated to an oligonucleotide adapter cassette (R Dpn 12/24). Subsequent to PCR amplification with the appropriate primer (R Dpn 24), the so-called representations are digested for removal of the adapter cassette. Only the tester amplicon is ligated to a new nonphosphorylated oligonucleotide adapter (J Dpn 12/24). (**B**) Outline of the difference enrichment procedure. Driver and tester are mixed at a ratio of 100:1, denatured, and reannealed for 20 h at 67°C. Three types of duplexes are formed: tester/tester homoduplexes, which have an adapter oligonucleotide on both 5'-ends; tester/driver hybrid duplexes, which have the adapter oligonucleotide on only

B   tester representation   driver representation

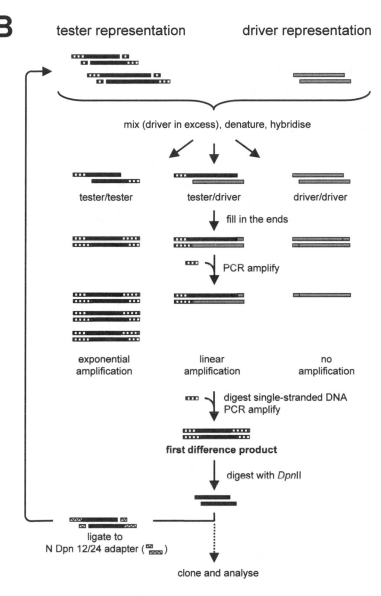

mix (driver in excess), denature, hybridise

tester/tester   tester/driver   driver/driver

fill in the ends

PCR amplify

exponential   linear   no
amplification   amplification   amplification

digest single-stranded DNA
PCR amplify

first difference product

digest with *Dpn*II

ligate to
N Dpn 12/24 adapter (▨▨▨)

clone and analyse

one end, and driver/driver homoduplexes without adapter. The 3'-recessed ends are filled in with *Taq* DNA polymerase, and tester/tester homoduplexes are selectively amplified in a PCR using tester-specific PCR primers (J Dpn 24). Note that driver duplexes are denatured during PCR and therefore are targets for the subsequent mung bean nuclease digest. The double-stranded products of exponential amplification are reamplified in order to obtain enough material of the first difference product. After the change of the adapters, the procedure is repeated using the difference product as tester and driver at a ratio of 1:800 for generation of DP2 and 1:400,000 for generation of DP3.

is cleaved and removed from tester and driver amplicons. A new unphosphorylated adapter is then ligated only to the tester representation.

1.1.2. Enrichment of Differences

This part of the procedure results in the isolation of target sequences owing to the subtraction of tester sequences, which are present in both tester and driver populations, and the kinetic enrichment of the remaining tester-specific sequences. After mixing tester with a large excess of driver, the fragments are denatured to separate the strands. The following reassociation results in the formation of hybrid tester/driver duplexes and self-reannealed driver and tester sequences. These fragments are treated with *Taq* polymerase in the presence of dNTPs at 72°C, which leads to the dissociation of the 12mer oligonucleotide from the 3' end of each tester fragment and the filling in of the 5' overhangs left by the covalently bound 24mer (note that the 12mer has not become covalently attached owing to a lack of phosphate group on its 5' end). PCR is then performed with the 24mer as primer, resulting in selective amplification. Driver/tester hybrid duplexes result from fragments that are present in both populations. Driver/tester hybrids are predominantly formed owing to the excess of driver. These fragments have primer sequences on only one end and are subject only to linear amplification. Self-reannealed tester fragments are formed in the absence of complementary driver strands and should predominantly represent differentially expressed sequences. These duplexes have primer sequences on both ends and are exponentially amplified. Self-reannealed driver fragments are not amplified owing to the lack of primer sequences.

After selective amplification, the driver strands and linear amplified tester strands are degraded by a single-strand specific mung bean endonuclease, whereas double-stranded products of the exponential amplification remain unaffected. These products are reamplified in order to obtain sufficient material of the so-called first difference product (DP1).

Enrichment of differences requires several rounds of reassociation followed by selective amplification. The tester:driver ratios are increased from 1:100 to up to 1:400,000. For each subsequent round, the difference product is digested with the initial restriction enzyme and ligated to a new adapter, before it is mixed with excess amounts of driver at the indicated ratios.

The final difference product obtained by cDNA RDA usually contains 2–10 cDNA fragments, which can be cloned in plasmid vectors for further characterization. All fragments should be verified for their differential expression on Northern blots with RNA of the starting material, which was used to generate driver and tester amplicons.

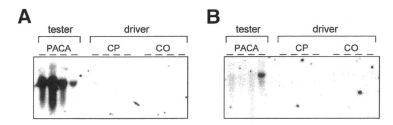

Fig. 2. Northern blots containing 30 µg of total RNA from human pancreatic cancer tissue (PACA), chronic pancreatitis (CP), and normal human pancreas (CO) were hybridized with gene fragments isolated by cDNA RDA *(3)*. As an example, the hybridization of cytokeratin 17 (**A**) and an unknown gene fragment (**B**) are shown. The method clearly identifies differentially expressed genes, which are absent in the driver and highly overexpressed in the tester.

1.2. Applications

1.2.1. Isolation of Genes Differentially Expressed in Cancer

One of the most exciting applications of cDNA RDA is to isolate genes overexpressed in an abnormal tissue as compared to its normal counterpart, because this offers the possibility of identifying new disease-related genes. In tumor diseases, the tester will usually represent a heterogeneous mixture of tumor, stromal, and inflammatory cells. Using cDNA RDA, a driver can be prepared, combining several different tissues or tissue components allowing subtraction of genes from unwanted components of the tumor tissue. This has been successful, e.g., in isolating genes with pancreatic cancer-specific expression *(3)*. In this approach, cDNA from normal pancreas and chronic pancreatitis tissue was combined to form the driver. Because chronic pancreatitis tissue contains a similar amount of fibrosis and inflammation as the tumor tissue, this allowed the subtraction of genes overexpressed in pancreatic cancer owing to the stromal reaction (**Fig. 2**).

1.2.2. Isolation of Growth-Factor Target Genes

A further interesting application is the isolation of target genes transcriptionally regulated by growth factors. In such an approach, cDNA from a growth factor–treated cell line would be used as tester and cDNA from untreated cells as driver to detect upregulated genes. In an inverse approach using the untreated cell as tester and the treated cell as driver, downregulated genes can be isolated in parallel (**Fig. 3**). This has been successfully used, e.g., to isolate transforming growth factor-β (TGF-β) target genes in pancreatic cancer cells *(4)*.

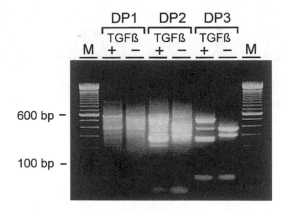

Fig. 3. Size fractionation of DP products obtained by standard cDNA RDA on 2.5% (w/v) agarose gels. (+), Products obtained using a TGF-β-treated pancreatic cancer cell line as tester and untreated cells as driver; (–), products obtained using untreated cells as tester and TGF-β-treated cells as driver. The following tester:driver ratios were used: DP1, 1:100; DP2, 1:800; DP3 1:400,000. The positions of the 600- and 100-bp marker bands are indicated.

1.2.3. Use of cDNA RDA for Generation of Subtracted Hybridization Probes

Standard cDNA RDA enables the isolation of a small number of differentially expressed genes with a high specificity. However, the yield is low and the standard protocol does not allow the study of complex alterations of gene expression. On the other hand, conventional differential hybridizations, which use radioactively or fluorescently labeled probes of complex mRNA populations to screen gridded cDNA libraries, are perfectly suited for expression profiling but have some disadvantages, such as high background, time-consuming image analysis, and the need for sophisticated equipment. These handicaps can be avoided by using subtracted hybridization probes generated by cDNA RDA (5). The difference product, used as hybridization probe on gridded cDNA filters, is usually DP2, which represents the best compromise between yield and specificity (**Fig. 4**). The use of cDNA RDA for generation of subtracted hybridization probes is therefore a powerful technique for the isolation of differentially expressed genes, combining the advantages of gridded library arrays and cDNA representational analysis.

2. Materials
2.1. cDNA Synthesis

1. Oligo-d(T)$_{25}$ coupled magnetic beads (DYNABEADS™, Dynal®, Oslo, Norway).
2. cDNA synthesis kit (e.g., cDNA Synthesis System; Gibco-BRL Life Technologies, Paisley, UK).

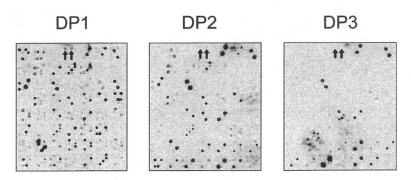

Fig. 4. Typical hybridization patterns on gridded cDNA filters obtained with cDNA RDA difference products (5). The first difference product (DP1), the second difference product (DP2), and the third difference product (DP3) of an RDA experiment, designed to isolate genes differentially expressed in pancreatic carcinoma, were labelled with ^{33}P and hybridized on a cDNA array. All clones were spotted in duplicate. For example, a housekeeping gene is highlighted by arrowheads. Note the strong signal in the DP1 hybridization, disappearing in the DP2/DP3 hybridization.

Table 1
Sequences of Oligonucleotides Used for RDA

Oligonucleotide for representations prepared with *Dpn*II	Sequence
R pair	
R Dpn 24	5' AGC ACT CTC CAG CCT CTC ACC GCA 3'
R Dpn 12	5' GAT CTG CGG TGA 3'
J pair	
J Dpn 24	5' ACC GAC GTC GAC TAT CCA TGA ACG 3'
J Dpn 12	5' GAT CCG TTC ATG 3'
N pair	
N Dpn 24	5' AGG CAA CTG TGC TAT CCG AGG GAA 3'
N Dpn 12	5' GAT CTT CCC TCG 3'

2.2. Oligonucleotide Adaptors

RDA experiments require three different adapters, each formed by one short and one long oligonucleotide (**Table 1**). The R pair is ligated to restriction-digested cDNA used for preparing the tester and driver amplicons, the J pair is ligated to the tester for the first round of difference enrichment, and the N pair is ligated to the difference product 1 for the second round of difference enrichment. The J and N pairs are alternated for odd- and even-numbered rounds of reassociation and selective PCR enrichment. Note that it is essential to use unphosphorylated oligonucleotides. The 12mer oligonucleotide provides a splint to allow the ligation of the 24 mer. Since the 12mer does not have a phosphate group on its 5'-end, it is not ligated itself and dissociates during the PCR preincubation step.

The oligonucleotides used during adapter ligation should be purified by high-performance liquid chromatography because T_4 DNA ligase is easily inactivated by traces of chemicals used in oligonucleotide synthesis, resulting in low yields of the tester and driver. Dissolve oligonucleotides in sterile water at a concentration of 1 μg/μL. They can be stored at −20°C indefinitely.

2.3. Solutions

PCR amplification steps in the RDA procedure are extremely sensitive to cross-contamination of reagents by tiny amounts of DNA. Therefore, all solutions should be prepared and maintained PCR clean. Use pipet tips with aerosol barriers for all manipulations.

1. *Dpn*II (10 U/μL) and corresponding 10X *Dpn*II buffer (New England Biolabs, Hitchin, Herts, UK).
2. 5X PCR buffer: 335 m*M* Tris-HCI, pH 8.8, 20 m*M* MgCI$_2$; 80 m*M* (NH$_4$)$_2$SO$_4$, 166 μg/mL BSA.
3. dNTP mix (4 m*M* each).
4. *Taq* DNA polymerase (5 U/μL, Perkin-Elmer, Warrington, Cheshire, UK).
5. T$_4$ DNA ligase (400 U/μL) and corresponding 10X T$_4$ DNA ligase buffer (New England Biolabs).
6. tRNA Solution: 5 μg/μL in 10 m*M* Tris-HCI, pH 7.5; 1 m*M* EDTA, pH 7.5 (TE).
7. Low TE: 2 m*M* Tris-HCI, pH 7.5; 0.2 m*M* EDTA, pH 7.5.
8. 3X EE buffer: 30 m*M* EPPS, pH 8.0 (Sigma-Aldrich, Poole, Dorset, UK); 3 m*M* EDTA, pH 8.0.
9. Mung bean nuclease (10 U/μL) and corresponding 10X mung bean nuclease buffer (New England Biolabs).
10. Phenol/chloroform/isoamyl alcohol (25:24:1).
11. Chloroform/isoamyl alcohol (24:1).
12. Mineral oil (Sigma-Aldrich).

2.4. Kits and Equipment

1. QIAquick PCR Purification Kit (Qiagen, Crawley, West Sussex, UK).
2. Thermal cycler (e.g., OmniGene; MWG-Biotech UK, Milton Keynes, UK).
3. Thin-walled PCR tubes (0.5 mL) (Rotec Scientific, Milton Keynes, UK).

3. Methods

3.1. Generation of Amplicons

3.1.1. Restriction of cDNA

It is important to keep the two cDNA populations to be compared separately throughout the procedure. However, both populations should be handled equally. Standard protocols start with 2 μg of cDNA, but the use of less material is also feasible (for smaller quantities 5 μg of tRNA should be added to the probe before digestion).

1. Prepare double-stranded cDNA (*see* **Note 1**) from poly(A)+ RNA (*see* **Note 2**).
2. Digest 2 μg of double-stranded cDNA in a volume of 100 μL with 20 U of *Dpn*II for 3 h at 37°C.
3. Extract each sample once with phenol/chloroform/isoamyl alcohol and once with chloroform/isoamyl alcohol, microcentrifuging for 2 min at 13,800g.
4. Precipitate each cDNA by adding 2 μg of 1 μg/μL glycogen (carrier) and 1/3 vol of 10 M ammonium acetate, mix, and add 3 vol of 100% (v/v) ethanol. After 5 min of incubation on ice, microcentrifuge at 13,800g for 5 min at 4°C, wash each pellet with 70% (v/v) ethanol, and vacuum dry.
5. Dissolve each digested cDNA in 20 μL of TE.
6. Analyze 3 μL of each sample on a 1.5% (w/v) agarose gel. Examine the size distribution, and ensure that both samples are digested to completion and look as similar as possible (*see* **Note 1**).

3.1.2. Ligation of Adapters

1. Prepare a ligation mixture for each digested cDNA by mixing 27 μL of double-distilled water (ddH$_2$O), 12 μL of 100 ng/μL digested cDNA, 6 μL of 10X T$_4$ DNA ligase buffer, 8 μL of 1 μg/μL R Dpn 24, and 4 μL of 1 μg/μL R Dpn 12.
2. Fill the holes of a heating block with glycerol and preheat to 50–55°C. Place the tubes of the ligation mixture in the heating block and transfer the block (without the heating device) into a cold room for approx 1 h to anneal the oligonucleotides.
3. As soon as the temperature has dropped to 10–15°C, place the tubes on ice and add 3 μL of 400 U/μL T$_4$ DNA ligase. Mix by pipetting and incubate overnight at 14°C.
4. Dilute each ligation mixture by adding 140 μL of TE (*see* **Note 3**).

3.1.3. PCR Amplification

Usually, four reactions will be needed for preparing the tester (*see* **Note 4**) and 20–30 reactions for preparing the driver (the expected yield of DNA is 10–20 μg/tube).

1. Set up 200-μL reactions by mixing 1 38 μL of ddH$_2$O, 40 μL of 5X PCR buffer, 17 μL of dNTP mix, 2 μL of 1 μg/μL R Dpn 24, and 2 μL of ligation mixture. Overlay each reaction mixture with two drops of mineral oil.

2. Preheat a thermal cycler to 72°C. Place the tubes in the thermal cycler for 3 min to allow the 12mer oligonucleotide to dissociate.

3. Fill in the 3'-recessed ends of the ligated DNA/adapters by adding 1 μL of 5 U/μL of *Taq* DNA polymerase to each tube in the thermal cycler, and mix by pipetting up and down. Incubate for 5 min at 72°C.

4. Thermocycle as follows: 95°C for 1 min and 72°C for 3 min for 20 cycles (*see* **Note 5**) and 72°C for 10 min, and cool the samples to room temperature.

5. Analyze 10 μL of each PCR product on a 1.5% (w/v) agarose gel to check the yield and quality of the amplicons. A smear ranging in size from 0.2 to 1.2 kb should be seen (*see* **Note 6**).

6. Combine the contents of four replicate reactions into one 1.5-mL microcentrifuge tube and extract twice with phenol/chloroform/isoamyl alcohol and once with chloroform/isoamyl alcohol, microcentrifuging for 5 min at 13,800*g*.

7. Precipitate the DNA with isopropanol by adding 1/10 vol of 3 *M* sodium acetate (pH 5.3), and 1 vol of isopropanol. After a 15-min incubation on ice, microcentrifuge the samples at 4°C for 15 min at 13,000*g* and wash the pellet with 70% (v/v) ethanol and dry under a vacuum.

8. Resuspend each pellet in approx 100 μL of TE and combine the driver amplicons into one tube.

9. To estimate the concentration of the samples, analyze 2 μL of both tester and driver DNA on a 1.5% (w/v) agarose gel, and include dilutions of an appropriate concentration standard, e.g., *Rsa*I-digested total human DNA.

3.1.4. Removing Adaptors from Amplicons

1. Using 5 U of *Dpn*II/μg of DNA, digest 200 μg of driver amplicon in a volume of 1.5 mL and 10 μg of tester amplicon in a volume of 100 μL. Digest for 3 h at 37°C.

2. Divide the driver digest into two tubes and extract twice with phenol/chloroform/ isoamyl alcohol and once with chloroform/isoamyl alcohol, microcentrifuging for 5 min at 13,800*g*.

3. Precipitate the DNA with isopropanol (as described in **Subheading 3.1.3., step 7**). to remove the adapters.

4. Dissolve each driver amplicon pellet in 150 μL of TE by vortexing at least twice for 1 min. Combine the content of the tubes and adjust to a final concentration of 0.5 μg/μL. This sample represents the cut driver, which will be used in all further hybridization steps.

5. Add 500 μL of buffer PB (QIAquick PCR purification kit) to the tester amplicon digest (100-μL vol), apply the sample to a QIAquick column, centrifuge at 13,800*g* for 1 min, and wash twice with 750 μL of buffer PE.

6. Elute DNA in 50 μL of TE and adjust to a final concentration of 100 ng/μL.

7. Analyze 1 μL of driver representation, 5 μL of tester representation, and appropriate concentration standards (e.g., *Rsa*I-digested total human DNA of known concentrations) on a 1.5% (w/v) agarose gel. Ensure a concentration and size range between 0.2 and 1.2 kb as expected.

3.1.5. Changing Tester Adapters

1. Ligate 2 μg of purified digested tester to oligonucleotide pair J by mixing 19 μL of ddH$_2$O, 20 μL of 100 ng/μL digested tester, 6 μL of 10X T$_4$ DNA ligase buffer, 8 μL of 1 μg/μL J Dpn 24, and 4 μL of 1 μg/μL J Dpn 12.
2. Continue the ligation by adding T$_4$ DNA ligase, as described in **Subheading 3.1.2.** (**steps 2** and **3**).
3. Dilute the ligated tester/adapter mixture to a concentration of 10 ng/μL by adding 140 μL of TE. This sample represents the tester, which will be used for the first round of hybridization (*see* **Note 7**).

3.2. Subtractive/Kinetic Enrichment

3.2.1. First Round of Hybridization

1. Mix 80 μL (40 μg) of digested driver representation (**Subheading 3.1.4., step 4**) and 40 μL (400 ng) of J-ligated tester representation (**Subheading 3.1.5, step 3**) (*see* **Notes 8** and **9**).
2. Extract once with phenol/chloroform/isoamyl alcohol and once with chloroform/isoamyl alcohol, microcentrifuging for 2 min at 13,800*g*.
3. Precipitate the DNA by adding 30 μL of 10 *M* ammonium acetate, mix, and add 380 μL of 100% (v/v) ethanol. Mix by inverting the tube several times. Place at –80°C for 10 min, followed by 37°C for 2 min (*see* **Note 10**).
4. Microcentrifuge the sample at 13,800*g* for 10 min at 4°C. Wash the pellet twice by adding 0.5 mL of 70% (v/v) ethanol and recentrifuging. Be careful not to lose the pellet, which becomes transparent and very difficult to see. Dry the pellet under a vacuum.
5. Resuspend the DNA very carefully in 4 μL of 3X EE buffer by vortexing for 2 min. Centrifuge briefly to collect the liquid at the bottom of the tube and pipet again for at least 2 min to ensure that the DNA is completely dissolved. Overlay with 35 μL of mineral oil.
6. Heat the sample at 98°C for 5 min in a heating block to ensure complete denaturation of the DNA.
7. Cool the sample to 67°C and immediately add 1 μL of 5 *M* NaCI directly to the drop of DNA under the oil on the bottom of the tube (*see* **Note 11**). Incubate at 67°C for 20 h to allow complete reassociation of the DNA strands.

3.2.2. Selective Amplification

1. Remove as much oil as possible and dilute the DNA stepwise, by adding 8 μL of tRNA solution and pipetting vigorously. Add 25 μL of TE and mix thoroughly. Add 362 μL of TE and mix by vortexing.
2. Set up two 200-μL reactions by mixing 120 μL of ddH$_2$O, 40 μL of 5X PCR buffer, 17 μL of dNTP mix and 20 μL of diluted reassociated DNA. Overlay each reaction with mineral oil.
3. Preheat a thermal cycler to 72°C. Place the tubes in the thermal cycler for 3 min to allow the 12mer oligonucleotide to dissociate.

4. Fill in the 3'-recessed ends of the reassociated DNA by adding 1 µL of 5 U/µL *Taq* DNA polymerase to each tube in the thermal cycler, and mix by pipetting up and down. Incubate for 5 min at 72°C.
5. Add 2 µL of 1 µg/µL J Dpn 24 to each tube in the thermal cycler and mix by pipetting up and down.
6. To amplify the self-reannealed tester DNA, thermocycle as follows: 95°C for 1 min and 72°C for 3 min for 10 cycles and 72°C for 10 min. Cool the samples to room temperature.
7. Combine the contents of the two PCR tubes in a 1.5-mL microcentrifuge tube and add 2 µL of tRNA solution.
8. Extract once with pheno/chloroform/isoamyl alcohol and once with chloroform/isoamyl alcohol, microcentrifuging at 13,800*g* for 5 min.
9. Precipitate the DNA with isopropanol (*see* **Subheading 3.1.3.**, **step 7**). Resuspend the pellet in 20 µL of low TE.
10. Eliminate single-stranded DNA by digesting with mung bean nuclease. Add 14 µL of ddH$_2$O, 4 µL of 10X mung bean nuclease buffer, and 2 µL of 10 U/µL mung bean nuclease. Incubate at 30°C for 30 min (*see* **Note 12**).
11. Add 160 µL of 50 m*M* Tris-HCI, pH 8.9, and inactivate the mung bean nuclease by incubating at 98°C for 5 min. Chill on ice.
12. Set up four 200-µL reactions by mixing 120 µL of ddH$_2$O, 40 µL of 5X PCR buffer, 17 µL of dNTP mix, 2 µL of 1 µg/µL J Dpn 24, and 20 µL of mung bean nuclease-treated DNA.
13. Incubate the tubes in a thermal cycler for 1 min at 95°C. Cool the temperature to 80°C and add 1 µL of 5 U/µL *Taq* DNA polymerase.
14. Thermocycle as follows: 95°C for min and 72°C for 3 min for 18 cycles and 72°C for 10 min. Cool the samples to room temperature.
15. Analyze 10 µL of the PCR products on a 2.5% (w/v) agarose gel to check the yield (usually 100–500 ng/10 µL) and the quality (usually 0.2–0.8 kb).
16. Combine the contents of the four reactions into one 1.5-mL microcentrifuge tube and extract twice with phenol/chloroform/isoamyl alcohol and once with chloroform/isoamyl alcohol, microcentrifuging at 13,800*g* for 5 min.
17. Precipitate the DNA with isopropanol (*see* **Subheading 3.1.3.**, **step 7**). Resuspend the pellet in 100 µL of TE. This sample is the DP1.
18. To estimate the concentration, analyze 2 µL of the first difference product on a 2.5% (w/v) agarose gel and include appropriate dilutions of a concentration standard, e.g., *Rsa*I-digested total human DNA. Adjust the concentration to 100 ng/µL with TE.

3.2.3. Changing of Adapters
for Subsequent Hybridization and Amplification

1. Digest 5 µg of the first difference product with 10 U of *Dpn*II in a volume of 100 µL for 3 h at 37°C.
2. Extract once with phenol/chloroform/isoamyl alcohol and once with chloroform/isoamyl alcohol, microcentrifuging at 13,800*g* for 2 min.

3. Precipitate the DNA by adding 1/10 volume of 3 M sodium acetate, pH 5.3, and 3 vol of 100% (v/v) ethanol. After 15 min of incubation on ice, microcentrifuge at 13,800g for 15 min at 4°C, wash the pellet with 70% (v/v) ethanol, and dry under a vacuum.

4. Dissolve the pellet in 50 μL of TE, leading to a final concentration of 100 ng/μL.

5. Ligate 200 ng of digested DNA to oligonucleotide pair N by mixing 37 μL of ddH$_2$O, 2 μL of 100 ng/μL digested DNA, 6 μL of 10X T$_4$ DNA ligase buffer, 8 μL of 1 μg/μL N Dpn 24, and 4 μL of 1 μg/μL N Dpn 12.

6. Continue the ligation by adding T4 DNA ligase (*see* **Subheading 3.1.2., steps 2 and 3**).

7. Dilute the N-ligated DP1 to a concentration of 1.25 ng/μL by adding 100 μL of TE.

3.2.4. Subsequent Hybridization and Amplification Steps

1. For generation of the DP2, mix 80 μL (40 μg) of digested driver representation (*see* **Subheading 3.1.4., step 4**) and 40 μL (50 ng) of N-ligated DP1 (*see* **Subheading 3.2.3., step 7**). Follow the procedure for reassociation and selective amplification as described in **Subheading 3.2.1.** and **3.2.2.** For selective amplification, use the N Dpn 24 oligonucleotide primer (*see* **Note 13**).

2. Change the adapter of the DP2 by using the J-pair oligonucleotides as described in **Subheading 3.2.3.** Adjust the concentration of the J-ligated DP2 to 2.5 pg/μL by diluting 30 μL of the ligation mixture (100 ng) with 370 μL of 20 μg/mL tRNA in TE, and diluting 4 μL of this solution with 396 μL of 20 μg/mL tRNA in TE.

3. For generation of the DP3, mix 80 μL (40 μg) of digested driver representation (*see* **Subheading 3.1.4., step 4**) and 40 μL (100 pg) of J-ligated DP2 (*see* **Subheading 3.2.4., step 2**). Follow the procedure for reassociation and selective amplification as described in **Subheadings 3.2.1.** and **3.2.2.** For selective amplification, use the J Dpn 24 oligonucleotide primer. To produce the final difference product, perform the final amplification for 22 cycles (*see* **Note 14**).

4. Remove the J adapters as outlined in **Subheading 3.2.3., steps 1–4**.

3.3. Analysis of Difference Products

3.3.1. Cloning of Individual Genes

1. Linearize 1–5 μg of an appropriate plasmid vector (e.g., pBluescript II SK) with a restriction enzyme producing compatible cohesive ends with the enzyme used to generate the representations (e.g., *Bam*HI or *Bgl*I).

2. Dephosphorylate the linearized vector with alkaline phosphatase (*6*).

3. Ligate the purified digested DP3 (*see* **Subheading 3.2.4., step 4**) into the plasmid vector and transform competent *Escherichia coli* (*6*).

4. Isolate plasmid DNA (*6*) from single colonies, and digest with appropriate restriction enzymes for isolation of the insert DNA.

5. Prepare Northern blots (*6*) with the RNA used for preparation of the tester and driver amplicons. Hybridize the labeled insert DNA and verify target

fragments that are present in the tester RNA population but not in the driver RNA population.

3.3.2. Use as Hybridization Probes

In addition to the standard cDNA RDA protocol, which is ideally suited to isolate a small number of individually cloned genes, cDNA RDA can be used to generate subtracted probes for hybridizations with gridded cDNA clones of known genes or gene libraries. All experiments done in this context have demonstrated that the use of the DP2 offers the best comprise between yield and sensitivity.

1. Prepare difference products by following the cDNA RDA protocol (*see* **Subheadings 3.1.** and **3.2.**). DP2 products are usually prepared at one of the following tester:driver ratios: 1:400,1:800,1:2000 (*see* **Note 15**).
2. Label 100 ng of the respective, digested DP2 product and 100 ng of the digested driver amplicon (*see* **Note 16**) by random hexamer priming using [α-^{33}P]dATP (*see* **Note 17**) and Klenow polymerase *(6)*.
3. Precompete each hybridization probe in a 100-µL reaction by mixing 45 µL of purified labeled DNA, 20 µL of 5 mg/mL sonicated human placenta DNA, 25 µL of 20X saline sodium citrate (SSC) *(6)* and 10 µL of 1% (w/v) sodium dodecyl sulfate (SDS).
4. Denature the DNA for 5 min at 95°C and incubate at 68°C for 2 h.
5. Hybridize cDNA arrays with the competed probes in 6X SSC, 5X Denhardt's solution *(6)*, 0.5% (w/v) SDS, 100 µg/mL yeast tRNA, 50 µg/mL sonicated human placenta DNA, and 50% (v/v) formamide at 42°C for 24 h.
6. Wash the cDNA arrays sequentially at room temperature in 2X SSC and 0.1% (w/v) SDS for 10 min, at 68°C for 30 min once with 2X SSC and 0.1 % (w/v) SDS, and once with 0.25X SSC and 0.1% (w/v) SDS.
7. Detect hybridization signals using X-ray film or a Phosphorimager.
8. Compare hybridization results obtained with the DP2 products and the driver. Verify the success of the selection (*see* **Note 18**) by Northern blot analysis *(6)*.

4. Notes

1. Use oligo-d(T) primers for reverse transcription, and ensure that the double-stranded cDNA generated has a size range of at least 200 bp to 10 kb and that the preparations to be subtracted are as similar as possible. If the quality of reverse transcription varies between subtracted populations, this can result in the detection of 5' fragments from long messages that are inefficiently transcribed in the driver population.
2. Check the integrity of the RNA samples and use only high-quality RNA to start RDA. Degraded RNA will result in the isolation of artificial bands. Regardless of the poly(A)$^+$ RNA purification protocol, the aim should be to obtain full-length transcripts and complete integrity of the RNA samples.

3. Sample leftovers obtained at each step should be stored at –20°C, to allow for repetition or modification of the experiment at any step in case of a mistake or failure.

4. For reciprocal subtractions (representations will be used as both tester and driver), prepare 20–30 reactions from each sample. A master mix may be used, however, it is imperative to avoid cross-contamination.

5. Under no circumstances increase cycle number; otherwise, artifacts will be produced. If more product is required, more reactions should be performed.

6. Insufficient quantities of fully active *Taq* DNA polymerase molecules or an exhaustion of one of the PCR reagents during the final PCR extension will generate single-stranded sequences. These appear as a smear of the PCR product toward the well of an agarose gel. Always use the stated amounts of PCR reagents or reduce the number of cycles.

7. Test the successful change of the adapters, performing a PCR reaction with the previous primers (R Dpn 24) and the new primers (J Dpn 24). Use 2 μL (20 ng) of diluted ligation mixture as a template in a 50-μL reaction and employ 25 thermocycles. The amplification with the previous primers usually generates small amounts of product. However, the amount of product obtained with the new primers should be significantly higher.

8. The purity and the use of the correct concentration of digested driver DNA are crucial at this stage. The DNA is resuspended at a maximum concentration, which is close to the limit of its solubility, to maximize the rate of DNA reassociation. Carefully determine driver and tester DNA concentrations using reliable concentration standards.

9. These proportions of driver representation and tester representation result in the following tester:driver ratios: first round of hybridization, 1:100; second round of hybridization, 1:800; third round of hybridization, 1:400,000.

10. Using these conditions, salt precipitation is minimized. Adenosine triphosphate (ATP) (present in the T_4 DNA ligase buffer) and residual proteins will dissolve in the ethanol solution and be efficiently removed in the subsequent centrifugation step.

11. NaCI is added to accelerate the reassociation of DNA strands. It must be added carefully, since the volumes are small and the expansion caused by the hot oil will force the NaCI out of the micropipet tip.

12. Mung bean nuclease removes tester and driver sequences, which are denatured during the selective PCR but cannot be exponentially amplified and, therefore, remain single stranded (linear-amplified products and driver DNA).

13. Usually 2–10 distinct bands are clearly visible in DP2, or at the latest in DP3.

14. The expected yield of DNA is 100–300 ng/10 μL. If the yield needs to be improved, add 1 μL of fresh 5 U/μL *Taq* DNA polymerase and perform three to five additional cycles and a final extension step.

15. Tester:driver ratios have to be adapted to the needs of the planned experiment. One would usually start with a DP2 tester:driver ratio of 1:800 and increase or decrease this ratio depending on the hybridization result. Always bear in mind

that increasing the tester:driver ratio (e.g., to 1:2000) will decrease the yield but will increase the specificity and the number of clones with a high degree of differential expression. Lowering tester:driver ratios (e.g., to 1:400) will increase yield at the expense of decreased specificity.

16. Although not absolutely necessary, when using RDA probes, it is helpful to perform a parallel hybridization of a second, identical clone array with a ^{33}P-labeled probe of the unsubtracted driver. Comparison of the hybridization results obtained with DP2 and the driver allows the identification of sequences present in the driver at high concentrations, which impede complete subtraction. Probes of the unsubtracted driver and of DP2 products should be handled identically.

17. The use of ^{33}P labeled nucleotides is strongly recommended because it avoids spreading of hybridization signals to neighboring clones on the grid.

18. Using this protocol, we usually achieve a specificity of about 80%.

Acknowledgments

We wish to acknowledge the participation of M. Geng, C. Wenger, H. Paul, S. Hahnel, and U. Lacher in the development of the protocols. Protocols originally developed by M. Hubank and D. G. Schatz were modified in the context of projects financed by grants by the European Union (BIOMED-2 programme: BMH4-CT98-3085), the German ministry for research and technology (BMBF: KBF GB 9401), and the German research society (DFG, SFB 518).

References

1. Lisitsyn, N. and Wigler, M. (1993) Cloning the differences between two complex genomes. *Science* **259,** 946–951.
2. Hubank, M. and Schatz, D. G. (1994) Identifying differences in mRNA expression by representational difference analysis of cDNA. *Nucleic Acids Res.* **22,** 5640–5648.
3. Gress, T. M., Wallrapp, C., Frohme, M., Muller-Pillasch, F., Lacher, U., Friess, H., Buchler, M., Adler, G., and Hoheisel, J. D. (1997) Identification of genes with specific expression in pancreatic cancer by cDNA representational difference analysis. *Genes Chromosomes Cancer* **19,** 97–103.
4. Geng, M. M., Ellenrieder, V., Wallrapp, C., Muller-Pillasch, F., Hendler, S., Adler, G., and Gress, T. M. (1999) Identification of TGFβ1 target genes in pancreatic cancer cells by cDNA representational difference analysis. *Genes Chromosomes Cancer* **26,** 70–79.
5. Geng, M., Wallrapp, C., Muller-Pillasch, F., Frohme, M., Hoheisel, J. D., and Gress, T. M. (1998) Isolation of differentially expressed genes by combining representational difference analysis (RDA) and cDNA library arrays. *Biotechniques* **25,** 434–438.
6. Sambrook, J., Fritsch, E. F., and Maniatis, T., eds. (1989) *Molecular cloning: A Laboratory Manual,* Cold Spring Harbor Laboratory, Cold Spring Harbor, NY.

20

Expression Profiling and Isolation of Differentially Expressed Genes by Indexing-Based Differential Display

Michael P. Starkey

1. Introduction

Profiling the expression status at the level of transcription is a starting point for delineation of the function of both known and unknown gene products. In addition, the identification of genes expressed in a regionally, temporally, or environmentally specific manner is fundamental to the understanding of processes such as development, differentiation, and disease.

Indexing represents a simple and reproducible general approach to expression profiling and for the isolation of differentially expressed genes (1). Digestion of cDNAs with a type IIs or interrupted palindrome restriction endonuclease produces fragments with every combination of possible bases in the cohesive ends. Under stringent conditions, the specific ligation of adapters with perfectly complementary overhangs partitions the cDNA fragments into nonoverlapping subpopulations. Internal cDNA restriction fragments are exponentially amplified by adapter primer polymerase chain reaction (PCR) and visualized by nondenaturing polyacrylamide gel electrophoresis (PGE). Because the subdivision of cohesive-ended cDNA restriction fragments is based on the sequence of their overhangs, indexing is not afflicted by the problem (common to approaches featuring subtractive hybridization, e.g., representational difference analysis [2]) that repetitive sequences shared by nonhomologous cDNAs may be responsible for the elimination of low-abundance cDNAs.

Indexing was initially utilized as a noncloning method for isolating specific DNA fragments from complex genomic digests, by selective ligation of defined adapters and PCR (3,4). The first example of this approach applied to cDNA

From: *Methods in Molecular Biology, vol. 175: Genomics Protocols*
Edited by: M. P. Starkey and R. Elaswarapu © Humana Press Inc., Totowa, NJ

populations demonstrated the power of selection by ligation to mixed adapter sets *(5,6)*. More recently, the profiles of genes expressed in mouse tissues have been generated by PCR-amplification of cDNA type IIs restriction enzyme fragments and recorded using an automated DNA sequencer *(7,8)*, a format incompatible with the isolation of differentially expressed transcripts.

In the simplified approach to indexing, adapted for the isolation of differentially expressed genes, described herein (and in **ref.** *1*), the fidelity of T_4 DNA ligase–catalyzed adapter ligation is the sole basis for the partitioning of internal type IIs cDNA restriction fragments into distinct subsets. This is in contrast to similar procedures *(9–11)* in which cDNA population subdivision is achieved by single base– or two base–specific reverse transcription and/or PCR. PCR amplification of indexed cDNA fragments is based on a single "long" PCR primer, ensuring that a fixed set of thermal cycling parameters is optimal. This is diametrically opposite of the low-stringency annealing of arbitrary primers that is associated with the differential display *(12)* and arbitrarily primed PCR *(13)* protocols. Consequently, indexing is not prone to the consequences of stochastic events during the first few cycles of low-stringency PCR. By contrast, indexing generates profiles that are highly consistent and reproducible. Furthermore, the isolation of internal cDNA restriction fragments avails the cloning of coding regions.

1.1. Indexing-Based Differential Display

A population of a cDNA molecule is digested with a type IIs restriction endonuclease, generating fragments with nonidentical cohesive ends (*[6]*; **Fig. 1**). The number of different end sequences is 4^n, in which *n* is the length of the overhang. An enzyme such as *Bbv*I generates fragments with 4-base 5'-overhangs. If two cohesive ends of a *Bbv*I fragment are considered, there are potentially $4^8/2$ (32,896) fragment classes, each with a different pair of cohesive ends. The ligation of adapters with perfectly complementary overhangs enables ordered partitioning of the restriction fragment classes as nonoverlapping subpopulations. For fragments with 4-base overhangs, 4^4 (256) different adapters are required. To access every internal cDNA fragment from a restriction digest, it is necessary to provide each cDNA fragment with every adapter in combination with ever other adapter. Employing single adapters in pairwise combinations, 32,896 reactions are required to isolate all the internal fragments in a *Bbv*I digest. However, division of the 256 adapters into 16 pools of 16 means that the number of ligation reactions is reduced to 136 (comprising 120 reactions featuring pairwise combinations of different adapter pools and 16 reactions effectively containing single adapter pools). Internal cDNA fragments, which have acquired an adapter at each end, may be exponentially amplified by an adapter primer and visualized by nondenaturing PAGE (**Fig. 1**).

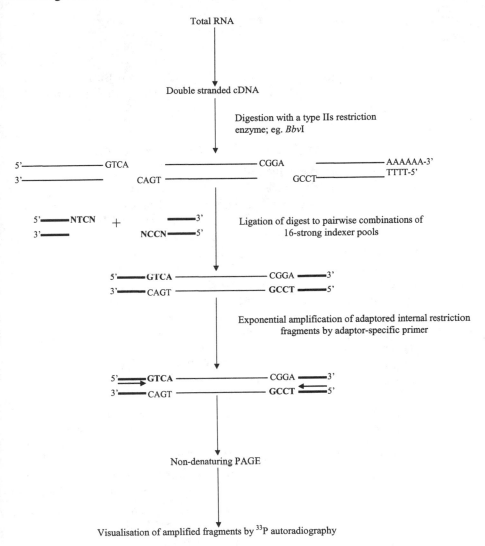

Fig. 1. Schematic illustrating indexing-based differential display.

2. Materials

2.1. cDNA Synthesis

1. SuperScript Choice System for cDNA Synthesis (Gibco-BRL Life Technologies, Paisley, UK), including 5X first-strand buffer (250 mM Tris-HCl, pH 8.3, 375 mM KCl, 15 mM MgCl$_2$) and 5X second-strand buffer (100 mM Tris-HCl, pH 6.9, 450 mM KCl, 23 mM MgCl$_2$, 50 mM (NH$_4$)$_2$SO$_4$, 0.75 mM β-NAD$^+$).
2. QIAquick PCR Purification Column Kit (Qiagen, Crawley, West Sussex, UK).

2.2. Restriction Digestion of cDNA

1. Type IIs restriction enzyme, e.g., *Bbv*I (New England Biolabs, Hitchin, Hertford-shire, UK).
2. 10X type IIs restriction enzyme buffer, e.g., *Bbv*I 10X NE Buffer 2 (500 mM NaCl, 100 mM Tris-HCl, pH 7.9, 100 mM MgCl$_2$, 10 mM dithiothreitol [DTT]) (New England Biolabs).
3. QIAquick PCR Purification Column Kit (Qiagen).

2.3. Specific Ligation of Adapters to cDNA Restriction Fragments

1. Sac adapter pools comprising the following:
   a. 5'-Phosphorylated Sac indexer: 5'-NXYNATGAGCTCTGAGTCGTGCTA-3' in which X and Y are specified bases representing 1 of 16 possible 2-base sequences, and N is an equimolar mixture of A, C, G, and T.
   b. Nonphosphorylated Sac primer: 5'-TAGCACGACTCAGAGCTCAT-3'. Prepare a 250 μL aliquot of a 100 nM Sac adapter by mixing 25 pmol of Sac primer and 1.56 pmol of each of 16X Sac indexers in 10 mM Tris-HCl, pH 8.0, and 1 mM EDTA. Heat the oligonucleotide mixture at 65°C for 5 min and allow to cool slowly to room temperature. Store each adapter at –20°C.
2. T$_4$ DNA ligase (1 U/μL) (Gibco-BRL Life Technologies).
3. 5X T$_4$ DNA ligase buffer: 250 mM Tris-HCl, pH 7.6, 50 mM MgCl$_2$, 5 mM adenosine triphosphate, 5 mM DTT; 25% (w/v) PEG-8000 (Gibco-BRL Life Technologies).
4. GeneAmp 9600 PCR machine (Perkin-Elmer, Warrington, Cheshire, UK).
5. Strips of 8 GeneAmp 9600 microtubes, held in a 96-well microtiter plate format (Perkin-Elmer).
6. QIAquick 8 PCR Purification Kit (Qiagen), QIAvac 6S vacuum manifold and Vacuum Regulator (Qiagen), and VP3 vacuum pump (Wolf, York, UK).

2.4. PCR Amplification of Adapted cDNAs

1. Nonphosphorylated Sac primer: 5'-TAGCACGACTCAGAGCTCAT-3'.
2. Reagents for PCR: AmpliTaq Gold (Perkin-Elmer); 10X PCR Gold buffer (150 mM Tris-HCl, pH 8.0, 500 mM KCl [Perkin-Elmer], 10X MgCl$_2$ (25 mM MgCl$_2$) (Sigma-Aldrich, Poole, Dorset, UK); 10X dNTPs (4X 2 mM dNTPs) (Ultrapure dNTPS, Amersham Pharmacia Biotech, Amersham, Buckinghamshire, UK); 1000–3000 Ci/mmol [^{33}P]dATP (Amersham Pharmacia Biotech).
3. Mineral oil (Sigma-Aldrich).
4. GeneAmp 9600 PCR machine (Perkin-Elmer).
5. Strips of 8 GeneAmp 9600 microtubes, held in a 96-well microtiter plate format (Perkin-Elmer).

2.5. Nondenaturing Polyacrylamide Gel Electrophoresis and Autoradiography

1. Vertical polyacrylamide gel apparatus; e.g., Model S2 Sequencing Gel Electrophoresis Apparatus (Gibco-BRL Life Technologies) + PowerPac 3000 (Bio-Rad, Hemel Hempstead, Hertfordshire, UK).

2. Page-Plus 40% (w/v) nondenaturing polyacrylamide gel mix (Anachem, Luton, Bedfordshire, UK).
3. 4X Nondenaturing loading dye: 20% (v/v) glycerol, 0.2% (w/v) bromophenol blue, 0.2% (w/v) xylene cyanol, 10 mM EDTA, pH 8.0.
4. Internal loading standard: A 1126-bp fragment of bacteriophage lambda DNA (100 ng) (Sigma-Aldrich) amplified by AmpliTaq Gold (Perkin-Elmer) in a 10-μL reaction in the presence of 0.1 μCi of [^{33}P]dATP (Amersham Pharmacia Biotech) using the following primers: 5'-CGACCATTGTGTATGAACGC-3' and 5'-TCATCATGGTAAACGTGCGT-3'.
5. *Bgl*I and *Hin*fI-digested pBR328 molecular weight markers (1 μg) (Roche, Lewes, East Sussex, UK) labeled sequentially with 4.67 μCi + 17.5 μCi of [^{33}P]dATP (Amersham Pharmacia Biotech) using terminal deoxyoucleotidyl transferase (Amersham Pharmacia Biotech) and Klenow fragment of DNA Polymerase I (Amersham Pharmacia Biotech) and resuspended at 20 ng/μL.
6. Gel drier, c.g., Model 583 Gel Dryer (Bio-Rad).
7. X-Ray film (Kodak X-OMAT AR 35 × 43 cm Scientific Imaging Film; Anachem), or Low Energy Storage Phosphor Screens 35 × 43 cm and Storm 860 PhosphorImager (Amersham Pharmacia Biotech).
8. Fragment analysis software, e.g., 1D software (Phoretix, Newcastle on Tyne, UK).

3. Methods

The protocol outlined requires 40 μg of total RNA from each of the RNA samples to be compared. This is sufficient for performing 1/3.4 of all the possible indexing reactions that may be derived from the use of a single type IIs restriction enzyme.

3.1. cDNA Synthesis

cDNA is synthesized utilizing a kit (*see* **Note 1**) featuring oligo (dT)$_{12-18}$-primed first-strand synthesis by cloned Moloney Murine Leukaemia Virus reverse transcriptase (RT) and second-strand synthesis via the extension of multiple RNase H-generated RNA fragments. The key component of the kit is the Superscript II RT, expressed by a cloned Moloney murine leukemia virus RT gene that has been engineered to eliminate intrinsic RNase H activity (which is detrimental to first-strand cDNA synthesis). The synthesis of cDNA from 30 μg of total RNA (in the presence of RT) and 10 μg of total RNA (in the absence of RT; *see* **Note 2**) is described. This provides sufficient material for the ligation in triplicate of +RT cDNA to each of 40 pairs of Sac adapter pools, and the single ligation of –RT cDNA to each of 40 pairs of Sac adapter pools.

1. Resuspend 30 μg of total RNA (+RT cDNA) and 10 μg of total RNA (–RT cDNA) in 10 μL of diethylpyrocarbonate (DEPC)-treated water (*see* **Notes 3–6**).
2. To each RNA sample add 2 μL of 0.5 μg/μL oligo (dT)$_{12-18}$ primer. Heat at 70°C for 10 min and chill on ice for 1 min.

3. Centrifuge each RNA sample briefly, and to each add 4 µL of 5X first-strand buffer, 2 µL of 0.1 M dithiothreitol and 1 µL of 4X 10 mM dNTPs. Mix by gentle vortexing and centrifuge briefly. Incubate at 45°C for 2 min to equilibrate the temperature.

4. Add 1 µL of 200 U/µL SuperScript II RT to the +RT cDNA and 1 µL of DEPC-treated water to the –RT cDNA. Mix gently and incubate at 45°C for 1 h. Terminate each reaction by placing on ice.

5. On ice, add the following in order to each of the first-strand reactions: 91 µL of DEPC-treated water, 30 µL of 5X second-strand buffer, 3 µL of 4X 10 mM dNTPs, 1 µL of 10 U/µL *Escherichia coli* DNA ligase, 4 µL of 10 U/µL *E. coli* DNA polymerase, and 1 µL of 2 U/µL *E. coli* RNase H. Mix each reaction mixture gently and incubate at 16°C for 2 h.

6. Add 2 µL of 5 U/µL T$_4$ DNA polymerase and continue incubating at 16°C for 5 min. Place on ice and add 10 µL of 0.5 M EDTA.

7. Store the cDNAs at –20°C until required.

8. Subdivide each cDNA sample into 2X 80.5-µL aliquots and add 5 volumes (402.5 µL) of Buffer PB to each. Mix before dispensing each sample into a QIAquick PCR purification column.

9. Bind each cDNA sample to the silica membrane in each QIAquick column by centrifuging at 13,800g for 1 min. Wash the silica membrane in each column with 750 µL of Buffer PE (diluted 1:4 with 96–100% [v/v] ethanol) and centrifuge two times at 13,800g for 1 min.

10. Elute the cDNA from each silica membrane by adding of 50 µL of filter-sterilized water (of confirmed pH 7.0–8.5) to each column, incubating at room temperature for 5 min, and centrifuging at 13,800g for 1 min.

11. Pool the 2X purified 50-µL aliquots of each cDNA sample and store at –20°C until required.

3.2. Restriction Digestion of cDNA

This section describes the restriction of cDNA with *Bbv*I. In principle, any type IIs restriction enzyme, which generates 4 base 5'-cohesive overhangs, may be utilized in conjunction with the Sac adapters.

1. Mix 100 µL of each cDNA with 12 µL of 10X NE Buffer 2, 2 µL of filter-sterilized water, and 6 µL of 2 U/µL *Bbv*I. Digest at 37°C for 2 h.

2. Incubate each reaction mixture at 65°C for 10 min to inactivate the *Bbv*I.

3. Purify each digested cDNA by silica membrane adsorption (*see* **Subheading 3.1.**), eluting each +RT cDNA in 600 µL of filter-sterilized water and each –RT cDNA in 200 µL of filter-sterilized water. Store each cDNA at –20°C until required.

3.3. Sequence-Specific Ligation of Adapters to cDNA Restriction Fragments

The ligation of *Bbv*I-digested cDNA to a single pair of Sac adapter pools is described. However, the procedure may be repeated for up to 135 other pairwise

combinations of Sac adapter pools. A single aliquot of each –RT cDNA is ligated to a pair of Sac adapter pools, while triplicate aliquots of each +RT cDNA (*see* **Note 7**) are ligated to a Sac adapter pool combination. The volumes of reagents quoted assume a comparison between two RNA samples; the reagent volumes can be scaled up according to the number of RNAs being compared and the number of adapter pool pair combinations utilized.

To increase the fidelity of T_4 DNA ligase–catalyzed adapter ligation, hot start ligation (an analog of hot start PCR *[14]*) is performed. By heating the components of the ligation reaction to 65°C, prior to the addition of the T_4 DNA ligase, the aim is to reduce the frequency of mismatch ligation by precluding preligation nonspecific base pairing.

The removal of unincorporated adapters and potential adapter dimers following ligation is essential, since such molecules would compete with adapted cDNAs for Sac PCR primer and (as a consequence of their size) would be amplified extremely efficiently.

1. Prepare a ligation reaction master mix by combining: 10 μL of 100 n*M* Sac adapter 1 (e.g., adapter with cohesive end of Sac indexer: 5'-NAAN-3'), 10 μL of 100 n*M* Sac adapter 16 (e.g., adapter with cohesive end of Sac indexer: 5'-NTTN-3'), 60 μL of 5X T4 DNA ligase buffer, and 145 μL of filter-sterilized water. Dispense 22.5 μL aliquots of the master mix into each of eight microtubes, held at 4°C.
2. Add 5 μL of a cDNA sample (3X +RT cDNA and 1X –RT cDNA for each of two RNAs) to each of the eight microtubes. Continue to maintain at 4°C.
3. Dispense 5μL of 1 U/μL T4 DNA ligase into each of eight new microtubes, held at 4°C.
4. Program a thermocycler as follows: 65°C for 5 min, 37°C for 2 min, 37°C for 1 h, 65°C for 10 min, and 4°C "forever." Start the thermocycler and when the thermocycler temperature reaches 65°C, "pause" the thermocycler. Place the eight microtubes containing the cDNA samples onto the thermocycler, and restart it.
5. When the thermocycler has completed the 37°C, 2 min step of the program, pause the thermocycler, and (using an eight channel pipet) add 2.5 μL of 1 U/μL T4 DNA ligase to each of the eight microtubes in a row (dispensing from the eight microtubes containing the T4 DNA ligase). Restart the thermocycler.
6. Remove unincorporated adapters by silica membrane adsorption (as described in **Subheading 3.1.**, except that vacuum filtration [200–600 millibars/150–450 mmHg of mercury] is employed as an alternative to centrifugation), eluting each adapted cDNA in 80 μL of filter-sterilized water. Store the adapted cDNAs at –20°C until required.

3.4. PCR Amplification of Adapted cDNAs

1. Amplify a 2.5-μL aliquot of each adapted cDNA in a reaction comprising 1 μL of 10X PCR Gold buffer, 1 μL of 10X MgCl₂, 1 μL of 10X dNTPs, 0.1 μL of 1000–3000 Ci/mmol [³³P]dATP, 1 μL of 5 μM Sac primer, 2.9 μL of filter-ster-

ilized water, and 0.5 μL of 5 U/μL AmpliTaq Gold. Cover each reaction mixture with mineral oil.

2. Thermocycle as follows: 95°C, 10 min; 95°C for 30 s, 60°C for 30 s, 72°C for 1 min 30 s for 30 cycles; 72°C for 10 min.

3. Ensure that a PCR negative control (2.5 μL of filter-sterilized water replacing adaptered cDNA) is included in every thermocycling run.

3.5. Separation and Visualization of Expressed cDNAs

1. Mix 10 μL of each ^{33}P-labeled PCR-amplified adaptered cDNA sample (and PCR negative control) with 1 μL of ^{33}P-labeled internal loading standard (*see* **Note 8**) and 3.25 μL of 4X nondenaturing loading dye. Electrophorese 3 μL of each sample through a 0.25 mm thick 4.8% (w/v) nondenaturing polyacrylamide gel.

2. To facilitate accurate sizing of visualized fragment, include on each gel, three aliquots (one on each end of the gel and one in the center) of 1 μL of ^{33}P-labeled molecular weight markers + 0.4 μL of 4X nondenaturing gel-loading dye.

3. Dry each gel for 45 min at 80°C. Expose each gel to a sheet of X-ray film at –70°C (overnight to 7 d), or to a phosphor screen at room temperature (3 h to 3 d) (*see* **Note 9–13**).

4. Notes

1. The protocol (**Subheading 3.1.**) describing the use of the SuperScript Choice System (Gibco-BRL Life Technologies) for cDNA synthesis may be employed for synthesizing cDNA from up to 1 60 μg of total RNA, employing 200 units of SuperScript II RT/30 μg of total RNA.

2. It is important to be aware of genomic DNA contamination of RNA samples, since adaptered genomic DNA fragments can be PCR amplified and visualized on a polyacrylamide gel. Because the occurrence of genomic DNA contamination will vary from RNA sample to RNA sample, genomic DNA fragments can be erroneously identified as differentially expressed mRNAs and prolonged effort wasted while attempting to validate their differential expression. To identify bands on a polyacrylamide gel derived from genomic DNA within a given RNA sample, "cDNA" may be prepared for indexing from the same RNA sample, but in the absence of reverse transcription.

3. The following are prerequisites for the manipulation of total RNA and the synthesis of cDNA:

    a. RNase-free water and RNase-free solutions should be prepared by adding DEPC (Sigma-Aldrich) to a final concentration of 0.1% (v/v), incubating overnight at room temperature, and autoclaving two times at 121°C for 30 min prior to use. Solutions containing Tris must be prepared in DEPC-treated water and filter-sterilized through a 0.2-μm filter.

    b. RNase-free antiaerosol micropipet tips (e.g., Aeroguard filters tips; Alpha, Eastleigh, Hants, UK) must be utilized.

c. Eppendorf tubes (in an RNase-free glass vessel) should be soaked in 0. 1% (v/v) DEPC at room temperature overnight, autoclaved two times at 121°C for 30 min, and dried prior to use.

d. New glassware (or glassware dedicated to RNA work) should be baked at 170°C for 4 h prior to use. Recycled glassware should be cleaned by rinsing with 0.5 M NaOH, prior to rinsing with copious amounts of DEPC-treated water, and (once dry) baking at 170°C for 4 h.

e. Presterilized disposable plasticware should be employed in preference to other labware.

f. Chemicals (molecular biology grade) reserved for RNA work must be utilized. The use of spatulas to dispense such chemicals should be avoided, but, if absolutely necessary, spatulas cleaned and baked at 170°C for 4 h maybe employed.

4. Total RNA may be prepared using a number of commercially available kits. Typically, the extraction of total RNA is based on the use of the chaotropic salt guanidinium thiocyanate in combination with phenol-chloroform extraction, at acid pH, to destroy ribonuclease activity and deproteinase nucleic acids *(15)*. The inclusion of detergents *(16)* in a guanidine thiocyanate/acid phenol lysis solution (Hybaid RiboLyser Kit; Hybaid, Teddington, Middlesex, UK) offers the added advantage of providing lubrication during the lysing step to prevent shearing of RNA. Total RNA may be further purified by selective adsorption to a silica membrane (RNeasy spin column; Qiagen). If RNA is to be prepared from isolated cells, or a cell line, one can isolate cytoplasmic RNA free from contaminating nuclear DNA and immature mRNA by selective lysis of the cell membrane (RNeasy kit; Qiagen).

5. RNA of high purity and integrity is a prerequisite for the generation of expression profiles. The purity of an RNA sample can be estimated by measuring the optical density (OD) at 260 and 280 nm, respectively, and calculating OD_{260nm}/OD_{280nm} (RNA giving a ratio of 1.8–2.0 is satisfactory). The integrity of the RNA can be assessed by agarose gel electrophoresis and ethidium bromide staining; sharp 28S and 1 8S ribosomal rRNAs (4.5 and 1.9 kb, respectively), whose the intensity of the 28S rRNA band is 1.5 to 2.5-fold that of the 1 8S rRNA band, are indicative of intact mammalian total RNA. An indication of the integrity of the mRNA isolated can also be demonstrated by RT-PCR assay, using gene-specific PCR primers that amplify either close to the entire length of a >1.5-kb transcript or a fragment close to the 5' end of a "long" transcript. Careful design of such gene-specific primers, to accommodate one or more introns, can also facilitate identification of contaminating genomic DNA.

6. Antiaerosol micropipet tips (e.g., Rainin Presterilised Aerosol Resistant Tips; Anachem) must be utilized at all times throughout the indexing procedure.

7. Triplicate ligation reactions are performed using each adapter pool pair for each RNA sample. Although the ligation reactions are derived from the same cDNA sample, they are nevertheless independent reactions. The presence of triplicate expression profiles derived by each adapter pool pair per RNA sample increases

confidence regarding the identification of putatively differentially expressed genes and also reduces the consequence of possible error in the processing of a single ligation reaction. The presence of triplicate reactions also facilitates statistical analysis (analysis of variance) of the likely significance of apparent quantitative differences in gene expression between one or more RNA samples. For a quantitative difference between the integrated intensity/volume of a given band between two or more RNA samples to be statistically significant, the extent of the difference between the RNAs must be compared to the magnitude of the differences within the replicates derived from each RNA.

8. Fragment analysis software is critical for the identification of quantitative differences in gene expression between RNA samples. To facilitate quantitative analysis, a given amount of a loading control (i.e., a labeled lambda DNA fragment) is added to each sample immediately prior to loading onto a polyacrylamide gel. Because the lambda DNA fragment should appear as a band of equal intensity in every sample, differences in band intensity reflect variable gel loading, and the extent of the differences can be employed to normalize the integrated intensities/volumes of all other bands in each sample. Fragment analysis software is also useful for the identification of bands that are present in one or more RNA samples and absent in one or more other RNA samples. Such software can generate tables in which bands are listed in rows according to their molecular weight/Rf value. Bands that are present in one sample (i.e., in one column of the table) and absent in another column/sample are thus readily identifiable.

9. The complexity of the transcriptional expression profiles derived by indexing is dependent on several variables:
    a. Number of different genes expressed in the RNAs under investigation.
    b. Mean length of the mRNAs transcribed.
    c. Length of the type IIs restriction enzyme recognition sequence and thus the frequency of restriction sites.
    d. Length of the cohesive overhangs generated by the type IIs restriction enzyme.
    e. Number of adapters in a ligation reaction.
    f. Sensitivity of the indexing procedure.
    A type IIs enzyme (e.g., *Bbv*I, *Bsm*AI, *Bsm*FI, *Fok*I, *Sfa*NI) recognizing a nonpalindromic 5-base recognition sequence cuts on average every $4^{5}/_{2}$ bp (512 bp). If the average size of an mRNA is 1500 bp, on average a type IIs enzyme such as BbvI cuts each mRNA twice, generating a single fragment with two cohesive ends for indexing. Widely quoted is the estimate that approx 15,000 different mRNAs are expressed by a single higher eukaryotic cell type. Consequently, an RNA sample representing a single cell type would yield 15,000 different fragments for indexing. There are potentially $4^{8}/_{2}$ (32,768) fragment classes, each with a different pair of cohesive ends, among the 15,000 fragments. In a ligation reaction featuring two pairs of adapter pools (i.e., 32 adapters), there are 528 different pairs of adapters, and, thus $528/32{,}768 \times 15{,}000 = 241$ different fragments may potentially be accessed. In a ligation reaction featuring a single adapter pool (i.e., 16 adapters), there are 136 different pairs of adapters and thus

$136/32,768 \times 15,000 = 62$ different fragments may potentially be accessed. These figures quoted obviously assume that the technology utilized is able to access every transcript, irrespective of transcript abundance. However, transcript abundance is an issue given it is estimated that, in a given cell type, "low-abundance" mRNAs are likely to represent 40–45% of the different mRNAs expressed *(17)*. The sensitivity of the indexing system using pairs of individual adapters has been demonstrated to be equivalent to the detection of transcripts expressed at the level of between 1 in 10,000 and 1 in 100,000 molecules *(1)*. The sensitivity of the indexing procedure using pairs of adapter pools, comprising 16 individual adapters, is likely to differ and will clearly significantly impact on the degree of mRNA representation attained by the indexing technology. The calculations outlined are clearly entirely hypothetical, are based on several assumptions (specifically the number of different mRNAs expressed), and are extremely difficult to verify in the absence of an extremely complex model system featuring species of known sequence and known but variable abundance.

10. Although the use of adapters in pairwise combinations of pools of 16 is described herein, the 256 individual 4-base 5'-overhang adapters may be employed in pairwise combinations of different complexity, i.e., 1×1, 4×4, or 8×8. There is some evidence (unpublished data) to suggest that a reduction in the complexity of a pair of adapters, which serves to lower the complexity of the cDNA population accessed by the adapter pair, increases the concentration of each cDNA in the population, thereby increasing the sensitivity of the procedure. However, the lower the complexity of each adapter, the larger the number of ligation reactions that must be performed to ensure that each cDNA restriction fragment is presented with every possible pair of 4-base 5'-cohesive end adapters; that is, 32,896 ligation reactions are required using pairs of individual adapters, pairwise combinations of 64 pools of four adapters require 2080 ligation reactions, and pairwise combinations of 32 pools of eight adapters require 528 ligation reactions.

11. On the assumption that the average length of an mRNA is 1500 bp, an approach based on the use of a type IIs enzyme recognizing a 5-base nonpalindromic recognition sequence is sufficient, in principle, to access the majority of cDNAs. However, cDNAs not accessible using a particular enzyme can be acquired using an alternative type IIs enzyme.

12. A prerequisite for using indexing for the identification of genes that display differential patterns of expression in one or more samples is that the samples are closely matched. Ideally the samples should be identical except regarding the syndrome under study. In this ideal situation, the only differences in transcriptional expression profile can be correlated with the syndrome being scrutinized. Given that it is invariably impossible to provide perfectly matched samples (i.e., there are often differences associated with genetic differences among different individuals), it is important to analyze multiple RNAs for each of the extremes being compared in order to identify conserved differences that are more likely to be correlated with the syndrome under investigation.

13. The differential expression of all cDNAs isolated by indexing-based differential display must be validated by an alternative technique, e.g., RT-PCR, Northern analysis, or reverse northern analysis.

References

1. Mahadeva, H., Starkey, M. P., Sheikh, F. N., Mundy, C. R., and Samani, N. J. (1998) A simple and effficient method for the isolation of differentially expressed genes. *J. Mol. Biol.* **284,** 1391–1398.
2. Hubank, M. and Schatz, D. G. (1994) Identifying differences in mRNA expression by representational difference analysis of cDNA. *Nucl. Acids Res.* **22,** 5640–5648.
3. Smith, D. R. (1992) Ligation-mediated PCR of restriction fragments from large DNA molecules. *PCR Methods Appl.* **2,** 21–25.
4. Unrau, P. and Deugau, K. V. (1994) Non-cloning amplification of specific DNA fragments from whole genomic DNA digests using DNA 'indexers.' *Gene* **145,** 63–169.
5. Sibson, D. R. (1992) Process for categorising nucleotide sequence populations. Patent application no. PCT/GB93/01452.
6. Sibson, D. R. and Starkey, M. P. (1997) Increasing the average abundance of low abundance cDNAs by ordered subdivision of cDNA populations, in *Methods in Molecular Biology, Vol. 69: cDNA Library Protocols* (Cowell, I. G. and Austin, C. A., eds.), Humana, Totowa, NJ, pp. 13–32.
7. Kato, K. (1995) Description of the entire messenger-RNA population by a 3'-end cDNA fragment generated by class IIS restriction enzymes. *Nucleic Acids Res.* **23,** 3685–3690.
8. Kato, K. (1996) RNA fingerprinting by molecular indexing. *Nucleic Acids Res.* **24,** 394–395.
9. Vos, P., Hogers, R., Bleeker, M., Reijans, M., van de Lee, T., Homes, M., Frijters, A., Pot, J., Peleman, J., Kuiper, M., and Zabeau, M. (1995) AFLP: a new technique for DNA fingerprinting. *Nucleic Acids Res.* **23,** 4407–4414.
10. Prashar, Y. and Weissman, S. M. (1996) Analysis of differential gene expression by display of 3'-end restriction fragments of cDNAs. *Proc. Natl. Acad. Sci. USA* **93,** 659–663.
11. Matz, M., Usman, Shagin, D., Bogdanova, E. and Lukyanov, S. (1997) Ordered differential display: a simple method for systematic comparison of gene expression profiles. *Nucleic Acids Res.* **25,** 2541–2542.
12. Liang, P. and Pardee, A. B. (1992) Differential display of eukaryotic messenger RNA by means of the polymerase chain reaction. *Science* **257,** 967–971.
13. Welsh, J., Chada, K., Dalal, S. S., Cheng, R., Ralph, D., and McClelland, M. (1992) Arbitrarily primed PCR fingerprinting of RNA. *Nucleic Acids Res.* **20,** 4965–4970.
14. Chou, Q., Russell, M., Birch, D. E., Raymond, J., and Bloch, W. (1992) Prevention of pre-PCR mix-priming and primer dimerisation improves low-copy-number amplifications. *Nucleic Acids Res.* **20,** 1717–1723.

15. Chomczynski, P. and Sacchi, N. (1987) Single-step method of RNA isolation by acid guanidinium thiocyanate-phenol-chloroform extraction. *Anal. Biochem.* **162,** 156–159.
16. Cheung, A. L., Eberhardt, K. J., and Fischetti, V. A. (1994) A method to isolate RNA from gram-positive bacteria and mycobacteria. *Anal. Biochem.* **222,** 511–514.
17. Davidson, E. H. and Britten, R. J. (1979) Regulation of gene expression: possible role of repetitive sequences. *Science* **204,** 1052–1059.

21

Expression Profiling by Systematic High-Throughput *In Situ* Hybridization to Whole-Mount Embryos

Nicolas Pollet and Christof Niehrs

1. Introduction

The genome of a given organism is considered in biology as the fundamental invariant *(1)*. It is virtually the same throughout lifetime and, to a lesser extent, over generations. By contrast, genetic information is expressed in complex and ever-changing temporal and spatial patterns throughout development and differentiation. The description and analysis of these patterns is crucial to elucidate the functions of genes and to understand the network of genetic interactions that underlies the process of normal development.

The study of the expression pattern of a gene is a prerequisite to understand its physiologic function, but the characterization of the expression of most known genes is incomplete. Consequently, it is almost impossible to compare gene expression patterns, and there are no specialized public databases available storing the data even though databases of gene expression are needed as a resource for the emerging field of functional genomics.

At the same time, genome science must bridge the gap between DNA sequence and function. To date, the study of cDNA copies of mRNAs has proven to be the most efficient way for large-scale gene identification and analysis. The additional information as to where and when an mRNA is present will be essential to help elucidate gene function.

The generation of the expression data for many genes should be a means of placing newly characterized sequences into context with respect to their sites of expression, of studying the correlation between gene expression and function, and of correlating the expression profiles with regulatory sequences.

From: *Methods in Molecular Biology, vol. 175: Genomics Protocols*
Edited by: M. P. Starkey and R. Elaswarapu © Humana Press Inc., Totowa, NJ

To identify all classes of developmentally important genes, expression-based and other molecular screens are needed to supplement classical genetic screens. Yet, most of the existing methodologies used to characterize gene expression have to be adapted to use in systematic studies using large numbers of samples. While the monitoring of gene expression using DNA arrays appears as a method of choice for high-throughput quantitative analysis, its spatial resolution is not as good as *in situ* hybridization (ISH).

An approach to study embryonic patterning at large scale is to use randomly isolated cDNAs and analyze the expression pattern of mRNAs by ISH, which allows direct access to the DNA sequence and reflects endogenous gene expression *(2–7)*. Different systems offer distinctive technical advantages for the study of particular aspects of development.

All ISH techniques involve the following steps: synthesis of probes, harvesting and preparation of embryos, tissue, and cells; pretreatment and permeabilization of embryos, tissue, and cells; hybridization; and washing and detection of hybridized probe. Detailed description of other ISH methods and discussions of theory can be found elsewhere *(8)*. The methods described here are based on several protocols *(9–11)* and have evolved for use on *Xenopus* embryos in a large-scale study.

2. Materials

All solutions should be prepared in clean sterile glassware.

1. Sterile bidistilled water (dH_2O).
2. Diethylpyrocarbonate (DEPC) treated dH_2O.
3. T3 primer: 5'-GCAATTAACCCTCACTAAAGGG-3' (12.5 μM).
4. T7 primer: 5'-GTAATACGACTCACTATAGGGC-3' (12.5 μM).
5. dNTPs (5 mM each) (MBI Fermentas, Immunogen International, Sunderland, Tyne & Wear, UK).
6. 10X Polymerase chain reaction (PCR) buffer (Gibco-BRL Life Technologies, Paisley, UK).
7. 5X Loading dye: 1.8 M sucrose, 5.25 mM cresol red.
8. *Taq* DNA polymerase (5 U/μL) (Gibco-BRL).
9. Multichannel pipet (Finnpipet; Life Sciences, Basingstoke, Hants, UK).
10. Replicator, 96- or 384-well microtiter plates for PCR (Advanced Biotechnologies, Epsom, Surrey, UK).
11. Thermocycler (MJ Research, Genetic Research Instrumentation, Braintree, Essex, UK).
12. Agarose (seakem grade; FMC BioProducts, Flowgen, Lichfield, Staffordshire, UK).
13. 1X TBE: 89 mM Tris, 89 mM boric acid, 2.5 mM EDTA, pH 8.3.
14. 5X Transcription buffer (MBI Fermentas).
15. DIG-RNA labeling mix (Roche, Lewes, East Sussex, UK).

16. RNA-guard (35 U/μL) (MBI Fermentas).
17. T7 RNA polymerase (20 units/μL) (MBI Fermentas).
18. Column loader (45 μL) (no. MACL09645[SE3P095V6]; Millipore, Watford, Herts, UK).
19. Multiscreen plate (sterile 0.45 μm hydrophilic, low protein binding Durapore membrane; no. MAHVS4510; Millipore).
20. Sephadex G50 DNA-grade resin (Amersham Pharmacia Biotech, Amersham, UK).
21. 1X STE buffer: 150 mM NaCl, 30 mM Tris-HCl, pH 8.0, 1 mM EDTA. Sterilize by autoclaving and store at 4°C.
22. Centrifuge with microtiter plate buckets (Sorvall, DuPont, Stevenage, Herts, UK).
23. Nile blue (no. N-0766; Sigma-Aldrich, Poole, Dorset, UK): 1% (w/v) in dH$_2$O, filtered through a 0.45-μm filter.
24. 1X Modified Danilchik buffer: 53 mM NaCl, 10 mM Na$_2$CO$_3$, 4.25 mM gluconic acid potassium salt, 1 mM MgCl$_2$, 1 mM CaCl$_2$, 6 mM bicine, pH 8.3; made as a 10X stock, filtered through a 0.2 μm filter and stored at –20°C.
25. 1X Modified Barth's Solution, pH 7.6: 88 mM NaCl, 1 mM KCl, 0.41 mM CaCl$_2$, 0.33 mM Ca(NO$_3$)$_2$, 0.82 mM MgSO$_4$, 2.4 mM NaHCO$_3$, 10 mM HEPES.
26. 3X Phosphate-buffered saline (PBS), pH 7.2: Mix 1:1 390 mM NaCl, 30 mM Na$_2$HPO$_4$ and 390 mM NaCl, 30 mM NaH$_2$PO$_4$. Filter through a 3-μm membrane and sterilize by autoclaving. Prepare 1X PBS by dilution using sterile dH$_2$O.
27. Proteinase K (1 mg/mL) (Roche) resuspended in 1X PBS (store at –20°C).
28. Collagenase A (40 mg/mL) (Roche) resuspended in 1X PBS (store at –20°C).
29. Hyaluronidase (20,000 U/mL) (Sigma-Aldrich) resuspended in 1X PBS (store at –20°C).
30. 10X MEMFA salts: 1 M MOPS, pH 7.4, 20 mM EGTA, 10 mM MgSO$_4$ (store at –20°C).
31. Formaldehyde (Fluke, Gillingham, Dorset, UK).
32. Rotator.
33. Glass vials (5 mL) and plastic Pasteur pipets.
34. PBSw: 0.1% (v/v) Tween-20 in 1X PBS.
35. Methanol (Fluke).
36. 6-Well plates (Falcon, Becton Dickinson, Cowley, Oxford, UK).
37. 4% (v/v) paraformaldehyde in 1X PBS. Dissolve by heating at 60°C. Filter through a 3-μm membrane and store at –20°C.
38. 10% (w/v) CHAPS (Roche) stock solution in dH$_2$O.
39. Formamide (Fluke). Formamide should be deionized before use. Add 5 g of a mixed-bed ion-exchange resin (e.g., no. AG501; Bio-Rad, Hemel Hempstead, Herts, UK) to 100 mL of formamide and stir for 1–2 h. Store at –20°C.
40. Hybridization buffer: 1% (w/v) Boehringer block (Roche), 50% (v/v) deionized formamide, 5X saline sodium citrate (SSC), 1 mg/mL of yeast RNA, 100 μg/mL of heparin, 0.1% (v/v) Tween-20, 0.1% (w/v) CHAPS, 5 mM EDTA.
41. 20X SSC: 3 M NaCl, 0.3 M sodium citrate. Adjust to pH 7.0 with NaOH. Filter through a 3-μm membrane and sterilize by autoclaving.
42. In Situ Pro reaction tubes and reagent tubes (Abimed, Germany).

43. 1X TNX: 50 m*M* NaCl; 100 m*M* Tris, 0.1% (v/v) Triton X-100, pH 7.0 (always use freshly prepared).
44. 1X TN: 50 m*M* NaCl; 100 m*M* Tris-HCl, pH 7.5 (made as a 20X stock and sterilized by autoclaving).
45. Blocking buffer: 1% (w/v) Boehringer Block (Roche) in TNX. Aliquoted and stored at –20°C.
46. Blocking buffer with antibody: 1% (w/v) Boehringer Block (Roche) in TNX. Anti-DIG Fab (Roche) 1/12,000. Titrate each batch of antibody.
47. BM purple solution (Roche). Use diluted 1:1 with dH$_2$O.
48. Microscope.
49. Color charge-coupled device camera (e.g., no. DXC-930P; Sony).
50. Image processing software (e.g., Adobe Photoshop software).

3. Methods

3.1. PCR Amplification of cDNA Inserts

The starting point is optimally a gridded cDNA library in a vector such as pBSKS+ (Stratagene, Cambridge, UK) containing different phage RNA polymerase promoters (*see* **Note 1**) on both sides of the inserts. **Figure 1** depicts the overall strategy.

1. Set up on ice a PCR reaction mix of 25 µL final volume per well for 96- or 384-well microtiter plates by mixing 9.2 µL of dH$_2$O, 1 µL of T3 primer, 1 µL of T7 primer, 2.5 µL of dNTPs, 2.5 µL of 10X PCR buffer, 2.5 µL of 25 m*M* MgO$_2$, 5 µL of 5X loading dye, and 0.3 µL of *Taq* polymerase (*see* **Notes 2–4**). Dispense 24 µL of PCR mix into each MTP well. Inoculate the PCR mix with 1 µL of bacterial suspension using either a replicator or a multichannel pipet. Mix well. Centrifuge the plate briefly.
2. Add 25 µL of mineral oil if needed. Thermocycle as follows: 95°C for 1 min, 55°C for 1 min, 72°C for 1.5 min for 35 cycles; 72°C for 5 min; cool to room temperature.
3. Check 2 µL of each PCR product by electrophoresis on a 2% (w/v) agarose gel. Identify clones with small (<500 bp) or no insert. These will not be used for cRNA synthesis.

3.2. Synthesis of Labeled cRNA Probe

1. Prepare a record sheet for a 96-well microtiter plate corresponding to the scheme of the ISH, taking into account positive and negative controls.
2. Set up a 10 µL/well *in vitro* transcription reaction mix as follow: 5.3 µL of DEPC-dH$_2$O, 2 µL of 5X transcription buffer, 1 µL of DIG-RNA labeling mix, 0.2 µL of RNA-guard, and 0.5 µL of T7 RNA polymerase. Dispense 9 µL of mix into each microtiter plate well. Add 1 µL of template (PCR product) according to the record sheet and mix well.
3. Incubate for 3 h at 37°C. Store at –80°C prior to purification.

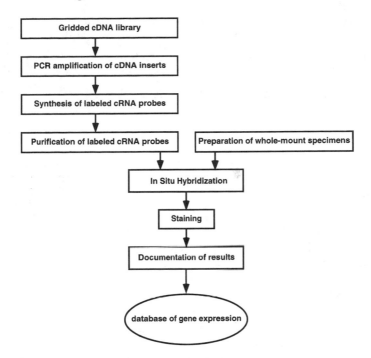

Fig. 1. Scheme of expression profiling by systematic high-throughput whole-mount ILSH.

3.3. Purification of Labeled cRNA Probe (see Note 5)

1. Set up Sephadex G50 columns in a Multiscreen 96-well plate by loading 45 µL of Sephadex G50 DNA-grade resin into each well using a column loader.
2. Remove the excess beads from the top of the column loader with the scraper supplied.
3. Place the Multiscreen plate upside down on the loader, invert both, and tap on the top to release the beads.
4. Add 300 µL of DEPC-dH$_2$O and incubate at room temperature for 3 h minimum (if the Multiscreen minicolumns are not immediately required, store at 4°C).
5. After removing the Multiscreen minicolumns from 4°C, equilibrate to room temperature before use.
6. Centrifuge the Multiscreen plate for 2 min, collecting the excess water into a 96-well microtiter plate, and then add 50 µL of 1X STE to the center of the minicolumns, and centrifuge for 2 min, collecting the excess of buffer into a 96-well microtiter plate.
7. Add 10 µL of DIG-labeled cRNA to the center of each minicolumn.
8. Add 40 µL of STE to the center of the minicolumns.
9. Centrifuge for 2 min, collecting the purified cRNA probes in a new 96-well microtiter plate.

10. Check a 10 µL aliquot of each probe by electrophoresis on a 1% (w/v) agarose gel in 1X TBE (*see* **Note 6**).

3.4. Preparation of Whole-Mount Xenopus Embryos Specimens

3.4.1. Vital Staining of Embryos with Nile Blue

We find it useful to stain *Xenopus* albino embryos in Nile blue to help sorting and staging *(12)*.

1. Dilute Nile blue to 0.005% (v/v) in 1X modified Danilchik buffer just prior to use.
2. Stain embryos for 5 min with gentle shaking, and wash three times in 0.3X Modified Barth's Solution.

3.4.2. Fixation of Xenopus Embryos

1. Prepare 100 mL of fresh MEMFA fixative by mixing in order 10 mL of 10X MEMFA salts, 10 mL of 37% (v/v) formaldehyde, and 80 mL of dH_2O.
2. Transfer selected embryos (without removing vitelline membrane) into a 30-mm Petri dish (do not put more than 200 embryos in a single dish) containing MEMFA fixative, and fix for 2 h on a rotator (*see* **Note 7**).
3. Transfer embryos into 5-mL glass vials (not more than 200 embryos per vial).
4. Wash three times for 10 min each in PBSw (at the lowest rotor speed).
5. Dehydrate by incubation for 5 min each in a series of methanol:PBSw solutions (1:3, 1:1, 3:1), and then five times with 100% (v/v) methanol.
6. Store at –20°C at least overnight, up to 3–6 mo.

3.4.3. Pretreatment of Embryos

1. Rehydrate by incubation for 5 min each in a series of methanol:PBSw solutions (3:1, 1:1, 1:3), finishing with two washes in PBSw. Always fill the glass vials to the brim.
2. Transfer the embryos (*see* Note 8) from the vials into the first well (of a 6-well plate) containing 2.5 mL of 10 µg/mL proteinase K, 2 mg/mL of collagenase A, and 20 U/mL of hyaluronidase in PBS. Mix well with a plastic pipet. Incubate for 9 to 10 min at room temperature. Shake the plate periodically by hand during incubation.
3. Transfer the embryos (*see* **Note 9**) into a second well containing 5 mL of PBSw and rinse briefly by shaking.
4. Transfer the embryos into a third well containing 5 mL of 10 µg/mL proteinase K. Incubate for 15 min (this should be adjusted for each batch of enzyme).
5. Transfer the embryos into a fourth well containing 5 mL of PBSw, rinse briefly, and transfer them into fresh glass vials.
6. Wash twice for 5 min each in PBSw (on a rotator).
7. Remove the PBSw and replace with 4% (v/v) paraformaldehyde in PBS, mix briefly, and incubate for 20 min. Move the vials from time to time by hand. The time for refixation should be watched carefully.

8. Wash four times for 5 min in PBSw (on a rotator).
9. Transfer the embryos into a Petri dish each PBSw, and using leftover glass injection needles puncture cavities in animal caps at stage 10,5, ventral of neural plate at stage 13, and though the first branchial arch at stage 30.
10. Transfer the embryos back into the glass vials containing PBSw.
11. Incubate for 3–5 min in 50% (v/v) PBSw, 50% (v/v) hybridization buffer (on a rotator), and for 5–10 min in hybridization buffer.
12. Renew the hybridization buffer and incubate for 1 h at 65°C (to effect inactivation of endogenous phosphatases). Invert the vials from time to time, to prevent the embryos from sticking together.
13. Store the embryos at –20°C. The embryos are now ready for ISH.

3.5. ISH Using the In Situ Pro

All steps from prehybridization to antibody washes are performed using the In Situ Pro robot (*[5]*; see **Notes 10–12**).

3.5.1. Preparation of the In Situ Pro

Before use, all reagent tubes are treated for 15 min at 65°C in 0.2 M NaOH to render them RNase free. Sterile dH_2O containing 0.02% (w/v) NaN_3 should be used to wash the needle (*see* **Note 13**). The water bath is filled with dH_2O.

3.5.2. Washing of Reaction Tubes for ISH

The XL_CN00 program is used to wash the reaction tubes (**Table 1**). It is used before any ISH program. The tubes will stay overnight in the hybridization buffer. The configuration is as follows: A is sterile dH_2O, B is hybridization buffer, C is 4% (v/v) paraformaldehyde in PBS, D is 0.2 M NaOH, ×0000000 is room temperature, and ×1000000 is 65°C. The reaction tubes are recycled by washing with dH_2O after a run, and stored in 0.2 M NaOH until next use.

3.5.3. Loading of the In Situ Pro

1. The embryos (not more than four) are loaded into the reaction tubes (washed using the XL_CN00 program) in the In Situ Pro using a pipet controlled by a screw system. Each embryo is separated from another by an air bubble to minimize the amount of buffer transferred.
2. Aliquot 150 µL of hybridization buffer into 500-µL PCR tubes in strips of eight.
3. Add 10 µL of purified RNA probe to each tube according to the record sheet.
4. Denature for 5 min at 95°C in a thermocycler and load into the robot.

3.5.4. Hybridization Programs

Two programs have been designed, one for week runs and another for weekend runs. It should be possible to reduce the time and number of washes, but

Table 1
XL_CN00 Method Overview

Step	Task	Time	Volume (μL)	Parameters
1	Rinse			5000/5000 μL
2	SetMultCon			×0000000
3	Incubate	30 min	300	C-Sample_A
4	Incubate	15 min	300	A-Sample_A
5	Incubate	15 min	300	A-Sample_A
6	SetMultCon			×1000000
7	Incubate	30 min	300	D-Sample_A
8	Incubate	15 min	300	A-Sample_A
9	Incubate	15 min	300	A-Sample_A
10	Incubate	15 min	300	A-Sample_A
11	Incubate	15 min	300	A-Sample_A
12	Incubate	15 min	300	A-Sample_A
13	Incubate	15 min	300	A-Sample_A
14	Incubate	15 min	200	B-Sample_A

the time schedule would become problematic. Solutions must be prepared in advance.

1. The XL_CN01 program (**Table 2**) is used to make ISH during the week. The time schedule is as follows: load embryos in the morning (d 0), add probes in the afternoon (d 0), add blocking solution and antibody in the afternoon of the next day (d 1), and the run is finished early on the morning of d 2.
2. The configuration is as follows: A is 150 mL of TNX, B is 35 mL of hybridization buffer; C is 35 mL of 2X SSC, 0.1% (w/v) CHAPS; from step 1 to 22 D is 35 mL of 2X SSC, 0.1% (w/v) CHAPS; from step 1 to 22 E is 35 mL of 0.2X SSC, 0.1% (w/v) CHAPS (35 mL); from step 23 onward D is 20 mL of blocking buffer (*see* **Note 14**); from step 23 onward E is 20 mL of blocking buffer containing antibody; F is TN; H is 15 mL of 2X SSC, 0.1% (w/v) CHAPS; I is 15 mL of 0.2X SSC, 0.1% (w/v) CHAPS; G, J, K, L, and M are empty. ×0000000 is room temperature, ×1000000 is 65°C, and ×1000001 is 60°C.
3. The XL_CN002 program (**Table 3**) is used to perform ISHs during the weekend. The time schedule is as follows: load embryos on the Friday afternoon and add probes in the afternoon during the prehybridization step or pause the robot, add blocking solution and antibody before leaving, and the run is finished early on Monday morning. Solutions must be prepared in advance.
4. The configuration is as follows: A is 150 mL of TNX; B is 35 mL of hybridization buffer; C is 35 mL of 2X SSC, 0.1% (w/v) CHAPS; D is 35 mL of 2X SSC, 0.1% (w/v) CHAPS; E is 35 mL of 0.2X SSC, 0.1% (w/v) CHAPS; F is 35 mL of TN; G is 35 mL of 2X SSC, 0.1% (w/v) CHAPS; H is 15 mL of 0.2X SSC,

Table 2
Overview of Method XL_CN01

Step	Task	Time	Volume (μL)	Parameters	Comments
1	Rinse			5000/5000 μL	# wash needle
2	SetMultCon			×0000000	# set temperature to 60°C
3	Incubate	2 h	150	B-SAMPLE_A	# prehybridization
4	WaitForKey				# installation of probes
5	SetMultCon			×0000000	# set temperature to 60°C
6	Incubate	16 h	150	Probe-SAMPLE_A	# add probes, hybridization
7	SetMultCon			×0000000	# set temperature to RT
8	Incubate	0 min	125	B-SAMPLE_A	# transfer to washing buffer
9	SetMultCon		125	H-SAMPLE_A	# transfer to washing buffer
10	Incubate	0 min	150	C-SAMPLE_A	# transfer to washing buffer
	Incubate			×0000000	# set temperature to 65°C
12	Incubate	40 min	150	C-SAMPLE_A	# first wash
	Incubate	40 min	150	D-SAMPLE_A	# second wash
14	Incubate	40 min	150	D-SAMPLE_A	# third wash
	Incubate	40 min	150	E-SAMPLE_A	# fourth wash
16	Incubate	40 min	150	E-SAMPLE_A	# fifth wash
17	SetMultCon			×0000000	# set temperature to RT
18	Incubate	0 min	75	I-SAMPLE_A	# transfer to TN buffer
19	Aliquot		75	F-SAMPLE_A	# transfer to TN buffer
20	Incubate	15 min	150	F-SAMPLE_A	# transfer to TN buffer
	Incubate	15 min	150	A-SAMPLE_A	# transfer to TN buffer
	WaitForKey				# installation of antibody
	Incubate	2 h	150	D-SAMPLE_A	# blocking
	Incubate	6 h	150	E-SAMPLE_A	# incubation antibody
	Incubate	20 min	150	A-SAMPLE_A	# first TNX wash
	Incubate	20 min	150	A-SAMPLE_A	# second TNX wash
	Incubate	20 min	150	A-SAMPLE_A	# third TNX wash
	Incubate	60 min	150	A-SAMPLE_A	# fourth TNX wash
	Incubate	60 min	150	A-SAMPLE_A	# fifth TNX wash
	Incubate	60 min	150	A-SAMPLE_A	# sixth TNX wash
	Incubate	60 min	150	A-SAMPLE_A	# seventh TNX wash
	Incubate	60 min	150	A-SAMPLE_A	# eighth TNX wash
	Rinse			5000/5000 μL	# wash needle
	SetMultCon			×0000000	# set temperature to RT

0.1% (w/v) CHAPS; I and J are each 15 mL of blocking buffer (*see* **Note 14**), L and M are each 15 mL of blocking buffer containing antibody; and K is empty. ×0000000 is room temperature, ×1000000 is 65°C, and ×1000001 is 60°C.

Table 3
Overview of Method XL_CN02

Step	Task	Time	Volume (μL)	Parameters	Comments
1	Rinse			5000/5000 μL	# wash needle
2	SetMultCon			×1000001	# set temperature to 60°C
3	Incubate	2 h	150	B-SAMPLE_A	# prehybridization
4	SetMultCon			×1000001	# set temperature to 60°C
5	Incubate	16 h	150	Probe-SAMPLE_A	# add probes, hybridizatio
6	SetMultCon			×0000000	# set temperature to RT
7	Incubate	0 min	125	B-SAMPLE_A	# transfer to washing buf
8	Aliquot		125	G-SAMPLE_A	# transfer to washing buf
9	Incubate	0 min	150	C-SAMPLE_A	# transfer to washing buf
10	SetMultCon			×1000000	# set temperature to 65°C
11	Incubate	40 min	150	C-SAMPLE_A	# first wash
12	Incubate	40 min	150	D-SAMPLE_A	# second wash
13	Incubate	40 min	150	D-SAMPLE_A	# third wash
14	Incubate	40 min	150	E-SAMPLE_A	# fourth wash
15	Incubate	40 min	150	E-SAMPLE_A	# fifth wash
16	SetMultCon			×0000000	# set temperature to RT
17	Incubate	0 min	75	H-SAMPLE_A	# transfer to TN buffer
18	Aliquot		75	F-SAMPLE_A	# transfer to TN buffer
19	Incubate	15 min	150	F-SAMPLE_A	# transfer to TN buffer
20	Incubate	15 min	150	A-SAMPLE_A	# transfer to TNX buffer
21	Incubate	15 min	75	I-SAMPLE_A	# blocking
22	Aliquot		75	J-SAMPLE_A	# blocking
23	Wait	2 h			# blocking
24	Incubate	15 min	75	L-SAMPLE_A	# incubation antibody
25	Wait		75	M-SAMPLE_A	# incubation antibody
26	Incubate	6 h		A-SAMPLE_A	# incubation antibody
27	Incubate	1 h	150		# first TNX wash
28	Incubate	2 h	150	A-SAMPLE_A	# second TNX wash
29	Incubate	3 h	150	A-SAMPLE_A	# third TNX wash
30	Incubate	4 h	150	A-SAMPLE_A	# fourth TNX wash
31	Incubate	4 h	150	A-SAMPLE_A	# fifth TNX wash
32	Incubate	4 h	150	A-SAMPLE_A	# sixth TNX wash
33	Incubate	4 h	150	A-SAMPLE_A	# seventh TNX wash
34	Incubate	5 h	150	A-SAMPLE_A	# eighth TNX wash
35	Incubate	5 h	150	A-SAMPLE_A	# ninth TNX wash
36	Rinse			5000/5000 μL	# wash needle
37	SetMultCon			×0000000	# set temperature to RT

3.6. Staining Reaction

1. Remove the reaction tubes containing the embryos from the robot, uncap them, and replace the needles by yellow plugs. Install the tubes on a 96-well rack and fill each up to the brim by adding 200 μL of TNX.
2. Aliquot 200 μL of TNX in each well of a 48-well plate and transfer the embryos (*see* **Note 15**) by inverting each reaction tube into the corresponding well.
3. Remove the TNX solution using a yellow tip connected to a vacuum pump. Add 800 μL of BM purple solution diluted 1:1 with dH$_2$O to each well. Stain at room temperature, at 37°C, or preferably at 4°C, with occasional gentle shaking. Monitor the staining by examination under the microscope.
4. When staining is optimal, stop the reaction by washing five times with 1X PBS (otherwise, the embryos will develop background within one week).
5. Fix the stained embryos in MEMFA fixative overnight. Transfer to 75% (v/v) glycerol via a series of increasing glycerol concentration (25% [v/v], 50% [v/v], 75% [v/v]), incubating for 20 min in each solution. Store at 4°C.

3.7. Interpretation and Presentation of Results

Careful interpretation of results is essential. Particular attention should be paid to the fact that no control sense strand probes are used for large-scale studies. Sectioning stained whole-mount embryos is a good method to help interpret the results. Rescreening should be made for probes giving restricted pattern of expression.

Photograph the embryos in 30-mm Petri dishes filled with 75% (v/v) glycerol, with substage illumination and a blue or yellow background. It is worth experimenting with different conditions to get the best possible pictures (*see* **Note 16**).

4. Notes

1. We have successfully used a chimeric primer introducing an SP6 promoter during PCR, enabling the use of gridded cDNA libraries in various vectors.
2. Adding betain (Sigma-Aldrich) to a final concentration of 1.5M can increase the yield of PCR amplification.
3. Different size criterias could be applied to select appropriate PCR products.
4. Positive and negative controls included at this step are no template and known template.
5. An alternative purification method can be performed by adding, to each PCR reaction, 5 μL of 7.5 *M* ammonium acetate and 30 μL of cold 100% (v/v) ethanol; precipitate overnight at –20°C, centrifuge for 1 h at 3000*g*, remove the supernatants (the plate of samples must be centrifuged inverted on paper for 10 s at 500*g*), wash the pellets with 100 μL of 70% (v/v) ethanol, stand for 5 min at room temperature, centrifuge for 1 h at 3000*g*, dry the pellets for 10 min at room temperature, resuspend each pellet in 10 μL of dH$_2$O, and check a 0.5-μL aliquot of each by agarose gel electrophoresis.

6. The efficiency of probe labeling can be checked using a dot-blot procedure. Template removal and reduction of probe length by hydrolysis were not found to give better ISH results.

7. Do not treat embryos at late tailbud stage with the cocktail of enzymes used to remove the vitelline membrane.

8. Embryos can be fixed overnight at 4°C. Dehydration should be soft to avoid loss of morphology. Alternatively, the vitelline membrane can be removed using watchmaker forceps. The embryos should never be left dry when exchanging liquids. To preserve morphology, particular care should be taken when transferring the embryos.

9. Embryos are fragile after the proteinase treatment and before the refixation.

10. An alternative to the robot is to use the same Multiscreen plate used for probe purification, together with a vacuum manifold to allow for the exchange of liquids.

11. Many problems can arise with the robot, most often drying in reaction tubes. Check that the inner needle is 8 mm distant from the tip of the outer needle, that the water bath is full at the start, and that reagents tubes are filled. Also, check the lids of reaction tubes.

12. Recycled tubes can be clogged, this would lead to a flood in the robot. It is safer to check the first step of incubation to monitor these clogging events and change the tubes accordingly.

13. Particular attention should be taken to use RNase-free vessels, and use NaN_3 in the water used to clean the needle.

14. The most common source of background seems to be contamination of the blocking reagent. This can be avoided by aliquoting and storage at –20°C, and operating the robot in a temperature-controlled room.

15. Some embryos can stick to the reaction tubes when transferred to the staining solution, use a pipet to detach them.

16. A database can be set up to allow for the storage of expression profiles and pictures, along with sequence and clone informations. An example using the acedb system can be found at <http://www.dkfz-heidelberg.de/abt0135/axeldb.htm>.

Acknowledgments

We thank Volker Gawantka for his introduction of ISH in frog embryos. Our many thanks to Ursula Fenger for her skillful technical assistance and to Nadja Muncke for her participation in the work. N. P. was supported by a Marie Curie fellowship.

References

1. Monod, J. (1970) *Le hasard et la necessité,* Editions du Seuil, Paris.
2. Bettenhausen, B. and Gossler, A. (1995). Efficient isolation of novel mouse genes differentially expressed in early postimplantation embryos. *Genomics* **28,** 436–441.
3. Gawantka, V., Pollet, N., Delius, H., Vingron, M., Pfister, R., Nitsch, R., Blumenstock, C., and Mehrs, C. (1998) Gene expression screening in *Xenopus*

identifies molecular pathways, predicts gene function and provides a global view of embryonic patterning. *Mech. Dev.* **77,** 95–141.

4. Kopczynski, C. C., Noordermeer, J. M., Serano, T. L., Chen, W.-C., Pendleton, J. D., Lewis, S., Goodman, C. S., and Rubin, G. M. (1998) A high throughput screen to identify secreted and transmembrane proteins involved in *Drosophila* embryogenesis. *Proc. Natl. Acad. Sci. USA* **95,** 9973–9978.

5. Plickert, G., Gajewski, M., Gehrke, G., Gausepohl, H., Schlossherr, J., and Ibrahim, H. (1997) Automated *in situ* detection (AISD) of biomolecules. *Dev. Gene. Evol.* **207,** 362–367.

6. Niehrs, C. (1997) Gene expression screens in vertebrate embryos: more than meets the eye. *Genes Funct.* **1,** 229–231.

7. Komiya, T., Tanigawa, Y., and Hirohashi, S. (1997) A large scale *in situ* hybridisation system using an equalised cDNA library. *Anal. Biochem.* **254,** 23–30.

8. Wilkinson, D.G. and Nieto, M.A. (1993) Detection of messenger RNA by *in situ* hybridization to tissue sections and whole mounts. *Methods Enzymol.* **225,** 361–373.

9. Harland, R. M. (1991) *In situ* hybridization: an improved whole-mount method for *Xenopus* embryos. *Methods Cell Biol.* **36,** 685–695.

10. Wang, K., Gan, L., Boysen, C., and Hood L. (1995) A microtiter plate-based high-throughput DNA purification method. *Anal. Biochem.* **226,** 85–90.

11. Islam, N. and Moss, T. (1996) Enzymatic removal of vitelline membrane and other protocol modifications for whole mount *in situ* hybridization of *Xenopus* embryos. *Trends Genet.* **12,** 459.

12. Nieuwkoop, P. D. and Faber, J. (1984) Normal table of *Xenopus laevis* (Daudin), 2nd ed., Garland Publishing Inc., New York and London.

22

Expression Monitoring Using cDNA Microarrays

A General Protocol

**Xing Jian Lou, Mark Schena, Frank T. Horrigan,
Richard M. Lawn, and Ronald W. Davis**

1. Introduction

As the Human Genome Project nears the completion of the first human sequence, the next great challenge is to elucidate the function of these genes. One route of exploring the function of a gene is by determining its pattern of expression. Various methods are available for detecting and quantitating gene expression levels, including Northern blots *(1)*, RNase protection assays *(2)*, differential display *(3)*, representational difference analysis *(1)*, and serial analysis of gene expression *(5)*. cDNA microarray technology *(6,7)* distinguishes itself from the other methods by allowing one to measure the expression levels of tens of thousands of genes in a single experiment. This capacity allows the expression of entire genomes to be monitored in parallel during different stages of embryonic development, disease progress, or drug response. Microarray technology has therefore attracted a great deal of interest from both academic and commercial sectors.

Microarray technology, like other hybridization-based techniques (Southern and Northern blot), is based on the principle that every nucleic acid strand carries the capacity to recognize complementary sequences through base pairing. Two key innovations also provide a foundation for microarray technology. The first is the use of a rigid and optically flat surface, which has facilitated miniaturization of DNA arrays and fluorescence-based signal detection. Microarrays contain discrete cDNA sequences at high spatial resolution in precise locations on a small surface such as a microscope slide. Fluorescence-based detection provides a sensitive, high-resolution

From: *Methods in Molecular Biology, vol. 175: Genomics Protocols*
Edited by: M. P. Starkey and R. Elaswarapu © Humana Press Inc., Totowa, NJ

measurement of molecular binding events on arrays. The second key innovation is the simultaneous hybridization of microarrays with two pools of fluorescence-labeled cDNA probe, representing total RNA from test and reference samples. In addition to providing information on the expression pattern in each sample, the ratio of these measurements provides a direct and quantitative comparison of message abundance in the test and reference samples.

There are two principle methods of constructing DNA microarrays. One is by printing or jetting cDNA clones onto microscope slides using a robotic arraying device capable of three-dimensional movement (cDNA microarrays). The other is to synthesize single-stranded polynucleotides directly onto a glass substrate (represented, e.g., by Affymetrix's GeneChip). In this chapter, we focus on the protocols developed in our laboratories for printed cDNA microarrays. The cDNA clones that are printed may have known or unknown sequences representing some or all of the genes in a given genome. Synthetic oligonucleotides made from expressed sequences (e.g., expressed sequence tags) have also been used.

Figure 1 illustrates the general strategy and procedures for the fabrication and use of cDNA microarrays. In brief, templates representing genes of interest are amplified by the polymerase chain reaction (PCR). After purification, aliquots of the PCR products (0.2–1.0 nL) are printed onto pretreated microscope slides using a robotic arrayer. To compare the expression of each gene in the test and reference samples, mRNA isolated from each of these samples is labeled with a different fluorescent dye such as Cy3 (green) and Cy5 (red), by reverse transcription. The two pools of labeled cDNA probes are then mixed and hybridized to a microarray. After hybridization, measurements are made with a high-resolution laser scanner that illuminates each DNA spot (at two wavelengths) and measures the fluorescent intensity of each dye separately. Following background subtraction, a ratio measurement of the absolute and relative abundance of each specific gene in the test and reference samples can be obtained.

There are many possible variations on the basic principles illustrated in **Fig. 1**, from the choice of surface chemistry to the analysis of signals. The following protocol is provided as an example of the cDNA microarray methods. In this protocol, silylated microscope slides were used to provide active aldehyde groups that covalently link to amine groups that have been introduced into the 5' end of cDNA molecules by PCR primers (*see* **Note 1**). This silane-based coupling chemistry is extremely stable. The microarrays used in these experiments were printed approximately 2 yr prior to processing and use. Hybridization was carried out with probes labeled with Cy3- or Cy5-coupled nucleotide analogs.

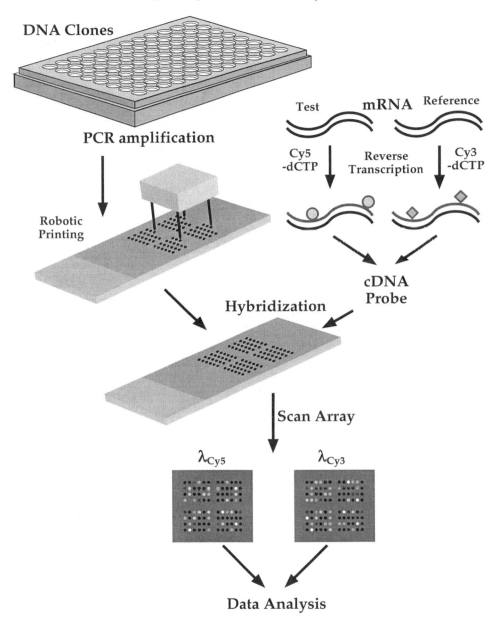

Fig. 1. Overview of a microarray assay. cDNA clones are amplified and purified and then deposited onto microscope slides with a robotic printing device. Two sources of mRNA are labeled with two different fluors, mixed and hybridized to the microarray. Fluorescent scanning of the microarray generates images that represent quantitative measurements of gene expression in the two samples. Analysis of the expression data provides biologic information.

2. Materials

For the following materials alternative vendors can be used, but pay special attention to selection of microscope slides, reverse transcriptase, and Cy3- and Cy5-labeled oligonucleotides.

1. PCR primers modified with a 5'-amino-modifier C6 (Glen Research, Sterling, VA).
2. 96-Well thermal cycler (Perkin-Elmer, Norwalk, CT).
3. 96-Well PCR plates (Perkin-Elmer).
4. *Taq* DNA polymerase and 10X PCR buffer: 500 mM KCl; 100 mM Tris-HCl, pH 8.3, 15 mM MgCl$_2$, 0.1% (w/v) gelatin (Stratagene, La Jolla, CA).
5. PCR Purification Kit (TeleChem, Sunnyvale, CA).
6. Flat-bottomed 384-well plates (Nunc, Naperville, IL).
7. Robotic arrayer (built in-house, based on a Synteni design).
8. ChipMaker Micro-spotting device (TeleChem).
9. Micro-Spotting solution (TeleChem).
10. Microscope slides coated with amine-reactive groups (e.g., silylated slides from CEL, Houston, TX) (*see* **Note 1**).
11. Sodium borohydride (98%) (J. T. Baker, Phillipsburg, NJ).
12. TRIZOL Reagent (Gibco-BRL, Grand Island, NY).
13. Oligotex mRNA Midi Kit (Qiagen, Valencia, CA).
14. RNA transcription kit (Stratagene).
15. Oligo-dT 21mer (treated with 0.1% [w/v] diethyl pyrocarbonate to inactivate ribonucleases).
16. 100 mM dATP, dCTP, dGTP, dTTP (Gibco-BRL).
17. 1 mM Cy3-dCTP (Amersham, Arlington Heights, IL).
18. 1 mM Cy5-dCTP (Amersham).
19. SuperScript II RNase H-Reverse Transcriptase (Gibco-BRL).
20. RNase inhibitor (Gibco-BRL).
21. Chromaspin-TE-30LC (Clontech, Mountain View, CA).
22. Hybridization cassettes (TeleChem).
23. Staining dishes (Wheaton, Millville, NJ) or Microarray wash station (TeleChem).
24. Speed Vac (Savant, Farmingdale, NY).
25. ScanArray 3000 microarray scanner (General Scanning, Watertown, MA).
26. ImaGene array analysis software (BioDiscovery, Los Angeles, CA).
27. Excel software (Microsoft, Seattle, WA).
28. TE buffer: 10 mM Tris-HCl, 1 mM EDTA, pH 8.0.

3. Methods

3.1. Making cDNA Microarrays

3.1.1. Preparation of cDNA Clones

All the following steps are performed in 96-well plates. Generic PCR primers (~21mers) complementary to vector sequences are commonly used.

1. Set up a PCR reaction by adding 1 μL of plasmid DNA (10 ng/μL; *see* **Note 2**) into 99 μL of master PCR mix containing 10 μL of 10X PCR buffer, 10 μL of 4X 2 mM dNTPs, 1.0 μL of 100 μM amino-modified 3' end primer, 1.0 μL of 100 μM amino-modified 5' end primer, 76 μL of H_2O, and 1 μL of 5 U/μL *Taq* polymerase.
2. Denature DNA at 94°C for 4 min (this step should not be eliminated if PCR is performed directly with bacterial culture or phage lysate) and then thermocycle for 30 cycles of 94°C for 30 s, 55°C for 30 s, and 72°C for 60 s.
3. Purify the PCR products using a 96-well PCR Purification Kit (*see* **Note 3**).
4. Elute each PCR product with 100 μL of 0.1X TE buffer (*see* **Note 4**).
5. Dry the products to completion in a Speed Vac.
6. Resuspend each PCR product in 7.5 μL of 1X Micro-Spotting solution.
7. If the arrayer only accepts 384-well plates, transfer the samples to 384-well plates before arraying. Because most of the currently available arrayers are very sensitive to subtle differences in plates, it is best to use the type of plates suggested by the arrayer's manufacturer.

3.1.2. Microarraying and Slide Processing

1. Scan a random sample of slides from the batch before arraying to confirm that the coating is uniform and the autofluorescence of the slides is low (*see* **Note 5**).
2. Print the purified PCR products onto the slides, using a robotic arrayer according to manufacturer's instructions (*see* **Note 6**).
3. Allow printed microarrays to dry overnight in a slide box (several days or more is acceptable). Drying increases the crosslinking efficiency. The printed slides are stable at room temperature for >20 mo.
4. Soak the slides twice in 0.2% (w/v) sodium dodecyl sulfate (SDS) for 2 min at room temperature with vigorous agitation. This step removes salt and unbound DNA.
5. Wash the slides twice in ddH_2O for 2 min at room temperature with vigorous agitation.
6. Transfer the slides into ddH_2O at 95–100°C for 2 min to allow DNA denaturation.
7. Allow the slides to dry thoroughly at room temperature (~5 min).
8. While drying the slides, prepare 400 mL of sodium borohydride (NaBH$_4$) solution by dissolving 1.0 g of NaBH$_4$ in 300 mL of phosphate buffered saline, and adding 100 mL of 100% (v/v) ethanol to reduce bubbling.
9. Transfer the slides into the freshly made NaBH$_4$ solution for 10 min at room temperature to reduce and inactivate free aldehydes.
10. Rinse the slides three times in 0.2% (w/v) SDS for 1 min each at room temperature.
11. Rinse the slides once in ddH_2O for 1 min at room temperature.
12. Submerge the slides in ddH_2O at 95–100°C for 2 s.
13. Allow the slides to air-dry and store in a dark box with desiccant at 25°C (stable for >1 yr).

3.2. Using cDNA Microarrays

3.2.1. Purification of PolyA⁺ mRNA from Test and Reference Samples

1. Isolate total RNA using the TRIZOL Reagent one-step guanidinium thiocyanate acid-phenol extraction method (*see* **Note 7**). Add an additional phenol:chloroform extraction before the final precipitation of RNA to improve the quality of the fluorescent signals after hybridization.
2. Purify polyA⁺ mRNA from total RNA using a Qiagen Oligotex mRNA Kit, according to the manufacturer's instructions, but with the following modifications:
   a. Preheat the elution buffer to 75°C.
   b. Elute the mRNA from the oligotex resin in the spin column 3 times with 33 µL aliquots of elution buffer preheated to 75°C. Each time, after adding elution buffer, heat the Eppendorf tube containing the spin column to 75°C for 30 s to assist in mRNA elution (failure to do so may decrease mRNA yield, because the elution buffer is in a very small volume, and it cools quickly).
   c. Pool the three 33-µL mRNA elutions. Precipitate mRNA by adding 10 µL of RNase-free 3 *M* sodium acetate and 250 µL of 100% (v/v) ethanol. Add 1 µL of 10 mg/mL glycogen to assist the precipitation.
3. Keep mRNA at –80°C as a precipitate until required (mRNA can be stored under such conditions for several years).

3.2.2. Generating Control mRNAs by In Vitro Transcription

1. Choose heterologous cDNA clones in pBluescript vectors (*see* **Note 8**).
2. Linearize 10 µg of each plasmid DNA in a 25-µL reaction with a restriction enzyme (e.g., *Bam*HI), such that the in vitro transcript will contain the polyA⁺ tract, but as little vector sequence as possible.
3. Extract each linearized plasmid once with phenol, once with phenol/chloroform/isoamyl alcohol (25:25:1 [v/v]), and three times with ether. The extractions remove trace ribonucleases and prevent degradation of the in vitro transcripts.
4. Incubate each extraction for 5 min at 65°C and vortex gently to drive off the residual ether.
5. To each 25 µL of linear plasmid, add 0.1 volume of 3 *M* sodium acetate and 2 vol of 100% (v/v) ethanol. Mix by vortexing.
6. Pellet each linearized plasmid by centrifuging at 13,000*g* in a microfuge for 5 min at room temperature.
7. Remove and discard each supernatant and dry each DNA pellet in a Speed Vac.
8. Resuspend each linearized plasmid DNA in 10 µL of TE buffer for a final concentration of approx 1.0 µg/µL.
9. To a microfuge tube add 20 µL of 5X transcription buffer, 4 µL of a linearized plasmid, 16 µL of 4X 2.5 m*M* rNTPs, 4 µL of 0.75 *M* dithiothreitol (DTT), 3 µL of 20 U/µL RNase inhibitor, and 52.5 µL of H₂O. Mix by tapping the microfuge tube gently.

10. Add 0.8 µL of 50 U/µL T3 or T7 RNA polymerase. Mix by tapping the microfuge tube gently.
11. Incubate the reaction for 30 min at 37°C.
12. Add 10 µL of 3 *M* sodium acetate.
13. Extract the 110-µL reaction once with phenol/chloroform/isoamyl alcohol (25:25:1 [v/v]) and three times with ether.
14. Incubate the extraction for 5 min at 65°C and vortex gently to drive off the residual ether.
15. Add 220 µL of 100% (v/v) ethanol and pellet the in vitro transcripts by centrifuging at 13,000g for 5 min in a microfuge.
16. Remove and discard the supernatant and dry the RNA pellet at 37°C for 5 min.
17. Resuspend the in vitro transcript in 10 µL of RNase-free TE buffer for a final concentration of ~4.0 µg/µL (*see* **Note 9**).

3.2.3. Fluorescent Probe Synthesis Using Reverse Transcription

1. To an RNase-free microcentrifuge tube add 5.0 µL of 1.0 µg/µL purified polyA$^+$ mRNA (*see* **Note 10**), 1.0 µL of 0.5 ng/µL control mRNA cocktail (*see* **Note 11**), 4.0 µL of 1.0 µg/µL oligo-dT 21mer, and 17.0 µL of RNase-free H$_2$O. Mix by pipetting up and down, and heat at 65°C for 3 min to disrupt the secondary structure of the mRNA.
2. Incubate the mixture at room temperature (25°C) for 10 min to let the oligo-dT anneal to the mRNA.
3. Add 10.0 µL of 5X first-strand buffer; 5.0 µL of 0.1 *M* DTT, 1.5 µL of 20 U/µL RNase inhibitor; 1.0 µL of dATP, dGTP, dTTP cocktail (25 m*M* each); 2.0 µL of 1 m*M* dCTP; 2.0 µL of 1 m*M* Cy3-dCTP (if Cy3-dCTP is used to label the reference sample, use Cy5-dCTP to label the test sample); and 1.5 µL of 200 U/µL SuperScript II reverse transcriptase for a total reaction volume of 50 µL.
4. Mix by tapping the microcentrifuge tube or pipetting gently.
5. Incubate the reaction at 42°C in the dark for 2 h.
6. Add 10 µL of TE buffer and 2.5 µL of 1 *M* NaOH and incubate for 10 min at 65°C to degrade mRNAs.
7. Neutralize the cDNA mixture by adding 2.5 µL of 1 *M* Tris-HCl (pH 6.8) and 2.0 µL of 1 *M* HCl.
8. Run the fluorescently labeled cDNA probe through a Chromaspin-TE-30 LC column to remove unincorporated Cy3- or Cy5-dCTP.
9. To the eluent add 0.1 vol of 3 *M* sodium acetate and 2.5 vol of 100% (v/v) ethanol. Centrifuge for 15 min at 13,000g in a microfuge (4°C) to pellet the Cy3- or Cy5-labeled cDNA.
10. Remove and discard the supernatant. Wash the pellet with 0.5 mL of 80% (v/v) ethanol.
11. Spin for 5 min, and carefully remove the supernatant.
12. Dry the pellet in a Speed Vac and resuspend in 13.0 µL of H$_2$O. Resuspend thoroughly, since the product often smears up the side of the tube.
13. Add 5.0 µL of 20X saline sodium citrate (SSC) (3 *M* NaCl, 0.3 *M* sodium citrate, pH 7.0) and 2.0 µL of 2% (w/v) SDS.

14. Heat at 65°C for 30 s to dissolve the synthesized probe.
15. Centrifuge for 2 min in a microfuge at 13,000*g* to pellet trace debris (insoluble material can lead to elevated background fluorescence).
16. Transfer the supernatant to a new tube. The final probe concentration will be ~0.25 μg/μL per fluor in 20 μL of 5X SSC and 0.2% (w/v) SDS.

3.2.4. Microarray Hybridization and Washing

1. Place the microarray in a hybridization cassette. Add 5.0 μL of ddH$_2$O to the slot in the cassette to prevent drying of the sample.
2. Mix Cy3-labeled reference probe with Cy5-labeled test probe in a 1:1 ratio.
3. Boil the mixed probes for 2 min, and spin briefly at 13,000*g*. Immediately add 1.7 μL/cm^2 of the mixed probe onto the microarray (prepared in **Subheading 3.2.4., step 1**), place a cover slip onto the microarray using forceps (*see* **Note 12**), close the hybridization cassette containing the microarray, and submerge the hybridization cassette in a water bath set at 62°C.
4. Hybridize at 62°C for 6–12 h.
5. Wash the microarray for 5 min at room temperature in 1X SSC and 0.1% (v/v) SDS with stirring (*see* **Note 13**). The cover slip should slide off the microarray immediately during the wash step. If the cover slip does not slide off within 30 s, use forceps to gently remove it from the microarray surface. Failure to remove the cover slip immediately may lead to elevated background fluorescence.
6. Transfer the slides to 300 mL of a second wash solution containing 0.1X SSC, 0.1% (v/v) SDS. Wash the microarray for 5 min.
7. Rinse the microarray briefly in a third solution containing 0.1X SSC to remove the SDS.
8. Dry the microarray by spinning in a centrifuge at 500*g* for 5 min.

3.2.5. Image Scanning and Data Acquisition

1. Scan the microarray for fluorescence emission in both 632-nm red and 543-nm green channels using a default setting such as 90% of laser power and 60% of photomultiplier voltage for ScanArray 3000 (*see* **Note 14**).
2. Adjust the laser power and photomultiplier settings for both channels such that <5% of the signals in the brightest spots are saturated and the ratio of the signals at control spots or control slides in two channels is close to 1 (*see* **Note 15**).
3. Save images acquired in red and green channels corresponding to test and reference samples (**Fig. 2A**) (*see* **Note 16**).

Fig. 2. (*opposite page*) Gene expression analysis with a cDNA microarray. In this experiment, mRNA samples from untreated (reference) and interleukin-1β (IL-1β) treated (test) human umbilical vein endothelial cells (HUVECS) are compared. The total mRNA pool of the untreated HUVECS was reverse transcribed in the presence of Cy3-dCTP, and the total pool of IL-1β treated HUVECS was reverse transcribed in the presence of Cy5-dCTP. The two pools of the Cy3- and Cy5-labeled cDNA probes

A

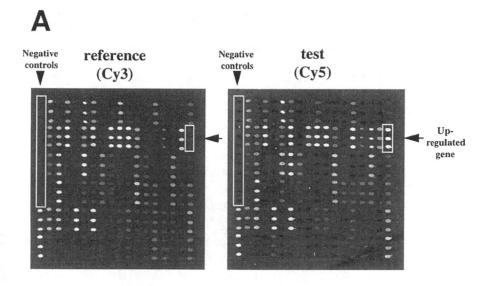

B

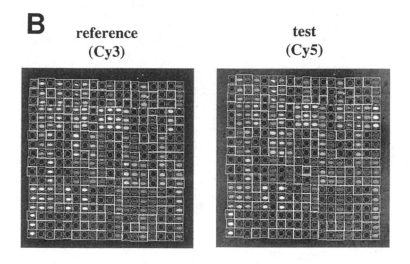

were then mixed and hybridized to a cDNA microarray that contained 104 human genes and 4 controls from *Arabidopsis thaliana*, with all 108 genes represented by three identical cDNA spots arranged as triplicates. **(A)** After washing, fluorescent images were acquired at 543 nm for the Cy3-labeled untreated HUVEC sample and at 632 nm for the Cy5-labeled IL-1β treated HUVEC sample with the ScanArray 3000 (General Scanning). Note that a few genes were strongly upregulated in the treated sample (examples shown by arrows). The negative control clones (*Arabidopsis* cDNA) are indicated by arrowheads. **(B)** Quantitation grids (BioDiscovery) were placed over the untreated (reference) image and the same location on the treated (test) image.

4. Open the pair of reference and test images in image analysis and data extraction software.
5. Place a grid to cover each spot according to the instructions of the software package (**Fig. 2B**, *see* **Note 17**).
6. Extract and save the data for data analysis.

3.2.6. Data Analysis

A variety of software tools have been developed for image and data analysis of microarrays (*see* **Note 17**). However, there is as yet no common method of signal identification and background subtraction that provides a universally acceptable measurement of data generated by different research groups using different conditions. At this time many groups are still writing custom software to fit their particular experimental conditions and purposes. For example, those who want to screen a large number of genes for changes in expression under a single condition may be most interested in the speed and the automation of the assay. Others who focus on quantitating the pattern of expression levels in a smaller set of genes under a variety of conditions may be more concerned with the sensitivity and accuracy of the measurements. The following is provided with the purpose of assisting readers in improving the accuracy and sensitivity of their microarray assay through data analysis. Analysis can be performed using Excel, if there is no suitable automated software available.

Accurate determination of expression ratios (R) requires measurement of the signal intensity in a DNA spot as well as an estimate of background fluorescence that may contribute to the signal. Expression levels of different genes and their corresponding signal intensities span a large dynamic range such that some are difficult to distinguish from the background whereas others are orders of magnitude brighter. The ratio of two bright signals will be relatively insensitive to background subtraction. However, some of the most biologically interesting responses involve a large increase or decrease in expression ($R \gg 1$ or $R \ll 1$) such that the signal in one channel is high whereas the other is low—approaching background levels. In such cases, the low-intensity signal and, therefore, the ratio measurement will be very sensitive to background subtraction.

Most data extraction programs provide measurements of the signal intensity within a DNA spot (S) as well as the background intensity in a local region of the slide surrounding the spot (B_L) (**Note 17**). B_L can often be used as an estimate of the background within the signal spot (B_S), but not always. The background fluorescence is likely to have both surface-specific and nonsurface-specific components. For example, dust deposited on the array would represent a nonsurface-specific background (B_{ns}) that contributes equally to B_L and B_S. However, because DNA and glass (or a coating on the glass) are different substances, it is also possible to observe background fluorescence that contributes differently to the glass surface (B_g) and DNA spot (B_d). Therefore, it is important to characterize these contributions before assuming that local background ($B_L = B_{ns} + B_g$) and signal background ($B_S = B_{ns} + B_d$) are equivalent. Under many experimental conditions (such as the example given later), negative controls (*see* **Note 6**) provided a better estimate of the signal-background than do local-background measurements.

The following protocols provide some guidelines for characterizing background fluorescence and evaluating the accuracy of ratio measurements. To illustrate the analysis, an array with 108 clones printed in triplicate (324 spots; representing one quadrant of a microarray) is used as an example. In this array, four control clones of *Arabidopsis* cDNA are printed along the left side of the array (12 spots) and used as negative controls (**Fig. 2**). The remaining 104 clones represent human cDNAs. All 108 clones are printed in triplicate so that the variability of the ratio measurements can be assessed. Although replicate measurements are generally useful for any assay, they are often not possible when using a commercial microarray or when space on the array is limiting. Nonetheless, this analysis illustrates some criteria that can be used to reject potentially unreliable ratio measurements in cases in which replicates are unavailable.

3.2.6.1. CHARACTERIZE BACKGROUND FLUORESCENCE

Plot the fluorescent intensities of all the DNA spots in the array (S) and compare them to the local background (B_L) measured around each spot (*see* **Note 17**) (**Fig. 3**). If B_L varies across the array while the lowest intensity signals do not follow the same trend (as in **Fig. 3**), then B_L may not provide a good estimate of B_S. Other indications that B_L may not represent B_S are if B_L is significantly greater than the lowest intensity signals or the intensity of negative controls (S_{nc}), or if B_L is significantly less than S_{nc}. In such cases, S_{nc} should be used as an estimate of B_S (*see* legend to **Fig. 3**).

3.2.6.2. CALCULATING RATIOS

The ratio (R) of expression in test vs reference samples is calculated from the following expression:

$$R = \frac{[S(Cy5) - B_S(Cy5)]}{[S(Cy3) - B_S(Cy3)]}$$

B_S is approximated by B_L or S_{nc} based on the characterization in **Subheading 3.2.6.1.** (also *see* **Fig. 4A** and **Note 20**).

3.2.6.3. IDENTIFYING POTENTIALLY UNCERTAIN RATIOS MEASUREMENTS

Variable ratio measurements are generated when one or both of the signals in each channel are weak. In our experience, the standard deviation (SD) of the

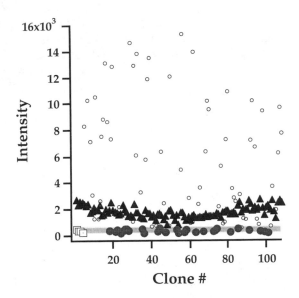

Fig. 3. Plot of the flourescent signal ($\bigcirc$) and the local-background ($\blacktriangle$) intensity for the Cy5 channel of the array in **Fig. 2** representing the means of triplicate measurements for each clone. Signals spanned a large range of intensities, but the data points with the lowest intensity ($\bullet$) fall within a constant band (shaded bar) representing the intensities ($S_{nc} + 2$ SD; $n = 12$) of the negative controls ($\square$). By contrast, B_L was consistently greater than S_{nc} and changed across the microarray in a U-shaped pattern, suggesting that much of the local background is surface specific and does not apply to the signal. B_L did not always vary as in **Fig. 3**; however even when B_L was relatively constant, it was often greater or less than S_{nc}. For example, in the Cy3 channel of the array used in **Fig. 3**, B_L was less than S_{nc}. The observation that the lowest signal intensities matched that of the negative controls suggests that the signal background (B_s) did not change across the array and that the S_{nc} can be used as an estimate of this background.

Log(R) increases dramatically when the smallest signal of the ratio pair is less than two times the SD of the negative controls [SD(S_{nc})] (**Fig. 4B**). This behavior can be used to identify the most uncertain data in cases in which variability cannot be assessed directly with replicate measurements:

1. The most uncertain ratios can be eliminated by excluding those in which the signals in both channels are <2 SD[Snc] in that channel (open symbols in **Fig. 4A**; *see* **Note 18**).
2. When only one of the signals in the ratio pair is <2 SD(S_{nc}), the ratio is flagged as potentially uncertain but is not eliminated from analysis because the corresponding response may be very interesting (predominantly expressed in one of the two mRNA samples) (open symbols in **Fig. 4C**).

3. For the data that are flagged in (2), it is often the case that R is clearly large (i.e., Log[R] >1) even though the estimate of R is variable. In such a case, when a single measurement is made and the exact value of R is uncertain, it can be useful to estimate a lower bound for R. One way to do this is by adding 2 SD(S_{nc}) to the smaller of the two signals in the ratio pair (*see* **Note 21**). This procedure results in a distribution of R_{min} values (open diamonds in **Fig. 4C**) that is less variable than the estimate of R and approximates the lower range of R values. The alternative is to use other quantitative measurements of gene expression to verify the results.

4. Notes

1. Three companies currently sell microscope slides coated with amine-reactive groups on the glass surface. CEL and TeleChem manufacture reactive aldehyde-coated slides. SurModics (Eden Prairie, MN) provides slides coated with a hydrophilic polymer containing amine-reactive groups. The advantage of this end-linked approach is that most of the arrayed DNA molecule is free to hybridize with the fluorescently labeled target DNA *(6)*. In addition, at least in the case of the CEL and TeleChem products, the aldehyde surface is extremely stable. The microarrays used in the experiments described here were printed on CEL slides and stored for >20 months at room temperature under ambient conditions, and the signals obtained were comparable with those on newly printed slides (**Fig. 2A**) (data not shown). The aldehyde-amine bond is also extremely stable to harsh treatments including boiling for 2 min in H_2O. Corning, Sigma, and TeleChem are planning to release slides coated with silane that can be easily modified to be amine reactive through additional treatment.
2. Alternatively, a bacterial clone that contains a DNA insert or the lysate of a phage clone that contains a DNA insert can be added directly to the PCR mixture for amplification.
3. Unpurified PCR products can be evaporated, reconstituted in 0.1% (v/v) SDS in H_2O, and arrayed directly onto slides. However, solid printing pins must be used (e.g., BioRobotics, Woburn, MA) rather than microspotting "bubble pins" (e.g., TeleChem), because debris in the PCR reaction can clog the nonsolid pins.
4. A few purified PCR products should be randomly selected and run on an agarose gel to view their quality and quantity (the final yield of most will be 2–5 µg).
5. This step is currently important. As the consistency of coated microscope slide production improves, this step may become unnecessary.
6. Control DNAs such as plant (e.g., *Arabidopsis*) clones *(8)* or human total genomic DNA *(9,10)* or a set of human housekeeping clones *(11)* should be included in each quadrant of the array. Negative control spots (DNA sequences that do not bind to the test or reference probes) should also be included. The advantage of using *Arabidopsis* clones is that they can serve as either positive or negative controls in human expression monitoring experiments, depending on whether the corresponding mRNA samples (synthesized in vitro) are spiked into the probe synthesis reaction (also *see* **Subheading 3.2.5.**).

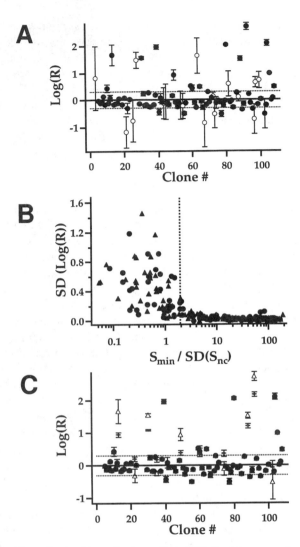

Fig. 4. Plots of Log-Ratio for each clone (Log[R]). In this example, the background (B_s) in each channel was approximated by the mean of the 12 negative control signals (S_{nc}). R was calculated as the ratio of the means of the 3 signals measured for each clone (*see* **Note 19**)

$$R = \frac{[S(Cy5)-S_{nc}(Cy5)]}{[S(Cy3)-S_{nc}(Cy3)]}$$

(A) The Log-Ratio for each clone (Log(R)). In addition to calculating the average ratio for each triplicate, ratios for the individual spots were determined and the standard deviation of the Log-Ratios {SD[Log(R)]} for each triplicate are plotted as error bars (*see* **Note 20**). Many ratios are close to 1[Log(R) = 0] and most fall within a range representing a twofold increase or decrease in expression (dashed lines). Several

7. When isolating RNA from low cell content tissues (e.g., human aorta), the $LiCl_4$ precipitation method should be used instead of TRIzol. Briefly, homogenize 1 g of tissue in 7 mL of tissue solubilization solution (5 M guanidine thiocyanate; 50 mM Tris-HCl; 10 mM EDTA, pH 7.5; 8% [v/v] 2-mercaptoethanol) using a Polytron homogenizer. Add 7 vol of 4 M LiCl and precipitate overnight at 4°C. Centrifuge at 11,000g at 4°C for 90 min. Discard the supernatant. Resuspend the pellets in 10 mL of 2 M LiCl and 4 M urea. Mix well. Spin at 11,000g at 4°C for 1 h. Resuspend the pellets in 10 mL of RNase-free RNA solubilization buffer (10 mM Tris-HCl, pH 7.5; 1 mM EDTA, 0.1% [w/v] SDS). Solubilize by freezing and allowing to thaw while vortexing. Vortex for 20 s every 10 min for 45 min. Extract two times with equal volumes of phenol:chloroform, pH 8.0. Precipitate with 0.1 vol of RNase-free 3 M sodium acetate, pH 5.2, and 2.5 vol of 100% (v/v) ethanol. Centrifuge at 13,000g for 30 min at 4°C, discard the supernatant, and wash the pellet with 70% (v/v) ethanol (in RNase-free water). Dry the pellet at 37°C for 5 min (avoid excessive drying), and dissolve the pellet in RNase-free water. Quantitate the RNA concentration by measuring the absorbance at 260 nm. The A_{260}/A_{280} ratio should be 1.9:2.0.
8. These in vitro synthesized mRNAs are used as controls for gene expression calibration. Clones should be as divergent from the mRNA source as possible. Plant (e.g., *Arabidopsis*) clones work well for human and yeast experiments. Clones should have a polyA$^+$ tract of 20–40 nucleotides to allow for priming by oligo-dT in the reverse transcription reaction (also *see* **Note 11**).
9. A Stratagene RNA transcription kit is often used. The in vitro transcription reaction is highly efficient. A large RNA pellet should be visible on centrifugation. Transcript integrity can be assessed with formaldehyde gels or by alkaline agarose electrophoresis of cDNAs generated from the mRNAs by oligo-dT priming and reverse transcription (*see* **Subheading 3.2.3.**).

---

increase more than 10-fold [Log(R) > 1]. Some ratio measurements are variable whereas others are highly reproducible. The open symbols represent the data that are eliminated by the criteria illustrated in (B), and they are generally the most variable measurements. **(B)** Plot of SD[Log(R)] vs the normalized amplitude of the smallest signal of the ratio pair (S_{min}). S_{min} was normalized by SD(S_{nc}) for that channel. SD[Log(R)] increases dramatically when $S_{min} < 2$ SD(S_{nc}) (dashed line). SD[Log(R)] provides an indication of the fractional variation of R. The most uncertain ratios can be eliminated by excluding those in which the signals in both channels are <2 SD(S_{nc}) in that channel (open symbols in **(A)**). **(C)** Plot of the data remaining after this filtering procedure. When only one of the signals in the ratio pair is <2 SD(S_{nc}), the ratio is flagged as potentially uncertain but is not eliminated from analysis because the corresponding response may be very interesting (predominantly expressed in one of the two mRNA samples). Data that are flagged by the 2 SD(S_{nc}) criteria are identified by triangles and include some of the highest ratios. Diamonds represents ratios calculated by adding 2 SD(S_{nc}) to the smaller of the two signals in the ratio pair (Log[R_{min}] or Log[R_{max}] ± SD (*see* **Note 21**).

10. This scale of synthesis generates enough probe for four hybridization reactions each covering an area of 22 × 22 mm. When fewer hybridization reactions are needed or less mRNA is available, this reaction can be scaled down.

11. In this cocktail, three different *Arabidopsis* control mRNAs from in vitro transcription are pooled in a ratio of 100:10:1, so that final molar ratios of 1:1000, 1:10,000 and 1:100,000 are achieved in the reverse transcription reaction (assuming an average mRNA length of 1.0 kb).

12. Cover slips must be free of oils, dust, and other contaminants. Lower the cover slip onto the microarray from left to right. Once it touches the liquid on the array, release it quickly so that the sample pushes out air bubbles as it forms a monolayer against the microarray surface. Small air bubbles trapped under the cover slip exit after several minutes at 62°C.

13. The microarray should be transferred quickly from the cassette to the washing buffer. Leaving the microarray at room temperature will lead to elevated background fluorescence. Either a microarray wash station (TeleChem) or staining dishes (Wheaton) can be used for this washing step. Note that permanent markers should not be used for labeling because the ink debris can deposit onto the array and cause elevated background fluorescence.

14. A number of microarray scanners are available *(12)*, including instruments from General Scanning, Molecular Dynamics (Sunnyvale, CA), Genetic MicroSystems (Woburn, MA) Virtek Vision (Woburn, MA), and Axon (Foster City, CA). Because the power of the lasers and the photomultiplier voltages used in different scanners are different, the laser and photomultiplier settings should be adjusted according to the manufacturer's recommendations.

15. The laser power and photomultiplier settings for limiting saturation to 5% in the brightest spots can be set using the microarray with the brightest signals. In cases in which the dynamic range of a scanner is not wide enough to linearly detect the signals for all the spots on the same array, an additional scan at a higher photomultiplier setting should also be performed to detect the weaker signals. The 1:1 ratio calibration can be obtained by using the set of control *Arabidopsis* clone spots (*see* **Notes 6** and **11**) or a slide containing hybridization of both Cy3- and Cy5-labeled reference probes. Alternatively, if an array contains many cDNA spots, and it can be assumed that the majority of the genes corresponding to these spots do not change their expression in the test and reference samples, the center of the distribution of the intensity ratios of the unchanged genes can be adjusted to 1:1.

16. Some scanners scan the red and green channels simultaneously (e.g., GenePix 4000 produced by Axon) In this case, a single composite image containing both red and green signals is saved.

17. During data extraction, a grid of target areas is aligned with each cDNA spot in the microarray image. Because distances between spots can vary, most commercially available array analysis software packages (e.g., ImaGene 2.031 from BioDiscovery; GenePix 1.0 from Axon; and MCID 4.0 from Imaging Research, St. Catharines, Ontario, Canada) require human intervention to ensure that grids

are properly aligned. Within each target area, a target circle is superimposed on the signal spot and used to determine the signal intensity (S), and an area outside of the circle is used to measure the local background (B_L). Because cDNA spots are not perfectly round, there can be some misalignment between the shape of the spot and the target circle. When this misalignment is significant, some local background will be included in the signal area and may need to be accounted for if the local- and signal-background are not equivalent (*see* **Subheading 3.2.6.**). For the example in **Fig. 2**, spots were elliptical but represented a constant fraction of the target circle area ($f_S = 0.58 \pm 0.02$; mean $\pm$ SD; $n = 10$). Therefore the signal (S) was determined from the expression $S = I_T - B_L(1 - f_S)$, in which I_T is the mean intensity in the target circle and the second term represents the contribution of local background to I_T. Image-processing techniques also can be used to isolate noncircular signal areas (http://nhgri.nih.gov/DIR/LCG/lSK/HTML/img_analysis.html) and will probably become more widely available as commercial array analysis software is improved.

18. The 2 SD filtering procedure only addresses the uncertainty in estimating ratio values based on the variability in negative control intensities and the signal amplitudes for one pair of reference and test samples. Variability in expression ratios from sample to sample may need to be determined separately and could be caused by a variety of experimental and biologic factors. Usually, if the reference and test samples originate from the same tissue or cells, the distribution of ratios observed when one of the samples is labeled with both Cy3 and Cy5 dye should give a good estimate of the confidence in detecting changes in expression. Otherwise the distribution of ratios for a set of positive control clones (*8*) or housekeeping genes (*13*) can be used.

19. The ratio of two normally distributed variables is not normally distributed and the ratio of the mean of two sets of measurements is not equal to the mean of their ratios. Therefore, when multiple measurements are available, it is more accurate to take the ratio of the means of the two signals rather than the mean of their ratios.

20. When signals are small, the background-subtracted signal (S-S_{nc}) can vary around O such that R varies between positive and negative values. For such cases, R is clearly uncertain but Log(R) cannot be determined when $R <$ O. Therefore, we set $(S-S_{nc}) = |(S - S_{nc})|$ so that SD[Log(R)] can be roughly approximated. This procedure is likely to underestimate the variability of R and overestimates the value of $(S - S_{nc})$/SD(S_{nc}) in **Fig. 4B**. However, $|(S - S_{nc})|$/SD(S_{nc}) was always <2 when $(S - S_{nc}) <$ O; thus, these examples are correctly identified as small signals in **Fig. 4B**.

21. R_{min} was calculated by adding 2 SD(S_{nc}) to the lowest intensity background-subtracted signal (S_{Low}) of the ratio pair. This is based on the assumptions that uncertainty in the estimate of R arises mainly from variability in S_{Low} and that when S_{Low} is small, SD(S_{Low}) can be approximated by SD(S_{nc}). If the mean value of S_{Low} is μ_{Low}, then the ratio of mean signals is $R^* = (\mu_{High}/\mu_{Low})$, which can be approximated as $R^* \cong (S_{High}/\mu_{Low})$. Single measurements of S_{Low} may be greater

or less than m_{min} so that $R = S_{High}/S_{Low}$ is greater or less than R^*. However, if S_{Low} is normally distributed, then the quantity $S_{Low} + 2\ SD(S_{Low})$ will be $\geq \mu_{min}$ for 97.8% of S_{Low} measurements. Therefore, $R_{min} = \{S_{High}/[S_{Low} + 2\ SD(S_{Low})]\} \leq R^*$ provides a lower estimate of R^* (i.e., R^* is $\geq R_{min}$ with ~98% confidence). If $R^* = (\mu_{Low}/\mu_{High})$ (i.e., $R^* \ll 1$), then the above procedure will provide an upper limit for R^* $\{R_{max} = [S_{Low} + 2\ SD(S_{Low})]/S_{High}\}$.

References

1. Alwine, J. C., Kemp, D. J., and Stark, G. R. (1977) Method for detection of specific RNAs in agarose gels by transfer to diazobenzyloxymethyl-paper and hybridization with DNA probes. *Proc. Natl. Acad. Sci USA* **74,** 5350–5354

2. Zinn, K., DiMaio, D., and Maniatis, T. (1983) Identification of two distinct regulatory regions adjacent to the human β-interferon gene. *Cell* **34,** 865–879.

3. Liang, P. and Pardee, A. B. (1992) Differential display of eukaryotic message RNA by means of the polymerase chain reaction. *Science* **257,** 967–971.

4. Hubank, M. and Schatz, D. G. (1994) Identifying differences in mRNA expression by representational difference analysis of cDNA. *Nucleic Acids Res.* **22,** 5640–5648.

5. Velculescu, V. E., Zhang, L., Vogelstein, B., and Kinzler, K. W. (1995) Serial analysis of gene expression. *Science* **270,** 484–487.

6. Schena, M., Shalon, D., Davis, R. W., and Brown, P. O. (1995) Quantitative monitoring of gene expression patterns with a complementary DNA microarray. *Science* **270,** 467–470.

7. Fodor, S. P. A., Rava, R. P., Huang, X. C., Pease, A. C., Holmes, C. P., and Adams, C. L. (1993) Multiplexed biochemical assays with biological chip. *Nature* **364,** 555–556.

8. Schena, M., Shalon, D., Heller, R., Chai, A., Brown, P. O., and R. W. Davis. (1996) Parallel Human Genome Analysis: Microarray-Based Expression Monitoring of 1,000 Genes. *Proc. Natl. Acad. Sci USA* **93,** 10,614–10,619.

9. DeRisi, J. L., Iyer, V., and Brown, P. O. (1996) Exploring the metabolic and genetic control gene expression on a genomic scale. *Science* 278, 680–686.

10. Lashkari, D. A., DeRisi, J. L., McCusker, J. H., Namath, A. F., Gentile, C., Hwang, S. Y., Brown, P. O., and Davis, R. W. (1997) Yeast microarrays for genome wide parallel genetic and gene expression analysis. *Natl. Acad. Sci. USA* **94,** 13,057–13,062.

11. DeRisi, J., Penland, L., Brown, P. O., Bittner, M., Meltzer, P. S., Ray, M., Chen, Y., Su, Y. A., and Trent, J. M. (1996) Use of cDNA microarray to analyze gene expression patterns in human cancer. *Nature Genet.* **14,** 457–460.

12. Bowtell, D. D. L. (1999) Options available—from start to finish—for obtaining expression data by microarray. *Nature Genet.* **21,** 25–32.

13. Chen, Y., Dougherly, E. R., and Bittner, M. L. (1997) Ratio-based decisions and the quantitative analysis of cDNA microarray images. *J. Biomed. Opt.* **2,** 364–374.

23

Prediction of Protein Structure and Function by Using Bioinformatics

Yvonne J. K. Edwards and Amanda Cottage

1. Introduction

Proteins mediate virtually all biological processes. Understanding the mechanisms by which proteins function requires a knowledge of their three-dimensional (3D) structures. As a consequence of the genome and full-length cDNA sequencing projects, there are several orders of magnitude more protein sequences compared with experimentally determined protein structures. To bridge this information gap, there is a considerable impetus to predict accurately the structures of proteins from sequence information. Protein structure prediction using bioinformatics can involve sequence similarity searches, multiple sequence alignments, identification and characterization of domains, secondary structure prediction, solvent accessibility prediction, automatic protein-fold recognition, and constructing 3D protein structures to atomic detail (*see* **Fig. 1**). The bioinformatics techniques used in predicting protein structure depend on the outcome from the analysis outlined in **Fig. 1** and **Table 1**.

The first step in a typical protein structure prediction is to establish if a protein sequence or part of a protein sequence has any structural homologs present in the Protein Data Bank (PDB) *(1)* using sequence similarity searches. Typically, protein structures are experimentally determined and classified at the level of the domain *(1–3)* (*see* **Note 1**). Comparative molecular modeling is the most successful and accurate method for protein structure prediction (*see* **Notes 2** and **3**). Given the success of comparative modeling techniques, it is important to be able to tell if part or all of a newly determined sequence will adopt a known fold that exists in the PDB. If a protein structure prediction can

From: *Methods in Molecular Biology, vol. 175: Genomics Protocols*
Edited by: M. P. Starkey and R. Elaswarapu © Humana Press Inc., Totowa, NJ

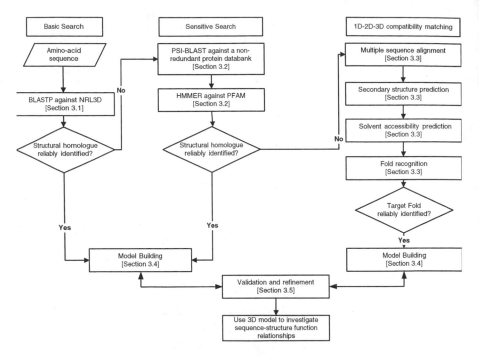

Fig. 1. Protein structure prediction flowchart highlighting the steps involved in constructing 3D structural models from protein sequences by using bioinformatics.

be carried out using well-understood and standard techniques; this should be the method of choice (*see* **Table 1** and **Fig. 1**).

In the absence of high sequence identity between sequence and structural homolog (*see* **Notes 4** and **5**), deciding what constitutes significant sequence similarity is not an easy task. This type of prediction project can be classed as "nontrivial". The most promising methods for solving this problem involve the characterizing of amino-acid sequence compatibility with the structural features of the local environments in the known tertiary structure and secondary structure of proteins. Such methods are useful in predicting common folds for proteins that share little or no sequence similarity. At low levels of sequence similarity, the structures of proteins sharing a common fold diverge to such an extent that the accuracy of models built by comparative techniques are significantly lower.

In this chapter, the protein sequence translated from the complete coding regions of the plasminogen related growth factor receptor 1 (PRGFR1) gene in the Japanese pufferfish, *Fugu rubripes* (Fugu) *(4)* is used to describe how to predict features of structure and function in protein sequences. PRGFR1 com-

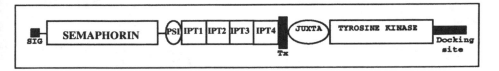

Fig. 2. Schematic representation of domains in Fugu PRGFR1. The PRGFR1 protein has an amino-terminal signal peptide (SIG). The semaphorin, domain occurs in semaphoring which are a large family of secreted and transmembrane proteins. The PSI domain contains a cysteine-rich repeat found in several different extracellular receptors. The PSI domain is located in **P**lexins, **S**emaphorins, and **I**ntegrins. The IPT domains are predicted to adopt an **Ig**-like fold also detected in **P**lexins and **T**ranscription factors. The transmembrane domain (Tx) is followed by a juxtamembrane domain (JUXTA). All PRGFR homologs have the conserved tyrosine kinase domain and a carboxyl-terminal docking site. The latter includes two conserved tyrosine residues known to be essential for intracellular signaling.

prises of 1425 amino acid residues. The PRGFR protein family has a role in embryogenesis, tissue regeneration, and neoplasia. Although some domains of this protein family have been well delineated at the sequence and structural level, many of the domains have only recently been characterized (*see* **Fig. 2**). The following text describes the methods that lead to protein domain characterization and structure prediction in the PRGFR1 orthologs (*see* **Note 6**). We predict, to atomic detail, two structures identified in the PRGFR1, i.e., the protein tyrosine kinase structure and one of the IPT domains (Immunoglobulin-like fold shared by domains in Plexins and some Transcription factors). We illustrate that the two predictions fall into the standard and nontrivial categories, respectively (*see* **Table 1**). The protein regions of PRGFR1 not considered fall into the virtually impossible category. At the time of writing, it is virtually impossible to predict their structures with confidence with the available tools. Methods are described regarding when and how to use the various protein structure prediction techniques (**Tables 1–6**). We describe some of the steps involved in validation and refinement of protein structural models (*see* **Table 7**), the expected accuracy and the weaknesses and strengths of some of the methods. The steps outlined will apply to many protein structure predictions.

2. Materials

We assume that you would like to predict structural features for a protein sequence, and do not necessarily possess all the computational resources. The time and resources you intend to invest on a protein structure prediction project

Table 1
Types of Protein Structure Prediction Projects*a*

Description of project based on the outcome of the following analysis	Standard	Nontrivial	Virtually impossible
Identification of sequence homolog	Yes	Yes	Yes/No
Identification of structural homolog	Yes	No	No
Mapped domain boundaries	Yes/No	Yes	No
Biochemical characterization	Yes/No	Yes/No	No

*a*A protein structure project can be classed as standard, nontrivial or virtually impossible, depending on the outcome of the analysis outlined. A standard project indicates that the protein fold can be predicted with a high degree of confidence. A nontrivial prediction requires much biochemical characterization such as site directed mutagenesis, circular dichroism and Fourier transform infrared to support and validate the fold recognition. Expect results, but do not expect accurate or reliable predictions from a project of the third type, deemed here as virtually impossible.

and the scientific questions to be addressed are not presumed. Therefore, the aim of this chapter is to outline the available choices so that the reader can make an informed decision about the tools used.

2.1. Internet Computing Systems for Protein Structure Prediction

Access to a computing system designed for bioinformatics analysis is required. For example, a user account on a computer system running a UNIX operating system (e.g., Solaris, Linux, or IRIX), sufficient memory, disk space, and applications (including an editor, a multiple sequence alignment program, a sequence similarity search program, and access to up-to-date biological sequence, structure, and biblographic data banks) are required. Such facilities are available to registered users of the UK Human Genome Mapping Project Resource Centre (HGMP-RC) bioinformatics facilities (*see* **Table 2**). An Internet connection and use of a Web browser such as Netscape or Internet Explorer are needed. The details of Web forms (the user interfaces to many bioinformatics tools) frequently change; so decide what is appropriate for your analysis and complete the forms accordingly. The fine details of form filling are not provided in this chapter. The URL of Web servers frequently change. Search the World Wide Web for sites hosting bioinformatics programs and servers by performing keyword searches using a Web search engine, such as Yahoo or Google. Various data banks and analysis tools are available for pro-

Table 2
URLs for Data Sets Useful
in Classifying Protein Structures, Domains, Folds, and Function[a]

Databank	Information	URL
Prodom	Sequence	http://protein.toulouse.inra.fr/prodom.html
Pfam	Sequence	http://www.sanger.ac.uk/Software/Pfam
		http://pfam.wustl.edu/
		http://pfam.wustl.edu/
		http://www.cgr.ki.se/Pfam/
SMART	Sequence	http://smart.embl-heidelberg.de
PDB	Structure	http://msd.ebi.ac.uk/
		http://www.rcsb.org/pdb/
CATH	Structure	http://www.biochem.ucl.ac.uk/bsm/cath/
SCOP	Structure	http://scop.mrc-lmb.cam.ac.uk/scop/
3Dee	Structure	http://jura.ebi.ac.uk:8080/3Dee/help/help_intro.html
FSSP	Structure	http://www.ebi.ac.uk/dali/fssp/
HSSP	Structure	http://www.sander.embl-heidelberg.de/hssp/
Prosite	Function	http://www.expasy.ch/prosite/
Prints	Function	http://www.biochem.ucl.ac.uk/dbbrowser/PRINTS/ PRINTS.html
Blocks	Function	http://www.blocks.fhcrc.org/
Rasmol	Visualization	http://www.umass.edu/microbio/rasmol/
BIDS	Bibliographic	http://www.bids.ac.uk/
PubMed	Bibliographic	http://www.ncbi.nlm.nih.gov/PubMed/

[a]A registered user of the HGMP-RC bioinformatics facilities (http://www.hgmp.mrc.ac.uk/) can access a program called PIX that identifies domains and functional features in protein sequences using many of the above bioinformatics tools.

tein database searching and predicting the secondary and tertiary structure over the internet (*see* **Tables 2–7**). With respect to building protein constructs to atomic detail, a protein modeling web server, SwissModel, is available (*see* **Table 6**).

2.2. Local Computing Systems for Protein Structure Prediction

Software such as Composer, Naomi, WhatIf, and Modeller are programs that can be downloaded and installed on local computer systems (*see* **Table 6**). These four programs are of value in protein structure modeling to atomic detail. Additional tools are required to visualize interactively and monitor the building process. Rasmol is an excellent macromolecule viewer, the correct mime-types, helper-applications, and user preferences need to be set in the

Table 3
Information Content
in Nonredundant Protein Sequence Data Banks[a]

Databank	Composite data banks
SPTR	SwissProt, SPTREMBL, TREMBLNEW
OWL	SwissProt, PIR, GenPept, NRL3D
NCBI's nr	SwissProt, nr-GenPept, PDB, PIR, PRF

[a]Entries with identical sequences are merged. GenPept is produced by extracting the translated coding regions in GenBank. PIR database is a protein sequence database founded by The Protein Information Resource, National Biomedical Research Foundation, Georgetown University Medical Center, US. PRF is the data bank of protein sequences created by the Protein Research Foundation, Osaka, Japan.

Table 4
URLs for Tools Used for Searching for Homologous Protein Families[a]

Software package	URL
BLAST (BLASTP)	http://www.hgmp.mrc.ac.uk/
PSI-BLAST	http://www2.ncbi.nlm.nih.gov/blast/psiblast.cgi
HMMER	http://pfam.wustl.edu/hmmsearch.shtml
	http://www.cgr.ki.se/Pfam/search.html
	http://www.sanger.ac.uk/Software/Pfam/search.shtml
SRS	http://srs.hgmp.mrc.ac.uk/
	http://srs.ebi.ac.uk/

[a]SRS is a valuable tool to retrieve sequences from respective data banks.

Table 5
URLs for Tools Used for Sensitive One-Dimensional
to Two-Dimensional and One-Dimensional
to Three-Dimensional Compatibility Matches

Software	URL
JPRED	http://circinus.ebi.ac.uk:8888/
Jalview	http://www2.ebi.ac.uk/~michele/jalview/contents.html
PHD	http://www.embl-heidelberg.de/predictprotein/predictprotein.html
GenThreader	http://insulin.brunel.ac.uk
3D-PSSM	http://www.bmm.icnet.uk
Server	

Table 6
URLs for Tools Used for Comparative Modelling of Protein Structures

Software	URL
Academic	
COMPOSER^	http://www-cryst.bioc.cam.ac.uk/
DRAGON*	http://mathbio.nimr.mrc.ac.uk/specinfo.html#dragon
Modeller*	http://guitar.rockefeller.edu/modeller/
Naomi*	http://www.psynix.co.uk/products/naomi/
WhatIf^	http://www.sander.embl-heidelberg.de/whatif/
SwissModel^	http://www.expasy.ch/swissmod/SWISSMODEL.html
Commercial	
Modeller*	http://www.msi.com/
Homology^	http://www.msi.com/
QUANTA	http://www.msi.com/
SYBYL	http://www.tripos.com/
COMPOSER^	http://www.tripos.com/

* = restraint-based molecular modeling techniques; ^ = rigid body fragment assembly techniques; DRAGON = Distance RegularisAtion for Geometry OptimisatioN.

Table 7
A List of URLs for Tools Useful
for Assessing Modeled Protein Structures

Software	URL
Biotech Validation Suite	http://biotech.embl-heidelberg.de:8400/
	http://biotech.ebi.ac.uk:8400/
Joy	http://www-cryst.bioc.cam.ac.uk/cgi-bin/joy.cgi
What If	http://swift.embl-heidelberg.de/servers2/

browser's preferences in order to view structures derived from the PDB (*see* **Table 2**). Rasmol enables manipulation of molecular viewing and representations. Rasmol was not designed to manipulate atomic stereochemistry. There are commercial packages for molecular modeling developed by companies such as Molecular Simulations Inc. (MSI) and Tripos. The commercial packages and WhatIf have very well-defined and -developed menu-driver interfaces for various modules for molecular modeling.

Having built a molecule, you may want to investigate complex molecular recognition processes like protein interaction networks and ligand-receptor binding with the aim of designing drugs, redesigning proteins, or understanding the etiology of disease states. If this is the case, control of visualizing and building accurately to atomic detail are important and as a result a custom-made molecular modeling computing system is required in order to provide modules to perform macromolecular editing with high-resolution, interactive viewing capability and energy minimization facilities. The commercial software molecular packages and the WhatIf suite provide such modules. Such programs need to be installed and maintained on local computer systems, which include a Silicon Graphics workstation on a network, plus a local copy of the PDB *(1)*. A local computer system of this type is an advantage to an intensive protein structure modeler. If you are affiliated with a nonprofit academic institution many computational resources will be available free or at lower prices compared to those available to commercial organizations.

3. Methods

Bioinformatics is a rapidly evolving science and new and improved versions of the software and data banks are released very frequently. As a result, this chapter is not a manual, it is a guide. It is important to have an understanding of the following: data bank search algorithms, information content of the data banks, retrieving sequences from the data banks, sequence alignments, a comprehensive introduction to protein structure, and basic Unix commands. We recommend reading some well-written, concise, and introductory reviews on this topic *(5–10)*. In this section, the methods to predict the structure and function of PRGFR1 by using bioinformatics are described.

3.1. Search for a Structural Homolog Using Basic Search Methods

A sequence similarity search tool should be used to perform a protein sequence search against the protein sequences derived from the 3D protein structures. If a structural homolog has been reliably identified for a significant fraction of the query sequence (*see* **Note 4**), a model can be built based on standard homology modeling methods.

BLASTP is used to detect sequence similarities in a data bank of protein sequences whose structures have been experimentally determined (*see* **Notes 7 and 8**. The results of the BLASTP *(11)* search against the protein sequences with their structures solved are shown in **Fig. 3**. Residues 1089–1352 in the PRGFR1 sequence match the protein tyrosine kinase structure of the human insulin receptor (PDB accession code: 1irk). As a result, this region in PRGFR1 should not be investigated using secondary structure predictions and automatic protein fold recognition methods (*see* **Subheadings 3.2.** and **3.3.**)

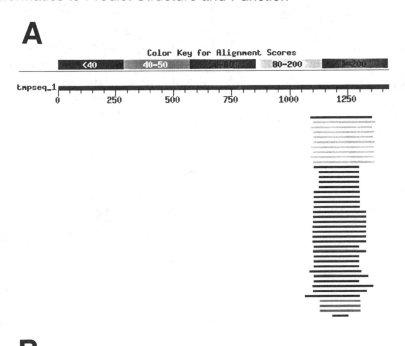

A

Color Key for Alignment Scores

| <40 | 40-50 | | 80-200 | -200 |

tmpseq_1

0   250   500   750   1000   1250

B

pdb|1IRK| Insulin Receptor (Tyrosine Kinase Domain) Mutant With Cys 981
             Replaced By Ser And Tyr 984 Replaced By Phe (C981s,
             Y984f)
             Length = 306

Score = 206 bits (518), Expect = 4e-53
Identities = 110/276 (39%), Positives = 171/276 (61%), Gaps = 18/276 (6%)

```
Query: 1089 IAREQLLLHLNQVIGRGHFGCVFHGTLLE--PDGQKQHCAVKSLNRITDLEEVSQFLKEG 1146
            ++RE++ L   + +G+G FG V+ G    +         AVK++N    L E +FL E
Sbjct: 14   VSREKITLL--RELGQGSFGMVYEGNARDIIKGEAETRVAVKTVNESASLRERIEFLNEA 71

Query: 1147 IIMKDFSHPNVLSLLGICLPPEGSP-LMVLPYMKHGDLRNFIRD---ESHN------PTV 1196
            +MK F+  +V+ LLG+     +G P L+V+  M HGDL++++R   E+ N       PT+
Sbjct: 72   SVMKGFTCHHVVRLLGVV--SKGQPTLVVMELMAHGDLKSYLRSLRPEAENNPGRPPPTL 129

Query: 1197 KDLMGFGLQVARGMEYLASKKFVHRDLAARNCMLDESYTVKVADFGLARDVYDKEYYSVH 1256
            ++++      ++A GM YL +KKFVHRDLAARNCM+   +TVK+ DFG+ RD+Y+ +YY
Sbjct: 130  QEMIQMAAEIADGMAYLNAKKFVHRDLAARNCMVAHDFTVKIGDFGMTRDIYETDYYRKG 189

Query: 1257 NKSGVKLPVKWMALESLQTHKFTSKSDVWSFGVLLWELMTRGAPPYSDVNSFDITVFLLQ 1316
            K    LPV+WMA ESL+    FT+ SD+WSFGV+LWE+ +        PY  +++  + F++
Sbjct: 190  GKG--LLFVRWMAPESLKDGVFTTSSDMWSFGVVLWEITSLAEQPYQGLSNEQVLKFVMD 247

Query: 1317 GRRLLQPEFCPDALYTVMIECWHPNPERRPSFSELV 1352
            G  L QP+ CP+ +  +M  CW  NP+ RP+F E+V
Sbjct: 248  GGYLDQPDNCPERVTDLMRMCWQFNPKMRPTFLEIV 283
```

Fig. 3. Results of a BLASTP search using the Fugu PRGFR1 protein sequence to query the data bank of protein sequences obtained from the PDB. (**A**) Schematic representation of the data bank matches aligned to the query. The score of each alignment is indicated by the different gray scales. Several proteins match the tyrosine kinase domain. (**B**) Pairwise sequence alignment of the tyrosine kinase structure of the insulin receptor and PRGFR1. The percentage sequence identity for this alignment is 39% spanning amino acid residues 1089–1352 of PRGFR1.

The significance of this search is to determine which region(s) of the sequence can be built to atomic resolution using standard homology modeling methods. For the regions of the protein sequence for which a structural homolog has not been reliably identified (*see* **Note 4**), further nontrivial probing of the data banks are required to establish possible links between other protein sequences and structural homolog(s) or analog(s) (*see* **Notes 5** and **6**, respectively).

3.2. Search for a Structural Homolog Using Sensitive Search Methods

3.2.1. Search Against the Databank of Pfam Profiles

Profile Hidden Markov Models (HMMs), built from the Pfam alignments, can be useful for automatically recognizing that a new protein contains an existing protein domain, even if the sequence similarity is weak *(12)*. Searching Pfam HMMs using the search package HMMER is intuitive to study multidomain proteins. Query sequences can be used to scan the Pfam HMMs. The query sequence should be in fasta format. Select whether you wish to scan Pfam-A or Pfam-B families (*see* **Note 9**) and the maximum cutoff value for the *E*-value (*see* **Note 8**). The type, the number, and the location of the Pfam domains identified by the search will be reported plus some annotation about the domain. If available, Pfam will provide references to homologous domains in protein structures deposited and classified in the PDB, CATH, and SCOP data banks. Our search identified three IPT domains in the PRGFR1 amino acid sequence (*see* **Table 8**). We provide further evidence for a fourth IPT domain between the PSI domain and the transmembrane region in the PRGFR family of sequences (*see* **Figs. 4–7**).

No structural homolog for either the semaphorin domain or the plexin repeat was identified from the HMMER search. Several homologous structures were identified for the protein tyrosine kinase domain. We proceed not with the plexin repeats or the semaphorin domains (*see* **Fig. 2**) as this has proved too involved for the purpose of this chapter, but with the IPT domains. At the time this chapter was written, the structure predictions obtained using the available data banks and tools (the secondary structures of folds predicted by fold recognition and secondary structure prediction) did not produce consistent results. The IPT domains were shown to share detectable but weak sequence similarity with the immunoglobulin-like fold in the cyclodextrin glucanotransferase protein structure (PDB accession code: 1cyg). By using similar techniques summarized in *(13)* we predict the fold for the IPT domain to illustrate how confidence can be gained in fold predictions by using different and complementary tools.

Table 8
Four Different Domain Types are Identified in Fugu PRGFR1
as a Result of a Standard Pfam-A Search[a]

Pfam domain name	Query start	Query end	Pfam start	Pfam end	Bits	E-value
Semaphorin	51	141	1	99	46.0	6.2e-13
Semaphorin	246	390	194	350	100.0	1.7e-27
Plexin repeat	528	571	1	67	39.3	3.2e-09
IPT	572	667	1	103	48.7	4.7e-12
IPT	669	752	1	103	76.8	1.6e-20
IPT	755	849	1	103	33.4	1.8e-07
Tyrosine kinase	1096	1353	1	274	289.3	1.7e-84

[a]A maximum E-value of 10 was used. For each domain identified in PRGFR1, the start and end points of the Pfam domain and query sequence are given, together with the statistical score and E-value of the sequence alignment of the representative pfam domain and PFRGR1. A semaphorin, a plexin-repeat (also known as the PSI domain), three IPT domains, and a tyrosine kinase were identified in PRGF1.

If a set of homologous sequences is identified but no homologous structure(s), the project categorically falls into the nontrivial category (*see* **Table 1**). If no homologous sequence or structure has been established, the project will be virtually impossible to complete with any degree of confidence. The residue numberings for the start and end for the three IPT domains in the PRGFR have been established from the HMMER search. The sequences defining the relevant IPT domains need to be extracted into separate files. It is a good practice to give your files meaningful names, as these sequences will form the basis of further analysis in the next stage.

3.2.2. Further Characterization of the IPT Superfamily

3.2.2.1. PSI-BLASTIPT2 Domain

Many members of the IPT domain superfamily were identified using the search program PSI-BLAST, the PRGFR1 IPT2 as input, and a nonredundant data bank of protein sequences to perform a search. **Figures 5** and **6** provide details of the parameters used in this search and some results. Some of the homologous IPT sequences were identified with copy numbers from 2–4 in homologous PRGFR sequences. **Note 10** provides a definition of a domain superfamily.

An experiment needs to devised to provide the evidence that PRGFR1 has four IPT domains. Two protein multiple sequence alignments need to be pro-

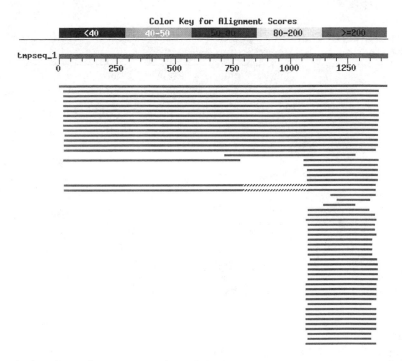

Fig. 4. A schematic representation of the BLASTP search using the amino acid sequence of Fugu PRGFR1 to query a nonredundant data bank of protein sequences. The score of each alignment is indicated by the different gray scales. Twelve unique proteins match the full-length amino acid sequence of the query (**Table 8**) and many more match the tyrosine kinase domain. The juxtamembrane domain is not present in mouse RON receptor sequences, and this large gap in the alignment is depicted by a striped line.

duced. The first alignment comprises the full-length PRGFR homologs and the second comprises the IPT-superfamily.

3.2.2.2. ESTABLISH THE MEMBERS OF THE PRGFR FAMILY

BLASTP was used to determine the homologous proteins to *Fugu* PRGFR1. The protein sequence of PRGFR1 is used to search a nonredundant protein sequence data bank (**Table 4**). Twelve unique proteins match the full length amino acid sequence (*see* **Table 9** and **Fig. 4**). PSI-BLAST was used to search a nonredundant protein sequence data bank, but in this case no new full-length homologs were established with further iterations. From a multiple sequence alignment, the percentage pairwise sequence identities range between 30 and 58% and common regions with highly conserved residues can

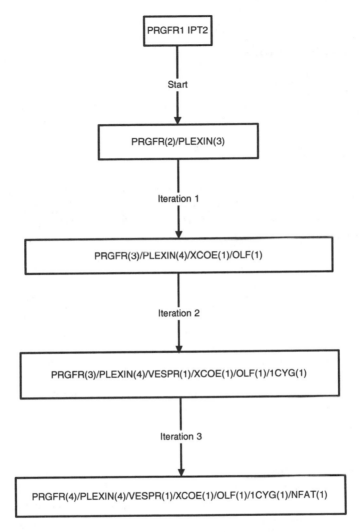

Fig. 5. PSI-BLAST results obtained from querying SPTR with the Fugu PRGFR1 IPT2 domain sequence. The IPT domain shares weak sequence similarity to the OLFl/ Ebf-like transcription factors (OLF), the nuclear factor of activated T-cell (NFAT) family of transcription factors, the transcription factor XCOE2 (XCOE), the viral encoded semaphorin receptor VESPR, and cyclodextrin glucanotransferase (the PDB accession code is 1cyg). The number of IPT domains identified in these proteins following consecutive iterations is given in parentheses. The E-value was set to 10 for all the PSI-BLAST iterations. Alignments were visually inspected, and matches to repeat sequences were excluded from succeeding iterations. The outcome of a PSI-BLAST search can be affected by the selected query sequence. Depending on which PRGFR1 IPT domain is used as the query, three or four IPT domains can be identified in the PRGFR homologs.

A

```
emb|CAA58863.1| (X84044) tyrosine kinase [Gallus gallus]
           Length = 1382


Score =  107 bits (266), Expect = 2e-23
Identities = 34/84 (40%), Positives = 54/84 (63%)

Query: 1    DPVVSEIFPTFGPKSGNTMLTIRGAFLDTGNKREVTVGKAACKIQSLSATMLTCKTPPHA 60
            +P+++ I PT+GPKSG T+LTI G +L++G  R + VG+   C ++S  S + + C TP
Sbjct: 656  NPIITSISPTYGPKSGGTLLTIAGKYLNSGKSRRIFVGEKPCSLKSTSESSVECYTPAQR 715

Query: 61   VPSKQPVRLTVDSVARDAPVLYTY 84
            +P + VR+ +D  RDA  +TY
Sbjct: 716  IPQEYRVRVGIDGAIRDAKGYFTY 739


Score = 42.4 bits (98), Expect = 8e-04
Identities = 18/65 (27%), Positives = 30/65 (45%), Gaps = 9/65 (13%)

Query: 1    DPVVSEIFPTFGPKSGNTMLTIRGAFLDTGNKREVTV--------GKAACKIQSLSATML 52
            DPVV +I P    SG + +T +G L++   + +           AC +S S+ ++
Sbjct: 742  DPVVLKIHPAKSFLSGGSTITAQGINLNSVCFPRMVITVPKLGMNFSVACSHRS-SSEII 800

Query: 53   TCKTP 57
            C TP
Sbjct: 801  CCTTP 805


Score = 41.6 bits (96), Expect = 0.001
Identities = 21/93 (22%), Positives = 32/93 (33%), Gaps = 11/93 (11%)

Query: 2    PVVSEIFPTFGPKSGNTMLTIRGAFLDTGN-------KREVTVGKAAC--KIQSLSATML 52
            P V EI P+  P  G T LT+ G          V +G   C +  +S +   L
Sbjct: 563  PRVYEILPSSAPLEGGTKLTLCGWDFGFSKNNRFELRNTVVHIGGQICALEAKSSNKNKL 622

Query: 53   TCKTPPHAVPS-KQPVRLTVDSVARDAPVLYTY 84
            C P    S      ++V  +       ++Y
Sbjct: 623  ECTAPAAKNASFNISSSVSVGHG-KTLFNTFSY 654


Score = 29.1 bits (64), Expect = 7.4
Identities = 15/62 (24%), Positives = 26/62 (41%), Gaps = 7/62 (11%)

Query: 1    DPVVSEIF-PTFGPKSGNTMLTIRGAFLDT----GNKREVTVGKAACKIQSLSATMLTCK 55
            +PV        P    +S  +L I+G  +D+     G  +V G  +C+   L +  + C
Sbjct: 839  NPVFKHFEKPVLISRSNPNVLEIKGNHIDSEAVKGEVLKV--GNKSCENLLLQSETILCT 896

Query: 56   TP 57
            P
Sbjct: 897  VP 898
```

Fig. 6. Four consecutive IPT domains identified in two homologous PRGFR sequences (chicken and mouse MET). The second PSI-BLAST iteration identified a match with 1cyg. The PDB identifier followed by the accession code (typically comprising four characters) indicates that this sequence has a structure deposited in the PDB. 1cyg contains 680 amino acids. IPT2 makes a match with the third domain of 1cyg, which is referred to 1cgy03 in the CATH data bank. 1cgy03 comprises residues 492–575 and adopts an Ig-like fold.

be established. For example, common regions including conserved cysteines, prolines, and glycines in the IPT2 domain are observed in the PRGFR family *(4,13)*. The methods in which a multiple sequence alignment can be obtained are described in the next section. The sequences for the fourth IPT domain are present in the alignment and we need to compare the fourth IPT domain sequences with the other three IPT domains.

B

```
ref|NP_032617.1|| met proto-oncogene >gi|125485|sp|P16056|MET_MOUSE HEPATOCYTE GROWTH
           FACTOR RECEPTOR PRECURSOR (MET PROTO-ONCOGENE TYROSINE
           KINASE) (HGF-SF RECEPTOR) >gi|91020|pir||S01254
           hepatocyte growth factor receptor precursor - mouse
           >gi|53059|emb|CAA68680.1| (Y00671) met proto-oncogene
           protein precursor (AA -24 to 1355) [Mus musculus]
           Length = 1379

 Score =  106 bits (263), Expect = 3e-23
 Identities = 30/84 (35%), Positives = 54/84 (63%), Gaps = 1/84 (1%)

Query: 1     DPVVSEIFPTFGPKSGNTMLTIRGAFLDTGNKREVTVGKAACKIQSLSATMLTCKTPPHA 60
             DPV++ I P +GP++G T+LT+ G +L++GN R +++G   C ++S+S ++L C TP
Sbjct: 655   DPVITSISPRYGPQAGGTLLTLTGKYLNSGNSRHISIGGKTCTLKSVSDSILECYTPAQT 714

Query: 61    VPSKQPVRLTVDSVARDAPVLYTY 84
                 + PV+L +D  R+   ++Y
Sbjct: 715   TSDEFPVKLKIDLANRETS-SFSY 737


 Score = 47.1 bits (110), Expect = 3e-05
 Identities = 21/79 (26%), Positives = 36/79 (44%), Gaps = 10/79 (12%)

Query: 1     DPVVSEIFPTFGPKSGNTMLTIRGAFLDTGNKREVTVG--------KAACKIQSLSATML 52
             DPVV NI PT    SG + +T G L++ + ++ +        AC+ +S S ++
Sbjct: 740   DPVVYEIHPTKSFISGGSTITGIGKTLNSVSLPKLVIDVHEVGVNYTVACQHRSNSE-II 798

Query: 53    TCKTPPHAVPS-KQPVRLT 70
               C TP      + P++
Sbjct: 799   CCTTPSLKQLGLQLPLKTK 817


 Score = 43.2 bits (100), Expect = 4e-04
 Identities = 22/93 (23%), Positives = 35/93 (36%), Gaps = 11/93 (11%)

Query: 2     PVVSEIFPTFGPKSGNTMLTIRG-------AFLDTGNKREVTVGKAACKIQS--SATML 52
             P V ++FPT  P  G T+LTI G          K +V +G  +C+ +    L
Sbjct: 562   PAVYKVFPTSAPLEGGTVLTICGWDFGFRKNNKFDLRKTKVLLGNESCTLTLSESTTNTL 621

Query: 53    TCKTPPHAVPSKQPVRLTV-DSVARDAPVLYTY 84
               C  P       V + + +S      ++Y
Sbjct: 622   KCTVGPAMS-EHFNVSVIISNSRETTQYSAFSY 653


 Score = 34.2 bits (77), Expect = 0.22
 Identities = 12/62 (19%), Positives = 22/62 (35%), Gaps = 7/62 (11%)

Query: 1     DPVVSEIF-PTFGPKSGNTMLTIRGAFLDT----GNKREVTVGKAACKIQSLSATMLTCK 55
             +PV       P    ++ I+G +D      G   +V G  +C+     + C
Sbjct: 837   NPVFEPFEKPVMISMGNENVVEIKGNNIDPEAVKGEVLKV--GNQSCESLHWHSGAVLCT 894

Query: 56    TP 57
             P
Sbjct: 895   VP 896
```

C

```
pdb|1CYG| Cyclodextrin Glucanotransferase (E.C.2.4.1.19) (Cgtase)
    Length = 680

    Score = 41.6 bits (96), Expect = 0.001
    Identities = 19/76 (25%), Positives = 26/76 (34%), Gaps = 4/76 (5%)

Query: 5     SEIFPTFGPKSG--NTMLTIRGAFLDTGNKREVTVGKAACKIQSLSATMLTCKTPPHAVP 62
             + I GP G    +TI G   T N   V GA+   S S +        P + P
Sbjct: 494   TPIIGHVGPMMGQVGHQVTIDGEGFGT-NTGTVKFGTTAANVVSWSNNQIV-VAVPNVSP 551

Query: 63    SKQPVRLTVDSVARDA 78
             K + +   S A
Sbjct: 552   GKYNITVQSSSGQTSA 567
```

Fig. 6B,C

```
      1                                                          60
{prgfr14} dPl...fqdP kltskdnksi velkG..... drmdreamkc qvltvsnh.. .sC....esl
{gg_met4} nPvfkhfekP vlisrsnpnv leikG..... nhidseavkg evlkvGnk.. .sC....enl
{prgfr13} dPiissiq.P srsfvsGgct vaahG..lfl qsglqpqmvl ttgqdaevfh vsC.....vy
{gg_met3} dPvvlkih.P aksflsGgst iTaqG..inl nsvcfprmvi tvpklGmnfs vaC.....sh
{prgfr12} dPvvseif.P tfgpksGntm lTirG.af.l dtgnkre... ..vtvGk... aaCki..qsl
{gg_met2} nPiitsis.P tygpksGgtl lTiaG.ky.l nsgksrr... ..ifvGe... kpCsl..kst
{prgfr11} tPvvtkvf.P tsgpirGstt vTmcGrnfgf dktesfkasl vtvevag... vpCklsrqdy
{gg_met1} lPrvyeil.P ssapleGgtk lTlcGwdfgf sknnrfelrn tvvhiGg... qiCal..eak
Consensus -P-------P ------G--- -T--G----- ---------- -----G---- --C-------

      61                                             109
{prgfr14} tlvgntleCT vPtelqttts kelqvewrq. aDsirhlgkv tlaqeqdyt
{gg_met4} llqsetilCT vPsdllksns .elniewkqe vlstv.igkv lirqdqnft
{prgfr13} genrtsiqCT tPslaklalq pPvvtkvafv lDgymteqwd li~~~~~~~
{gg_met3} rssseiicCT tPslkafnlq pPfvtkvffi fDgvsslyfd fd~~~~~~~
{prgfr12} sa..tmltCk tPpha..... vPskqpvrlt vDsvardapv lytyh~~~~
{gg_met2} se..ssveCy tPaqr..... iPqeyrvrvg iDgairdakg yftyr~~~~
{prgfr11} asrwteiqCs .Pmfsgn..f tPsghtvkvt sghkiatieg f~~~~~~~~
{gg_met1} ssnknkleCT aPa.aknasf niss.svsv. .ghgktlfnt f~~~~~~~~
Consensus --------CT -P-------- -P-------- -D-------- ---------
```

Fig. 7. A protein multiple sequence alignment of the IPT domains found in the chicken MET and Fugu PRGFR1 was obtained using Pileup. Pileup creates a multiple sequence alignment from the related sequences using progressive, pairwise alignments. The gap creation penalty was set to 4, the gap extension penalty was set to 1, and the Blosum 30 substitution matrix was used. A program called Pretty was used to produce the display of multiple sequence alignments and calculate a consensus sequence. The alignment shows highly conserved structurally important amino acid residues such as cysteines, prolines, and glycines. Hydrophobic and hydrophilic characteristics can be observed in equivalent positions. The alignment provides some evidence for the existence of the fourth IPT domain in the PRGFR family.

3.2.2.3. MULTIPLE SEQUENCE ALIGNMENT OF IPT DOMAINS

At the HGMP-RC Unix-based computing system, a multiple sequence alignment was performed using the Pileup program. The version of Pileup used is part of the Genetics Computer Group's Seqlab environment which in turn is part of the Wisconsin package (14). In the IPT alignment, the parameters such as the gap penalty, gap extension and substitution matrix were altered in a stepwise manner to optimize the number of equivalents (i.e., the length of the alignment is decreased, and the number of conserved positions increase). We then define invariant and highly conserved residues and positions of the alignment that comprise hydrophobic and polar residues. From the IPT alignment, the patterns of sequence divergence can be quantified (see **Fig. 7**).

The sequences of the fourth IPT domain has diverged so much it is likely that the function of the fourth domain has diverged considerably compared to the other three IPT domains. The four IPT domains are likely to share a similar

Table 9
The Names and Data Bank Accession Codes
for 12 Unique Homologous PRGFR Sequences[a]

	Organism	Protein	Accession Number
1	Mouse	RON	OWL:I48751
2	Human	RON	SPTR:Q04912
3	Chicken	SEA	SPTR:Q08757
4	Frog	SEA	OWL:JC4860
5	Fugu	PRGFR2	SPTR: Q9YGM5
6	Fugu	PRGFR3	SPTR: Q9YGN0
7	Rat	MET	SPTR:P97579
8	Mouse	MET	SPTR:Q62190
9	Human	MET	SPTR:P08581
10	Chicken	MET	SPTR:Q90975
11	Frog	MET	OWL:JC5148
12	Fugu	PRGFR1	SPTR:Q9YGM7

[a]PRGFRs can be grouped into two subfamilies. The MET subfamily includes PRGFR1. The SEA/RON family includes PRGFR2 and PRGFR3. MET was first identified as the activated oncogene in an N-methyl-*N'*-nitro-*N*-nitrosoguanidine (MNNG)-treated human osteosarcoma and *Xeroderma pigmentosa* cell lines. RON (**R**ecepteur d'**O**rigine **N**antaise) was isolated from a human foreskin keratinocyte cDNA library. It is a 1400 amino acid receptor tyrosine kinase protein and is homologous to the 1408 amino acid MET protooncogene. SEA was originally identified in the genome of the S 13 avian erythroblastosis retrovirus. This virus causes Sarcomas, Erythroblastoses, and Anemias in young chicks.

protein fold. Characterizing the properties of domains where the sequence identities are this low is a nontrivial exercise. This is an interesting example of *in silico* characterization of domains with low sequence identity. If the results of this step is wrong, analysis or conclusions based on the newly characterized domains are likely to be erroneous.

3.3. Search for a Structural Analog Using 1D–2D–3D Compatibility Matches

3.3.1. Prediction of Secondary Structure and Solvent Accessibility

There are many good secondary structure and solvent accessibility prediction packages available, for example, Jpred2 *(15)*. Jpred2 is an Internet web server that takes either a protein sequence or a multiple alignment of protein sequences, and predicts secondary structure and solvent accessibility. It works by combining 11 high-quality prediction methods to form consensus predictions. The server runs in two modes, single sequence and multiple sequence. If your input is an alignment, the alignment returned as part of the Jpred2 results will be modified so that it does not contain gaps in the first sequence. The first sequence should, therefore, always be your main sequence of interest. For single sequences submitted, Jpred2 uses PSI-BLAST to perform an automatic protein sequence similarity search, retrieves the subject protein sequences, and generates an alignment. The resulting alignments are automatically modified to have no gaps in the query sequence (*see* **Fig. 8**). Once an alignment has been generated and modified, the algorithms predict the secondary structure. Jpred2 will predict a consensus secondary structure and solvent accessibility profile. The immunoglobulin-like domain of lcyg is composed of nine beta strands. **Figure 8** shows the secondary strucutre predictions from alignments of PRGFR1 IPT2. Saver strands have been predicted with similar solvent accessibility profile to lcyg(03).

3.3.2. Automatic Protein Fold Recognition Methods

The protein fold recognition program Threader (*16*) is used to score protein sequence compatibility against known protein folds. Threader can be run from the UK HGMP-RC bioinformatics applications menu. Sequence threading against a structural data bank of 1902 known protein folds were performed for the 48 IPT sequences (the four IPT domains in each the 12 homologous PRGFR sequences). Threadings were computed in terms of (1) pairwise interaction energies, (2) solvation potential energies, and (3) their weighted sum, in order to evaluate the fit of each IPT sequence to a particular fold conformation, and represented as Z-scores (= (Energy − Mean)/Standard Deviation). Provided there is greater than 50% sequence and structure matching, the Z-scores were sorted for input into a program called SumThreader (*17*) in order to summarize the outcome of the searches. For each of the three Z-scores, the average value for each fold was calculated from the 48 values determined for the individual IPT domain sequence threadings. The average position of each fold in the sorted list of 1902 folds in the 48 searches were calculated. The IPT domains were matched favorably with protein structures (protein structure codes plus domain annotation are given and the average Z-score are given in parentheses): 1cgt03 (3.08), 1cyg03 (2.65), 1cdg03 (2.57), and 1vcaA1 (1.51). The first three domains are cyclodextrin glycosyltransferase from *Bacillus circulars*, *Bacillus stearothermophilus*, and *Bacillus circulars*, *respectively,* and the fourth is the N-terminal domain of the human vascular cell adhesion molecule-1. The top-ranked folds showing the average ranked positions are given in parentheses): 1cgt03 (44.79), 1cyg03 (67.96), 1vcaA1 (84.56), and 1cdg03 (85.92). These

```
OrigSeq    :DPVVSEIFPTFGPKSGNTMLTIRGAFLDTGNKREVTVGKAACKIQSLSATMLTCKTPPHAVPSKQPVRLTVDSVARDAPVLYTYH
AAF22147   :DPVLLSLNPQWGPQAGGTQLTIHGQYLQTGGNISVFVGDQPCPIQEPVPEAIICHTMPQTEPGEAVVLIVFGHVERKLLTPFRYT
MET_HUMAN  :DPVITSISPKYGPMAGGTLLTLTGNYLNSGNSRHISIGGKTCTLKSVSNSILECYTPAQTISTEFAVKLKIDLANRETS.IFSYR
PLX4_HUMAN :TPTFDQVSPSRGPASGGTRLTISGSSLDAGSRVTVTVRDSECQFVRRDAKAIVCISPLTLGPSQAPITLAIDRANISSPLIYTYT
P70206     :TPTFYRVSPSRGPLSGGTWIGIEGSHLNAGSDVAVSIGGRPCSFSWRNSREIRCLTPPHT.PGSAPIVININRAQLSNPVKYNYT
P70207     :NPSVLSLSPIRGPESGGTMVTITGHYLGAGSSVAVYLGNQTCEFYGRSMNEIVCVSPPSNGLGPVPVSVSVDRARVDSSLQFEYI
Q62555     :EPVLTSIKPDFGPRAGGTYLTLEGQSLSVGTSRAVLVNGTQCRLE.QV..QILCVTPPGAGTARVPLHLQIGGAEVPGSWTFHYK
O96681     :DPKILDFNPKFGPTSGGTEIHITGKHLNAGSRIQASINDHPCKILSTDSSQAICRTSASPGIIEGRLKMSFDNGPREFNYNFKYV
CAB56222   :DPKVHSIFPARGPRAGGTRLTLNGSKLLTGEDIRVVVGDQPCHLLPEQSEQLRCETSPRPTPATLPVAVWFGATERRLQGQFKYT
P79950     :EPAITSVEPNFGPLAGGTRLTLKGQNLTAGETQRVFIDGAECKTINGS.EVLCCVSPKSLSLGPLNVFALLDGAQIPSPEQFQYK
Q22222     :IP.IIEMTPSSSSLKGGQKMLVVGGYYRKGHEYKISFGRGMMPAVLIHAGVLSCVIPPSAKPEVVQIRVFCNGQAISTASEFTYE
Q91823     :LPSFNRVTPSRGPLSGGTWISIEGNYLNAGSDVSVAIGGRPCMFSWRTAKEIRCKTPQPS.TGKAEIQILINRATMNNSVHYNYT
O96682     :NVLLTGLYPTIGPRSGGTQLSLIGKFLNIGSTMRAFLDEYECHIDVTQSSQVSCTTSETQPEPIRSLHLVIDGANRTLE...CQI
Q9YGM5     :EPSITDIQPDYGPAFGGTTVTLTGRHLDSGFQRDVFFGEKQCRILSVSSSSIVCLPAVAEDVGSVPVKVLIDSFPVTATKMFFYK
Q9W650     :NPIITSIRPSYGPRAGRTLLTIKGHYLDSGKDRKVYIGKEMCNIKSVSSAAIVCLTPGQGTTGTYLVALKIDNANRESSTRFTYM
Q90975     :NPIITSISPTYGPKSGGTLLTIAGKYLNSGKSRRIFVGEKPCSLKSTSESSVECYTPAQRIPQEYRVRVGIDGAIRDAKGYFTYR
Q08757     :EPHISTLHPSFGPGQGGTLMSLYGTHLSAGSSWRVTINGSECLLDGQP.GEIRCTAPAATSLGAAPVALWIDGEEFLAPLPFEYR
RON_HUMAN  :EPVLIAVQPLFGPRAGGTCLTLEGQSLSVGTSRAVLVNGTECLLA.RV..QLLCATPPGATVASVPLSLQVGGAQVPGSWTFQYR
O45657     :RTSIFSAYPLYGPISGGTRITLYGQNLSSGSQTSVTVGGMPCPIERVNSTVLTCLTPSTRIGKSARVVVHVDHSQTQLDQPFEYR
Q9Y4D7     :LPLVHSLEPTMGPKAGGTRITIHGNDLHVGSELQVLVNDTPCTELMRTDTSIACTMPEGALPAPVPVCVRFERRGCVHGLTFWYM
O15031     :QPKPLSVEPQQGPQAGGTTLTIHGTHLDTGEDVRVTLNGVPCKVT..KGAQLQCVTGPQATRGQMLLEVSYGGSPVPNPIFFTYR
consv      :25-4-251-117612-371718--216-2-132163622-28-1------261--34-1------1-8-61531--2-1---1171
           :1---------11---------21---------31---------41---------51---------61---------71---------81---

OrigSeq    :DPVVSEIFPTFGPKSGNTMLTIRGAFLDTGNKREVTVGKAACKIQSLSATMLTCKTPPHAVPSKQPVRLTVDSVARDAPVLYTYH

dsc        :---EEEEE---------EEEEEEEEE-----EEEEEE----EEEE----EEEEE---------EEEEEEEE---------EEEEE
jalign     :-------------------EEEEEE---------EEEEE------EE-----EEEEE---------EEEEEE-----------
jfreq      :-----EEE---------EEEEEEEE------EEEEEE----EEE-----EEEEE---------EEEEEE--------EEEEE-
jhmm       :-----EEE---------EEEEEE----------EEEEEE----EE-----EEEEE---------EEEEEE------------
jnet       :---EEE---------EEEEEEEE---------EEEEEE----EEE----EEEEEE---------EEEEEEE---------EEEEE-
jpssm      :-----EEE---------EEEEEEE---------EEEEEE---------EEEEEEE---------EEEEEE---------EEEE--
mul        :---EEEE---------EEEE----------EEEE-----EE------EEEEE---------EEEEEEE----------EE-
nnssp      :---EEE---------EEEEEEEE---------EEEEEE----EEE----EEEEEE---------EEEEEE---------EEEEE
phd        :--EEEEE---------EEEEEE---------EEEEEE----EEEEE----EEEEE---------EEEEEE---------EEEEE
pred       :---------------EEEEE---------EEEEE---------EEEE---------EEEEE----------
zpred      :EEEEEEEE---------EEEEEEEEE-----EEEEE----EEE-----EEEEE---------EEEEEEE---------EEE

Jpred      :---EEE---------EEEEEEE---------EEEEEE----EEE----EEEEE---------EEEEEEE---------EEEE-

PHDHtm     :-----------------------------------------------------------------------------------
PHDacc     :---BB-BU--UB-------BB-B-BB-----BBBBB----B-B-BU-B-BBBBBB--------BBBBBBB-UB-B-B-BUB-U-
Jnet_25    :-B-B--B-B-BBB--BBBBBBBBB-B--B------B-BBB----B-B--------BBBB-BB-------BBB-B-B-B---B-B-B
Jnet_5     :-----------------B-B-BBB-B---------B-B-B---------B-B----------B-B-B-B----------B-B-
Jnet_0     :-----------------------B-B--------------B-----------------------------------------

PHD Rel    :97697753687877767179996231226871599974985666745875587743888887621699985076534641334549
Pred Rel   :00886608999999999769997887787997689998997766677776556709999999986556655677799976000
Jnet Rel   :9975466004565468659997425898734999758864364337617999726899997137899966888883478871

Key:
consv      - Conservation number (+) = 0; (-) = 10
phd        - PHD prediction
dsc        - DSC prediction
pred       - PREDATOR prediction
nnssp      - NNSSP prediciton
zpred      - Zpred prediction
mul        - Mulpred prediction
jnet       - Jnet prediction
jalign     - Jnet alignment prediction
jhmm       - Jnet hmm profile prediction
jpssm      - Jnet PSIBLAST pssm profile prediction
jfreq      - Jnet PSIBLAST frequency profile prediction
Jpred      - Consensus prediction over all methods

PHDacc     - Solvent Accessibility

PHD Rel   - PHD Reliability
PRED Rel  - Predator Reliability
NNSSP Rel - NNSSP Reliability
PHDHtm    - PHD transmembrane prediction
MCoil     - MultiCoil prediction (+ Dimer and trimer predictions)
Lupas     - Lupas Coil prediction (21,14,and 28 window sizes)

Note on coiled coil predictions - = < 50% probability
                        c = >50% <90% probability
                        C = >90% probability
```

Fig. 8. Consensus secondary structure prediction from Jpred2 using Fugu PRGFR1 IPT2 domain as the query.

four domains share a common fold. They are mainly all beta stranded proteins with a beta sandwich consisting of nine beta strands.

Similar results are obtained from GenThreader, PHD and the 3D-PSSM servers (*see* **Table 5**) with the input sequence of the IPT2 domain. Use these servers to predict the protein folds from sequence information. However, do not expect to enter a 1500 amino acid residue sequence through and expect to receive meaningful predictions. Submitting small-sized (i.e., less than 350 amino acids residues) and well-characterized sequence domains typically produce results that are more meaningful. Avoid submitting domains that make a significant match with sequences of known structure, sections of coiled coil, or known transmembrane regions.

3.4. Modeling Protein Structures to Atomic Detail

Automated procedures have been developed to facilitate the construction of a protein model based on the assembly of rigid fragments from existing known structures (*see* **Tables 6** and **10–12**). The methods generally encompass the following stages: determining the structurally conserved regions (SCRs) of the selected homologous protein structures, aligning the sequence of the unknown structure against the SCRs, and constructing the main chain for the SCRs of the unknown; adding structurally variable regions (SVRs) are determined by searching a data bank of fragments of crystal structures and selecting the fragment that is predicted to be most compatible with the amino acid sequence. The construction of side chains is achieved by using side-chain rotamer libraries and rules relating the conformations of amino acid side chains at equivalent positions in the homologous proteins. **Note 3** provides a short description of other methods.

3.4.1. Automatic Comparative Modeling Using the SwissModel Server

SwissModel is a commonly used automated comparative protein modeling server that employs a rigid body fragment assembly program (*18*). This server has many advantages as it hides the technical and tedious aspects of modeling procedure. The modeling server is fast, free, and available and performs some What If checks (*19*). The results of the analysis are sent to the user via E-mail. However, fully automated sequence alignment algorithms often misplace insertions and deletions when the overall sequence identity falls below 30%. Additionally, you have limited control over what features can be engineered in and out of the protein model.

SwissModel was used in the First Approach Mode. The following details were provided to the form: an E-mail address, a name, a request title, and the complete sequence of PRGFR1. The BLASTP P(N) limit for template

Table 10
A Summary of How the Protein Modeling Server SwissModel Works

Program	Database	Function
BLASTP2	ExNRL3D	Searches for target sequence with sequences of known structure
SIM	—	Searches for template groups and shows global alignment
		Selects template structures with pairwise sequence identity above 25% and projected model size larger than 20 amino acids
		Detects domains that can be modeled for target sequence
—	—	Generates ProModII input files
ProModII	ExPDB	Generates models with ProModII
Gromos96	—	Minimizes energy of all models

Table 11
Defined SCRs in the *Fugu* PRGFR1 IPT2 Domain[a]

SCR	1CYG(03)	IPT2	SCR length
SCR1	494–505	1–12	12
SCR2	510–518	19–27	9
SCR3	522–545	32–55	24
SCR4	552–559	65–72	8
SCR5	569–575	79–85	7
Total number of framework residues in IPT2 model			60

[a]The SCRs are based on the atomic coordinates of the crystal structure of the Ig-like domain of cyclodextrin glucanotransferase. The five defined SCRs form the framework for the model of the PRGFR1 IPT2 domain.

selection was set to 0.0001 (*see* **Note 8**). SwissModel was used in the normal mode and returns the final model coordinates file in PDB format and a log file tracing all the actions taken by the server. A WhatCheck report of the final model was requested. The WhatCheck report of protein analysis is performed by the WhatIf program. Other parameters were set to the default values.

The kinase model contains two domains (*see* **Figs. 9–11**). The domains have been described and classified in the CATH and SCOP data banks. The N-terminal domain comprises a two-layer sandwich. The beta-sheet is fairly flat and the architecture is described in terms of secondary structural layers *(2,3)*. The N-terminal domain comprises a two-layer alpha+beta sandwich,

Table 12
Modeling of the Four SVRs in Fugu PRGFR1 IPT2 Domain[a]

SVRs	SVR start and end position	IPT2 SVR length	C_{SCR_i}—N_{SCR_i} (Å)	Loop type (9,23)	SVR source	Flex residues	Deviation (Å)	RMS deviation tail/no tails
SVR1	13–18	6	10.1	BB β-hairpin	1rsy (196)	3,3	0.39	0.52/N
SVR2	28–32	4	6.1	BB β-arch	1vba (3:102)	3,3	0.43	1.27/N
SVR3	54–64	9	14.6	BB β-hairpin	1kit (367)	4,4	0.42	1.87/N
SVR4	73–78	6	14.2	BB β-arch	1uae (63)	4,4	0.63	0.61/N
Total residues in SVR		25						

[a]For each SVR, the comprising amino acid residues and distance between the main-chain C-atom of the preflex (the ith SCR) and the main-chain N-atom of the first residue in the postflex (the $i + l$th SCR), C_{SCR_i}—N_{SCR_i}, are described. All SVRs are located in the solvent-accessible loops, i.e., regions not defined as regular repeating secondary structure in the analogous Ig-like domain of cyclodextrin glucanotransferase by DSSP (27). The residue numbers of the first amino acid residue of the selected fragment are specified in parentheses in the SVR source column. The numbers of amino acid residues in the pre- and postflex regions used to screen the protein database for suitable fragments to interconnect the ith SCR and the $i + l$th SCR and the RMS deviation of the selected flex region with equivalent residues in the respective pair of SCRs are given. BB, a loop enclosed by two B-strands.

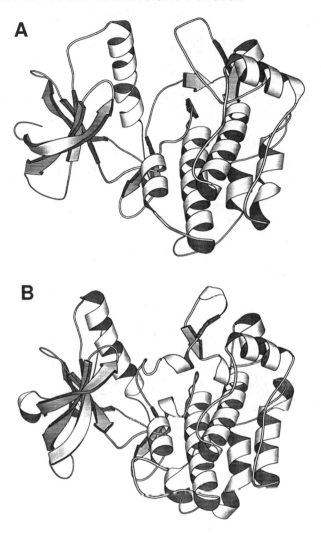

Fig. 9. Protein structures of tyrosine kinase. (**A**) 3D model of the Fugu PRGFR1 tyrosine kinase produced by SwissModel. This model is based on the atomic coordinates of five homologous tyrosine kinase structures. The PDB accession codes are 1irk, 1ir3, 1fgi, 1agw, and 1fgk. The PRGFR1 tryosine kinase model contains 273 amino acids (i.e., residues 1091–1363 of PRGFR1). The model consists of two domains. The C-terminal domain is mostly alpha helical. The secondary structure of the model is calculated by DSSP *(27)* from the model coordinates. The diagram was created by Molscript *(28)*. (**B**) The experimentally determined crystal structure of human insulin receptor tyrosine kinase (1irk) is in the same orientation as the model. The model and the template structure were superimposed in Insight (MSI) and are shown in the same orientation. Most of the differences between the two molecules lie in the crevice in between the two domains of the protein structure.

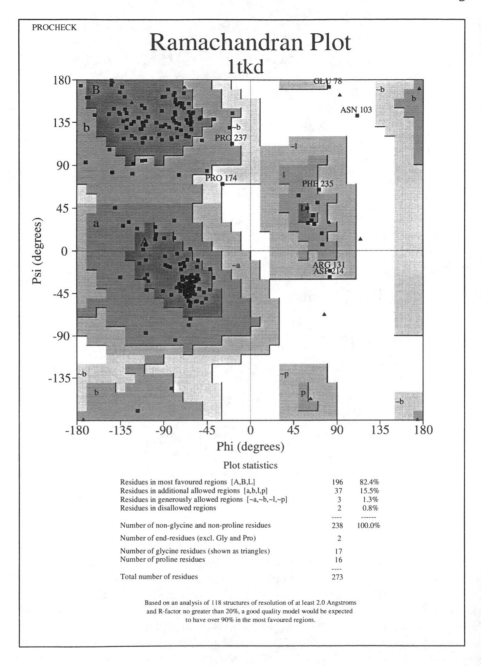

Fig. 10. A Ramachandran plot of the Fugu PRGFR1 tyrosine kinase model. This plot is created by Procheck based at the Biotech validation site (**Table 7**).

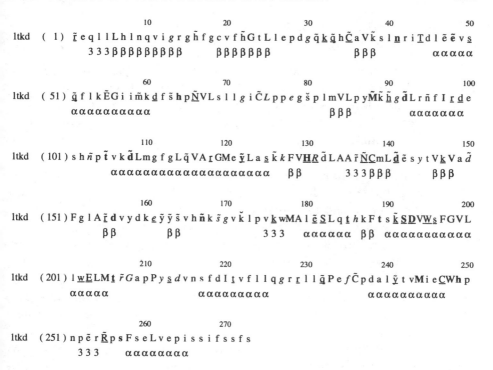

Fig. 11. A Joy output highlights the structural aspects of the model of the PRGFR1 tyrosine kinase. The key to the Joy feature formatting is as follows: solvent inaccessible (uppercase), solvent accessible (lowercase); alpha helix (α); beta strand (β); 3–10 helix (3); hydrogen bond to main-chain amide (bold); hydrogen bond to main-chain carbonyl (underlined); hydrogen bond to side chain (tilde); *cis*-peptide (breve); disulfide bond (cedilla); and positive phi (italics).

in which one layer is a beta sheet (with five strands) and the second layer is a long alpha helix. The C-terminal domain is mostly alpha-helical described as a nonbundle fold. The nonbundle architecture is a general architecture that groups together helical proteins which cannot be classified as bundles *(2,3)*.

The secondary structure and solvent accessibility calculated from the homology model will be about 70–90% accurate on a residue per residue level if the sequence similarity between the model and the template is significant (*see* **Note 4**). Run the program Joy to define the secondary structure and calculate the solvent accessibility as well as other structural features using the coordinates of the 3D model as input (*see* **Fig. 11**). **Table 7** provides the details of where this analysis can be performed.

3.4.2. Interactive Comparative Modeling
Using MSI's Homology Package

Based on sensitive sequence searches and automatic protein fold recognition methods, an association with the IPT sequences with an experimentally determined structure has been established. We build a 3D model of the IPT2 domain in the pufferfish PRGFR1 based on the atomic coordinates of the crystal structure of the immunoglobulin-like domain in cyclodextrin glucanotransferase.

All the following computations were performed on a Silicon Graphics workstation that operates under IRIX. Three-dimensional properties of protein structures were visualized and examined on the Silicon Graphics machines using the molecular modeling and visualization software package Insight II (MSI). The coordinates of protein structures were obtained from the PDB (*1*). The rigid-body fragment assembly method implemented in the commercial software package Homology was used to construct an atomic 3D model for the PRGFR1 IPT2 domain. Four stages were used in the modeling procedure: (1) the construction of a 3D framework from the consideration of known structures, (2) selection of suitable fragments from a data bank of fragments to interconnect consecutive fragments of the framework, (3) building side-chain coordinates, and (4) refinement of the model using manual modeling with interactive computer graphic techniques and energy refinement to improve covalent geometry and minimize bad contacts.

The sequence of the IPT2 domain was aligned with the third domain of cyclodextrin glucanotransferase (1cyg03). This alignment was initially extracted from the threading alignment and was modified by eye to optimize the equivalences and minimize the number of gaps in the sequence alignment. The percentage sequence identity between 1cyg03 and Fugu PRGFR1 IPT2 domain is 22.6%. The topological equivalences, identities, and conservative amino acid exchanges between the sequence of the template structure and the sequence of the IPT2 domain were optimized and nongap regions were essentially defined as the structurally conserved regions (SCRs), which formed the framework of the homology model (*see* **Table 11**). The insertions and deletions in the alignment were mainly positioned in the loops of the known structure and were designated as the structurally variable regions (SVRs). The framework of SCRs used to build the model of the IPT2 domain of PRGFR1 contains five peptide fragments, which comprise a total of 60 residues and is described in (**Table 11**). Fragments of the backbone from the template structure were least-squared fitted to the average Cα positions of the immunoglobulin-like domain in cyclodextrin glucanotransferase framework in order to construct the core of the model.

Peptide fragments of a predefined length from known protein structures from the PDB were selected and used in the modeling the SVRs of the model. A precalculated Cα distance matrix for all known proteins is used to search for regions of proteins that best fit the Cα distance matrix for a predefined number of residues flanking the SCRs that have the same number of flanking and intervening residues. **Table 12** describes the modeling of four SVRs for the IPT2 domain. The RMS (root mean squared) deviation for Cα atoms between the IPT2 model and flanking, or preflex and postflex peptide fragments of the selected data bank proteins is shown (*see* **Table 12**).

The SVRs for the IPT2 domain in PRGFR1 comprise 25 amino acids from the total of 85. The SVRs comprise less than 30% of the total model constructed. This is a significant proportion of the structure and will inevitably introduce a higher degree of uncertainty in the 3D model. The loops that comprise SVRs are all typical of loop-length distribution in protein structures (*see* **Table 12**). The side-chain atoms were placed automatically for both the SCRs and SVRs using information from the template structure and general rules for residue exchanges. The model was refined by using energy minimization. As a general rule of thumb, use energy minimization refinements and molecular dynamics simulations very sparingly in this type of modeling. In this example, six hundred steps of steepest-descent minimization were performed using the program Discover (MSI) at the splice sites (i.e., where the SCRs and SVRs join) and all the other side-chains. After refinement, the covalent geometry of regions joining SCRs and SVRs and bad contacts were significantly improved as assessed by the program Procheck (*20*).

3.5. Validation of Protein Structure Models

Previously defined SCRs and SVRs can be altered to remove unfavorable geometric or stereochemical features. Alignments may need to be altered manually, especially if the sequence similarity between the sequence of the unknown structure and the sequence of the structural template is low (*see* **Note 4**). If the selection of the template structures is wrong, the model based on it will be wrong. If your alignment is incorrect, local features of the model will be incorrect. If the protein is well characterized biochemically use this information to validate the model. For example, information that certain residues are known to coordinate metal ion binding can be of value. Use such information to ensure that the relevant amino acid side chains are in close proximity in 3D space and in the correct orientation for metal coordination. If the alignment is wrong, the residues for coordinating residues could end up on opposite sides of the molecule. Similarly, the knowledge that two cysteine residues involved in disulfide bridge formation can provide useful indicator that a protein structure has

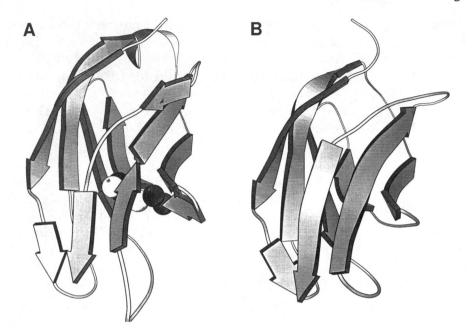

Fig. 12. Protein structures of Ig-like folds. **(A)** 3D model of the IPT2 domain in Fugu PRGFR1. The atomic coordinates are created by using Homology and Discover (MSI). The model is based on 1cyg(03) as the template structure. The model consists of 85 amino acid residues and adopts a β-sandwich architecture. These structures have two small β-sheets packed together in a layered arrangement. The side chains of two cysteines (residues 42 and 54) are shown. These are close in 3D space and are likely to form a disulfide bridge. **(B)** The 3D structure of the template 1cyg(03) in the same orientation as the model. *See* legend to **Fig. 9**.

been modeled correctly (**Fig. 12A**). Such information can be used to check the geometry of formed disulfide bridges in your model. It is important to visually inspect various features of models built, e.g., well-defined secondary structure and main-chain conformation (*see* **Figs. 10** and **13**), strands and helices, the globular nature of protein folds, and 3D clusters of interacting side chains. Tools to help point to regions of the model that might need correcting are cited in **Table 7**. To determine the secondary structure and solvent accessibility of a protein structure (either predicted or experimentally solved), submit the protein coordinates to the Protein Analysis server on the WhatIf Website (*see* **Table 7**).

3.5.1. Checks Performed by the Biotech Protein Structure Validation Suite

A model of a protein structure built to atomic details requires validation of the stereochemistry and assessment of the biological viability (**19,20**). Checks

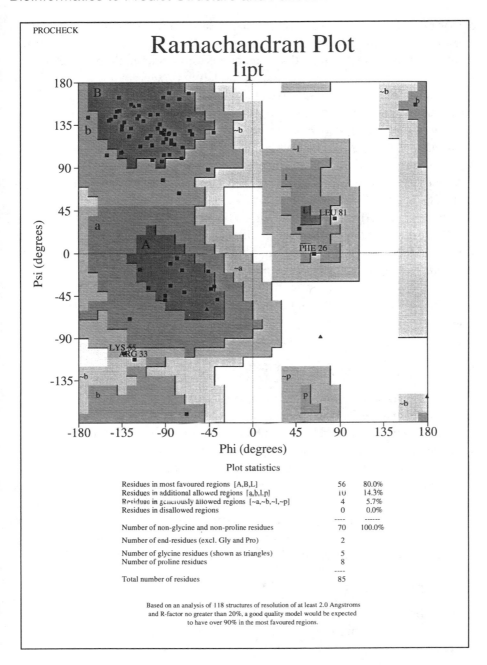

Fig. 13. Ramachandran plot of the Fugu PRGFR1 IPT2 created by Procheck. *See* legend to **Fig. 10**.

performed by Procheck on a given protein structure are as follows: covalent geometry, planarity, dihedral angles, chirality nonbonded interactions, main-chain hydrogen bonds, disulfide bonds, stereochemical parameters, and residue-by-residue analysis. Molecular modeling process of atomic detail typically constitutes part of an iterative cycle, having obtained initial models. Properties such as bad stereochemistry, bad van der Waals contacts, and parts of the model not supporting known experimental evidence should be engineered out of the model. Interactive molecular modeling tools are required for this (*see* **Subheadings 2. and 3.4.2.**). In correcting undesirable features of models, some parameters that can be altered in remodeling process are the alignment, definition of SCRs, and the selection of SVRs.

WhatIf can perform the following checks: bond angle deviations, bond lengths, buried unsatisfied hydrogen bond donors and acceptors, bumps (bad van der Waals contacts), peptide bond flip, amino acid handedness, his-gln-asn side-chain conformation, atom nomenclature, side-chain planarity, proline puckering, directional atomic contact analysis, directional atomic contact analysis, amino acid side-chain rotamer analysis, symmetry, torsion angle evaluation, isolated water clusters, and atomic occupancy. The server provides detailed descriptions of all these features.

3.5.2. Checks Performed by Joy

Joy is a program to annotate protein sequence alignments with 3D structural features (*see* **Table 7**). It was developed to display 3D structural information in a sequence alignment and help understand the conservation of amino acids in their specific local environments *(21)*. For instance, it has been recognized that a side chain hydrogen bonded to a main-chain amide plays an important role in stabilizing the 3D structure and is generally well conserved during evolution. Such a residue is shown in a boldface letter in the formatted alignments. Another example is the importance of solvent-inaccessible residues, which are shown in uppercase letters. These features conserved in families of protein structures can also be monitored in model building (*see* **Figs. 11** and **14**).

3.6. Where Next?

A predicted protein structure can only be validated in its entirety by comparison it with its experimentally determined 3D structure. One way to improve the decision-making processes in a protein structure prediction project is to investigate assessments of protein structure predictions in the light of their structures being solved *(17,22–24)*. If the bioinformatics tools are used intuitively, such analysis can provide very useful indicators of function. Even though the rate of determination of protein structures is larger in comparison to

```
              10              20              30              40              50
ipt2  ( 1)  d P v v s̲ e i f p̆ t f g p k s̲ g ñ t m̃ L t I r̄ Ga f Ld̲ t g n k ī e V t Vg k a a C̰ k i q̃ s̃ L s a t
            β β β β β β    β β β              β β β β β β  3 3 3        β β β β    β β β  β β β β

              60              70              80
ipt2  (51)  m̃ L ī C̰ k t P p h a v p s k q̆ p v r L T V d̄ s v a r̲ d̲ a p v l Y ī Y̲ h̃
            β β β β              β β  β β β β        β β        β β β β
```

Fig. 14. Joy output of the Fugu PRGFR1 IPT2 model. *See* legend to **Figs. 11–13**.

10 years ago, some proteins may never have their 3D structures determined experimentally. As the bioinformatics techniques improve and data banks grow, these approaches to structure predictions may be the method of choice for studying the 3D structure and functions of globular proteins.

4. Notes

1. A domain is a polypeptide chain or part(s) of a polypeptide chain that can independently fold into a stable tertiary structure. Domains need not be formed from contiguous regions of an amino acid sequence. Typically, they have distinctive secondary structure content and a hydrophobic core. In small disulfide-rich and metal-ion binding domains the core may be provided by cysteines and metal ions, respectively. Domains can be defined in terms of a unit of function. Proteins may comprise a single domain or as many as several dozens. At the sequence level, homologous domains with common functions usually show sequence similarities. Structural domains typically comprise 35–350 amino acid residues.

2. Many proteins, particularly those sharing a common evolutionary origin, have been shown to possess similar backbone structures, that is, they share similar 3D folds. It is this property that is exploited in the approach known as comparative modeling. The aim is to base a 3D model for a protein sequence on a homologous structure (*see* **Note 5**) or analogous protein structure (*see* **Note 6**). The most reliable indicator that a pair of proteins share a common fold is provided by amino acid sequence comparisons. If the target protein has a sequence with detectable sequence similarity with the sequence of a protein of known structure (*see* **Note 4**), then a model can usually be built that is as accurate as a medium resolution X-ray or nuclear magnetic resonance (NMR) structure. A large number of structural parameters are considered when modeling a structure. To minimize subjective decisions, specially written computer algorithms have been developed to exploit our knowledge of protein structures in a systematic way and make this task more manageable.

3. A description of comparative modeling using rigid-body, fragment-based methods have been described in the main text. Other comparative modeling approaches have been described in which 3 D models are constructed by satisfaction of spa-

tial restraints using methods similar to those used in NMR protein structure determinations. The restraints are obtained from a consideration of homologous or analogous structures *(25)*. Restraint-based approaches are, perhaps, more automated than fragment assembly approaches and produce models with better stereochemistry. Fragment assembly-based methods, on the other hand, are significantly less computationally intensive than restraint-based methods. Both techniques can produce models with similar overall accuracy.

4. If a protein sequence has 30% sequence identity or higher (over a region of 70 amino acid residues or more) to another protein sequence of known structure, then the two proteins can safely be described as homologous (*see* **ref.** *[26]*) for more details). This type of relationship infers that the sequences are highly likely to perform a similar function.

5. Homologous sequences share a common evolutionary ancestor and are have arisen by gene duplication followed by gene divergence. There are no degrees of homology. Sequences are either homologous or they are not. Paralogs and orthologs are homologs. Orthologous sequences are homologous proteins that perform the same function in different species. Paralogous sequences are homologous proteins that perform differing function in the same species.

6. Analogous sequences are nonhomologous proteins that have a similar protein 3D fold or similar functional sites believed to have arisen through convergent evolution.

7. Version 2 of NCBI's BLAST (Basic Local Alignment Search Tool) program performs gapped alignments *(11)*. BLAST is the heuristic search algorithm employed by the five programs (BLASTP, BLASTX, BLASTN, TBLASTN, and TBLASTX). BLASTP compares an amino acid query sequence against a protein sequence data bank. Databank search algorithms are based on mathematical models. Two general models view alignments as sequence similarity across the full length (global alignments) and regions of similarity in parts of the sequence (local alignments). For the purpose of protein structure prediction and domain characterization and identification, performing local alignments to search data banks is more desirable.

8. The E-value is the expected value. For a given score, the E-value is the number of hits in a data bank search that we expect to *see* by chance with this score or better. The E-value takes into account the size of the data bank searched. The lower the E-value, the more significant the match is. If the E-value is 10, we expect 10 matches to be found by chance. If the statistical significance ascribed to a match is greater than the E-value, the match will not be reported. The lower the E-value, the more stringent the search, this leads to fewer chance or false positive matches being reported. The P-value is similar to an E-value, but it is the probability of a match occurring by chance with this score or better as opposed to the expected number of hits. The P-value has a maximum value of 1.0. The E-value can have the maximum value of the number sequences in the data bank searched. Version 2 of NBCI'S BLAST program quotes E-values, whereas version 1 of the same package quoted P-values. HMMER also reports E-values *(12)*.

9. Pfam is a data bank of protein multiple sequence alignments and Hidden Markov Models (HMMs) *(12)*. A HMM is a probabilistic model that is suited for providing a mathematical scoring scheme for profile analysis. The HMMs describe the propensity of amino acid exchange in common protein domains and conserved regions. The HMMER software uses the multiple sequence alignment to build an HMM profile of the family. The profiles incorporate position specific scoring information derived from the amino acid frequency observed in equivalent positions in a protein sequence alignment. Families known as Pfam-A are generated by the HMM package from well-annotated, high-quality families that comprise accurate human crafted multiple alignments. Families known as Pfam-B are generated using an automatic clustering of the rest of SWISSPROT and TrEMBL, derived from the Prodom data bank. Pfam-B families are not of consistent quality and little may be known of their function.

10. A superfamily is composed of two or more homologous families. Not all of the different proteins are detectable sequence similarity with all the members of the other families.

Acknowledgments

We thank our project supervisors Greg Elgar, Melody Clark, and Martin Bishop, the editors, Mike Starkey and Ramnath Elaswarapu, and our partners, Peter Keller and Tim Cottage, for their encouragement whilst this chapter was being written.

References

1. Keller, P. A., Henrick, K., McNeil, P., Moodie, S., and Barton, G. J. (1998) Deposition of macromolecular structures. *Acta Crystallogr.* **54,** 1105–1108.

2. Bray, J. E., Todd, A. E., Pearl, F. M., Thornton, J. M., and Orengo, C. A. (2000) The CATH Dictionary of Homologous Superfamilies (DHS): a consensus approach for identifying distant structural homologues. *Protein Eng.* **13,** 153–165.

3. Lo Conte, L., Ailey, B., Hubbard, T. J., Brenner, S. E., Murzin, A. G., and Chothia C. (2000) SCOP: a structural classification of proteins database. *Nucleic Acids Res.* **28,** 257–259.

4. Cottage, A., Clark, M., Hawker, K., Umrania, Y., Wheller, D., Bishop, M., and Elgar, G. (1999) Three receptor genes for plasminogen related growth factors in the genome of the puffer fish Fugu rubripes. *FEBS Lett.* **443,** 370–374.

5. Trends Guide to Bioinformatics. (1998) Trends Supplement. Elsevier Science.

6. Attwood, T. K. and Parry-Smith, D. J. (1999) *Introduction to Bioinformatics. Cell and Molecular Biology in Action Series.* Addison Wesley Longman, Harlow, Essex, UK.

7. Barton, G. (1996) Protein sequence alignment and database scanning, in *Protein Structure prediction: A Practical Approach* (Sternberg, M. J. E., ed.), IRL, Oxford University Press, Oxford, UK, pp. 31–63.

8. Bishop, M. J., ed. (1999) *Genetics Databases*, Academic Press, San Diego, CA.
9. Branden, C. and Tooze, J. (1998) *Introduction to Protein Structure,* 2nd ed., Garland, New York and London.
10. Sternberg, M. J. E., ed. (1996) *Protein Structure Prediction: A Practical Approach.* IRL, Oxford University Press, Oxford, UK.
11. Altschul, S. F., Madden, T. L., Schaffer, A. A., Zhang, J., Zhang, Z., Miller, W., and Lipman, D. J. (1997) Gapped BLAST and PSI-BLAST: a new generation of protein database search programs. *Nucleic Acids Res.* **25,** 3389–3402.
12. Sonnhammer, E. L., Eddy, S. R., Birney, E., Bateman, A., and Durbin, R. (1998) Pfam: multiple sequence alignments and HMM-profiles of protein domains. *Nucleic Acids Res.* **26,** 320–322.
13. Bork, P., Doerks, T., Springer, T. A., and Snel, B. (1999). Domains in plexins: links to integrins and transcription factors. *Trends Biochem Sci.* **24,** 261–263.
14. Butler, B. A. (1998) Sequence Analysis Using GCG, in *Bioformatics. A practical Guide to the Analysis of Genes and Proteins.* (Baxevanis, A. D. and Ouellette, B. F. F., eds.), John Wiley, New York, pp. 74–97.
15. Cuff, J. A., Clamp, M. E., and Barton, G. J. (1998) JPred: A consensus secondary structure prediction server. *Bioinformatics* **14,** 892–893.
16. Jones, D. T., Taylor, W. R., and Thornton, J. M. (1992) A new approach to protein fold recognition. *Nature* **358,** 86–89.
17. Edwards, Y. J. K. and Perkins, S. J. (1996) Assessment of protein fold predictions from sequence information—the predicted alpha/beta doubly wound fold of the von Willebrand factor type A domain is similar to its crystal-structure. *J. Mol. Biol.* **260,** 277–285.
18. Guex, N., Diemand, A., and Peitsch, M. C. (1999) Protein modelling for all. *Trends Biochem Sci.* **24,** 364–367.
19. Vriend, G. (1990) What If: A molecular modeling and drug design program. *J. Mol. Graph.* **8,** 52–56.
20. Laskowski, R. A., Rullmann, J. A., MacArthur, M. W., Kaptein, R., and Thornton, J. M. (1996) AQUA and PROCHECK-NMR: programs for checking the quality of protein structures solved by NMR. *J. Biomol. NMR* **8,** 477–486.
21. Mizugochi, K., Deane, C. M., Blundell, T. L., Johnson, M. S., and Overington, J. P. (1998) Joy: protein sequence-structure representation and analysis. *Bioinformatics* **14,** 617–623.
22. Benner, S. A., Cannarozzi, G., Gerloff, D., Turcotte, D., and Chelvanayagam, M. (1997) Bona fide predictions of protein structure using transparent analyses of multiple sequence alignments. *Chem. Rev.* **97,** 2725–2843.
23. Johnson, M. S., Srinivasan, N., Sowdhamini, R., and Blundell, T. L. (1994) Knowledge-based protein modeling. *Crit. Rev. Biochem. Mol. Biol.* **29,** 1–68.
24. Sippl, M. J., Lackner, P., Domingues, F. S., and Koppensteiner, W. A. (1999) An attempt to analyse progress in fold recognition from CASP1 to CASP3. *Proteins,* **37(3),** 226–230.
25. Brocklehurst, S. M. and Perham, R. N. (1993) Prediction of the three-dimensional structures of the biotinylated domain from yeast pyruvate carboxylase and of the

lipoylated H-protein from the pea leaf glycine cleavage system: a new automated method for the prediction of protein tertiary structure. *Protein Sci.* **4,** 626–639.
26. Sander, C. and Schneider, R. (1991) Database of homology-derived protein structures and the structural meaning of sequence alignment. *Proteins* **9,** 56–68.
27. Kabsch, W. and Sander, C. (1983) Dictionary of protein secondary structure: pattern recognition of hydrogen-bonded and geometrical features. *Biopolymers* **12,** 2577–2637.
28. Kraulis, P. J. (1991) MOLSCRIPT: a program to produce both detailed and schematic plots of protein structures. *J. Appl. Crystallogr.* **24,** 946–950.

24

Identification of Novel Genes
by Gene Trap Mutagenesis

Anne K. Voss and Tim Thomas

1. Introduction

Functional analysis of the mammalian genome will be a major task of biologic science in the future. Gene trap is a method designed to provide functional information for novel genes *(1–3)*. It offers tagging of a gene (facilitating subsequent cloning), analysis of the expression pattern by a simple staining technique, and generation of a mutant mouse strain in one experimental approach. According to our experience *(4)*, about two thirds of the genes isolated by this method are either completely unknown or published only as expressed sequence tags. The reporter gene reflects the expression pattern of the endogenous gene faithfully in about three quarters of all cases. Overt phenotypic abnormalities can be expected in about half of the mutant mouse lines generated by gene trap. However, note that frequently the trapped allele is not a null allele, but rather a hypomorphic allele. This issue is discussed in **ref.** *4* and *5*). This may be beneficial in cases in which preimplantation lethality would ordinarily preclude the analysis of functions of the gene later in development or in adult life. The most serious criticism to date is that there is little possibility to direct mutagenesis by gene trap to a specific organ system, although attempts in that direction have been made.

In this chapter, we describe methods used in producing mouse lines containing genes tagged by gene trap construct insertions. The approach used involves electroporation into murine embryonic stem ES cells. Readers interested in the widely used alternative, retroviral gene trap vectors, are referred to **refs.** *1* and *3*.

From: *Methods in Molecular Biology, vol. 175: Genomics Protocols*
Edited by: M. P. Starkey and R. Elaswarapu © Humana Press Inc., Totowa, NJ

2. Materials

2.1. ES Cell Culture

1. Dissection instruments: scissors and forceps.
2. Petri dishes: 15, 10, and 3.5 cm (Falcon).
3. 24 and 96-Well plates (Falcon).
4. Erlenmeyer flask with 100-mL glass beads.
5. Wire meshes.
6. Stirring rod.
7. General cell culture glassware.
8. 0.1 % Gelatin (G-1890; Sigma). Make up the stock in H_2O and autoclave.
9. Feeder medium: Dulbecco's modified Eagle's medium (DMEM) (Gibco), 10% fetal bovine serum (FBS), virus and mycoplasma screened.
10. Primary embryonic fibroblasts isolated from embryonic day 13.5 (e13.5) murine embryos or SNL cells.
11. Mitomycin C (M-0503; Sigma): Dissolve 1 vial (2 mg) in 4 mL of phosphate-buffered saline (PBS), filter sterilize, and store protected from light at 4°C. Use within 1 wk; check for precipitates before use.
12. PBS (10X stock): 80 g/L of NaCl, 2 g/L of KCl, 11.5 g/L of Na_2HPO_4 2 g/L of KH_2PO_4. Sterilize by autoclaving. Dilute 10X PBS 1:10 with water, check pH (7.2–7.4), and autoclave again for storage.
13. Trypsin/EDTA (5X stock): 8 g/L of NaCl, 0.4 g/L of KCl, 0.1 g/L of Na_2HPO_4, 1 g/L of glucose, 3 g/L of Tris-base, 0.4 g/L of Na_2-EDTA, 5 g/L of trypsin (Seromed 1:250). Adjust the pH to 7.6 and sterilize by filtration (0.2 µm). Store at 4°C and use within 1 wk (or freeze aliquots at –20°C). Dilute the stock 1:5 with sterile PBS, store at 4°C, and use within 1 wk.
14. ESC medium: DMEM (high glucose, 4.50 mg/L; Gibco), 0.1 mM β-mercaptoethanol (Sigma 47522), 1X nonessential amino acids (Gibco), 1X L-glutamine (Gibco), 1X sodium pyruvate (Gibco), 20% FBS (Gibco offers FBS tested for ES cell culture), 1000 U/mL of mLIF (Gibco).
15. Incubator, 37°C and 5% CO_2.
16. Sterile laminar flow hood that fits a dissection microscope.
17. Inverted microscope, magnification ×50–×320, phase-contrast optics.
18. Cell culture centrifuge.
19. Liquid nitrogen container to store cells.
20. 2X Freezing medium: mix 30 parts ESC medium, 9 parts dimethylsulfoxide (DMSO) (D-8779; Sigma), and 6 parts FBS. The final concentration after treatment of cells for freezing is 10% DMSO, 20% fetal bovine serum and 16.7% trypsin/EDTA.
21. 2–20 µL micropipet plus tips; 20–200 µL micropipet plus tips.

2.2. Generation of Gene Trap ES Cell Clones

1. Gene Pulser electroporator (Bio-Rad).
2. Electroporation cuvet: 4-mm electrode distance, 0.8-mL vol (Bio-Rad).

3. G418 (Geneticin[R], Gibco).
4. Dissection microscope, magnification ×6–×40 (Wild-Leitz).

2.3. β-Galactosidase Staining

1. 37–39% Formalin (Fluka).
2. 5-Bromo-4 chloro-3-indolyl-β-D-galactopyranoside (X-gal).
3. 25% Glutaraldehyde.
4. $K_3Fe(CN)_6$ (0.5 M stock in water).
5. $K_4Fe(CN)_6$ (0.5 M stock in water).
6. $MgCl_2$ (0.1 mM stock in water).
7. NP40 (10% stock solution in water).
8. Sodium deoxycholate (1% solution in water).
9. 30°C Incubator.
10. 20X PBS buffer.
11. Glycerol stocks (20, 40, 60, and 80% glycerol in PBS).

2.4. Generation of Chimeras

1. 70% Ethanol.
2. Avertin: Prepare the stock by dissolving 1 g of 2,2,2-tribromo ethyl alcohol in 1 mL of tertiary amyl alcohol. Keep the stock protected from light at 4°C. Dilute to 2.5% in 42°C, 0.9% sterile saline for use (injection solution). Observe complete mixing. Cool the injection solution down to room temperature slowly. Keep protected from light at 4°C, and use within 4 wk.
3. Acid Tyrode's solution: 0.8 g of NaCl, 0.02 g of KCl, 0.024 g of $CaCl_2·2H_2O$, 0.01 g of $MgCl_2·6H_2O$, 0.1 g of glucose, and 0.4 g of polyvinylpyrrolidone. Make up the volume to 100 mL, filter, and aliquot. Store at –20°C.
4. M2 and M16: Prepare from stock solutions stored at –20°. Prepare medium for one week and store at 4°C. Replace stocks after approx 3 mo. For a more extensive description see **ref. 6.** For 10 mL:

    M2: 1 mL Stock A, 160 µL Stock B, 100 µL Stock C, 100 µL Stock D, 840 µL Stock E, 7.8 mL H_2O, 40 mg BSA. Sterile filtrate.

    M16: 1 mL Stock A, 1 mL Stock B, 100 µL Stock C, 100 µL Stock D, 7.8 mL H_2O, 40 mg serum bovine albumin (BSA). Sterile filtrate.

5. 10X Solution A: 5.534 g/100 mL NaCl, 0.356 g/100 mL KCl, 0.162 g/100 mL KH_2PO_4, 0.293 g/100 mL $MgSO_4·7 H_2O$ 2.610 g/100 mL sodium lactate, 1 g/100 mL glucose, 0.060 g/100 mL penicillin, and 0.05 g/100 mL streptomycin.
6. 10X Solution B: 2.101 g/100 mL $NaHCO_3$ and 0.01 g/100 mL phenol red.
7. 100X Solution C: 0.036 g/10 mL sodium pyruvate.
8. 100X Solution D: 0.252 g/10 mL $CaCl_2·2 H_2O$.
9. 100X Solution E: 5.958 g/100 mL HEPES and 0.01 g/100 mL phenol red. Adjust the pH to 7.4 with 0.2 N NaOH.
10. BSA, Fraction V, minimum 96% (A-9647; Sigma).

11. Light mineral oil (M-8410; Sigma).
12. Surgical swabs.
13. Aluminum foil.
14. 1-mL Syringes.
15. 2-mL Syringes.
16. Short 27-gage injection needles.
17. Flushing needle, 33-gage needle with the tip cut off and slightly bent.
18. 3.5-cm Petri dishes.
19. 10-cm Petri dishes.
20. Mouth pipet assembled from a mouthpiece. Soft silicon tubing, a sterile filter inserted between two parts of the tubing, and a pipet tip for 200–1000 μL (cut off the tip and invert; the wide opening will fit the wide opening of a Pasteur pipet).
21. Short Pasteur pipets.
22. Medium tapestry needles to make depressions in the bottom of a 3.5-cm Petri dish: For aggregation wells, try several to find a suitable needle, and then equip with a handle of either metal or plastic (heated and formed in place).
23. Bunsen burner.
24. Tissue culture incubator, 37°C and 5% CO2 in air.
25. Low-magnification binocular microscope.
26. Cold fiberoptic light source.
27. Fine clippers.
28. Dissection instruments: large scissors (for cutting skin), small scissors, blunt small forceps, and no. 5 watchmaker's forceps.
29. Surgery instruments: small surgical forceps, small blunt forceps, small scissors, small Serrefine clamp, small wound clips (Michel's clips), and wound clip applicator.

3. Methods

3.1. Gene Trap Constructs

We used two splice acceptor trap (pGTl.8geo and pKCl99βgeo) and two exon insertion trap constructs (pEIT2 and pElT3). All four constructs were promoterless. pGTl.8geo *(7)* consists of intron and exon sequences spanning a splice acceptor of the murine engrailed-2 gene fused in frame to codon 8 of the β-galactosidase coding sequence and in frame to codon 2 of the neomycin phosphotransferase coding sequence. The neomycin resistance coding region is concluded by an SV40 polyadenylation signal. pKCl99βgeo contains an Hoxc9 splice acceptor fused in frame to the βgeo fusion of the β-galactosidase coding region and a mutated neomycin phosphotransferase coding region as in pSAβgeo *(1,8)*. pEIT2 and pElT3 are derivatives of pGTl.8geo. Instead of the intron sequences of the engrailed-2 splice acceptor, they contain base 865–905 (pEIT2) and base 490–905 (pEIT3) of the microtubule-associated protein 4 coding region fused in frame to the engrailed-2 exon of pGT1.8geo resulting in 259- and 634-bp buffer sequence 5' of the β-galactosidase coding region for pEIT2 and pEIT3, respectively *(4)*. A more specialized gene trap construct has been designed to select for insertions into genes coding for secreted molecules *(7)*.

Promoterless constructs rely on activation by an endogenous promotor and reliably integrate into bona fide transcriptional units. To generate G418-resistant ES cell colonies, the trapped endogenous gene must be active in ES cells. Our data suggest that genes with very low transcriptional activity in ES cells can be trapped. However, the population of genes that can be targeted by this method is almost certainly limited by the need to be expressed in ES cells. Initially, gene trap constructs were designed containing a splice acceptor fused to the *lacZ* gene with a polyadenylation signal followed by a promotor driving a neomycin phosphotransferase gene concluded by a polyadenalytion signal. Although eliminating the need to insert into a transcriptionally active locus in ES cells, these constructs produced G418-resistance inserting outside of transcriptional units, and, therefore, actual gene trap events were rare (2–5%). To overcome this problem, polyadenylation trap constructs were designed (*see* **Note 1**).

Polyadenylation trap constructs do not contain polyadenylation signals at the end of the neomycin phosphotransferase gene and rely on linking up to an endogenous polyadenylation signal to produce a stable mRNA. This alone is thought to select for insertions into transcriptional units allowing the use of a promotor. A polyadenylation trap construct may consist of a splice acceptor, an internal ribosomal entry site (IRES), a β-galactosidase coding region, a polyadenylation signal, and a promotor driving a neomycin phosphotransferase gene concluded by a splice donor *(9,10)*. Such a construct will allow integrations into genes silent in ES cells. In this case, the ES cells will be G418 resistant but will not exhibit β-galactosidase activity. Only on activation of the endogenous locus will the *lacZ* gene be activated. This could be achieved by an in vitro differentiation procedure. One drawback of this type of gene trap construct is that in the case of multiple copy tandem integrations, the splice donor 3' of the neomycin phosphotransferase gene will be spliced to the splice acceptor 5' of the *lacZ* gene of the following copy of the gene trap construct. Thus, the *lacZ* gene can be driven by the promotor meant to drive the neomycin phosphotransferase alone. The IRES will render such an artificial transcriptional unit polycistronic so that functional β-galactosidase is produced in every case.

Splice acceptor trap constructs such as pGT1.8geo or pKC199βgeo function when inserted into intron or exon sequences. In the case of an intron insertion, the splice donor of the preceding endogenous exon is spliced to the splice acceptor of the gene trap construct. In the case of an exon insertion the splice donor of the endogenous exon preceding the exon carrying the insertion is spliced to the splice acceptor of the gene trap construct. In our hands, insertion into exons seem to be more likely to mutate the endogenous locus functionally. A gene trap construct inserted into an intron can be spliced out apparently without affecting the function of the endogenous locus (*5; see* **Note 2**).

3.2. ES Cell Culture

3.2.1. Feeder Cell Monolayers

Murine ES cells can be cultured on gelatin-coated tissue culture plasticware or on monolayers of feeder cells. We prefer to culture ES cells on feeder cells, because, in our hands, the rate of germline chimera production is higher after culture on feeder cells. For the last three passages of ES cells before chimera production, we prefer primary embryonic fibroblast feeder cell monolayers over SNL feeder cells *(11)*.

3.2.1.1. Isolation and Routine Culture of Primary Embryonic Fibroblasts

Primary embryonic fibroblasts (PEFs) are isolated from e12.5 to e14.5 mouse embryos. Transgenic mice carrying a neomycin resistance gene have to be used if PEFs are intended for G418 selection.

1. Kill one to two pregnant mice by cervical dislocation, and open the abdominal cavity by changing scissors between the skin layer and muscle layer.
2. With a sterile pair of forceps and scissors, dissect out the uterus, and wash with three changes of sterile PBS.
3. Transfer into a sterile laminar flow hood and wash again by passing through three Petri dishes containing sterile PBS.
4. Dissect embryos from uterus and wash 3X with PBS.
5. Remove the head, heart, liver, and other internal organs and wash the remainder three times in PBS.
6. Cut into small pieces with fine scissors in a small volume of PBS (5 mL).
7. Transfer to a prewarmed (37°C) sterile Erlenmeyer flask containing 50 mL of 1X trypsin/EDTA solution, a stirring rod, and 100 mL of glass beads.
8. Stir the solution gently at 37°C for 30 min.
9. Recover the first 50 mL of trypsin solution by passing through a wire mesh, and add an equal volume of feeder medium. Keep this batch at room temperature until the second digest is recovered.
10. For the second digest, add 50 mL of prewarmed trypsin solution to the tissue pieces in the Erlenmeyer flask and incubate at 37°C with gentle stirring for 30 min.
11. Pass the second digest through a wire mesh and add feeder medium.
12. Spin both digests at 200*g* at for 10 min.
13. Discard the supernatant and resuspend the pellet in 20 mL of feeder medium per six embryos.

14. Plate the cells at three to six embryos per 15-cm dish. Change the medium the next day.
15. Carefully examine the cells for signs of contamination and cells without fibroblast morphology.

3.2.1.2. FREEZING OF CELLS

Freeze the clean preparations of PEF when confluent at three vials per 15-cm plate.

1. For freezing, wash PEFs twice with PBS.
2. Add 5 mL of 1X trypsin/EDTA and incubate at 37°C for 3 min.
3. Add 5 mL of feeder medium, centrifuge at 200g for 5 min, and remove supernatant.
4. Resuspend the pellet in 1.5 mL of feeder medium and add an equal volume of 2X freezing medium.
5. Mix the cells carefully and transfer to cryovials (1 mL each).
6. Slowly freeze to –70°C, and transfer quickly to liquid nitrogen. In liquid nitrogen, they can be kept for years. Defrost frozen vials in a 37°C water bath, no longer than it takes for the last ice crystals to disappear. Pipet out the contents slowly into 10 mL of feeder medium, mix by inverting, centrifuge at 200g for 5 min, and remove supernatant.
7. Disrupt the pellet carefully by tapping and resuspend in 20 mL of feeder medium.
8. Plate onto a gelatin-coated 15-cm Petri dish. PEFs should not be passaged more than once before cleavage inactivation and use.

3.2.1.3. ROUTINE CULTURE OF SNL CELLS

SNL cells can be obtained from A. Bradley *(11)*. They are a permanent fibroblast cell line (STO) transfected with neomycin phosphotransferase and leukemia inhibitory factor (LIF) expression vectors.

1. Defrost frozen vials in a 37°C water bath, no longer than it takes for the last ice crystals to disappear.
2. Pipet the content of a cryovial slowly into 10 mL of feeder medium, mix by inverting slowly, centrifuge at 200g for 5 min, and remove supernatant.
3. Disrupt the pellet carefully by tapping, and resuspend in the appropriate volume of feeder medium.
4. Plate onto 15-cm tissue culture dish (*see* **Note 3**).

3.2.2. Inactivation of Feeder Cells

PEF or SNL cells are grown under sterile conditions in feeder medium. SNL cells have to be passaged before they reach confluence. PEFs are passaged only once before use.

1. To cleavage inactivate feeder cells, treat approx 80% confluent cells with medium containing 10 μg/mL of mitomycin C for 2 h.

2. Meanwhile, coat tissue culture dishes with 0.1% gelatin solution for 30 min.
3. Wash mitomycin C–treated feeders twice with PBS.
4. Trypsinize as in **Subheading 3.2.1.2., steps 1** and **2** for 3 min and transfer to feeder medium.
5. Centrifuge, remove supernatant, and resuspend 20 mL of feeder medium per 15-cm Petri dish.
6. Count and plate at a density of 5×10^4 cells/cm^2. Medium is changed the next day and from then on twice a week. Feeders should be used within 1 wk (*see* **Note 4**).

3.2.3. Defrosting and Plating of ES Cells

1. To defrost ES cells, place a cryovial into a 37°C water bath for as long as it takes to dissolve the last ice crystals.
2. Carefully transfer the cells to a centrifuge tube containing 10 mL of ESC medium and centrifuge at 200*g* for 2 min.
3. Discard the supernatant and resuspend carefully in 2 mL of ESC medium.
4. Plate onto freshly inactivated feeders (e.g., 3.5-cm dish). Vigorous pipetting at this stage will kill cells and result in low plating efficiency. Change the medium daily, and keep it from turning acidic (i.e., yellow).

3.2.4. Passaging of ES Cells

1. To passage the ES cells, wash the dishes twice with PBS.
2. Incubate in 1X trypsin/EDTA at 37°C for approx 5 min (each batch of trypsin/EDTA solution has to be checked for the appropriate time of ES cell dissociation).
3. Pipet the cells in trypsin/EDTA about three times.
4. Add 3 vol of ESC medium.
5. Centrifuge at 200*g* for 2 min.
6. Discard the supernatant and disrupt the cell pellet carefully.
7. Resuspend in an appropriate volume of ESC medium.
8. Plate the cells onto a monolayer of inactivated feeder cells (*see* **Note 5**).

3.2.5. Freezing of ES Cells

1. For freezing, trypsinize ES cells (0.2 mL trypsin/EDTA per well of a 24-well plate, 0.5 mL per 3.5-cm dish, or 2 mL per 10-cm dish) as described in **Subheading 3.2.4.**
2. After dissociation of the cells in trypsin/EDTA solution, add twice the volume of ESC medium and mix by pipetting (0.4 mL per 24-well, 1 mL per 3.5-cm dish, or 4 mL per 10-cm dish).
3. Finally, add an equal volume of 2X freezing medium (0.6 mL per 24-well, 1.5 mL per 3.5-cm dish or 6-mL per 10-cm dish).
4. Mix the cell suspension by gentle pipetting, and transfer 1 mL of each to prelabeled cryovials.
5. Cool the cryovials slowly in a styrofoam box to –70°C, and transfer quickly to liquid nitrogen (*see* **Note 6**).

3.3. Generation of Gene Trap ES Cell Clones

3.3.1. Electroporation

1. Wash exponentially growing ES cells (usually two 10-cm plates will yield 4 to 6×10^7 ES cells) twice in PBS solution.
2. Trypsinize and add to ESC medium.
3. Centrifuge at 200g for 5 min, remove supernatant and resuspend in PBS.
4. Count and centrifuge again at 200g and remove supernatant.
5. Resuspend in PBS to a density of 10^7 cells/0.8 mL for each electroporation cuvet (*see* **Note 7**).
6. Add 20 μg of DNA to the cells and mix by gentle pipetting avoiding the formation of air bubbles.
7. Incubate the cell suspension plus DNA for 5 min at room temperature.
8. Resuspend and transfer to an electroporation cuvet (4-mm electrode distance, 0.8-mL vol) avoiding the formation of air bubbles, and expose to a pulse of 250 V and 500 μF.
9. Add 1 mL of ESC medium immediately after electroporation.
10. Incubate for 5 min at room temperature and resuspend in 4 mL of medium.
11. Plate onto a 15-cm plate of feeder cells.

3.3.2. Selection

Usually gene trap constructs contain a neomycin phosphotransferase gene that confers neomycin resistance. As the selection, Geneticin® (G418) is used. G418 can be kept in aliquots as a sterile filtered 1000X stock solution at –20°C. Repeated defrosting and freezing of G418 reduces activity.

1. Select stable integration events with 250 μg/mL of G418 (by weight, corresponding to approx 125 μg/mL of active substance) in ESC medium starting 24 h after electroporation for 7–12 d.
2. Change the medium daily.
3. To test the activity of a new batch of G418, subject sham electroporated ES cells (without DNA) to 250 μg/mL of G418 (*see* **Note 8–10**).

3.3.3. Picking of ES Cell Clones

1. Pick colonies of a 500-μm diameter or larger starting after 7 days of selection using a 2–20 μL pipet set to 2 and a dissection microscope placed in a laminar flow hood.
2. Transfer the colonies to 100 μL of 1X trypsin solution in a 96-well plate.
3. Incubate at 37°C for 5 min.
4. Dissociate the cells by pipetting up and down using a 20–200 μL pipette.
5. Transfer to 24-well dishes of feeder cells with 1 mL of ESC medium.
6. Incubate for 24 h and change medium to 0.5 mL of fresh ESC medium.
7. Propagate the individual colonies as individual cell lines.

3.3.4. Freezing

After 2–3 d either freeze (*see* **Subheading 3.2.5.**) one cryovial per well of a 24-well plate or passage each well onto a 3.5-cm dish (*see* **Note 11**). Freeze three cryovials from each confluent 3.5-cm dish. After freezing add more ESC medium and grow remaining cells for β-galactosidase staining.

3.3.5. Basic Differentiation Protocol

1. After aliquots of each G418-resistant ES cell clone are frozen, grow remaining cells in each well at very low cell density for 14 d maintaining G418 levels at 250 μg/mL and 200 U/mL of LIF (*see* **Note 12**).
2. Stain the cultures after 14 d for β-galactosidase activity.
3. Evaluate the cultures microscopically at ×100 and ×320 magnification. Cell clones with a variety of morphologic features will be observed (undifferentiated, neuron-like, epithelioid, mesenchymal, fibroblast-like, endoderm-like, vesicle forming, and tubule forming). Clones exhibiting the cell type of interest can be selected for further studies.

3.4. β-Galactosidase Staining of Cells and Embryos

3.4.1. Fixing Cells or Embryos

1. Wash the cells once in PBS.
2. Fix cells for 2 min in 1% formaldehyde and 0.2% glutaraldehyde in PBS, and wash twice in PBS. Fix embryos in 1% formaldehyde, 0.2% glutaraldehyde, 0.02% NP40, and PBS for 10 (e8.5) to 60 min (e15.5).
3. Wash in two changes of PBS for 10–60 min (*see* **Note 13**).

3.4.2. Staining of Cells

1. Transfer the cells to staining solution (PBS containing 1 mg/mL of X-gal, 5 mM $K_3Fe(CN)_6$, 5 mM $K_4Fe(CN)_6$, 2 mM $MgCl_2$).
2. Stain overnight at 37°C.
3. Wash stained cells in PBS. They can be kept in PBS at 4°C for a few days. If later reference is needed, sodium azide can be added to the PBS to prevent fungal growth (*see* **Note 14**).

3.4.3. Staining of Embryos

1. Transfer the embryos to staining solution as for cells (PBS containing 1 mg/mL of X-gal, 5 mM $K_3Fe(CN)_6$, 5 mM $K_4Fe(CN)_6$, 2 mM $MgCl_2$. (Add 0.2% NP40 and 0.1% sodium deoxycholate for embryos older than e 11.5.)
2. Incubate overnight at 30°C.
3. After staining, wash the embryos in PBS briefly (*see* **Notes 14** and **15**).

3.4.4. Clearing of Embryos

Embryos are either processed for histologic sections or cleared in ascending concentrations of glycerol in PBS (20, 40, 60, and 80%). When first placed into the next higher glycerol concentration, the embryos float in the solution. Once an equilibrium is reached, the embryos sink to the bottom of the dish and can be transferred to the next higher concentration of glycerol. If embryos are transferred to higher concentrations of glycerol too quickly, some parts of the embryos shrink, e.g., the roof of the hindbrain.

3.5. Generation of Chimeras

3.5.1. Recovery of Morulae

Fertile females of the mouse strains NMRI, CD1, or C57Bl6 (coat color of embryo donor mouse strain must be distinguishable from that of the mouse strain from which the ES cells were derived) are superovulated by ip injection of pregnant mares' serum gonadotropin (PMSG) (7.5 IU for NMRI and CD1; 5 IU for C57B16) followed by an injection of human chorionic gonadotropin hCG (5 IU) 46 h later (e.g., PMSG at 3:00 PM, hCG at 1:00 PM 2 d later; *see* **Notes 16** and **17**). Hormone-treated females are mated 1:1 with stud males of the same mouse strain overnight. Successful matings are recognized by the presence of a vaginal plug the next morning. Noon on the day of the vaginal plug is called e0.5. Eight-cell stage embryos are recovered between 9:00 AM and 11:00 AM on e2.5 from the oviduct. We usually use between 10 and 20 females per operator.

1. Before starting to flush the oviducts, fill a 3.5-cm Petri dish with 2 mL of M16.
2. Place 6 µL drops of M16 in another 3.5-cm Petri dish (10–20 drops) and cover with mineral oil.
3. Push six to nine depressions through the mineral oil into the plastic of the bottom of the Petri dish within each drop of M16 using a tapestry needle (sterilize in 70% ethanol and allow to dry before use).
4. Leave three drops without depressions for ES cell clump selection. This is the aggregation dish.
5. Place both dishes containing M16 into a 37°C, 5% CO_2 in air tissue culture incubator for equilibration.
6. Warm M2 to room temperature before use in subsequent steps.
7. For collection of embryos and further manipulations, use finely drawn out Pasteur pipets (*see* **Note 18**).
8. Kill superovulated and plugged female mice by cervical dislocation.
9. Open the abdominal cavity and hold the uterus with a pair of blunt forceps.
10. Remove the mesometrium from the uterus by perforating it with a pair of small scissors and opening the scissors parallel to the uterine horn and oviduct.

11. Excise the oviducts leaving 0.5 cm of uterus, and cut carefully between the ovary and oviduct in order to prevent damage to the oviduct and the infundibulum.
12. Transfer the oviducts to drops of M2 in a 10-cm dish, one drop per animal.
13. When all oviducts are collected, transfer to fresh drops of M2 in a 10-cm dish, this time one drop per oviduct.
14. Flush the oviducts under a low magnification microscope. Load a 2-mL syringe with M2 and attach a 33-gage flushing needle. Fix the infundibulum using no. 5 watchmaker's forceps. Insert he flushing needle into the infundibulum and hold with the forceps in place.
15. Flush about 200 μL of M2 through the oviduct with little pressure. Leave the uterine end of the oviduct in the drop of M2. During this flushing procedure embryos can be observed exiting the oviduct through the remaining uterine stump.
16. Attach a pipet to the mouth pipet and preload with M2. Collect embryos (10–20) by gently sucking into the pipet, and transfer them to a fresh 3.5-cm Petri dish filled with 2 mL of M2. During collection, good 8-cell stage or morulae embryos should be counted vs degenerated embryos, embryos delayed in development, and unfertilized eggs to assess success of superovulation and mating. Usually similar numbers of embryos can be expected from each of the two oviducts recovered from one animal. Eight-cell stage embryos and more or less compacted morulae can be used for the following steps of the procedure (*see* **Note 19**).

3.5.2. Removal of Zona

1. To remove zona pellucida, collect the embryos with a pipet preloaded with acid Tyrode's solution and transfer to a 3.5-cm Petri dish filled with 2 mL of acid Tyrode's solution (*see* **Note 20**).
2. Monitor the process of zona disappearance closely under the low-magnification microscope. The zona disappears within 1 to 2 min. To avoid damage to the zonaless embryos, collect them swiftly with a pipet preloaded with M2.
3. Wash zonaless embryos twice through 3.5-cm Petri dishes containing 2 mL of M2.
4. Wash the embryos (zonaless) again through the equilibrated dish containing 2 mL of M16; and then place singly into the depressions in the previously prepared aggregation dish.
5. Return the aggregation dish to the incubator.

3.5.3. Preparation of ES Cells for Aggregation

1. Passage the ES cells for aggregation at least two times after defrosting, and keep in logarithmic growth phase throughout culture to enrich for healthy undifferentiated cells. The optimal time for aggregation is about 20–24 h after the last passage.
2. Change medium on the cultures on the morning of the aggregation, i.e., several hours before aggregation, to ensure that the cells are growing under optimal conditions.
3. Wash a 3.5-cm Petri dish of ES cells twice with PBS and partially trypsinize in 0.5 mL of 1X trypsin/EDTA solution. The trypsinizing time will be similar to that for passaging the ES cells, but mechanical dissociation is reduced so that

small numbers of ES cells stay loosely attached to each other in small clumps or branching chains, whereas all the feeder cells fall off the ES cells.

4. Add 1.5 mL of ESC medium to the cells and check the number of ES cells per clump or chain. If the clumps are still too large, pipet once or twice again with a 2-mL pipet and check the cell number.
5. Dilute partially trypsinized ES cells with 4–6 mL of ESC medium.

3.5.4. Aggregation

1. Select ES cell clumps or chains under ×40 magnification and transfer to the depression-free drops of aggregation dish (*see* **Note 21**).
2. Select the ES cells again and transfer single clumps or chains of the cells to each zonaless embryo, and position such that a maximal contact between the embryo and the ES cells is achieved.
3. After supplying all embryos with ES cells, check again that they are in contact with ES cells and carefully transfer to the incubator (*see* **Note 22**).

3.5.5. Transfer of Embryos

After about 26 h of culture most of the aggregates will have developed into blastocysts and are ready for embryo transfer into the uterus of pseudopregnant recipient mice. Aggregates that did not develop to the blastocyst stage can still be transferred after a further 24 h of culture (*see* **Note 23**).

Pseudopregnant embryo transfer recipient mice are generated by mating fertile females (e.g., NMRI or CD1, best at 8–12 wk of age) to vasectomized males. After successful mating, a vaginal plug can be observed the next morning. The pseudopregnant females are used on e2.5, but minus 24 h asynchronous to the aggregated embryos that were recovered on e2.5 and then cultured for 1 d.

1. Transfer blastocysts from the aggregation dish to a 3.5-cm dish containing 2 mL of M2.
2. Transfer again to a 3.5-cm dish containing five 20-μL drops of M2. Transfer all embryos (four to eight) for one side of a recipient uterus to one drop. From these they can easily be recovered for embryo transfer during surgery.
3. Keep the embryos (in drops) outside the incubator at room temperature. In initial experiments, embryos for only one transfer should be transferred to drops because the embryos should not be kept outside of the incubator for too long.
4. Put the recipients into general anaesthesia by injecting approx 20 μL of the injection solution of avertin 1 g of body weight. Avertin is more potent the first 2 d after the preparation of the final solution. Each new preparation of avertin may vary and has to be tested for best results.
5. Shave the lateral body walls between the last ribs and pelvis with fine clippers. Disinfect the surgical instruments with 70% ethanol and allow to dry. Make "surgery tray" by folding aluminum foil (four layers, 10 × 6 cm) and place it under the low-magnification microscope.
6. Place the anesthetized mouse onto the surgery tray.
7. Disinfect surgery area of mouse with 70% ethanol.

8. Cut a small incision, roughly halfway between the last rib and the tuber coxae of the pelvis and about 1.5 cm below the spine, into the skin in an angle of 45° at the last rib with small scissors while holding the skin with surgical forceps. In this area, almost always the fat pad of the ovary forms a small mound that is visible through the skin. This can be used for orientation. The incision can be made on top of this mound. The opening is bluntly widened by inserting the scissors and opening them.

9. Cut the muscle layers of the abdominal wall. Make the incision in an area lacking blood vessels and nerves. This cut will often include the peritoneum. For initial experiments, it is advisable to cut a larger opening to facilitate a better view of the organs. Experienced operators will cut an opening of <1 cm. The ovarian fat pad is usually substantial and found easily. It can be used as a handle to expose the fat pad, ovary, the oviduct, and cranial part of the attached uterine horn through the body wall opening. A Serrefine clamp can now be attached to the fat pad and placed onto the back of the animal to weigh down the fat pad and hold the uterine horn in place. The animal can be moved out of the field of view for the next step by moving the aluminum surgery tray.

10. Collect four to eight embryos into a drawn-out Pasteur transfer pipet attached to mouth pipetting tubing preloaded with two drops of M2 with an intermediate air bubble and an air bubble at the end. In the end, the pipet should contain from the tip: four to eight embryos in a minimal amount of M2, air, M2, air, M2, air. The loaded pipet is carefully set aside so that it can be picked up easily.

11. Move the animal back into the view field, and adjust the focus to the surface of the uterine horn about 1 cm from the oviductal-uterine connection.

12. Hold the uterine horn with small blunt forceps at the oviductal end.

13. Perforate the uterine wall with a 27-gage injection needle near the forceps.

14 Make a note of this place, pick up the transfer pipet carefully, and insert it into the uterus. Gently blow the embryos into the uterine cavity with minimal medium while avoiding blowing air into the uterus.

15. Under microscopic control, suck M2 into the pipet and blow out again to check, that the embryos are successfully transferred.

16. Release the Serrefine clamp from the fat pad, and replace the organs into the abdominal cavity. Now the peritoneum and the musculature of both sides of the abdominal wall opening are juxtaposed such that peritoneum touches peritoneum and is held together using two pairs of forceps.

17. Use one pair of forceps to hold the tissues in this position while using the other to pull the skin of both sides of the wound over the musculature. The resulting wound ridge consists of six layers (skin, muscle, peritoneum, peritoneum, muscle, and skin) and is fixed using small surgical wound clips.

18. Repeat this procedure on the contralateral side.

19. Wrap the mouse in paper tissue and place onto a warm plate at 37°C to prevent hypothermia. As the animal starts to recover from anesthesia, place it into a clean cage.

20. Examine the animal and the surgery wounds the next day (*see* **Notes 24** and **25**).

3.6. Mouse Breeding and Genotyping

3.6.1. Mouse Breeding

An estimate of the overall contribution of the ES cells to the chimera can be made from the ES cell contribution to the pigment cell population (i.e., percentage of coat color chimerism). In our experience, all mice with about 90–100% ES cell contribution, as assessed by coat color, were germline chimeras, if they were fertile. About half of the lower percentage chimeras were germline chimeras with no correlation to the contribution to the pigment cell population (*see* **Note 26**). Very low percentage chimeras were rarely germline chimeras. The resulting chimeras are bred to females of a mouse strain chosen such that the phenotype of the coat color genes of the ES cells can be recognized. This first mating is to test for germline transmission of the ES cell genome. Once germline transmission is established, we routinely cross chimeras back to the mouse strain that was used for ES cell production (in our case 129/SvPas). This mating will generate mutant mice on a defined genetic background. Coat colors are no indication in this mating. The inbred mice are usually less fertile but always much more consistent in all parameters of interest. Therefore, we usually perform an initial phenotypic analysis on a mixed genetic background and then repeat these experiments on an inbred background for better consistency. Unlike in homologous recombination experiments, gene trap only generates one ES cell clone per mutation of a specific gene. Therefore, care must be taken to eliminate the possibility of an unrelated mutation in the genome of the ES cells causing the observed phenotype. The final phenotypic analysis should be performed after backcrossing the gene trap allele to wild-type mice for several generations. This will help remove unlinked mutations. We recommend that 100 meioses should be checked for cosegregation of the gene trap allele and the phenotype. Tightly linked mutations are not likely to segregate. However, the most likely linked mutation would be a rearrangement at the insertion site. This possibility can be eliminated by testing for the integrity of the endogenous locus outside of the gene trap insertion by Southern analysis of regions outside of the insertion site. *Also see* **Note 27**.

3.6.2. Genotyping by PCR

DNA is isolated from tail biopsies *(12)*. To genotype offspring of heterozygous by wild-type matings, polymerase chain reaction (PCR) amplification of 508 bp of the *lacZ* gene can be performed. The PCR buffer consists of: 50 mM KCl, 10 mM Tris-HCl, 2 mM MgCl$_2$, 0.1% Triton X-100, and 0.2 mM dNTPs.

1. Perform PCR using 5' TTGGCGTAAGTGAAGCGAC3' as a forward and 5' AGCGGCTGATGTTGAACTG3' as a reverse primer to delete *LacZ* gene.

2. PCR cycle: Denaturing at 94°C for 5 min, 30 cycles of 94°C for 1 min, 60°C for 1 min 30 s, and 72°C for 1 min; final extension 72°C, 10 min. Separate the PCR products on a 2% agarose gel and visualize with ethidium bromide.

3.6.3. Quantitative Southern Hybridization

During the initial screen for mutant phenotypes, an endogenous probe for a gene-specific Southern analysis may not be available. Because only about 50% of the gene trap mouse lines exhibit a mutant phenotype, it may be advisable to postpone laborious cloning procedures until after an interesting phenotype has been observed.

To genotype offspring of heterozygous by heterozygous matings in the absence of a specific probe, we use a quantitative Southern analysis distinguishing one and two copies (or multiples of these) of the gene trap construct per genome (*see* **Note 2**).

1. Cut the DNA with appropriate restriction enzyme.
2. Separate by agarose gel electrophoreses and transfer onto nylon filters *(13)*.
3. Hybridize with [α-^{32}P] dCTP-labeled cDNA probes for the β-galactosidase or the neomycin phosphotransferase gene and an endogenous murine gene as an internal control for two copies per genome *(14)*.
4. Compare the intensity of the *LacZ* or the *neomycin phosphotransferase* gene signals and the endogenous gene signals on the same filter to each other and among animals to determine animals with one or two copies of the gene trap vector per genome.
5. Test suspect homozygous males by mating with the wild-type females for their ability to transmit the trapped allele to 100% of their offspring.

3.7. Identification of Tagged Gene

The quickest way to obtain sequence information from the tagged locus is to use a 5'-RACE technique. We have used two different methods for this and both have worked well *(15,16)*. Both these methods are also available as kits from Gibco-BRL and Clontech. When only a small number of 5'-RACE products are required, using one of these kits is probably the most cost-effective option. In general, we have found 5' RACE on RNA purified from ES cells more successful than from adult tissues. This is probably because the sequence complexity is lower and we routinely select the cells in G418-containing medium first, which selects for cells expressing the fusion mRNA in case of promoterless gene trap constructs. We use the repeated differential precipitation RNA purification method *(17)*. It is important to use an RNA purification method that gives low DNA contamination.

1. Synthesize first-strand cDNA using *lacZ* gene–specific primer (5'-ATTCAGGC-TGCGCAACTGTTGG-3').

2. Amplify by two rounds of PCR using nested oligonucleotide primers (5'-CTG-CAAGGCGATTAAGTTGG-3' and 5'-TAACGCCAGGGTTTTCCCAG-3') from the *lacZ* sequence. Size select the products of the first PCR by agarose gel electrophoresis before second round of PCR.

3. After ligation into a plasmid vector, perform bacterial colony hybridization on filter lifts *(13)* probing with a nested primer complementary to sequences in the gene trap construct 5' of the *lacZ* gene, e.g., the engrailed–2 exon (5' AAACTCAGCCTTGAGCCTCTGGAGCTGCTCAGCAGTGAAGGC 3') in the case of *pGT1.8geo*. This last step greatly increases the number of specific clones.

4. Confirm 5'-RACE products by reverse transcriptase PCR.

4. Notes

1. Low functional mutation efficiency depends on the gene trap construct used. Each new gene trap should construct, therefore, be tested sufficiently before use in a large-scale screen.

2. We have no indication that multiple tandem copy integrations increase the chance of producing a functional mutation. They are problematic when using certain types of polyadenylation trap gene trap constructs (*see* **Subheading 3.1.**).

3. STOs should not be allowed to reach confluence; instead, they should be passaged before they reach confluence by washing them twice with PBS, adding 1X trypsin/EDTA, incubating them at 37°C for 3 min, adding feeder medium (4–9 vol of trypsin/EDTA), and plating them onto gelatin-coated tissue culture plastic. SNL cells can be frozen as described above for PEFs (*see* **Subheading 3.2.1.2.**).

4. Mitomycin C is very unstable and should be stored in the dark. Different batches from the same supplier can vary in activity, resulting in feeders that continue to proliferate or feeders that are so damaged that they start dying after plating. Ideally, feeders should not proliferate, but otherwise look healthy the day after inactivation. The presence of large numbers of dead cells may indicate that mitomycin C is more active than usual and poor-quality feeders will result.

5. The split ratio depends on the density of cells in the original dish and can vary between 1:3 and 1:12 (if there are only very few colonies present in a dish, they may have to be passed 1:1 into a fresh dish of the same size as the previous well). The cells should be split in such a ratio that they can be passaged every other day with daily medium change in between. The cell density should be maintained such that the medium does not turn yellow before the next 48-h cell passage is due. It is important to keep track of the passage number, since it becomes increasingly difficult to produce germline chimeras efficiently with ES cell lines of higher passage numbers (more than 16 passages).

6. ES cells can be kept for years in liquid nitrogen without affecting their potential to form germline chimeras.

7. Low plating efficiency may result if ES cells have not been in maximal growth phase before electroporation or the gene trap construct DNA contains bacterial

endotoxins. In our hands, using $CsCl_2$ gradient purified DNA for electroporation yielded the most consistent results.

8. After 7–9 d all colonies should have died. After 3 to 4 d of selection, the death of nonresistant cells is clearly visible. The dead cells lose the usually tight contact to neighboring cells in their colony, detach from the feeder cells, and float in the medium.

9. G418 concentration will have a significant effect on the number of resistant clones. G418 is known to vary from batch to batch in active component. It may be advisable to test the minimum concentration that will kill ES cells that have not been electroporated in 7 d. Avoid repeated thawing and freezing of G418.

10. We obtain an average of about 25 G418-resistant colonies electroporating 10^7 ES cells with 20 μg of pGT1.8geo and 10 colonies using pKC199βgeo.

11. In cases where insufficient colonies have grown after picking, it may be necessary to passage the cells 1:1 onto fresh feeders.

12. These culture conditions favor the cell type that expressed the selection gene very strongly while allowing slow differentiation into this cell type. Differentiation by complete LIF withdrawal is not as successful, because the cells tended to differentiate rapidly along the pathways of least resistance and a complex culture does not develop.

13. For embryos older than e11.5 0.2% NP40 and 0.1% sodium deoxycholate should be added to the fixative. Embryos older than e12.5 must be cut into halves longitudinally.

14. Whole-mount β-galactosidase staining gives satisfactory results only up to e11.5. In older embryos, the fixative and stain do not penetrate well, giving irregular staining. This is normally sufficient for a rough overview, but for detailed histologic analysis, β-galactosidase staining of cryostat sections is necessary.

15. Background staining can occur because of endogenous β-galactosidase activity. Usually, ensuring that the glutaraldehyd component has been store correctly and/or lengthening the fixation time solves the problem. However, low intensity real staining can be abolished by overfixation. It is important that the volume of fixative is at least 10X the tissue volume and that the embryos are gently rocked so all surfaces are exposed to the fixative.

16. The described superovulation protocol may need to be adjusted when using other mouse strains. For this protocol, we prefer postpubertal females to prepubertal females. Prepubertal females produce high numbers of fertilized oocytes but the embryos frequently do not develop well.

17. If the stud males are too old very few healthy embryos will be obtained. When using our males two to three times a week, we exchange them three times a year. Despite the use of a controlled environment (light cycle, temperature, and humidity control), we observed seasonal changes in reproductive performance of our mouse colonies, with a low in the coldest month and the hottest month.

18. Pasteur pipets are finely drawn out by hand after heating their thin section above the small flame of a Bunsen burner such that the diameter of the pipet is slightly larger than the diameter of an embryo including the zona pellucida. The fine part

of the pipet is broken such that it is about 4 cm long and the broken edge is straight. We usually prepare a large number to choose from, which are kept upside down in a glass beaker.

19. When very different numbers of embryos are often obtained from both oviducts within animals, this is an indication of lack of skill on the part of the operator.

20. When too much M2 is transferred with the embryos into the acid Tyrode's solution, zona removal will take much longer.

21. We use associations of 12–20 cells for aggregation with embryos of the strains NMRI and CD1 and 2–6 cells for C57Bl6. These numbers may vary with ES cell lines and with mouse strains used and have to be established empirically.

22. For best results, our aggregations have to be finished by 11:00 PM, but this time point may vary with the superovulation schedule and mouse strain used. However, embryos that are developed too far will not incorporate ES cells. Four hours after aggregation, the success can be assessed by examining the aggregates under the microscope. The ES cells should be incorporated into the embryos, which should be compacted morulae by this time.

23. If you notice problems with in vitro development of aggregates, check the water used to make up M2 and M16, the M16, the mineral oil, and the incubator. We regularly test new batches of autoclaved Milli-Q water, first M16 made from new stock solutions, and mineral oil on unmanipulated embryos. The aggregates also will have problems developing when too much ESC medium was introduced to their M16 while supplying them with ES cells. Embryos may also fail to develop if they are left too long in acid Tyrode's solution or not handled carefully.

24. Swellings at the site of abdominal surgery occur if the peritoneum and musculature are not closed properly.

25. If low implantation rates are observed, check surgery techniques by transferring unmanipulated embryos.

26. Low ES cells contribution to chimeras may result if either ES cell culture before aggregation or the parental ES cell line is suboptimal. Check that the parental ES cell lines produce germline chimeras with high efficiency before proceeding further.

27. We observed multiple integrations in 2 of 26 mouse lines crossed to homozygosity. They were unlinked and segregated within one generation of mouse breeding.

References

1. Friedrich, G. and Soriano, P. (1991) Promoter traps in embryonic stem cells: a genetic screen to identify and mutate developmental genes in mice. *Genes Dev.* **5,** 1513–1523.

2. Gossler, A., Joyner, A. L., Rossant, J., and Skarnes, W. C. (1989) Mouse embryonic stem cells and reporter constructs to detect developmentally regulated genes. *Science* **244,** 463–465.

3. von Melchner, H., DeGregori, J. V., Rayburn, H., Reddy, S., Friedel, C., and Ruley, H. E. (1992) Selective disruption of genes expressed in totipotent embryonal stem cells. *Genes Dev.* **6,** 919–927.

4. Voss, A. K., Thomas, T., and Gruss, P. (1998) Efficieny assessment of the gene trap approach. *Dev. Dynam.* **212,** 171–180.
5. Voss, A. K., Thomas, T., and Gruss, P. (1998) Compensation for a gene trap mutation in the microtubule associated protein 4 locus by alternative polyadenylation and alternative splicing. *Dev. Dynam.* **212,** 258–266.
6. Hogan, B. L. M., Constantini, F., and Lacy, E. (1986) *Manipulating the Mouse Embryo: A Laboratory Manual,* Cold Spring Harbor Laboratory, Cold Spring Harbor, NY.
7. Skarnes, W. C., Moss, J. E., Hurtley, S. M., and Beddington, R. S. (1995) Capturing genes encoding membrane and secreted proteins important for development. *Proc. Natl. Acad. Sci. USA* **92,** 6592–6596.
8. Thomas, T., Voss, A. K., Chowdhury, K., and Gruss, P. (2000) A new gene trap construct enriching for insertion events near the 5'end of genes. *Transgenic Res.* **9,** 395–404.
9. Salminen, M., Meyer, B. I., and Gruss, P. (1998) Efficient poly A trap approach allows the capture of genes specifically active in differentiated embryonic stem cells and mouse embryos. *Dev. Dynam.* **212,** 326–333.
10. Niwa, H., Araki, K., Kimura, S., Taniguchi, S., Wakasugi, S., and Yamamura, K. (1993) An efficient gene-trap method using poly A trap vectors and characterization of gene-trap events. *J. Biochem.* **113,** 343–349.
11. McMahon, A. P. and Bradley, A. (1990) The *Wnt-1* (int-1) proto-oncogene is required for development of a large region of the mouse brain. *Cell* **62,** 1073–1085.
12. Laird, P. W., Zijderveld, A., Linders, K., Rudnicki, M. A., Jaenisch, R., and Berns, A. (1991) Simplified mammalian DNA isolation procedure. *Nucleic Acids Res.* **19,** 4293.
13. Sambrook, J., Fritsch, E. F., and Maniatis, T. (1989) *Molecular Cloning: A Laboratory Manual.* Cold Spring Harbor Laboratory, New York.
14. Church, G. M. and Gilbert, W. (1984) Genomic sequencing. *Proc. Natl. Acad. Sci. USA* **81,** 1991–1995.
15. Frohman, M. A., Dush, M. K., and Martin, G. R. (1988) Rapid production of full-length cDNAs from rare transcripts: Amplification using a single gene-specific oligonucleotide primer. *Proc. Natl. Acad. Sci. USA* **85,** 8998–9002.
16. Chenchik, A., Diachenko, L., Moqadam, F., Tarabykin, V., Lukyanov, S., and Siebert, P. D. (1996) Full-length cDNA cloning and determination of mRNA 5' and 3' ends by amplification of adaptor-ligated cDNA. *BioTechniques* **21,** 526–534.
17. Chirgwin, J. M., Przybyla, A. E., MacDonald, R. J., and Rutter, W. J. (1979) Isolation of biologically active ribonucleic acid from sources enriched in ribonucleases. *Biochemistry* **18,** 5294–5299.

25

Determination of Gene Function by Homologous Recombination Using Embryonic Stem Cells and Knockout Mice

Ahmed Mansouri

1. Introduction

A decade ago the first alteration of a gene using embryonic stem (ES) cells was performed in the mouse *(1)*. Since then ES cells have become a powerful tool to generate mutant mice for the analysis of gene function. These mutant mice (also called knockout mice) have provided new insights into normal and pathologic development to improve our knowledge and open new avenues into diagnostic and therapeutic fields.

ES cells are derived from the inner cell mass of the blastocyst and can be perpetuated in vitro. The appropriate maintenance of ES cells in vitro keeps them in an undifferentiated and pluripotent state. When reintroduced into the early embryo, ES cells contribute to all embryonic tissues, including the germline. Thus, they constitute an ideal vehicle for the introduction of foreign genetic information into the germline of the mouse.

The combination of ES cells with gene targeting by homologous recombination has created a new transgenic technology, to produce any desired genome alteration in the mouse *(2)*, ranging from point mutations to chromosomal translocations.

In this chapter, I describe a basic protocol for the use of ES cells to create knockout mice and explain the generation of the targeting vector, ES cell culture, introduction of the targeting construct into ES cells, screening for targeted clones, and the use of the aggregation procedure to produce chimeric mice to transmit the mutation to the mouse germline.

From: *Methods in Molecular Biology, vol. 175: Genomics Protocols*
Edited by: M. P. Starkey and R. Elaswarapu © Humana Press Inc., Totowa, NJ

2. Materials

1. 100X Antibiotics (penicillin/streptomycin) (Gibco-BRL Life Technologies GmbH, Karlsrahe, Germany).
2. Qiagen endotoxin-free kit (Qiagen, Crawley, West Sussex, UK).
3. Dulbecco's modified Eagle's medium (DMEM) (Gibco-BRL Life Technologies).
4. Fetal calf serum (FCS) (Gibco-BRL Life Technologies). Thaw in a water bath at 37°C and heat inactivate by incubating at 56°C for 30 min. Store in 50-mL aliquots at −20°C.
5. Gelatin (Sigma, Taufkirchen, Germany).
6. Geneticin (G418) (Gibco-BRL Life Technologies).
7. Gancyclovir (supplied by any pharmacy).
8. Glucose (Mallinckrodt Baker Deutschland Zweigniederlassung der Mallinckrodt Chemical GmbH, Griesheim, Germany).
9. Glutamine (Gibco-BRL Life Technologies).
10. Leukemia inhibitory factor (LIF) (Gibco-BRL Life Technologies).
11. β-Mercaptoethanol (Sigma).
12. Mitomycin C (Sigma).
13. Nonessential amino acids (Chemicon).
14. Phenol red (Sigma).
15. Proteinase K (La Roche Diagnostics GmbH, Mannheim, Germany).
16. Na pyruvate (Mallinckrodt Baker).
17. Trypsin (Difco, 1 :250) (Gibco-BRL Life Technologies).
18. Dissecting microscope.
19. 500-mL Erlenmeyer flask containing 50 mL of glass beads (3 mm diameter) and a stirring bar.
20. Tissue culture dishes (3.5, 6, 8.5, and 14.5 cm) (Becton Dickinson, Cowley, Oxford, UK).
21. V-bottomed 15- and 50-mL Falcon tubes (Becton Dickinson).
22. Embryonic day 13–15 (e13–e15) embryos.
23. Tweezers and scissors.
24. Gene Pulser and electroporation cuvets (Bio-Rad, Munchen, Germany).
25. Darning needle.
26. 37 C Warming plate (Minitüb Afüll und Labortechnik GmbH und CoKG, Tiefenbach, Germany).
27. Pasteur pipets.
28. Hemocytometer.
29. Mineral oil (cat. no. M-8410; Sigma).
30. Phosphate-buffered saline (PBS): 8.0 g of NaCl, 0.2 g of KCl, 1.15 g of $Na_2HPO_4 \cdot 2H_2O$, and 0.2 g of KH_2PO_4. Dissolve in H_2O, adjust the pH to 7.2, and adjust the volume to 1000 mL. Autoclave and store at room temperature.
31. Saline/EDTA: 8.0 g of NaCl, 0.2 g of KCl, 1.15 g of $Na_2HPO_4 \cdot 2H_2O$, 0.2 g of KH_2PO_4, and 0.2 g of EDTA (disodium salt). Dissolve in distilled water, adjust the pH to 7.2 and add H_2O to a total volume of 1000 mL. Autoclave and store at room temperature.

32. Trypsin solution: 8.0 g of NaCl, 0.4g of KCl, 0.1 g of $Na_2HPO_4·2H_2O$, 1.0 g of glucose, 3.0 g of Trizma base, 0.01g of phenol red, and 2.50 g of trypsin; dissolve in H_2O, adjust the pH to 7.6, and add H_2O to 1000 mL. Filter sterilize and keep in 10-mL aliquots at –20°C. For use, dilute 1:4 with saline/EDTA and store ready for use 10-mL aliquots at –20°C.

33. ES medium: DMEM containing 4.5 g/L of glucose, 2 mM β-mercaptoethanol, 2 mM glutamine, 1 % (v/v) stock solution of non essential amino acids, 1 mM Na pyruvate, 15% (v/v) FCS, and 500 U/mL of LIF.

34. Fibroblast medium or Emfis medium: DMEM containing 2 mM glutamine and 10% (v/v) serum. Prepare 500 mL by adding 5 mL of glutamine and 50 mL of FCS to 445 mL of DMEM. For convenience, the same medium but with the addition of 4.5 g of glucose is used for fibroblast culture.

35. Fibroblast medium containing antibiotics: Mix 440 mL of DMEM, 5 mL of glutamine, 5 mL of 100X antibiotics, and 50 mL of FCS.

36. Gelatin solution: Add 1000 mL of H_2O to 1 g of gelatin, autoclave, and store at 4°C.

37. Inactivation medium for fibroblasts (mitomycin C): Resuspend 2 mg of mitomycin C in PBS and filter sterilize. Add 1 mL of mitomycin solution to 100 mL of Emfis medium (final concentration 100 µg/mL), and store the inactivation medium in 20-mL aliquots at –20°C.

38. Freezing medium: Add 1 mL of FCS and 1 mL of dimethylsulfoxide to 8 mL of ES medium.

39. G418 solution: Resuspend G418 in PBS containing 10 mM HEPES (pH 7.2) at a concentration of 250 mg/mL, sterilize by filtration, and store in 1-mL aliquots at –20°C. The G418 potency varies between batches and should be checked before use to find the minimal concentration needed to kill untransfected ES cells.

40. Gancyclovir: Dissolve in distilled water at a concentration of 2 mM, sterilize by filtration, and store in 1-mL aliquots at –20°C. For selection, add to ES medium at a 1:1000 dilution (working concentration of 2 µM).

41. Lysis buffer: 100 mM Tris-HCl, pH 8.5; 5 mM EDTA; 0.2% (w/v) sodium dodecyl sulfate (SDS), 200 mM NaCl; and 100 µg/mL of proteinase K.

42. Proteinase K: Resuspend at a concentration of 10 mg/mL in 10 mM HCl and store at –20°C.

43. Acidic Tyrode solution: 8 g of NaCl, 0.2 g of KCl, 0.24 g of $CaCl_2·2H_2O$, 0.1 g of $MgCl_2·6.H_2O$, 1 g of glucose, and 4 g of polyvinylpyrrolidone. Adjust the pH to 2.5 with 1 M HCl, filter sterilize, and store at 4°C.

44. M2 and M16 media (Sigma); *see* also **ref. 3**.

3. Methods

3.1. Targeting Construct

The targeting construct consists of two domains with homology to the gene to be targeted, one at the 5' end and the other at the 3' end. A selection marker is inserted between these parts (**Fig. 1**). The neomycin resistance gene (*neo*) is

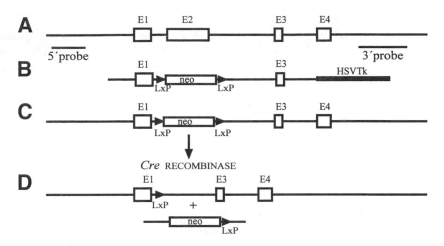

Fig. 1. Basic targeting construct using the positive-negative selection procedure (PNS). **(A)** Genomic organization of the normal allele. **(B)** Targeting construct. The second exon is replaced by the neomycin resistance gene (*neo*). *neo* is flanked by LoxP sites and can be excised by the Cre recombinase in ES cells or in mice. The HSVtk as a negative selection marker is placed outside of the homologous region on the 3' end of the construct. **(C)** Knockout allele, where *neo* is still present. **(D)** Knockout allele where the *neo* has been excised by the Cre recombinase. The final knockout allele carries a deletion of exon 2 and one remaining LoxP site. 5' and 3' external probes are indicated.

usually used, which allows selection with Geneticin (G418) to kill all the cells that have not stably integrated the targeting construct. In the first generation of targeting vectors, the *neo* gene was inserted to interrupt or replace deleted coding sequences in order to abolish gene function *(2)*. However, it turned out recently that the *neo* promoter/enhancer of the PGKneo may act on neighboring genes and, hence, may interfere with the phenotype *(4)*. Therefore, it is advisable to remove the *neo* gene, once homologous recombination has occurred.

The second generation of targeting vectors is designed to introduce the desired mutation into the locus of interest and to remove the selection marker in a subsequent step (**Fig. 1**). This is accomplished by the site-specific recombination system of the phage P1. DNA sequences that are flanked by LoxP sites (34 bp) can be recognized by the Cre recombinase of the phage P1 and are excised (**Fig. 1**). The Cre recombinase has been shown to perform recombination at LoxP sites in bacteria and eukaryotic cells and has already been successfully used in ES cells *(5,6)*.

The targeting frequency varies between loci and is influenced by at least two factors: the size of the genomic fragments included in the construct *(7)* and the origin of the DNA *(8)*. Optimal frequencies are achieved by including not less than 10 kb as the length of homology to the endogenous locus. In addition, the length of the genomic DNA on either side should not be <1.5 kb. Furthermore, the generation of the targeting construct by using isogenic DNA isolated from the 129 Sv genomic library, the mouse strain that from which most ES cell lines are derived, results in higher targeting frequencies.

To optimize further the homologous recombination frequency, the positive-negative selection (PNS) procedure may be used *(9)*. It is designed to select against random integrations. Basically, the herpes simplex thymidine kinase gene (*tk*) is added on either side of the homologous domains of the construct (**Fig. 1**). When homologous recombination occurs, sequences outside of the regions of homology are excluded from the integration into the locus. Therefore, a second selection with gancyclovir will kill all the cells that have retained the *tk* gene (random integration events). However, in practical terms only enrichment factors of optimize- to 10-fold are achieved.

1. Prepare targeting construct DNA using the Qiagen endo-free kit, according to the manufacturer's instructions.
2. Linearize the targeting construct by digestion with a restriction enzyme cleaving outside the region of homology, or excise it and separate it from the cloning vector by agarose gel electrophoresis.
3. Purify the DNA by extraction with an equal volume of phenol/chloroform, precipitate with 1/10 vol of 3 M sodium acetate and 2.5 vol of 100% (v/v) ethanol, and resuspend in 10 mM Tris-HCl (pH 8.0) 1 mM EDTA at 0.5 µg/µL. Before electroporation, confirm DNA quality by agarose gel electrophoresis.

3.2. Embryonic Fibroblasts (Emfis)

1. Prepare e13–e15 mouse embryos (*see* **Note 1**) in PBS, and using tweezers pull out soft tissues including liver and intestine leaving only the carcasses. Wash the carcasses in PBS to remove blood.
2. Mince the carcasses into small pieces in 5 mL of trypsin and transfer into a 500-mL Erlenmeyer flask containing glass beads and a magnetic stirring bar. Add trypsin to a total volume of 50 mL.
3. Trypsinize for 30 min at 37°C and gently agitate using the magnetic stirrer.
4. Remove the cell suspension using a wide-poured 25-mL pipet and transfer to a 50-mL tube, leaving the cell clumps in the flask.
5. Add 50 mL of trypsin to the flask containing the remaining cell clumps and repeat **step 3**.
6. Centrifuge the cell suspension from **step 4** at 160*g* for 10 min, and resuspend the cell pellet in 40 mL of fibroblast medium containing antibiotics.
7. Collect the second cell suspension (**step 5**) from the flask and centrifuge for 10 min at 160*g*. Resuspend the pellet in 40 mL of fibroblast medium.

8. Pool the cells from **steps 6** and **7** and plate in 14.5-cm tissue culture dishes (cells from two embryos/dish). Incubate overnight at 37°C.

9. Aspirate the medium and replace with 20 mL of fresh fibroblast medium containing antibiotics. Incubate at 37°C.

10. When confluent (usually after 2 d) trypsinize the cells by adding 12 mL of PBS to each tissue culture dish to wash the cells and remove the remaining medium. Remove the PBS, add 5 mL of trypsin, and incubate for 5 min at room temperature until the cells start to detach from the surface of the tissue culture dish. Using a 10-mL pipet, pipet the cells up and down until a homogeneous suspension (without lumps) is produced. Add 7.5 mL of fibroblast medium, mix well, and transfer to a 50-mL tube. Add an additional 7.5 mL of fibroblast medium to each dish to take up the remaining cells, and transfer to the 50-mL tube.

11. Take a 1-mL aliquot of trypsinized cells and culture fibroblasts for three passages (*see* **Note 2**) in a 6-cm tissue culture dish to ensure that the prepared batch is not contaminated.

12. Harvest the remaining trypsinized cells (from **step 10**) by centifugation at 160*g* for 5 min. Resuspend the contents of each 50-mL tube in 5 mL of freezing medium and store five 1-mL aliquots of each at –20°C.

3.3. Inactivation of Embryonic Fibroblasts by Mitomycin C

Before being used as a feeder layer for ES cell culture, embryonic fibroblasts should be inactivated with mitomycin C.

1. For routine culture of ES cells, thaw one vial of fibroblasts in an 8.5-cm tissue culture dish and incubate at 37°C. When confluent, treat the cells with trypsin (as described in **Subheading 3.2., step 10**) subdivide between four 8.5-cm tissue culture dishes, and culture at 37°C. When confluent, trypsinize the cells in each of the four dishes, and subdivide the contents of each into one 14.5-cm tissue culture dishes, and incubate at 37°C. When the cells reach confluence proceed to **step 2**.

2. Thaw fibroblast inactivation medium (10 mL for each 14.5-cm confluent dish of cells).

3. For each dish of confluent cells, replace the fibroblast medium with 10 mL of fibroblast inactivation medium and incubate the cells at 37°C for 2.5 h.

4. Remove the inactivation medium from each dish, and wash the cells (attached to the tissue culture dish) carefully twice with 10 mL of PBS. Add 20 mL of fresh fibroblast medium to each dish, or proceed directly to **step 6**.

5. Gelatinize (*see* **Note 3**) 8.5-cm tissue culture dishes by covering their surface with gelatin solution for at least 15 min at room temperature. Remove the gelatin solution and leave the coated surfaces to air-dry.

6. Trypsinize the cells (**Subheading 3.2., step 10**), resuspending the contents of each tissue culture dish (4.5×10^6 cells) in 10 mL of fibroblast medium, and plate in a gelatinized dish at a density of 8×10^4 cells/cm^2 (*see* **Note 4**). Freeze the inactivated fibroblasts in liquid nitrogen (*see* **Note 5**).

3.4. Culture of ES Cells

To keep the ES cells in an undifferentiated pluripotent state, it is necessary to maintain them routinely on a fibroblast feeder layer and in medium containing LIF. Inactivated embryonic fibroblasts should be used within 1 wk after plating. ES cells are usually subcultured every second or third day (we subculture our cells on Mondays, Wednesdays, and Fridays). When the cells reach 50–60% confluency, 1/5 or 1/8 of the cells are plated on a new dish. To avoid differentiation, it is recommended to get an almost single cell suspension after trypsin treatment. Most of the ES cell lines are cultured in medium with 15% heat-inactivated (*see* **Subheading 2., item 4**) FCS, except for RI cells (provided by Dr. A. Nagy, Mount Sinai Hospital in Toronto), which are cultured in 20% inactivated FCS.

3.4.1. Trypsinization of ES Cells

1. Aspirate ES medium from the plate when ES cells have grown to 50–60% confluency and wash once with PBS.
2. Add trypsin/EDTA solution (2, 1, and 0.5 mL for 8.5-, 6-, and 3.5-cm tissue culture dishes, respectively) and incubate at 37°C for 5 min.
3. After 5 min of incubation, cells should detach from the bottom of a dish. Add 1, 0.5, and 0.3 mL of ES medium per 8.5-, 6-, and 3.5-cm tissue culture dishes, respectively, and pipet up and down with a plugged Pasteur pipet, to get a homogeneous cell suspension that is mostly single cells.
4. Add 7, 4, and 3 mL of ES medium per 8.5-, 6, and 3.5-cm tissue culture dishes, respectively) to stop trypsinization. Then resuspend and centrifuge for 5 min at 160*g*.
5. Remove the supernatant and resuspend the cells in fresh ES medium.
6. Remove 1/5 or 1/8 of the cells (this may vary with the ES cell line used and serum batches) and plate on freshly inactivated feeder cells (**Subheading 3.3.**).
7. On the following day, replace half of the medium with fresh ES medium.
8. On the second day, process the cells again as described in **steps 1–6**.

3.5. Gene-Targeting Experiment

3.5.1. Electroporation

One week before electroporation, thaw fibroblast feeder cells and passage (*see* **Note 2**) twice as described in **Subheading 3.3., steps 1–6**. The ES cell culture should be started early enough in order to have at least one plate of ES cells ready for electroporation, 1 or 2 d after feeder inactivation. One 8.5-cm plate of ES cells is usually enough for one electroporation.

1. After inactivation of the fibroblasts (*see* **Subheading 3.3., steps 1–4**), prepare five to six 8.5-cm feeder plates (*see* **Subheading 3.3., step 6**), which are needed for each electroporation. The feeder cells should be prepared from embryo carry-

ing a neomycin phosphotransferase transgene to confer resistance to the selection drug G418 (*see* **Note 1**).

2. On the morning of the day of electroporation, aspirate the medium from the ES cell plate and add fresh ES medium.

3. Remove the medium from the 8.5-cm feeder plates and add 6 mL of ES medium to each plate.

4. Four hours later, trypsinize the ES cells as described in **Subheading 3.4., step 2**, but wash the cells twice with PBS before adding trypsin/EDTA solution. Stop trypsin action by adding ES medium to 10 mL, and centrifuge the cell suspension at 160g for 5 min.

5. Remove the supernatant and resuspend the cells in 30 mL of PBS. Take an aliquot to determine cell number (should be 1 to 1.5 × 10^7 cells). Centrifuge again for 5 min at 160g.

6. Resuspend the cell pellet in 0.85 mL of PBS and add 25–30 μg of targeting construct (see **Subheading 3.1.**) and stand for 5 min at room temperature.

7. Resuspend the cells again by pipetting carefully up and down and transfer 0.8 mL to one electroporation cuvet avoiding the creation of air bubbles.

8. Electroporate with one pulse of 500 μF and 250 V at room temperature (pulse time is about 7 ms). Stand at room temperature for 5 min.

9. With a plugged Pasteur pipet, transfer the cells to a 50-mL tube containing 20 mL of ES medium. Resuspend thoroughly and distribute into five 8.5-cm feeder plates. Use plate 6 for control ES cells (electroporated without DNA) at the same cell density.

10. Twenty-four hours after electroporation, start selection by replacing the medium with ES medium containing G418, or G418 plus gancyclovir (*see* **Note 6**) if using the PNS procedure (*see* **Subheading 3.1.** and **ref. 9**). In the latter case, select one plate of electroporated cells containing DNA with ES medium containing only G418 to check the enrichment factor.

11. Change the medium daily.

12. Three days after electroporation, thaw new fibroblast feeder cells in order to have enough fibroblasts for inactivation to seed the clones generated from electroporation.

13. In the case of the PNS procedure, on the fifth day after starting selection replace the medium with fresh ES medium plus G418.

14. Inactivate fibroblast feeder cells (*see* **Subheading 3.3.**) and prepare several 24-well microtiter plates (*see* **Subheading 3.3., step 6** and **Note 4**) for seeding the picked ES colonies.

3.5.2. Picking ES Clones

1. On d 8 of selection, check the selection plates for resistant colonies, and mark them. In the control plate, there should be no ES cells left.

2. Prepare two 96-well microtiter plates, one with 40 μL of trypsin/EDTA in each well and the other with 250 μL of ES medium in each well (**Fig. 2**).

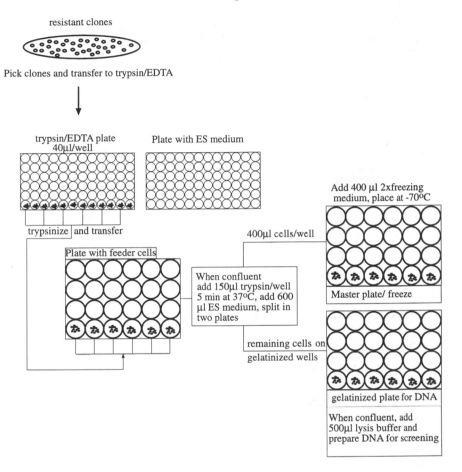

Fig. 2. Scheme of how clones are picked and further processed until freezing and screening.

3. Add 1 mL of ES medium containing 100 µg/mL of G418 to each well of the 24-well plates (from **Subheading 3.5.1., step 14**) containing inactivated fibroblast feeder cells.

4. Clean a dissecting microscope with 70% (v/v) ethanol and place under a flow hood.

5. Using a micropipet with 10-µL micropipet tips, pick every marked colony (*see* **Note 7**) and transfer to one well of the 96-well plate containing trypsin/EDTA (handle 24 colonies in one step). Incubate for 5 min at 37°C.

6. Using a 12-channel micropipet, add 40 µL of ES medium (from the second 96-well plate) to each well of the trypsinized colonies, pipet up and down to desegregate the cells, and transfer to the 24-well plate containing the inactivated

fibroblast feeder cells. Use only six channels of the multichannel pipet (every second channel is left empty) to ensure the transfer of trypsinized cells from alternate wells of the 96-well plate into one row of 6 wells of the 24-well plate. Repeat the procedure two times to ensure the transfer of most of the cells, before proceeding to transfer another six trypsinized colonies to the second row of the 24-well inactivated fibroblast feeder cell plate. Mix well and place at 37°C.

7. Replace the medium with fresh ES medium the next day.
8. When the cells are confluent, prepare 24-well gelatinized plates (as described in **Subheading 3.3., step 5**) and add 500 μL of ES medium to each well.
9. To trypsinize the cells, aspirate the medium and wash each well with 500 μL of PBS. Add 150 μL of trypsin/EDTA to each well and incubate for 5 min at 37°C.
10. When cells start to detach from the surface, add 600 μL of ES medium to each well and mix thoroughly using a 2-mL pipet. Remove 400 μL from each well and transfer to separate wells in a new 24-well plate. Add the remaining trypsinized cells in each well to a separate well of a gelatinized plate (this plate will serve to make DNA for the analysis for recombinant clones) (**Fig. 2**).
11. To the nongelatinized plate containing 400-μL aliquots of trypsinized cells, add 400 μL of 2X freezing medium to each well, mix carefully to homogeneity, cover with a plastic bag and paper, and place in a box at –70°C (this plate henceforth becomes the master plate).

3.6. Preparation of Genomic DNA for Screening

Prepare DNA from confluent ES cells that have been grown on the gelatinized plates.

1. Aspirate the medium from each well and add 500 μL of lysis buffer containing 100 μg/mL of proteinase K.
2. Leave overnight or for at least 6 h at 37°C.
3. Transfer the 500 μL of DNA from each well to a 1.5-mL Eppendorf tube, and add 500 μL of isopropanol for DNA precipitation. Mix well and let stand for a few minutes at room temperature.
4. Centrifuge at 13,000g for 10 min at room temperature and aspirate the supernatants.
5. Add 500 μL of 70% (v/v) ethanol to wash each DNA pellet, and centrifuge at 13,000g for 5 min at room temperature.
6. Aspirate the supernatants and air-dry the pellets. Resuspend each pellet in 100 μL of 1 mM Tris-HCl (pH 8.0) and 0.1 mM EDTA. Incubate at 37°C overnight.
7. Digest 20 μL of each DNA with an appropriate restriction enzyme in a total volume of 40 μL (*see* **Note 8**) and prepare a Southern blot.
8. Screen the Southern filter with probes (*see* **Note 9**) external to the targeting construct (**Fig. 1**). Homologous recombinant clones should be confirmed by both 5' and 3' external probes in order to exclude insertions. Further hybridizations with *neo* and internal probes are also recommended to exclude additional integrations.

3.7. Removal of neo Cassette from the Targeted Locus by the Cre-Recombinase in ES Cells

Once positive clones are confirmed, the neomycin resistance gene can be removed in ES cells.

1. Electroporate (*see* **Subheading 3.5.1.**) 10^7 ES cells with 25 µg of supercoiled Cre plasmid (we used PGK-Cre driven by the PGK promoter), and plate onto one 14.5-cm tissue culture dish containing inactivated feeder cells.
2. After 48 h, trypsinize the cells (*see* **Subheading 3.4.1.**) and plate 10^3 cells onto each of four 8.5-cm tissue culture dishes containing inactivated feeder cells. Freeze the remaining cells. Pick colonies when they become visible and of reasonable size (it takes about 4 d), and proceed as described in **Subheading 3.5.2.**
3. Check the positive clones (*see* **Note 10**) for their sensitivity to G418, by culturing one aliquot in a 96-well plate containing ES medium plus G418.
4. Prepare DNA (**Subheading 3.6.**) from the positive clones, digest with an appropriate restriction enzyme, and screen a Southern blot using a probe external to the targeting construct and a *neo* cassette.
5. Proceed to aggregation or blastocyst injection to generate chimeric mice.

3.8. Generation of Chimeric Mice

3.8.1. ES Cells

Chimeric mice may be generated by blastocyst injection (*10*) or morulae aggregation. However, aggregation is less complicated and less expensive. In my hands, R1 ES cells are the most suitable for aggregation.

1. Prepare 3.5-cm plates with inactivated fibroblast feeder cells (*see* **Subheading 3.3.**).
2. Prewarm ES medium at 37°C.
3. Remove the 24-well master plate (*see* **Subheading 3.5.2.**, **step 11**) containing the positive clones from the –70°C freezer and place under a flow hood (*see* **Note 11**).
4. Quickly add 1 mL of prewarmed ES medium to the well containing a positive clone, carefully pipet up and down four times and put into a 15-mL tube. Add a further 1 mL of ES medium to the appropriate well of the master plate, pipet up and down until all the remaining cells are thawed, and transfer to the 15-mL tube. Wash the well twice with 1 mL of ES medium, and add to the cells in the 15-mL tube.
5. Add ES medium to a total volume of 10 mL and mix well.
6. Centrifuge at 160*g* for 5 min.
7. Carefully aspirate the medium (the pellet is very small), resuspend the cells in 2 mL of ES medium, and plate onto a 3.5-cm feeder plate.
8. When confluent, process the cells as described in **Subheading** 3.4. Freeze some stocks by adding an equal volume of 2X freezing medium.

3.8.2. Aggregation to Generate Chimeric Mice

Before starting aggregation, prepare the following plates and store them at 37°C.

3.8.2.1. AGGREGATION PLATE

1. Spot 13 8 μL microdrops of aggregation medium (M16 medium + 2% [v/v] ES cell medium for C57B1/6 and 4% [v/v] ES cell medium for CD-1 or NMRI embryos) onto the bottom of a 3.5-cm tissue culture dish and cover with mineral oil.
2. Leave the 2 upper drops for the cells (*see* **Fig. 3**), and using the darning needle, make six holes (depressions in the plastic) under each of the remaining 11 drops. Each depression is designed for one embryo.

3.8.2.2. WASHING PLATES

Spot 15 10 μL microdrops of aggregation medium onto the bottom of two 3.5-cm tissue culture dishes and cover with mineral oil (**Fig. 3**).

3.8.2.3. ZONA-REMOVING PLATE

Subdivide a 3.5-cm tissue culture into three parts (*see* **Fig. 3**). In the top third, spot four to five 10-μL microdrops of M2 medium. In the middle third, spot three rows of 10-μL microdrops of acidic Tyrode solution, and in the bottom third, spot three 10-μL microdrops of M2 medium.

3.8.2.4. PREPARATION OF THE EMBRYOS FOR AGGREGATION

We use superovulated mice (C57B1/6 or CD–1) to prepare eight-cell embryos. Normally 10–15 mice are hormone-treated for each day of aggregation (4 d/wk) so that 80 embryos can be aggregated every day.

1. Kill the mice by dislocation.
2. Using a dissecting microscope and a 37°C warming plate, dissect out the oviducts and place in PBS.
3. Flush out eight-cell embryos into a new dish using M2 medium and a syringe with a small needle (minimum 33 gage) suitable for the infundibulum (*see* **Note 12**).
4. Collect the embryos using a forged Pasteur pipet (*see* **Note 13**). Wash the embryos in M2 medium by moving from one drop to another.

3.8.2.5. REMOVAL OF THE ZONE PELLUCIDA

1. Transfer the embryos to the lower row of M2 medium microdrops in the zona-removing plate. Process 5–10 embryos rapidly through consecutive rows of the tyrode solution. Stop at the last drop and wait (~10 s) until the zone is gone (*see* **Note 14**) before transferring (immediately) to the upper rows containing M2

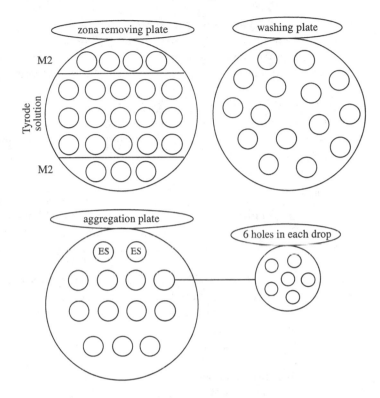

Fig. 3. Scheme of the aggregation procedure to generate chimeric mice.

medium. Pass the embryos through two to three drops of the M2 medium to wash away the acidic Tyrode solution.

2. Transfer the embryos without zone to a washing plate and wash three to four times through aggregation medium (by transferring embryos from one drop to the next).
3. Transfer six embryos to each drop in the aggregation plate, and place them beside the holes created with the darning needle. Incubate at 37°C.

3.8.2.6. PREPARATION OF THE ES CELLS FOR AGGREGATION

ES cells are normally thawed and subcultured once before being used in aggregation. Confluent cells are not suitable for aggregation. About 40% confluence is recommended. I use 3.5-cm plates for aggregation cultures.

1. Wash ES cells with PBS.
2. Add 0.5 mL of trypsin/EDTA and incubate for 3 to 4 min, depending on the desired size of the ES cell aggregates.
3. Check the size of the cell clumps under the microscope, keeping in mind that clumps of 2–5 cells are required for C57Bl/6 and clumps of 10–15 cells are

required for CD-1 or NMRI embryos. Add 6 mL of ES medium and mix gently enough to retain clumps of appropriate cell number (2–5 or 10–15).

4. Under the dissecting microscope and using a 100-μm pulled Pasteur pipet (for collection of embryos), select cell aggregates of suitable size (according to the host embryo.

5. When sufficient ES cell aggregates are collected, transfer them to one washing plate and transfer successively through three to four drops of aggregation medium.

6. Transfer all the washed ES cell aggregates to an aggregation plate, and place them in the upper two drops (**Fig. 3**) of aggregation medium that do not have holes beneath them.

3.8.2.7. AGGREGATION

1. In the aggregation plate, transfer (using a forged Pasteur pipet) at least six ES cell aggregates to each drop of aggregation medium containing embryos. Drop each cell aggregate softly into one of the six holes beneath each microdrop so that they sink into the middle of a hole.

2. Carefully bring each embryo (*see* **Subheading 3.8.2.5., step 3**) to one hole, and softly place an ES cell aggregate into the hole so that the ES cell aggregate gets attached to the embryo. Use a forged Pasteur pipet to softly push the embryo down into the hole and ensure that the embryos and cells get attached.

3. Check that all the embryos are still in the holes and well attached to the ES cells. Incubate overnight at 37°C (*see* **Note 15**).

4. Transfer the embryos to pseudopregnant females.

5. At d 19.5 of gestation (day of transfer is referred to as d 2.5) check mice for delivery. Mice that are pregnant and do not deliver should be opened by Caesarean **Subheading** and the embryos transferred to a second foster mother for nursing (*see* **Note 16.**).

3.9. Genotyping of Knockout Mice

To genotype knockout mice, a tail biopsy must be performed. For the first generation of mice, check by Southern blot hybridization using probes external to the targeting construct. Once the knockout line is established polymerase chain reaction (PCR) screening, is advisable.

1. Cut 0.5 cm off a tail of a 3-wk-old mouse. Cover the tail with 500 μL of lysis buffer containing 100 μg/mL of proteinase K and incubate at 55°C overnight.

2. Centrifuge for 5 min and carefully transfer the supernatant to a tube containing 500 μL of isopropanol. Mix thoroughly and let stand at room temperature for a few minutes.

3. Using a micropipet tip, transfer the pellet to a new tube containing 600 μL of 70% (v/v) ethanol. Centrifuge at 13,000g for 5 min at room temperature.

4. Aspirate the supernatant and air dry the pellet. Resuspend in 100 μL of 1 mM Tris-HCl (pH 8.0) and 0.1 mM EDTA. Incubate overnight at 37°C, and use 10 μL for digestion with the appropriate restriction enzyme (*see* **Note 17**).

3.10. Fast Protocol for Preparing DNA from Tails for PCR Screening

DNA prepared using this fast protocol (Beier, D. and Rabeler, R., personal communication) is not suitable for Southern blot analysis.

1. Cut 0.5 cm off a tail of a 3-wk-old mouse and transfer to 600 μL of 50 mM NaOH.
2. Heat at 95°C for 10 min, vortex, and neutralize with 50 μL of 1 M Tris-HCl, pH 8.0.
3. Centrifuge at 13,000g for 6 min, and transfer the supernatant to a fresh tube.
4. Employ 5 μL of the supernatant in a 50-μL PCR reaction featuring primers flanking the targeting construct.

4. Notes

1. I use NMRI outbred strain for normal ES culture and NMRI females that have been mated to a homozygous male carrying a neomycin resistance transgene when ES cells are electroporated and selected with G418.
2. The term *passage* (or *subculture*) means to treat cells with trypsin and when confluent, or have achieved a certain density, subdivide them among new tissue culture dishes. Three passages represents a repetition of this process three times.
3. Tissue culture dishes are gelatinized to enable optimal attachment of fibroblasts. Gelatinized 3.5-cm dishes are used for routine culture of ES cells, being processed for aggregation. Gelatinized 8.5-cm dishes are used to culture ES cells prior to electroporation, or to make stocks for freezing.
4. Alternatively, plate each aliquot of 4.5 × 10^6 trypsinized inactivated fibroblasts in 32 wells of gelatinized 24-well plates by resuspending the trypsinized inactivated fibroblasts in 16 mL of fibroblast medium and adding 0.5 mL to each of 32 wells of gelatinized 24-well plates.
5. I usually freeze inactivated cells from one 14.5-cm tissue culture dish in one vial. To thaw frozen inactivated feeder cells, quickly warm the vial at 37°C, add 10 mL of fibroblast medium, mix well, take a small aliquot to count cells. Centrifuge the cells for 10 min at 160g. Plate the fibroblasts at 8 × 10^4 cells/cm^2, taking into account that about 15–20% are killed by the freezing procedure.
6. Gancyclovir selection is only necessary for the first 4 d.
7. About 200–300 colonies (depending upon the gene) should be picked to ensure enough homologous recombinant clones. In most cases, I find that between one quarter and one half of the clones are double selected clones (having survived both G418 and gancyclovir selection). Big ES cell colonies should be picked immediately, because if left to get too large, they tend to differentiate.
8. Two clones can be screened simultaneously by pooling 15 μL of each of the two DNAs.
9. The external probes for Southern hybridization should be screened for repetitive sequences by screening wild-type genomic DNA restricted with the same restriction enzyme as that used to digest the DNA prepared from the positive ES cells. Repetitive sequences can ultimately be blocked with denatured mouse genomic DNA.

10. Usually about 10% of the clones are positive.
11. Sometimes when the ES-positive clones are thawed, only a few colonies are detected in the dish after a few days of culture. In this case, do not subculture the cells—just trypsinize the cells and leave them in the same dish for another passage. In this way you can recover clones from a few cells.
12. The infundibulum is the part of the oviduct in which there is a natural opening; the needle of a syringe can be inserted and embryos flushed through the uterus for collection in a dish.
13. Soften the narrow end of a Pasteur pipet by rotating in a flame and pull out quickly to make a tube with an internal diameter of 150–200 μm. Break the end with a diamond point, and quickly pass the end through a flame for 2 s to round off the tip. Plug a 1-mL pipetting tip (mouthpiece) onto one end of a 30-cm piece of silicon tubing, and attach the forged Pasteur pipet at the other end.
14. Zona removal is very fast (10–15 s), and you should keep monitoring the embryos until transfer to M2 medium.
15. We usually get 90% of the embryos developed to the blastocyst stage by 2:00 PM the next day.
16. Second foster matings should always set up in parallel to the aggregation experiments.
17. When resuspending DNA from tail preparations, do not worry if a pellet is still present. The DNA can be digested with all the restriction enzymes that we have used (*Eco*RI, *Hin*dIII, *Bam*HI, *Xba*I, *Sac*I, *Pst*I, *Kpn*I).

Acknowledgments

I would like to thank Prof. P. Gruss for constant support and D. Treichel for reading the manuscript. This work was supported by the Max-Planck Society.

References

1. Schwartzberg, P. L., Goff, S. P., and Robertson, E. J. (1989) Germ-line transmission of a *c-abl* mutation produced by targeted gene disruption in ES cells. *Science* **246,** 799–803.
2. Capecchi, M. R. (1989) Altering the mouse genome by homologous recombination. *Science* **244,** 1288–1292.
3. Hogan, B., Beddington, R., Constantini, F., and Lacy, E., eds. (1994) In vitro culture. In: *Manipulating the Mouse Embryo: A Laboratory Manual,* 2nd ed., Cold Spring Harbor Laboratory, Cold Spring Harbor, NY, pp. 389–397.
4. Olson, E. N., Arnold, H. H., Rigby, P. W. J., and Wold, B. J. (1996) Know your neighbors: three phenotypes in Null mutants of myogenic bHLH gene MRF4. *Cell* **85,** 1–4.
5. Sauer, B. (1993) Manipulation of transgenes by site-specific recombination: use of Cre recombinase, in *Methods in Enzymology* (Wasserman, P. M. and DePamphilis, M. L., eds.), Academic, New York, pp. 890–900.

6. Hirota, H., Chen, J., Betz, U. A. K., Rajewsky, K., Gu, Y., Ross Jr., J., Muller, W., and Chien, K., R. (1999). Loss of a gp130 cardiac muscle cell survival pathway is a critical event in the onset of heart failure during biomechanical stress. *Cell* **97**, 189–198.

7. Deng, C. and Capecchi, M. R. (1992) Reexamination of gene targeting frequency as a function of the extent of homology between the targeting vector and the target locus. *Mol. Cell. Biol.* **12**, 3365–3371.

8. Riele, H. T., Maandag, E. R., and Berns, A. (1992) High efficiency gene targeting in embryonic stem cells through homologous recombination with isogenic DNA constructs. *Proc. Natl. Acad. Sci. USA* **89**, 5128–5132.

9. Mansour, S. L., Thomas, K. R., and Capecchi, M. R. (1988) Disruption of the protoncogene ins-2 in mouse embryo-derived stem cells: a general strategy for targeting mutations to non-selectable genes. *Nature* **336**, 348–352.

10. Robertson, E. J. (1987) Embryo-derived stem cell lines, in *Teratocarcinomas and Embryonic Stem Cells. A Practical Approach* (Robertson, E. J., ed.), IRL, Oxford, pp. 71–112.

26

Genomic Analysis Utilizing the Yeast Two-Hybrid System

Ilya G. Serebriiskii, Garabet G. Toby, Russell L. Finley, Jr., and Erica A. Golemis

1. Introduction

As the completion of genomc sequencing efforts leads to the definition of increasing numbers of genes, the need to reliably assign function to identified coding sequences becomes paramount. One means of gaining initial insight into the function of an undefined protein is to develop a map of other defined proteins with which it physically or functionally interacts. There are several approaches to assigning interacting protein groups. In suitable model organisms such as yeast, a traditional approach has been to create null mutations in the gene encoding the novel protein of interest, and to use suppressor analysis to identify genetically (functionally) interacting proteins. Alternatively, copurification of complexes of interest followed by use of mass spectrophotometry to assign identity of individual component protcins has been used to define interacting groups based on physical interactions. The genetic approaches offer speed and low cost; the physical approaches offer the certainty that copurified proteins physically function together on the protein level, rather than being connected via indirect regulatory pathways. A third approach, the yeast two-hybrid system, combines the advantages of working with yeast while targeting proteins that physically associate.

The idea of a yeast two-hybrid system was first proposed as a model for detecting protein-protein interactions in 1989 *(1)*; **Figure 1** presents a schematic representation of the system. In its most basic manifestation, two "hybrid" proteins are created. The first is a translational fusion of a known DNA-binding domain (DBD) to a protein of interest (bait). The second is a translational fusion of a transcriptional activation domain (AD) to either a

From: *Methods in Molecular Biology, vol. 175: Genomics Protocols*
Edited by: M. P. Starkey and R. Elaswarapu © Humana Press Inc., Totowa, NJ

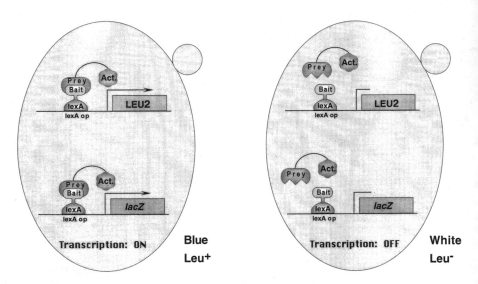

Fig. 1. Schematic of two-hybrid assay. Paradigm for two-hybrid system, in which interaction between AD-fused protein Y and DBD-fused protein X causes activation of a reporter gene under transcriptional control of binding sites for the DBD *(1)*. In the case of the Interaction Trap *(4)*, the activation domain is provided by the "acid blob" B42 *(20)* while the DBD is provided by the bacterial protein LexA *(21,22)*; activated reporter genes are LacZ, and *LEU2*.

library or a second known protein (prey). Both hybrids are expressed in a yeast strain that encompasses two or more reporter genes in which a DNA-binding site cognate to the utilized DBD serves as UAS (enhancer) sequence. Interaction between the two hybrid proteins, and binding of the DBD fusion protein to the reporters, moves the AD sequences in proximity to the reporter gene promoter, allowing transcription of the reporter gene.

From 1991 to 1993, several variants of the system were developed and shown to be suitable for identifying novel proteins from libraries based on physical interaction with bait proteins of interest *(2–5)*. The initial interest in these systems was on the part of individual investigators seeking to find partners for proteins of specific interest to their laboratories, and in the period of 1991–1998, more than 1000 articles appeared in the scientific literature demonstrating the suitability of the systems for such a goal. Beginning in 1994, with the description of an interaction mating strategy that allowed the rapid examination of interactions between sets of baits and preys, the two-hybrid system began to be adapted for genomic application *(6)*. In the last several years, demonstration projects have shown that large-scale application of the two-hybrid system can be used to solve the interactions of proteins within a (small) genome *(7)* or a functionally linked group of proteins *(8)*. Ongoing studies utilize two-hybrid techniques to generate interaction maps for *S. cerevisiae, C. elegans*, and *D. melanogaster.*

The system described below is based on the Interaction Trap two-hybrid system *(4)*. In this system, the DBD derives from LexA, a bacterial repressor protein; and the AD from the bacterial artificial activating sequence B42. The two reporter genes are LacZ and *LEU2*. The provided protocols first describe the execution of a directed two-hybrid library screen utilizing a single bait protein. These protocols divide the execution of an interaction trap/two-hybrid screen into three stages, as illustrated in **Fig. 2**. In the first, characterization of a novel bait is described, with attention to controls to increase the likelihood that it will function effectively in a two-hybrid screen. In parallel, transformation of a cDNA library is also delineated. In the second, interaction mating with a pretransformed library and selection of positive interactors is detailed. In the third, a number of control experiments aimed to establish significance of interaction are outlined. Subsequently, a discussion of the manner in which these basic screening tools can be adapted to genomic level applications is provided (**Subheading 3.4.** and **Note 1**).

2. Materials

Interaction Trap reagents represent the work of many contributors: many of the original basic reagents were developed in the Brent laboratory *(4)*, with contributions by J. Kamens (pJK plasmids), Steve Hanes (pSH plasmids), J. Gyuris (pJG plasmids, libraries), R. Finley (pRF plasmids, RFY strains), and E. Golemis (pEG plasmids, EGY strains), and subsequently in the Finley and Golemis (SKY strains; pGKS3 *[9]*) laboratories. Plasmids with altered antibiotic resistance markers (all pMW plasmids) were constructed at Glaxo, in Research Triangle Park, NC *(10)*. pNLexA was developed through the cumulative efforts of I. York, Dana-Farber Cancer Center, Boston; and M. Sainz and S. Nottwehr, University of Oregon. pGilda was developed by D. A. Shaywitz, MIT Center for Cancer Research, Cambridge. The majority of these reagents are available commercially, through sources including Invitrogen (Carlsbad, CA), Clontech (Palo Alto, CA), Origene (Rockville, MD), and DisplaySystems Biotech (Vista, CA). Some reagents can be acquired by request from the Golemis laboratory at Fox Chase Cancer Center (phone: 215-728–2860; fax: 215-728–3616; e-mail: ea_golemis@fccc.edu).

All the protocols utilize an overlapping set of reagents. Thus, all materials necessary for the three basic protocols are presented here.

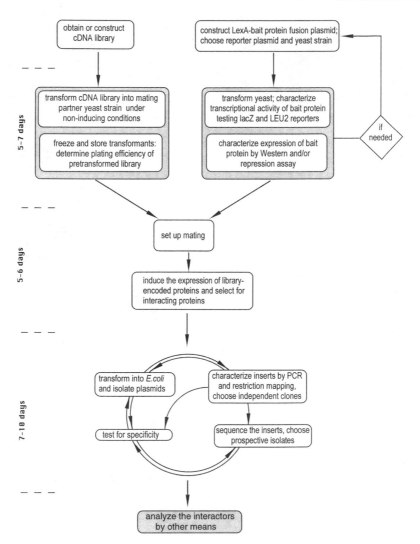

Fig. 2. Flowchart of the two-hybrid screen done by interaction mating. Direct transformation requires a different order of steps. Stage 3 allows flexibility in step order, shown in greater detail in **Fig. 5**. *See* text for details.

2.1. Plasmids

1. pJK202 and pMW103, *HIS3* plasmids for making LexA fusion protein with (JK202) or without (pMW103) an incorporated nuclear localization sequence. Expression is from the constitutive ADH promoter. The bacterial selective marker is ampicillin resistance (Ap^R) for pJK202 and kanamycin resistance (Km^R) for MW103.

2. pJG4-5, *TRP1* plasmid for making a nuclear localization sequence (AD) hemagglutinin epitope tag fusion to a unique protein or a cDNA library. Expression is from the GAL1 galactose-inducible promoter. The bacterial selective marker is Ap^R.

3. pMW111, pMW109, or pMW112: *URA3* plasmids containing 1, 2, or 8 LexA operators upstream of the LacZ reporter gene, respectively. The bacterial selective marker is Km^R.

4. pJK101: *URA3* UAS_{GAL}/LexA-operator/LacZ-reporter plasmid for repression assay. The bacterial selective marker is Ap^R.

5. pSH17-4: *HIS3* plasmid encoding LexA-GAL4, a strong positive control for activation. The bacterial selective marker is Ap^R.

6. pEG202-hsRPB7: *HIS3* plasmid encoding LexA-hsRPB7, a weak positive control for activation. The bacterial selective marker is Ap^R.

7. pRFHM1: *HIS3* plasmid encoding LexA-bicoid, a negative control for activation and positive control for repression. The bacterial selective marker is Ap^R.

8. pGKS3: *HIS3* plasmid, to complement yeast *his3* marker for positive control part of repression assay. The bacterial selective marker is Ap^R. Any *HIS3* yeast plasmid not expressing LexA can be substituted for this plasmid.

9. (Optional) pJK202: pGilda, pNLexA: plasmids related to pEG202 that incorporate a nuclear localization sequence into the LexA-fusion construct, are expressed from the inducible GAL1 promoter, or fuse LexA to the carboxy-terminal end of the test protein, respectively.

2.2. Strains

1. Yeast strain EGY48 *(MATα ura3 trpl his3 3LexAop-leu2)*.
2. Yeast strain EGY191 *(MATα ura3 trpl his3 1LexAop-leu2)*.
3. Yeast strain SKY473 *(MATa ura3 trpl his3 2LexAop-leu2 3cIop-lys2)*.
4. Yeast strain RFY206 *(MATa his3 D200 leu2-3 lys2D201 ura3-52 trplD: :hisG)*.
5. *Escherichia coli* strain KC8 *(pyrF leuB600 trpC hisB463)*.

2.3. Reagents for Lithium Acetate Transformation of Yeast

1. Sterile filtered 10 mM Tris-HCl, pH 8.0; 1 mM EDTA; 0.1 M lithium acetate.
2. Sterile filtered 10 mM Tris-HCl, pH 8.0; 1 mM EDTA, 0.1 M lithium acetate; 40% (w/v) PEG 4000.

2.4. Reagents for Minipreps/PCR from Yeast

1. STES lysis solution: 100 mM NaCl; 10 mM Tris-HCl, pH 8.0, 1 mM EDTA, 0.1% (w/v) SDS.
2. Acid-washed sterile glass beads, 0.15–0.45 mm diameter (e.g., cat. no. G-1145, Sigma, St. Louis, MO).
3. TE: 10 mM Tris-HCl, pH 8.0; 1 mM EDTA.
4. 1:50 β-glucuronidase type HP-2 (crude solution from *Helix pomatia*, Sigma): 50 mM Tris-HCl, pH 7.5; 10 mM EDTA; 0.3% (v/v) 2-mercaptoethanol (prepare fresh).

5. Reagents for polymerase chain reaction (PCR) (*see* **Subheading 3.3.1., step 4**):
   5 U/μL of *Taq* DNA polymerase, dNTP mix, PCR buffer, and $MgCl_2$ buffer (MBI
   Fermentas, Amherst, NY).
6. Reagents for PCR (*see* **Subheading 3.4.2., step 4**): 2.5 U/μL of high-fidelity
   thermostable *Pfu* DNA polymerase, dNTP mix and 10X PCR buffer including
   20 m*M* $MgCl_2$ (Stratagene, La Jolla, CA).

2.5. Reagents for β-Galactosidase Overlay Assays

X-Gal-agarose: 1% (w/v) low melting temperature agarose in 100 m*M*
$KHPO_4$, pH 7.0. Add 5-bromo–4-chloro–3-indolyl-β-D-galactopyranoside
(X-Gal) to 0.25 mg/mL when cooled to approx 60°C.

2.6. Solid Media Plates (100 mm diameter) for Growing Bacteria

1. Luria Bertani (LB) broth plus 1.5% (w/v) bacto-agar (cat. no. 0140-01; Difco;
   BD Biosciences, Sparks, MD) supplemented with 50 μg/mL of ampicillin.
2. KC8 plates for selecting library plasmids:
   a. Autoclave (121°C, 20 min) 1 L of dH_2O containing 15 g of bacto-agar (Difco),
      1 g of $(NH_4)_2SO_4$, 4.5 g of KH_2PO_4, 10.5 g of K_2HPO_4, and 0.5 g of sodium
      citrate·$2H_2O$. Cool to 50°C.
   b. Add 1 mL of sterile filtered 1 *M* $MgSO_4·7H_2O$; 10 mL of sterile filtered 20%
      (w/v) glucose; and 5 mL each of 40 μg/mL sterile filtered stocks of L-histidine,
      L-leucine, and uracil. Pour the medium into plates.

2.7. General Directions for Defined Minimal Yeast Media

Leaving out one or more nutrients selects for yeast able to grow in its
absence, i.e., containing a plasmid that covered the deficiency. Thus, "dropout
medium" lacking uracil (denoted -Ura in recipes given in **Subheadings 2.8.–2.10**)
would select for the presence of plasmids with the *URA3* marker, and so on.
The quantities of nutrients listed produce a quantity of dropout powder sufficient to make 40 L of medium; it is advisable to scale down this volume for
most of the dropout combinations listed in **Subheadings 2.8.–2.10**. Premade
dropout mixes are available from some commercial suppliers.

1. All minimal yeast media, liquid, and plates are based on the following three
   ingredients: 6.7 g/L of Yeast Nitrogen Base amino acids (cat. no. 0919-15; Difco),
   20 g of glucose (Glu) or 20 g of galactose (Gal) + 10 g of rafinose (Raff), and 2 g
   of appropriate nutrient "dropout" mix (*see* **item 2**). For solid media, 20 g of
   bacto-agar (Difco) is also added.
2. A complete minimal (CM) nutrient mix consists of the following: 2.5 g of
   adenine, 1.2 g of L-arginine, 6.0 g of L-aspartic acid, 6.0 g of L-glutamic acid,
   1.2 g of L-histidine (His), 1.2 g of L-isoleucine, 3.6 g of L-leucine (Leu), 1.8 g of
   L-lysine, 1.2 g of L-methionine, 3.0 g of L-phenylalanine, 22.0 g of L-serine,

12.0 g of L-threonine, 2.4 g of L-tryptophan, 1.8 g of L-tyrosine, 9.0 g of L-valine, and 1.2 g of uracil (Ura).

2.8. Solid Media Plates (100 mm diameter) for Growing Yeast

1. Defined minimal dropout plates with glucose as a carbon source: -Ura; -Trp; -Ura-His; -Ura-His-Trp; -Ura-His-Trp-Leu.
2. Defined minimal dropout plates with galactose + raffinose as a carbon source: -Ura-His-Trp-Leu.
3. YPD (rich medium): 10 g/L of yeast extract, 20 g/L of peptone, 20 g/L of glucose, 20 g/L of bacto-agar (Difco). Autoclave at 121°C for approx 18 min, and pour approx 40 plates.

2.9. Liquid Medium for Growing Yeast

1. Defined minimal dropout medium with glucose as a carbon source: -Ura-His; -Trp.
2. YPD: 10 g/L of yeast extract, 20 g/L of peptone, 20 g/L of glucose. Autoclave at 121°C for approx 15 min.

2.10. Solid Media Plates (240 × 240 mm) for Growing Yeast Library Transformations

Defined minimal dropout plates with glucose as a carbon source: -Ura-His-Trp. Each plate requires approx 250 mL of medium.

2.11. X-Gal Plates

In 900 mL of dH$_2$O, dissolve 6.7 g of Yeast Nitrogen Base-amino acids (Difco), 20 g of glucose or 20 g of galactose + 10 g of raffinose, 2 g of appropriate nutrient dropout mix (*see* **Subheading 2.7.**). Autoclave at 121°C for 20 min and allow to cool to approx 65°C. Add 100 mL of sterile filtered 10X BU salts (10X stock = 70 g/L of Na$_2$HPO$_4$·7H$_2$O, 30 g/L of NaH$_2$PO$_4$, with pH adjusted to 7.0, and filter sterilized), and 2 mL of 40 mg/mL X-Gal in dimethylformamide. After pouring, plates should be stored at 4°C and protected from light. Required X-Gal plates: -Ura-His, made with glucose; -Ura-His, made with galactose + raffinose.

2.12. Miscellaneous

1. Sterile glass beads, 3 to 4 mm (cat. no. 3000; Thomas Scientific, Swedesboro, NJ, or cat. no. 11-312A; Fisher, Pittsburgh, PA).
2. Sterile glycerol solution for freezing transformants: 65% (v/v) sterile glycerol; 0.1 *M* MgSO$_4$; 25 m*M* Tris-HCl, pH 8.0.
3. Insert grid from a rack of 200-μL micropipet tips (Rainin RT series; Alpha, Eastleigh, Hampshire, UK).
4. Metal frogger with 96 spokes in a 12 × 8 configuration (e.g., cat. no. MC48; Dankar, Reading, MA).

5. Plastic replicators with 48 spokes in a 6 × 8 configuration (e.g., Bel-Blotter cat. no. 378776-0002; Bel-Art, Pequannock, NJ; or cat. no. 1371213; Fisher Scientific).
6. 96-Well cluster tubes (Costar; Corning, Acton, MA).
7. 50 mL Polypropylene tubes (Falcon; Fisher).
8. Velvet replica plating pad (Clontech Laboratories Inc.).
9. *Hae*III (10 U/μL) (New England Biolabs, Beverly, MA), *Eco*RI (10 U/μL), and *Xho*I (10 U/μL) (MBI Fermentas).

3. Methods

3.1. Defining a Functional Bait

3.1.1. Constructing and Transforming a Bait Protein

A prerequisite for an interactor hunt is a construction of a plasmid that expresses the protein of interest as a fusion to the bacterial protein LexA (a pBait). This plasmid is cotransformed with a *lexAop-lacZ* reporter plasmid into a yeast strain containing a chromosomally integrated *lexAop-LEU2* reporter gene. The suitability of the bait protein for library screening is then established: controls allow determination of whether the bait is appropriately synthesized, not transcriptionally active, and expressed in the cell nucleus (*see* **Fig. 3**). If any of these conditions is not met, strategies for modifying bait or screening conditions are suggested (**Table 1**). To minimize the chance of artifactual results or other difficulties, it is a good idea to move rapidly through the suggested characterization steps before undertaking a library screen. Although plasmids will be retained for extended periods in yeast maintained at 4°C on stock plates, variable protein expression and transcriptional activation results will be more likely to be obtained in yeast left for approximately 10 d to 2 wk in the refrigerator.

1. Clone the DNA encoding the protein of interest into the polylinker of pMW103 (**Fig. 4**) to enable synthesis of an in-frame protein fusion to LexA (*see* **Note 2**).
2. Select a colony of EGY48 (*see* **Note 3**) and grow a 20-mL culture in liquid YPD medium overnight at 30°C in a shaking incubator.
3. Dilute the 20-mL overnight culture into 300 mL of YPD liquid medium such that the diluted culture has an OD_{600nm} of approx 0.15. Incubate at 30°C on an orbital shaker until the culture has reached an OD_{600nm} of 0.5–0.7.
4. Transfer 50 mL of culture to a sterile 50-mL Falcon tube, and centrifuge for 5 min at 1000–1500g at room temperature. Gently resuspend the pellet in 5 mL of sterile water.
5. Recentrifuge the cells for 5 min at 1000–1500g. Pour off the water and resuspend the yeast in 0.5 mL (sufficient for 10 transformations) of TE/0.1 M lithium acetate.

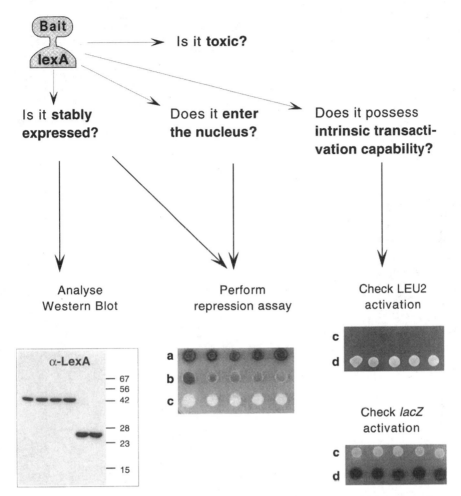

Fig. 3. Bait characterization. Representative data for Western blot, repression, and activation assays. **(Left)** The Western blot was probed with anti-LexA antibodies; lanes 1–4 contain lysates from four independent colonies expressing a stable bait fusion, lanes 5 and 6 are LexA alone. **(Center)** for a repression assay, a Gal-Raff/CM-ura X-Gal plate is shown; **(Right)** for an activation assay: Glu/CM-ura-his-leu and Glu/CM-ura-his X-Gal overlay plates are shown. Five independent clones of each of the following EGY48 transformants are shown on repression and activation assay plates: a, pJK101 alone; b, pJK101 + pRFHMI (LexA-bicoid); c, pRFHMI + pSH18-34; d, pSH18-34 (LexA-GAL4) + pSH18-34. An optimal bait would be well expressed and behave similarly to pRFHMI in these assays.

6. Add 50 μL of competent yeast cells to each of seven microfuge tubes containing a mix of 1 μg of freshly sheared, denatured salmon sperm DNA with the following combinations of LexA fusion and *lexAop*-LacZ plasmids (100–500 ng each) (*see* **Note 4**):

Table 1
Possible Modifications to Enhance Bait Performance in Specific Applications[a]

Response bait problem	Truncate/modify bait	Use more stringent strain/reporter combination	Fuse to nuclear localization sequence pJK202	Put LexA-fused protein under Gal1-inducible promoter pGilda	Fuse LexA to the carboxy-terminal end of the bait pNLexA	Integrate bait, reduce concentration pEG2021
Bait is strongly activating	+	−	−	−	−	−
Bait is weakly activating	+	+	−	−	+?	+?
Bait has low expression level or is not transported to the nucleus.	−	−	+	−	−	−
Continuous expression of LexA fusion is toxic to yeast.	+	−	−	+	+?	+?
Bait protein requires unblocked N-terminal end for function.	−	−	−	−	+	−
Bait protein is expressed at high levels, unstable or interacts promiscuously.	+?	−	−	+?	+?	+
Potential new problem[b]	It may be necessary to subdivide bait into two or three overlapping constructs and test independently.	Use of very stringent interaction strains may eliminate detection of biological is relevant interactions.	.	GAL-dependence of reporter phenotype can no longer be used to indicate cDNA-dependent interaction	Generally, LexA poorly tolerates attachment of the N-terminal fusion domain. Only ~60% of constructs are expressed correctly.	Reduced bait protein concentration may lead to reduced assay sensitivity.

[a]Would usually help; +?, may help; −, will not help.

[b]All of the alternative bait expression vectors remain on an Amp^R selection for bacteria. If using them as is, the investigator may need to use a KC8 bacteria to isolate the library plasmid after a library screen.

a. pBait + pMW109 (test for activation).
b. pEG202-hsRPB7 + pMW109 (weak positive control for activation).
c. pSH17-4 + pMW109 (strong positive control for activation).
d. pRFHM1 + pMW109 (negative control for activation).
e. pBait + pJK101 (test for repression)
f. pRFHM1 + pJK101 (positive control for repression).
g. pGKS3 + pJK101 (negative control for repression).
7. Plate each transformation mixture on Glu/CM -Ura-His dropout plates, and maintain at 30°C for 2 to 3 d to select for yeast colonies containing transformed plasmids (*see* **Note 4**).

3.1.2. Replica Technique/Gridding Yeast: Assessing Bait Activation of Reporters, and Repression Assay

For each combination of plasmids, assay at least six independent colonies for activation phenotype of *lacZ* and *LEU2* reporters (*see* **Note 6**). Assessment of transcriptional activation requires the transfer of yeast from master plates to a variety of selective media. This transfer can be accomplished simply by using a sterile toothpick to move cells from individual patches on the master plate to each of the selective media. However, in cases in which large numbers of colonies and combinations of bait and prey are to be examined, and particularly in genomic-scale applications, it is useful to use a transfer technique that facilitates high-throughput analysis. The following technique, based on microtiter plates, is an example of such an approach.

1. Add 25–50 μL of sterile water to each well of one-half (wells A1–H6) of a 96-well microtiter plate (e.g., using a syringe-based repeater). Place an insert grid from a rack of micropipet tips over the top of the microtiter plate and attach it with tape: the holes in the insert grid should be placed exactly over the wells of the microtiter plate (this is not essential but will stabilize the tips in the plate, and allow simultaneous removal, speeding the replica process).
2. Using sterile plastic micropipet tips, pick six yeast colonies (1 to 2 mm diameter) from each of the transformation plates a–d (**Subheading 3.1.1., step 8**), and insert the tips into the first 4 rows of water-filled wells (A1–D6) of the microtiter plate. Leave the tips supported in a near-vertical position by the insert grid until all the colonies have been picked. Resuspend the yeast in the water (at this point 4 rows [$^1/_4$ of the plate] will be filled with yeast suspension and the remaining 4 rows will just contain water).
3. Swirl the plate gently to mix the yeast into suspension, remove the sealing tape, and lift the insert grid, thereby removing all the tips at once.
4. Place a plastic replicator into the plate; if the yeast has already sedimented, shake the replicator in a circular movement (or vortex the whole plate at medium speed). Lift the replicator (which will now carry drops of liquid on its spokes), turn it 180°, and reinsert it into the plate in wells A1–H6, making an approx 1:20 dilu-

DBD-fusion (bait) vectors' polylinkers:

pEG202 (aka pLexA, displayBait)

```
                         SalI              NotI            SalI
  EcoRI         BamHI       NcoI*        XhoI
GAA TTC CCG GGG ATC CGT CGA CCA TGG CGG CCG CTC GAG TCG AC
```

pLexZeo

```
EcoRI                              ApaI          NotI        SalI
          SacI              PvuII       KpnI          XhoI        PstI
GAA TTC AAG CTT GAG CTC AGA TCT CAG CTG GGC CCG GTA CCG CGG CCG CTC GAG TCG ACC TGC AG
 E   F   E   L   R   S   Q   L   G   P   V   P   R   P   L   E   S   T   C
```


AD-fusion (library) vectors' polylinkers:

pJG4-5 (aka pB42AD, displayTarget)

```
                                    EcoRI          XhoI
ATG GGT GCT CCT CCA AAA AAG AAG ... CCC GAA TTC GGC CGA CTC GAG AAG CTT ...
 M   G   A   P   P   K   K   K  ...  P   E   F   G   R   L   E   K   L  ...
```

pYesTrp2

```
                     KpnI              BamHI
           HinDIII        SacI
ATG GGT AAG CCT ... AAG CTT GGT ACC GAG CTC GGA TCC ACT AGT AAC GGC
 M   G   K   P       K   L   G   T   E   L   G   S   T   S   N   G
```

```
           EcoRI                              NotI              SphI
     BstXI                      BstXI              XhoI
CGC CAG TGT GCT GGA ATT CTG CAG ATA TCC ATC ACA CTG GCG GCC GCT CGA GGC ATG C
 R   Q   C   A   G   I   L   Q   I   S   I   T   L   A   A   R   G   M   H
```

Fig. 4. Polylinkers of two-hybrid basic vectors. Maps and sequences are available at <http://www.fccc.edu/research/labs/golemis/InteractionTrapInWork.html>. Only restriction sites that are available for insertion of coding sequences are shown; those shown in bold type are unique. (**Top**) LexA fusion vectors. The strong ADH promoter is used to express bait proteins as fusions to the DNA-binding protein LexA. Multiple restriction sites are available for insertion of coding sequences; the sequence CGTCAGCAGAGCTTCACCATTG can be used to design a primer to confirm the correct reading frame for LexA fusions. The pEG202 plasmid contains the *HIS3* selectable marker and the 2-μm origin of replication to allow propagation in yeast, and an ampicillin (Ap^R) resistance gene and the pBR322 origin of replication to allow propagation in *E. coli*. In pMW101 and pMW103 (*10*), Ap^R was replaced with chloramphenicol (Cm^R) and kanamycin (Km^R) resistance genes, respectively. All alternative bait plasmids (**Table 1**) have the same polylinkers as pEG202. In pMW103 the *Nco*I site is not unique and cannot be used for cloning. In Invitrogen's pLexZeo, both the HIS3 marker and antibiotic resistance markers have been replaced with the

tion of the primary suspensions, with the original transformation plate colony order abed now converted to dcba (mirror image) (*see* **Note 7**).

5. Use a plastic replicator to plate (*see* **Note 8**) yeast suspensions (each spoke will leave a drop approximately equal to a 3-μL vol) on the following plates:

    a. To assess activation (for six transformants from each of reactions a–d): Glu/CM -Ura-His (a new master plate); Gal-Raff/CM -Ura-His-Leu, and Gal-Raff/CM -Ura-His, X-Gal (direct plate X-Gal assay; see **Note 9**). Incubate the plates at 30°C for up to 4 d, and save the Glu/CM -Ura-His master plate at 4°C.

    b. To assess repression (*see* Notes 9 and 10) (for six transformants from each of reactions e–g): Glu/CM -Ura-His, X-Gal and Gal-Raff/CM -Ura-His, X-Gal. Incubate the plates at 30°C for up to 2 d.

6. Inspect daily the Gal/CM -Ura-His-Leu plates on which the transformants from reactions with a–d have been plated. Yeast containing the strong positive control (from reaction c) should be detectably growing within 1 to 2 d, yeast containing the weak positive control (from reaction b) should exhibit growth within 4 d, and yeast containing the negative control (from reaction d) should not grow. If the yeast containing the bait under test (from reaction a) shows no growth in this period, it is probably suitable for library screening; if it gives a profile similar to the transformants from reaction b, it may be suitable but is likely to have a high background in library screening, suggesting that the use of a different screening strain may be appropriate; if it is similar to the transformants from reaction c, it must be reconfigured (*see* **Notes 5** and **11**).

7. Inspect the X-Gal plates on a daily basis. In assessing the transformants from reactions a–d, strongly activating baits will be detectable as medium dark blue colonies in 1 to 2 d, whereas negative controls should remain as faint blue or white colonies out to 4 d; an optimal bait would either mimic the negative control or only develop faint blue color after 3 d (*see* **Note 12**).

8. Twelve to 24 h after plating, inspect the X-Gal plates containing the transformants from the reactions (e–g) designed to assess the ability of a bait to repress transcription/bind DNA. A good result (i.e., real repression) will generally reflect a two- to threefold reduction in the degree of blue color detected for JK101 + bait vs JK101 + pGKS3, on plates containing galactose (*see* **Note 11**).

Zeocin-resistance gene, which can be selected in both yeast and bacteria. (**Bottom**) Activation domain (AD) fusion vectors. The library plasmids express cDNAs as translational fusion to a nuclear localization sequence (NLS), the activation domain, and the epitope tag. Expression of sequences is under the control of the GAL1 galactose-inducible promoter. Library plasmids contain the *TRP1* selectable marker and the 2-μm origin to allow propagation in yeast, and an Ap^R gene and the pUC origin to allow propagation in *E. coli*. The pJG4-5 fusion cassette consists of the SV40 NLS, the acid blob B42, and the hemagglutinin (HA) epitope tag *(4)*. Invitrogen's pYesTrp2 AD vector has a cassette that incorporates a V5 epitope tag, followed by an NLS and the acid blob B42.

3.1.3. Detection of Bait Protein Expression

One excellent confirmation that a bait is correctly expressed would be its specific interaction with a known partner, expressed as an AD fusion protein. In the absence of such confirmation, Western analysis of lysates of yeast containing LexA-fused baits is helpful in characterizing of the bait's expression level and size. Some proteins (especially in which the fusion domain is 60–80 kDa or larger) may either be synthesized at very low levels or be post-translationally clipped by yeast proteases. Proteins expressed at low levels and apparently inactive in transcriptional activation assays can be upregulated to much higher levels under the leucine- selection and suddenly demonstrate a high background of transcriptional activation. When proteins are proteolytically clipped, screens might inadvertently be performed with LexA fused only to the amino-terminal end of the larger intended bait. Either of these two problems can lead to complications in library screens. Western analysis should be performed as follows (*see* also **ref. *11***).

1. From the Glu/CM -Ura -His master plate (**Subheading 3.1.2., step 5**), inoculate at least two primary bait/reporter transformants for each bait to be tested into Glu/CM -Ura -His liquid medium (including pRFHMI transformants as a positive control for protein expression). Grow overnight cultures on an orbital shaker at 30°C. Dilute the saturated cultures into fresh tubes containing 3 mL of Glu/CM -Ura -His to the density at OD_{600nm}, approx 0.15, and grow at 30°C.
2. After the OD_{600nm} of the cultures reaches 0.45–0.7 (after about 4–6 h), harvest cells from 1.5 mL of each culture by centrifuging at 13,000*g* for 3–5 min. When each cell pellet is visible (should be 2–5 µL of packed cell volume), carefully remove each supernatant (*see* **Note 12.**).
3. Add 50 µL of 2X Laemmli sample buffer (0.125 *M* Tris-HCl (pH 6.8), 4% (w/v) SDS, 20% (v/v) glycerol, 10% (v/v) 2-mercaptoethanol, and 0.002% (w/v) bromophenol blue) to each pellet, and rapidly vortex to resuspend each pellet. Heat the samples at 100°C for 5 min for immediate assay, or freeze at –70°C (use dry ice) for subsequent use (such samples will be stable for at least 4–6 mo, and should be heated at 100°C for 5 min before use).
4. After heating, chill the samples on ice and centrifuge for 30 s at 13,000*g* to pellet large cell debris. Load 10–25 µL of each sample onto a 0.1% (w/v) SDS-polyacrylamide gel electrophoresis gel.
5. Prepare a western blot and screen *(12,13)* LexA fusions using an antibody to LexA (*see* Note 14), allowing comparison of expression levels of the bait protein under test with other standard bait proteins, e.g., RFHMI. Alternatively, screen using an antibody to the fusion domain.
6. Note which colonies on the master plate express bait appropriately (*see* **Note 15**), and use one of these colonies as a founder to propagate for library transformation/mating.

3.2. Transforming and Characterizing Interactors from a Library

A partial list of available libraries compatible with the Interaction Trap can be found at <http://www.fccc.edu/research/labs/golemis/InteractionTrapInWork. html>. Currently, the most convenient source of libraries suitable for the interaction trap is commercial; the broadest selection is found at Invitrogen, Origene, Clontech, and DisplaySystems and can be viewed at each of these companies' Web sites. If one wishes to make your own library, it should be cloned in a vector such as pJG4-5 or a related vector such as pYesTrp2 (Invitrogen; the polylinker sequence at the site of cDNA insertion is shown in **Fig. 4**).

The following protocols are designed with the goal of saturation screening of a cDNA library derived from a genome of mammalian complexity. Fewer plates will be required for screens with libraries derived from organisms with less complex genomes, and researchers should scale down accordingly. Separate protocols are provided for mating in the library against the bait of interest or directly transforming the library into yeast containing the bait. The advantage of the former approach is that if the investigator wishes to use the same library to screen multiple baits, only a single large-scale transformation is required.

In a subsequent characterization of potential interactors a positive control is usually quite useful. While you set up your library transformation or interaction mating, it is useful to use the same technique to get a pair of interacting proteins, expressed in bait and library plasmids, in the same strain background with matching *LEU2* and LacZ reporters. Normally, these positive controls (referred to as pBait-control and pPrey-control) are provided with each two-hybrid kit, if reagents were obtained from a company.

3.2.1. Transforming the Library

3.2.1.1. TRANSFORMING THE LIBRARY INTO MATING PARTNER YEAST STRAIN

1. Select a colony of an appropriate mating partner yeast strain (such as SKY473), and grow a 20-mL culture in liquid YPD medium overnight at 30°C in an orbital shaker (*see* **Note 3**).
2. Dilute the 20-mL overnight culture into approx 300 mL of YPD liquid medium such that the diluted culture has an OD_{600nm} of 0.15. Incubate at 30°C on an orbital shaker until the culture has reached an OD_{600nm} of 0.5–0.7.
3. Subdivide the culture among six sterile 50-mL tubes, and centrifuge at 1000–1500g for 5 min at room temperature. Gently resuspend each pellet in 5 mL of sterile water, and combine all the slurries in a single tube. Add sterile water to the top of the tube and mix.
4. Recentrifuge the cells at 1000–1500g for 5 min at room temperature. Pour off the water and resuspend the yeast in 1.5 mL of TE/0.1 M lithium acetate.

5. Mix 30 µg of library DNA and 1.5 mg of freshly denatured sheared salmon sperm DNA, and add the DNA mix to the yeast. Mix gently and dispense 60-µL aliquots of DNA/yeast suspension into 30 microfuge tubes (*see* **Note 16**).

6. To each tube, add 300 µL of sterile 40% (w/v) PEG 4000/0.1 *M* lithium acetate/ TE buffer, pH 7.5. Mix by gently inverting the tubes several times (do not vortex). Place the tubes at 30°C for 30–60 min.

7. To each tube, add 40 µL of dimethylsulfoxide, and again mix by inversion. Place the tubes in a heat block set to 42°C for 10 min.

8. Pipet the contents of each tube onto a separate 240 × 240 mm Glu-Trp dropout plate, and spread the cells evenly using 12–24 sterile glass beads (*see* **Subheading 2.12., item 1**) (*see* **Note 17**). Invert the plates and incubate at 30°C until colonies appear.

9. Select two representative transformation plates, draw a 23 × 23 mm square (1% of the plate bottom surface) over an average density spot, count the colonies in each grid section, and recalculate for the whole transformation. A good transformation performed according to this protocol should yield approx 20,000–40,000 colonies per plate.

3.2.1.2. DIRECTLY TRANSFORMING THE LIBRARY INTO YEAST CONTAINING THE BAIT

Proceed as described in **Subheading 3.2.1.1.**, except start with a yeast colony expressing the bait and *lexAop*-LacZ reporter (*see* **Note 18**) determined to be optimal in the initial control experiments and grow it in Glu/CM -Ura -His liquid dropout medium. Plate the library transformants on Glu/CM -Trp -Ura-His dropout plates.

3.2.2. Harvesting and Pooling Primary Transformants

In the next step, a homogenized slurry is prepared (*see* **Note 19**) from the pool of primary transformants (approx 3×10^5–10^6 colonies), aliquoted, and frozen. Each of these aliquots is representative of the complete set of primary transformants and can be used in subsequent mating (or simply plated on leucine-selection medium in the case of direct transformation into a bait-expressing strain).

1. Pour 10 mL of sterile water onto each of five 240 × 240 mm plates containing transformants. Stack the five plates on top of each other. Holding on tightly, shake the stack horizontally until all the colonies are resuspended (1 to 2 min). Using a sterile pipet, collect yeast slurry from each plate (by tilting the plates) and pool in a sterile 50-mL conical tube.

2. Repeat for two further sets of five plates of transformants, resulting in a total of 150 mL of suspension split between three 50-mL tubes (*see* **Note 20**).

3. Fill each tube containing yeast to the top with sterile TE or water, and vortex/ invert to suspend the cells. Centrifuge the tubes at 1000–1500*g* for 5 min at room

temperature, and discard the supernatants. Repeat this step. After the second wash, the cumulative pellet volume should be approx 25 mL of cells derived from up to 10^6 transformants.

4. Resuspend each packed cell pellet in 1 vol of glycerol solution. Combine the contents of the three tubes and mix thoroughly. Disperse as 0.2 to 1.0-mL aliquots in a series of sterile Eppendorf tubes and freeze at –70°C (stable for at least 1 yr).
5. If the library is to be used for mating, proceed to the procedure outlined in **Subheading 3.2.3.** If the library was directly transformed against the bait, an option is to proceed directly to plating on selective medium (approx 5 h is required to complete the process). In this case, leave one aliquot unfrozen and proceed directly to the protocol outlined in **Subheading 3.2.4.**, assuming that the viability of the culture is 100% (*see* **Note 21**).

3.2.3. Mating the Bait Strain and the Pretransformed Library

Once the bait strain has been made and characterized and the library strain has been transformed and frozen in aliquots, the next step is to mate the two strains. To mate the two strains, the bait strain is grown in liquid culture and mixed with a thawed aliquot of the pretransformed library strain. The mixture is plated on rich media and grown overnight. During this time individual cells of the bait strain will fuse with individual cells of the library strain to form diploid cells. The diploids, along with unmated haploids, are collected and plated on media to select for interactors (as described in **Subheading 3.2.4.**). In practice, the diploid/haploid mixture is generally frozen in a few aliquots to allow titering and repeated platings at various dilutions.

It is generally a good idea to additionally mate new bait strains with a control strain. The control strain is the same strain used for the library but containing the library vector with no cDNA insert. Mating with the control strain can be performed at the same time as the library mating, and both matings can be treated identically in the next step, selecting interactors. This control will provide a clear estimate of the frequency of cDNA-independent false positives, a frequency that is important to know when deciding how many positives to pick and characterize.

1. Start a 30-mL Glu/CM -Ura-His liquid culture of the bait strain (EGY48/pBait/p*lacZ*) from the Glu/CM -Ura-His master plate. Grow with shaking at 30°C to mid- to late-log phase ($OD_{600nm} = 1.0$–2.0).
2. Collect the cells by centrifuging at $1000g$ for 5 min at room temperature. Resuspend the cell pellet in 1 mL of sterile water and transfer to a sterile 1.5-mL microfuge tube. Measure the OD of a dilution to ensure that the OD_{600nm} of the undiluted suspension is 30–50. This will correspond to about 1×10^9 cells/mL.
3. Thaw an aliquot of the pretransformed library strain at room temperature. Mix 200 μL of the bait strain with approx 10^8 colony-forming units (CFU) of the pretransformed library strain (*see* **Subheading 3.2.2., step 5**).

4. Centrifuge the mixture of cells at 1000*g* for 5 min and discard the supernatant. Resuspend the cell pellet in 200 µL of YPD medium. Plate on a single 100-mm-diameter YPD plate and incubate at 30°C for 12–15 h.

5. Add 1 to 2 mL of sterile water to the surface of the YPD plate and suspend the cells using sterile glass beads. Transfer the suspension to a sterile tube and vortex gently for 2 min. Collect the cells by centrifugation at 1000*g* for 5 min and resuspend in 1 vol of sterile glycerol solution. Distribute into 200 µL aliquots and freeze at –80°C (*see* **Note 22**).

6. Titer the mated cells by thawing an aliquot and plating serial dilutions on Glu/CM -Trp-His-Ura plates (unmated haploids will not grow on this medium). Count the colonies that grow after 2 to 3 d, and determine the titer of the frozen mated cells.

3.2.4. Screening for Interacting Proteins

This section describes how interactors are selected by plating the mated cells onto selection plates lacking leucine. It is important to know how many viable diploids were plated onto these selection plates to gain a sense of how much of the library has been screened and to determine the false positive frequency (*see* **Note 23**). This information is provided by the titer (colony-forming units per milliliter) of the frozen mated cells (*see* **Subheading 3.2.3., step 6**).

If the protocol described in **Subheading 3.2.3.** was followed, perform the following steps with the frozen mated cells (from both matings of the bait strain with the library strain and with the control strain). However, if the bait strain was transformed directly with library DNA (*see* **Subheading 3.2.2., step 5**), perform the following steps with an aliquot of the frozen transformants.

1. Thaw an aliquot of the mated yeast (or cells containing pbait that were transformed directly with the library DNA). Dilute 100 µL into 10 mL of Gal-Raff/CM -Ura-His-Trp liquid dropout medium and incubate with shaking at 30°C for 5 h. If the frozen culture was not previously titered, plate serial dilutions onto Glu/CM -Ura-His-Trp plates.

2. On the assumption that a culture at $OD_{600nm} = 1.0$ contains 2×10^7 cells/mL, plate 10^6 cells on each of an appropriate number of 100-mm Gal-Raff/CM-Ura-His-Trp-Leu plates. For each original transformant obtained, plate three to five cells. Avoid plating more than 10^6 cells/plate, because this results in higher levels of background growth.

3. Incubate for 5 d at 30°C. Depending upon the individual bait used, good candidates for positive interactors will generally produce LEU+ colonies over this time period, with the most common appearance of colonies at 2–4 d.

4. Inspect the plates on a daily basis. Mark the location of colonies visible on d 1 with dots of a given color on the plate. Each day, mark further colonies arising with different colors. At d 4 or 5, streak colonies (*see* **Notes 23 and 24**) in a microtiter plate format onto a solid master plate (Glu/CM-Ura-His-Trp), in which

colonies are grouped by day of appearance (*see* **Note 25**). If many apparent positives appear, pick separate master plates for colonies arising on d 2, 3, and 4, respectively.

5. Include the positive control colonies (pbait-control and pPrey-control) on each of the master plates.
6. Incubate the master plates at 30°C until patches/colonies form.

3.2.5. First Confirmation of Positive Interactions

The following steps test for galactose-inducible transcriptional activation of both the *lexAop-LEU2* and *lexAop-lacZ* reporters. Simultaneous activation of both reporters in a galactose-specific manner generally indicates that the transcriptional phenotype is attributable to expression of library-encoded proteins, rather than derived from mutation of the yeast. Testing for β-galactosidase activity and for Leu requirement is the same as described in **Subheading 3.1.2.** For interpretation of the results, refer to **Table 2**.

1. Invert a frogger on a flat surface and place a master plate upside down on the spokes, making sure that the spokes and colonies are properly aligned. Remove the plate and insert the frogger into a microtiter plate containing 50 μL of sterile water in each well. Let the plate sit for 5–10 min, shaking from time to time to resuspend the cells left on the spokes. When all yeast are resuspended, print (*see* **Note 8**) on the following plates: Glu/CM -Ura-His-Trp, Glu/CM -Ura-His-Trp X-Gal (*see* **Note 9**), Gal-Raff/CM -Ura-His-Trp X-Gal (*see* **Note 9**), Glu/CM (-Ura-His-Trp)-Leu, Gal-Raff/CM (-Ura-His-Trp)-Leu.
2. Repeat for each master plate (from **Subheading 3.2.4., step 6**).
3. Incubate the plates at 30°C for 3 to 4 d. After 1 d of incubation, take out all three -Ura-His-Trp plates. Retain the Glu/CM -Ura-His-Trp plate as a fresh master plate. Score growth on the -Leu plates 48–72 h after plating.

3.3. Library Plasmid Isolation, and Second Confrmation of Positive Interactions

Execution of the previous protocols for a given bait will result in the isolation of between zero and hundreds of potential "positive" interactors. These positives must next be evaluated for reproducible phenotype, and specific interaction with the bait used to select them, using a strategy as shown in **Fig. 5**. If a large number of positives are obtained, these subsequent characterizations require prioritization and careful storage of clones while tests are being performed. In general, a first workup of putative positives will select up to approx 24–48 independent colonies with robust phenotype (i.e., appeared within the first 2–3 d after plating on selective media; strong blue color with X-Gal, good growth on -Leu medium), while maintaining a master plate of additional positives at 4°C. This first analysis set should be tested for specificity and screened by PCR/restriction analysis and/or sequencing to determine whether clusters

Table 2
Interpretation of β-Galactosidase and Leu Testing

Phenotype					Suggestion/explanation	
Leu growth		X-Gal color			Traditional	Optimistic
Glu	Gal	Glu	Gal			
–	+	–	+			Very good sign
(+)	+	(+)	+		Bait is upregulated/mutated to a high back ground of transcriptional activation	GAL1 promoter is slightly leaky.
						Both proteins are very stable.
						Interaction occurs with high affinity.
–	+	–	–		Yeast mutation occurred that favors growth or transcriptional activation on galactose medium.	Some bait-interactor combinations are known to prefentially activate $lacZ$ vs $LEU2_1$ or vice versa.
All other phenotypes					They have contamination/plasmid rearrangements/mutations.	They are something really new

434

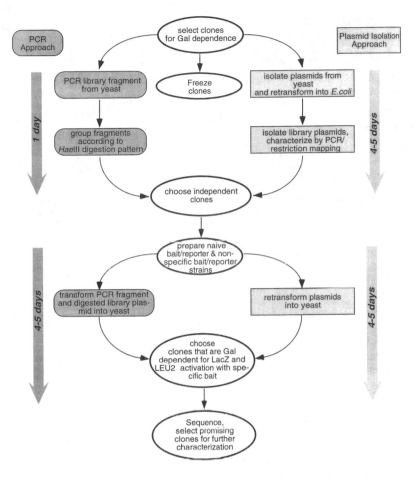

Fig. 5. Detailed library screening flowchart. *See* text for details.

of frequently isolated cDNAs are obtained: such clusters are generally a good indication for a specific interaction. Two strategies for analyzing positives are provided below and are summarized in the flowchart in **Fig. 5**. Both utilize similar methods, but the order with which techniques are applied differ; the choice between strategies depends on whether the individual investigator would rather spend time and money doing bulk yeast plasmid recovery or bulk PCR. The latter protocol is generally 1–3 d faster, but some investigators have difficulties obtaining reliable results in PCRs from yeast using the protocol (*see* **Subheading 3.3.1.**) outlined, whereas the plasmid recovery protocol (*see* **Subheading 3.3.2.**) described is generally quite trouble free.

A major strength of the protocol described in **Subheading 3.3.1.** is that it will identify redundant clones prior to plasmid isolation and bacterial transformation, which in some cases greatly reduces the amount of work required. However, accurate records should be maintained as to how many of each class of cDNA are obtained; and if any ambiguity is present as to whether a particular cDNA is part of a set or unique, investigators should err on the side of caution.

A further time-saving approach is to conduct the specificity test by interaction mating *(6)*. In this approach, each PCR product is transformed along with the digested pJG4–5 vector into just one strain (e.g., RFY206); the transformants can then be mated with any number of baitexpressing strains, including a strain expressing the original bait (*see*, e.g., **Subheadings 3.4.2.** and **3.4.3.**).

In some cases, no positives are obtained from library screens. The reasons for this might include inappropriate library source; an inadequate number of screened colonies (<500,000); a bait that in spite of production at high levels is nevertheless incorrectly folded or posttranslationally modified; or, alternatively, a bait that does not interact with its partners with a sufficiently high affinity to be detected. In addition, be aware of such simple explanations as a wrong batch of plates. In such cases, it may be worth trying screens again with a different variant of bait, screening strain, and/or library, although success is not guaranteed. It is rarely if ever profitable to continue to rescreen the same bait/strain/library combination through >3–5,000,000 primary transformants.

3.3.1. PCR Approach: Rapid Screen for Interaction Trap Positives

1. Starting from the Glu/CM -Ura-His-Trp master plate (*see* **Subheading 3.2.5., step 5**) (*see* **Note 26**), resuspend each yeast colony in 25 µL of β-glucuronidase solution in a well of a 96-well microtiter plate. Seal the wells using tape, and incubate on a horizontal shaker at 37°C for 1.5–3.5 h.
2. Remove the tape, add about 25 µL of glass beads (*see* **Subheading 2.4., item 2**) to each well, and seal again. Attach (e.g., using rubber bands) the microtiter plate to a vortex with a flat top surface and mix vigorously for 5 min.
3. Add 100 µL of sterile distilled water to each well. Take 0.8–2 µL as a template for each PCR reaction (*see* **Note 27**). Reseal the plate with tape, and store the remaining suspensions at 70°C.
4. Using primers specific for the library plasmid employed (*see* **Note 28**) and 0.1 U/µL of *Taq* DNA polymerase, and thermocycle 30-µL PCR amplifications *(14)* as follows: 94°C for 2 min; and 94°C for 45 s, 56°C for 45 s, and 72°C for 45 s for 31 cycles (*see* **Note 29**).
5. Analyze 20 µL of each PCR product by electrophoresis through a 0.7% (w/v) agarose gel. Identify fragments that appear to be the same. Put the gel in a refrigerator until you are ready to isolate fragments (*see* **Note 30**).

6. Digest 10 μL of each PCR product with *Hae*III in a total volume of 20 μL. Load the digestion products on a 1.5% (w/v) agarose gel, rearranging the loading order such that the *Hae*III digests representing nondigested PCR products of equivalent size (**step 5**) are run side by side. Run out the DNA a sufficient distance to get good resolution of DNA products in the 200- to 1000-bp size range (*see* **Note 31**).

7. Purify fragments from the agarose gel *(15)*, and in cases where a very large number of isolates representing a small number of cDNA classes have been obtained, directly sequence the PCR products (*see* **Note 27**).

The next step is to determine whether isolated cDNAs reproduce interaction phenotypes specifically with the pBait of interest, and to exclude library-encoded cDNAs that interact with the pBait in a nonspecific manner and clones isolated because of mutations in the initial EGY48 strain that result in growth and transcriptional activation nonspecifically. This can be done using a PCR-recombination approach (derived from **ref.** *15*) in a single step, after which confirmed specific positive clones can be worked up through conventional plasmid purification.

8. Digest an empty library plasmid with two incompatible enzymes in the polylinker region (e.g., *Eco*RI and *Xho*I for JG4-5 plasmid). Ensure that the restriction enzyme sites are in the region flanked by the priming sites.

9. Perform a PCR from a pPrey-control plasmid (*see* **Subheading 3.2.1.**) using the FP1 and FP2 primers (*see* **Note 28**) and purify the PCR-amplified cDNA *(13)*.

10. Transform (*see* **Subheading 3.1.1.**) EGY48 containing pBait-control and pMW109 with the following:
    a. Digested library plasmid.
    b. Digested library plasmid (50–100 ng) and pPrey-control PCR product (0.5–1 μg).
    c. Uncut library plasmid (*see* **Note 32**).

11. Plate the transformations on Glu/CM -Ura-His-Trp dropout plates and incubate at 30°C until colonies grow (2 to 3 d). Store at 4°C.

When transformed together, the PCR-amplified cDNA fragment from a pPrey-control plasmid and the digested library plasmid will undergo homologous recombination in vivo in up to 97% of the transformants that acquired both vector and insert. This is owing to the identity between the cDNA PCR fragment and the plasmid at the priming sites. If the transformation efficiency of reaction b is 5–20-fold higher than that of reaction a, proceed to the next step.

12. Use digested library plasmid (50–100 ng) in combination with selected PCR products (0.5–1 μg; from **step 7**) to transform the following:
    a. EGY48 containing pMW109 and pBait.
    b. EGY48 containing pMW109 and pRFHM-1.
    c. EGY48 containing pMW109 and pBait-control.

d. EGY48 containing pMW109 and a nonspecific bait (*see* **Note 34**). In parallel, transform the digested library plasmid (50–100 ng) and the pPrey-control PCR product (0.5–1 µg) into a–d (*see* **Note 34**).

13. Plate each transformation mix on Glu/CM -Ura, -His, -Trp dropout plates and incubate at 30°C until colonies grow (2 to 3 d).

14. Prepare a master plate for each library plasmid being tested. Each plate should contain at least 10 colonies from each of the transformations a–d for each of the transformed PCR-insert/digested plasmid combinations.

15. Test for β-galactosidase activity and for leucine requirement as described in **Subheading 3.1.2.** True positives should show a LEU+ LacZ+ phenotype with transformation a, but not with transformations b–d.

16. Proceed with sequencing and biologic characterization. Transform (*[13]* **Note 35**) selected positive cloned cDNAs into *E. coli,* using 2–4 µL of the β-glucuronidase-treated frozen yeast (from **step 3**).

3.3.2. Plasmid Isolation Approach: Isolation of Plasmids, and Transfer to Bacteria

The following option is suggested as an alternative to the basic protocol in case PCR technology is not readily available for use, or in case of failure to obtain a specific PCR product using the library vector primers. This protocol can also be scaled up if many colonies are to be assayed. It is based on lysing the cells with glass beads and phenol-chloroform extraction of the plasmid DNA (*see* **Note 36**), bacterial transformation followed by plasmid isolation, and plasmid retransformation into yeast.

1. Grow the colonies with the appropriate phenotype in 2 mL of Glu/CM -Trp overnight at 30°C. (It is advisable to omit the -Ura-His selection in this case to enrich for library plasmids at the expense of the bait and reporter plasmids.)

2. Centrifuge 1 mL of each culture at 13,000g for 1 min. Resuspend each pellet in 200 µL of STES lysis buffer. To each add approx 100 µL of 0.45-mm-diameter sterile glass beads (**Subheading 2.4., item 2**) and vortex vigorously for 1 min.

3. Extract the mixtures first with buffer-saturated phenol (without removing the glass beads) and then with phenol/chloroform. Transfer each aqueous phase to a fresh microfuge tube.

4. Precipitate the plasmid DNAs with 2 vol of 100% (v/v) ethanol and resuspend each pelleted DNA in 5–10 µL of TE.

5. If plasmids (e.g., pMW103, pMW111, pMW109, or pMW112) with a Km^R bacterial selective marker has been employed in combination with Ap^R library plasmid pJG4-5, transform (*[13]* and *see* **Note 35**) *E. coli* strain DH5α (suitable for plasmid DNA isolation and sequencing) and select on medium containing ampicillin, since only bacteria that have taken up a library plasmid will grow (*see* **Note 37**).

6. Prepare a small quantity of plasmid DNA (*13*) from each bacterial clone.

7. Use digested library plasmid (50–100 ng; (*see* **Subheading 3.3.1., step 8**) in combination with each recombinant library plasmid DNA (0.5–1 µg) to transform the following:
   a. EGY48 containing pMW109 and pBait.
   b. EGY48 containing pMW109 and pRFHM-1.
   c. EGY48 containing pMW109 and pBait-control.
   d. EGY48 containing pMW109 and a nonspecific bait (*see* **Note 33**).
   In parallel, transform the digested library plasmid (50–100 ng) and the pPrey-control plasmid (0.5–1 µg) into a–d (*see* **Note 34**).
8. Plate each transformation mix on Glu/CM -Ura, -His, -Trp dropout plates and incubate at 30°C until colonies grow (2–3 d).
9. Prepare a master plate for each library plasmid being tested. Each plate should contain at least 10 colonies from each of the transformations a–d for each of the transformed recombinant library plasmid/digested plasmid combinations.
10. Test for β-galactosidase activity and for leucine requirement as described in **Subheading 3.1.2.** True positives should show a LEU+ LacZ+ phenotype with transformation a, but not with transformations b–d.
11. Proceed with sequencing and biologic characterization.

3.3.3. Follow-Up for Library Screening

Following completion of the above specificity tests, the next step is to leave work with the two-hybrid system and proceed to biologic characterization of the interaction in the appropriate organism for the bait. Such characterization will be necessarily bait specific and should serve to further eliminate interactions of dubious physiologic relevance. A database of common false positives, along with salient discussion of issues related to false positives, is available at: <http://www.fccc.edu/research/labs/golemis/interactiontrapinwork.html>.

3.4. Large-Scale Two-Hybrid Approaches to Characterize Protein Networks and Whole Genomes

The success of yeast two-hybrid systems in understanding how individual proteins function has led to its application for studying whole networks of interacting proteins, and even to attempts at genome wide surveys of protein interactions. The value of such approaches is based on the fact that many important biologic processes are mediated by networks of interacting proteins. The best-described examples of protein networks may be the signal transduction pathways that lead from a cell surface receptor to, frequently, a nuclear transcription factor. By an ordered series of protein-protein interactions, the many proteins in the pathway transduce the initial signal, binding of a ligand to a cell-surface receptor, to a downstream output, e.g., activation or inactivation of a transcription factor governing gene expression. The best-characterized signal transduction pathways of this variety consist of a series of protein kineses

in which the upstream kineses activate the downstream kineses by phosphorylation. There are many examples of studies in which the interactions have been
detected by the yeast two-hybrid assay. By screening cDNA libraries as
described previously in this chapter, researchers have found new members of
signal transduction pathways, discovered new interactions between previously
identified members, ordered members of the pathway, and confirmed interactions and epistatic relationships that had been suggested by genetic experiments. Such results have demonstrated the potential of two-hybrid technology
to find and characterize most of the proteins of any protein network, starting
with an individual component of interest. By contrast, the following section
discusses two-hybrid-based approaches to study large sets of proteins and
whole networks. We conclude with a brief discussion of efforts to map protein
interactions on a genome-wide scale.

3.4.1. Reiterative Scaleup

One approach to elaborating a protein network is to perform reiterative
interactor hunts (e.g., *see* **ref. 8**). Such hunts can start with one or several different baits known to be involved in the biology under study; in some cases,
the starting point may be just one partially characterized protein presumed to
belong to a network. Subsequent interactor hunts can then be performed using
the newly cloned proteins as baits. Such a protein "interaction walk" can be
performed using standard protocols like those described earlier in this chapter.
If the goal is to elaborate a large protein network that may require many
interactor hunts, the rate-limiting step can become subcloning and characterizing new baits. This process can be streamlined by making new bait-expressing
plasmids from newly isolated library clones by PCR and in vivo recombination. In this approach, a single set of primers that has homology to the library
vector immediately upstream and downstream of the cDNA insertion site and
that also has 5' tails that are homologous to the bait vector is used. Amplification of library clones with these primers results in a product that can be
cotransformed along with a linearized bait vector. The PCR product will be
recombined into the bait vector by homologous recombination in the yeast, as
described in **Subheading 3.4.2.** The resulting yeast strain can be used directly
in an interactor hunt by mating with an aliquot of frozen pretransformed library
strain, as described in **Subheading 3.2.3.**

Before the new bait strain is used, it should be tested to ensure that it
expresses the new bait. The most efficient way to accomplish this is to mate the
new bait strain (expressing bait B) with a strain expressing the original bait
protein (bait A) as an AD fusion (AD-A). This will require subcloning the
original bait into the library plasmid. For each subsequent iteration of the pro-

Bait A → **AD-B** → Bait B → **AD-C** → Bait C → **AD-D**

library | *in vivo* | library | *in vivo* | library
screen | subclone | screen | subclone | screen
 | *Test mate* | | *Test mate* |
 | *with AD-A* | | *with AD-B* |

Fig. 6. Flowchart for reiterative screening. See text for details.

tein walk, the new bait strain can be tested by mating it with strains expressing the previously isolated library clones, as shown in **Fig. 6**.

An added benefit to this approach is that each interaction gets tested twice, each time with the two proteins expressed with different fusion moieties. Although there are documented cases in which a two-hybrid interaction is not detectable when the DBD and AD are swapped, it is more common that the interaction can be detected in both orientations. To facilitate a rapid walk through a network, some researchers may choose to streamline the approach by dispensing with some of the bait characterization steps. For example, rather than performing the western and repression assays to show that a bait is expressed and transported to the nucleus, it may be satisfactory to show that the new bait interacts with the AD version of the protein that was used as the bait to isolate it.

3.4.2. Making and Testing New Bait Plasmids by Recombination Cloning

1. Construct a pJG4-5 derivative expressing an AD-fused version of a protein that will interact with the new bait to be constructed. For example, if protein A was used as a bait in an interactor hunt to isolate the cDNA for protein B (which is now going to be made into a bait), construct a plasmid for expressing an AD-fused version of A (*see* **Note 38**).
2. Transform (*see* **Subheading 3.1.1.**) yeast strain RFY206 with the new AD fusion vector, and separately with pJG4-5. Select transformants on Glu/CM -Trp. Streak three to six colonies from each transformation in parallel lines on a 100-mm Glu/CM -Trp plate. Grow at 30°C for 1 to 2 d.
3. Prepare DNA from each colony by β-glucuronidase treatment (*see* **Subheading 3.3.1.**).
4. Perform 20 µL PCR amplifications (thermocycling for 25 cycles of 96°C for 45 s, 55°C for 45 s, and 72°C for 90 s) using 1 to 2 µL of each yeast DNA, 0.025 U/µL of *Pfu* DNA polymerase, and one of the following primer pair (50 n*M* each) combinations. To transfer a cDNA from pJG4–5 to pEG202 (*see* **Note 39**), use these primers:
   a. Forward primer: 5'-GGGCTGGCGGTTGGGGTTATTCGCAACGGCGA CTGGCTG<u>GTGCCAGATTATGCCTCTCCCG</u>-3'.
   b. Reverse primer: 5'-GAGTCACTTTAAAATTTGTATACAC-3'.

To transfer a cDNA from pJG4–5 to pNLex (fusion introduced amino-terminal to LexA) (*see* **Note 40**).

   a. Forward primer: 5'-GACTGGCTGGAATTGGCCCCCAAGAAAAAGAGAA AG<u>GTGCCAGATTATGCC TCTCCCG</u>-3'.
   b. Reverse primer: 5'-GAGTCACTTTAAAATTTGTATACAC-3'.

5. Digest pEG202 or pNLex to completion with *Eco*RI and *Xho*I. Dilute the digested plasmid DNA to 20 ng/μL.

6. For each RFY206 transformant (**step 2**), transform (*see* **Subheading 3.1.1.**) EGY48 containing one of the *URA3 lacZ* reporter plasmids (e.g., pMW112, pMW109, or pMW112) with 200 ng of the double-digested pEG202/pNLex along with 20–200 ng of PCR product from **step 4**. In parallel, perform separate control transformations with 200 ng of the double-digested pEG202/pNLex alone, and with 200 ng of uncut pEG202/pNLex (*see* **Note 32**). Select transformants on Glu/CM -Ura-His plates.

7. Streak six colonies from each transformation on parallel lines across a 100-mm Glu/CM -Ura-His plate and incubate at 30°C for 1 to 2 d. Record which streaks came from which colonies so that they can be saved after testing. To save, streak part of the picked colonies to new Glu/CM -Ura-His master plates.

8. Press the bait strain plate and the AD fusion plate (**step 2**) to the same velvet replica-plating pad so that the two sets of parallel streaks of yeast are perpendicular and cross each other. Lift the print of yeast from the velvet with a single YPD plate. Incubate at 30°C for 12–15 h to allow the two strains to mate.

9. Replica plate the YPD plate to the following plates: Glu/CM -Ura-His-Trp (two times), Gal-Raff/CM -Ura-His-Trp, Glu/CM (-Ura-His-Trp) -Leu, Gal-Raff/CM (-Ura-His-Trp) -Leu.

10. Only the mated diploid yeast at the intersections of the two sets of parallel lines will grow on these plates. Test for β-galactosidase activity and for leucine requirement (as described in **Subheading 3.1.2.**) (*see* **Note 41**).

3.4.3. Arrayed Panels of Baits and Preys

Reiterative hunts can lead rapidly to large collections of yeast strains expressing bait proteins and AD fusions. Such collections can be supplemented with additional clones thought or known to be involved in a relevant biologic process to create panels that can be easily screened for interaction with any newly identified protein or collection of proteins. For example, clones isolated by some other means can be subcloned into the AD vector and tested for interaction with a panel of baits using a simple replica plating technique (*see* **Subheading 3.4.4.**).

Screening arrayed panels of bait or prey strains by mating *(6)* has several advantages over screening entire libraries. First, this approach obviates the need to screen through potentially large numbers of nonspecific false positives that are selected when screening a whole library. For example, some bait proteins interact nonspecifically with many other proteins. By screening these against a defined panel of AD-fused proteins, the search for relevant interactions can be focused. Second, baits that activate transcription of the yeast reporters can be included in the bait panels to be screened with particular AD fusions. Because the position of each bait strain in the panel is well defined, the level of background reporter activation can be assessed and screens with AD fusion strains can detect increases in reporter activation when an interacting AD fusion is expressed. For example, if a strain with an activating bait results in dark blue X-Gal staining when mated with an AD fusion strain, but only light blue X-Gal staining when mated against a strain without the AD fusion, an interaction is indicated. Third, yeast expressing toxic AD fusion proteins can be included in the panels. Because the AD fusion proteins are conditionally expressed from the GAL1 promoter, yeast strains bearing their expression vectors can be maintained in glucose where they are repressed and only shifted to galactose to induce expression when testing for interaction. When mated and replica plated to the galactose indicator plates, β-galactosidase activity can be detected in the cells even if they fail to thrive. Such toxic AD fusions are rarely isolated in library screens that demand selection of interactors by growth on Leuplates. Fourth, interactions between proteins that are toxic when expressed together in yeast can be detected. Like toxic AD fusions, toxic combinations of bait fusions can be tested for interaction by testing for β-galactosidase in nongrowing mated cells. Fifth, new variants and mutated versions of proteins can be tested against panels of known interactors without the need for a labor-intensive rescreening of a library. For example, yeast expressing mutated libraries of a bait protein can be mated with a panel of yeast expressing AD fusions to simultaneously identify bait mutants that fail to interact with one or more AD proteins or that differentially interact with members of the panel.

3.4.4. Testing an AD Fusion Protein for Interaction with a Panel of Bait Strains

1. Array bait strains (e.g., EGY48/pBait/placZ) in a 48- or 96-well format. This can be conveniently accomplished by inoculating 96-well cluster tubes each containing 2 mL of Glu/CM -Ura-His liquid medium, with colonies of EGY48/placZ transformed with pBait plasmids. Cover and grow at 30°C with light shaking for 2 d, or until saturated (*see* **Note 42**).

2. From fresh 2-d cultures, print a plate of the arrayed bait strains for each AD fusion to be tested. Ensure that the yeasts in the cluster tubes are thoroughly suspended, dip a frogger into the cultures, place it on the surface of the plate, and allow it to drain. Incubate the plate at 30°C for 1 to 2 d until uniform round colonies form.

3. Grow a 50-mL Glu/CM -Trp culture of strain RFY206 transformed with the vector expressing the AD fusion protein to an OD_{600nm} of approx 2. Pour the culture into a sterile lid from a 96-micropipet tip rack or a similarly shaped container.

Use a frogger to transfer some of the culture to a Glu/CM -Trp plate. Incubate at 30°C for 1 to 2 d until uniform round colonies form (this creates a plate on which every array spot has the same AD fusion–expressing strain).

4. Mate the two strains by pressing the bait strain plate (from **step 2**) and the AD fusion plate (from **step 3**) to the same replica-plating velvet so that the colonies overlap. Lift the print of yeast from the velvet with a single YPD plate. Incubate at 30°C for 12–15 h to allow the two strains to mate.

5. Replica plate the mated yeast from the YPD plate to the following plates: Glu/CM -Ura-His-Trp (two times), Gal-Raff/CM -Ura-His-Trp, Glu/CM (-Ura-His-Trp) -Leu, Gal-Raff/CM (-Ura-His-Trp) -Leu.

6. Test for β-galactosidase activity and for leucine requirement as described in **Subheading 3.1.2.** (*see* **Note 43**).

3.5. Conclusions

In the 10 yr since it was first described, the yeast two-hybrid system has become a mature and robust technology. False positives and false negatives, although not eliminated, have been minimized to the point that a two-hybrid interaction can often provide an important clue about protein function. Hundreds of new proteins and new protein interactions have been identified. Comprehensive high-throughput two-hybrid systems promise to begin providing genomewide protein linkage in the near future. Such interaction maps, particularly when combined with data from other genomewide and functional genomics approaches such as gene sequence and expression profiles, will be a rich source of data for generating testable hypotheses about protein and pathway function.

4. Notes

1. The value of two-hybrid data for understanding protein and pathway function has led a number of researchers to begin developing scaled-up two-hybrid approaches to map very large numbers of protein interactions. The ultimate goal of such efforts is to map all the protein interactions encoded by a genome. However, as with genome-wide sequencing efforts, it is likely that protein interaction maps will be generated from the smaller genomes first. The first such genome-wide two-hybrid interaction map was generated by Bartel et al. (*7*) for the bacteriophage T7 genome. Random fragments of the T7 genome were used to generate libraries in the AD and DBD vectors and transformed two different yeast strains with the two libraries. Bartel et al. (*7*) used a combination of three approaches to test for interactions between members of the two libraries. In one approach, they performed several interactor hunts by mating individual bait strains with the entire AD library. In the second approach, they mated pools of 10 bait strains against the entire AD library. Because many DBD-fused proteins can activate transcription on their own, they first tested random members of the DBD library for their ability to activate the reporter (*HIS3*) and removed those that activated from their pools. In the third approach, they mated individual bait and individual AD fusion

strains to test all the possible interactions between the proteins they had identified in the first two approaches. In principle, these approaches could be used for any large set of proteins. The resulting protein linkage map revealed 25 interactions between the 55 proteins encoded by the T7 genome, including several interactions not previously suspected. More important, the protein linkage map provided new insights into the biology of the T7 phage. Approaches similar to those taken with the T7 genome could be used to map the interactions encoded by a larger genome, though some modifications may be necessary. For example, larger random pools of strains expressing bait and AD fusions could be mated and then diploids expressing interacting pairs could be selected on reporter selection plates; the identity of the interacting pair of proteins in each diploid might be determined by sequencing PCR products. One problem that must be overcome in such an approach is the high frequency of baits that activate transcription of the reporters on their own. This could be solved by depleting yeast containing activating baits from a library using a toxic reporter such as *URA3*, as described by Vidal et al. *(18)*. A potentially more serious problem with mating libraries and selecting interactors at random is that this would lead to selection for nonspecific false positives. The high frequency of these false positives in routine interactor hunts *(19)* suggests that they would be responsible for the bulk of the positives from a mating of two random libraries. One approach to overcoming these problems is to array both the DBD and AD libraries. As the arrays are screened, the positions of the nonspecific false positives become apparent and they can be ignored. As already discussed, baits that activate transcription could also be tested for interactions in an array approach; the positions of activating baits can be readily identified in the arrays so that their interactions can be assayed by scoring for increases in reporter activation.

2. It is a good idea to include a translational stop sequence at the carboxy-terminal end of the bait sequence. In some cases (e.g., if a bait is known not to localize well to the nucleus), it may be desirable to use an alternative LexA-fusion plasmid as a starting point, as outlined in **Table 1**. In choosing how to construct a bait, it is important to remember that the assay depends on the ability of the bait to enter the nucleus and requires the bait to be a transcriptional *nonactivator*. Therefore, if the chosen protein has obvious sequences that confer attachment to membranes, or sequences that are transcriptional activation domains, these should be removed.

3. It is important to use a fresh (thawed from −70°C and streaked to a single colony less than 7 d previously) colony and maintain sterile conditions throughout all subsequent procedures.

4. Plasmids a–d allow you to determine whether your bait protein directly activates transcription; to be suitable for two-hybrid screening, a bait must be a weak or nonactivator of transcription. Plasmids e–g are used in a "repression assay," to gage whether the bait in question is actually binding DNA sequence (*see* **Fig. 7**).

5. An efficient transformation would yield approx 10^4 transformants/µg of DNA (when two plasmids are being simultaneously transformed). Therefore, this

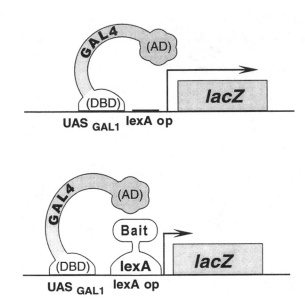

Fig. 7. Repression assay for DNA binding. The plasmid JK101 contains the upstream activating sequence (WAS) from the *GAL1* gene followed by LexA operators upstream of the *lacZ* coding sequence. Thus, yeast containing pJK10 1 will have significant β-galactosidase activity when grown on medium in which Gal is the sole carbon source because of binding of endogenous yeast GAL4 to the UAS$_{GAL}$ **(top)**. LexA-fused proteins that are made enter the nucleus and bind the lexA operator sequences, which will block activation from the UAS$_{GAL}$, repressing β-galactosidase activity three- to fourfold **(bottom)**. On glucose X-Gal medium, yeast containing JK101 should be white because UAS$_{GAL}$ transcription is repressed. Adapted from **ref. 23**.)

experiment also provides a good chance to assess transformation efficiency, which will be much more important by the time of library transformation. Thus, if only a very small number of colonies are obtained, or colonies are not apparent within 3 to 4 d, it would imply that transformation is, for some reason, very inefficient, and results obtained in characterization experiments may not be typical. In this case, all solutions, media, and conditions must be double-checked or prepared fresh and the transformation repeated. Sheared salmon sperm DNA (sssDNA), which is most often used as carrier, must be of very high quality; using a poor-quality preparation can reduce transformation frequencies one to two orders of magnitude. sssDNA is available commercially from several companies or can be easily homemade *(16)*. If very few transformants containing the bait plasmid appear (compared to the controls), yeast expressing the bait protein grow noticeably more poorly than control yeast, or the bait plasmid-containing colony population appears much more heterogeneous (e.g., presents a mix of large and small colonies) than the control colony population, this would suggest that the bait protein is somewhat toxic to the yeast (*see* **Note 11**).

6. This is important, because for some baits, protein expression level is heterogeneous between independent colonies, with accompanying heterogeneity of apparent ability to activate transcription of the two reporters.

7. This strategy will produce both relatively heavy and diluted spots of each yeast colony suspension, on subsequent replating to selective media. The value of having both high and low dilutions stems from the nature of the assays for transcriptional activation. If yeast are plated too densely on -Leu plates, cross-feeding can occur between cells that results in growth even in the absence of activation of the reporter, thereby obscuring a true positive result. In addition, since yeast growth is suboptimal on X-Gal plates owing to their neutral pH (7.0 to optimize β-galactosidase activity, compared with pH 5.0–5.5 for normal media), it will be easier to determine a blue-white phenotype of the initially heavier spots, because fewer cell divisions are required.

8. When making prints on a plate, put the replicator on the surface of the solidified medium and tilt slightly in a circular movement, lift the replicator, and put it back in the microtiter plate (retaining the correct orientation). Make sure all the drops left on the surface are of approximately the same size. If only one or two drops are missing, it is easy to correct by dropping 3 µL of yeast suspension on the missing spots from the corresponding wells. If many drops are missing, make sure that all the spokes of the replicator are in good contact with the liquid in the microtiter plate (it may be necessary to cut off the side protrusions on the edge spokes of a plastic replicator) and redo the whole plate. Continue replicating by shuttling back and forth between the microtiter and media plates. Let the liquid absorb to the agar before putting a plate upside down in an incubator.

9. An alternative approach to assessing activation or repression of the LacZ reporter is to use a chloroform overlay technique (adapted from **ref. *17***). This technique is much more sensitive than a standard X Gal plate assay, can be done within 24 h of plating on appropriate medium, and is generally preferred in high-throughput analysis.

    a. Gently overlay Gal/CM -Ura-His and Glu/CM -Ura-His plates with chloroform, pipetting slowly in from the side so as not to smear colonies. Leave colonies completely covered for 5 min.

    b. Briefly rinse the plates with another 5 mL of chloroform (optional), drain, and let dry for another 5 min at 37°C or for 10 min in a fume hood.

    c. Overlay the plates with 10 mL of X-Gal-agarose, making sure that all the yeast spots are completely covered (plates will be chilled after chloroform evaporation, so it will be difficult to spread less than 7 mL of top agarose).

    d. Incubate the plates at 30°C and check for color changes after 20 min, and again after 1–3 h.

    For the activation assay, strong activators such as the LexA-GAL4 control (pSH 17-4) will produce a blue color in 5–10 min, and a weak activator control will produce a blue color within approx 1 h. Such weakly activating baits have been used successfully in library screens (in a less sensitive strain and with a less sensitive LacZ reporter), albeit not without trouble. A bait protein that activates more strongly than the weak activator control is unsuitable and should be modified; one that activates in a comparable fashion or weaker (also compare vs negative control pRFHMI) may be suitable. The repression assay should be monitored within 1 to 2 h because the high basal LacZ activity will make differential activation of JK101 impossible to see with longer incubations.

10. The repression assay provides an indirect gage of bait binding to LexA operators, based on its ability to interfere with GAL4 transcriptional activation (*see* **Fig. 7**).

11. Three basic problems that can be identified and potentially corrected before screening are bait activation of transcription, bait toxicity, and inappropriate bait protein expression. Because all of these can cause difficulties in performing library screening, it may be necessary to modify the bait or conditions of screening (as described in **Table 1**).

12. In an optimal result, all six colonies assayed within a transformation group (e.g., all the colonies from reaction a) would possess approximately equivalent phenotypes for a given assay. For a small number of baits, this is not the case. The most typical deviation is that of six colonies, assayed for a new bait, of which some fraction are white on X-Gal and do not grow on -Leu medium, and the remaining fraction display some degree of blueness and growth. Do *not* select the white, nongrowing colonies as a starting point in a library screen; generally, these colonies possess the phenotypes they do because they are synthesizing little or no bait protein (as can be assayed by Western blot; *see* **Subheading 3.1.3.**). The reasons for this are not clear; however, it appears to be a bait-specific phenomenon and may be linked to some degree of toxicity of continued expression of particular proteins in yeast. It will probably be necessary to adjust sensitivity levels or use an inducible bait to allow work with blue/growing colonies.

13. Many LexA-fusion proteins exhibit sharp decreases in detectable levels of protein with the onset of stationary phase. Therefore, saturated cultures may not necessarily have an increasing yield of protein to assay. It may be a good idea to freeze duplicate samples at this stage for later use.

14. An antibody to LexA is commercially available from Invitrogen, Clontech or Santa Cruz Biotechnology (Santa Cruz, CA).

15. A high percentage of the colonies not appropriately expressing the bait protein, although containing the bait plasmid, may be indicative that the bait is toxic in the yeast (*see* **Note 11**).

16. A good library transformation efficiency should be approx 10^5 transformants/µg of library DNA (for a single transformation). Transformation of yeast in multiple small aliquots in parallel helps reduce the likelihood of contamination; further, it frequently results in significantly better transformation efficiency than that obtained by using larger volumes in a smaller number of tubes. Finally, do not use excess transforming library DNA per aliquot of competent yeast cells because this may take up multiple library plasmids, complicating subsequent analysis. Under the

conditions described here, less than 10% of yeast will contain two or more library plasmids.

17. While it is possible to throw away the beads after spreading, it is acceptable and efficient to keep the glass beads on the lids while incubating the plates; glass beads are needed to harvest the library transformants (**Subheading 3.2.2.**).

18. The bait and *lexAop*-LacZ reporter plasmids should have been transformed into the yeast less than 7–10 d prior to supertransformation with the library.

19. If molds or other contaminants are observed on the plates, carefully excise them and a region around them using a sterile razor blade prior to beginning harvest of library transformants.

20. This technique allows you to minimize the time the plates are open and thus avoid contamination from airborne molds and bacteria. About one third of the yeast slurry will be left on the plates; a second wash (add a further 10 mL of sterile water, shake again, and transfer the slurry to an unwashed plate) can greatly improve the yield. However, in a direct library transformation no more than 2% of the collected slurry is normally used; thus, the only important thing is to ensure approximately the same wash-off rate for all the plates.

21. In general, for yeast frozen for <1 yr, viability will be >90%. Refreezing a thawed aliquot results in the loss of viability; therefore, many frozen aliquots (0.2–1.0 mL) should be made (especially if multiple hunts will be conducted by Interaction Mating). A series of limiting dilutions on Glu/CM -Trp (or Glu/CM -Trp-His-Ura for a direct library transformation) should be performed.

22. As with the frozen pretransformed library strain, the mated yeast should not be thawed and refrozen; because only one or a few of the aliquots will be needed to represent the library, thawed aliquots can be discarded after use.

23. The number of Leu+ colonies to pick and characterize should be based on the number of cDNA-independent false positives that arise on the Leu+ plates for the control mating. The higher the frequency of false positives, the more Leu+ colonies that should be picked to find rare true positives. Since the frequency of true positives will be unknown at this step, the goal will be to pick all the false positives that are expected in the number of library transformants being screened. For example, if the number of library transformants was 10^6, the goal be to pick the number of false positives expected in 10^6 diploids. If the cDNA-independent false positive frequency were 1 Leu+ colony in 104 CFU plated, it would be necessary to pick at least 100 Leu+ colonies to find a true positive that exists at a frequency of 1 in 10^6.

24. If contamination occurred at an earlier step and results in the growth of many (>500) colonies per plate, this will interfere with screening. In the case of bacterial contamination, the situation can be retrieved by adding 15 µg/mL of tetracycline to the selective plates and repeating library induction/plating. However, if the contamination is fungal, there is little to be done; hence, transformation must be repeated.

25. If colonies do not arise within the first week after plating, colonies appearing at later time points are not likely to represent bona fide positives. True interactors

tend to come up in a window of time specific for a given bait, with false positives clustering at a different time point; hence, pregrouping by date of growth facilitates the decision of which clones to analyze first.

26. Transfer approximately the volume of one middle-sized yeast colony (a 2 to 3-μL packed pellet); do *not* take more, or the quality of the isolated DNA will suffer. The master plate does not need to be absolutely fresh; plates that have been stored for 5 days at 4°C have been successfully used. If appropriate, a multicolony plastic replicator/frogger can be used.

27. PCR product can be obtained directly from the yeast colonies even without β-glucuronidase treatment (e.g., by introducing a 10 min, 94°C step at the beginning of the PCR program).

28. For the plasmid JG4-5; forward primer, (FP1) is 5'-CTGAGTGGAGATGCC TCC-3', and the reverse primer, (FP2) is 5'-CTGGCAAGGTAGACAAGCCG-3'. FP1 works well in the sequencing of PCR fragments, but the FP2 will only work in sequencing purified plasmids. In general, the TA-rich nature of the ADH terminator sequences downstream of the polylinker in the pJG4-5 vector makes it difficult to design high-quality primers in this region.

29. Modified versions of this protocol with extended elongation times were also found to work; the variant described has amplified fragments of as much as 1.8 kb in fair quantity.

30. To interpret the results of the PCR, it is helpful to have the following control templates: Empty library plasmid (diluted); yeast from the positive control colonies, treated alongside the experimental clones; and the same amounts of diluted library plasmid and positive control yeast, mixed together. For analysis of results, *see* **Table 3**.

31. This will generally yield distinctive and unambiguous groups of inserts, confirming whether multiple isolates of a small number of cDNAs have been obtained. Sometimes a single yeast will contain two or more different library plasmids. If this happens, it will be immediately revealed by PCR; hence, after bacterial transformation an increased number of clones should be checked to avoid the loss of the "real" interactor.

32. Transformation a is a control experiment providing an indication of the degree of digestion of the library plasmid. The background level of colonies transformed with digested empty library plasmid should be minimal; if the background is high, ensure complete digestion of the empty library plasmid by increasing the digestion incubation time or the restriction enzyme concentration. Transformation c is a positive control for the transformation.

33. In the event that the pBait used in the screen shows weak transcriptional activity on its own, it is highly advisable to choose a nonspecific control bait that can weakly activate transcription on its own in order to set up the background level of transcription activation, because baits that have transcriptional activation capacity have greater difficulties with false positive background in general.

34. Clones transformed with pPrey-control cDNA provide both positive and negative controls: transformations a, b, and d should be negative whereas transformants

Table 3
Interpretation of PCR Results

Template	Possible outcomes			
Plasmid[a]	−	+	+	+
Yeast pPrey-control[b]	−	−	−	+/−
Plasmid + yeast pPrey-control	−	+	−	+/−
Clone 1 . . . to n	−	−	−	+/−
Interpretation	Bad master mix, wrong settings, faulty amplifier.	Not enough template.	Lysed yeast inhibited PCR.	Too much yeast; uneven template load.
Recommendation	Double-check, repeat.	Add more template, improve lysis.	Add less template.	Adjust template, load, re-PCR from obtained bands.

[a]PCR from the empty vector yields a product of ~130 bp for JG4-5 (FP1 and FP2 primers), and ~185 bp for YesTrp (YesTrp forward and reverse primers).

[b]Consult kit description/manufacturer for predicted fragment size.

451

from c should be positive when assayed for β-galactosidase and growth on -Leu plates.

35. The use of electroporation is highly recommended.

36. Crude yeast lysate obtained following β-glucuronidase treatment can also be used as a source of plasmid for electroporation into *E. coli* (**Subheading 3.3.1., step 3**). In addition, a number of kits for yeast minipreps are commercially available (e.g., from Clontech). Some companies (e.g., Bio101, Vista, CA; http://www.bio101.com/serviceslhybrid.html) will isolate plasmid from the yeast cells, transform, and amplify the plasmid in *E. coli* to produce a sequencing template.

37. If using ampicillin-resistant bait and reporter plasmids in combination with Ap^R library plasmid pJG4–5, it will be necessary to select specifically for transformants containing a library plasmid by the ability of the yeast *TRP1* gene to complement the *E. coli trpC* mutation.

    a. Electroporate *(13)* 1 μL of each plasmid DNA into *E. coli* KC8 *(pyrF leuB600 trpC hisB463)*, and plate on LB/ampicillin. Incubate overnight at 37°C.

    b. Restreak or replica plate colonies from the LB/ampicillin plates to bacterial defined minimal medium KC8 plates supplemented with uracil, histidine, and leucine but lacking tryptophan. Colonies that grow under these conditions contain the library plasmid, since the *TRP1* gene contained on this plasmid efficiently complements the bacterial *trpC9830* mutation. It is also feasible to plate *E. coli* KC8 transformants directly onto bacterial minimal medium, although it may take 2 d for colonies to grow.

38. This is only necessary for the first step in a protein interaction walk; for subsequent steps, the AD version of the previous bait will already be available from the previous hunt.

39. In the forward primer sequence, the overlined section is from pEG202, up to but not including the *Eco*RI site. The underlined section is from pB42AD. The 3' G is the first G in the *Eco*RI site of pB42AD. The reading frame for pEG202 and pB42AD are the same.

40. In the forward primer sequence, the overlined section is from pNLex, up to but not including, the *Eco*RI site. The underlined section is from pB42AD. The GTG is from both vectors. The 3' G is the first G in the *Eco*RI site of pB42AD. The reading frame for pNLex and pB42AD are the same.

41. Most of the streaks of the new bait strain should produce an interaction phenotype (galactose-dependent Leu+*lacZ*+) when crossed with the strain expressing the interacting AD fusion protein, but not with the strain containing the library vector alone. About 1 in 10 of the new bait strain colonies will fail to produce the expected interaction phenotype. Some of these failures result from bait vectors that did not receive an insert and others result from incorrect recombination events, e.g., between the *lacZ* vector and the bait vector; the former class will result in Leu-*lacZ*- phenotype when mated, whereas the later class can lead to galactose-independent *lacZ*+ yeast. Bait strain colonies that result in the correct positive interaction phenotype can be used in subsequent interactor hunts by

mating with frozen pretransformed library (as described in **Subheadings 3.2.3.–3.2.5.**).

42. The culture can be used to inoculate additional culture arrays and to freeze as a stock culture. To inoculate another array of cluster tubes, resuspend the cells either by covering and inverting or by pipetting up and down with a multichannel pipettor. Insert a frogger into the cluster tubes and draw out slowly allowing excess liquid to drip back into the tubes, and insert it into a new set of cluster tubes containing 2 mL of Glu/CM -Ura-His liquid medium. Grow with shaking at 30°C for 2 d. Each culture can be used to perform multiple matings or can be frozen for future use. To freeze, add 1 mL of glycerol solution and mix by covering and inverting or pipetting up and down. Freeze at –80°C.

43. Each panel of bait strains should be mated once with a strain containing the AD fusion vector (e.g., pJG4-5) with no insert as a control to reveal the background transcriptional activation potential of the baits. Increases in reporter activation in matings with strains expressing AD fusion proteins relative to this control mating will be interpreted as interactions.

References

1. Fields, S. and Song, O. (1989) A novel genetic system to detect protein-protein interaction. *Nature* **340,** 245, 246.
2. Chien, C. T., Bartel, P. L., Steruglanz, R., and Fields, S. (1991) The two-hybrid system: a method to identify and clone genes for proteins that interact with a protein of interest. *Proc. Natl. Acad. Sci. USA* **88,** 9578–9582.
3. Durfee, T., Becherer, K., Chen, P. L., Yeh, S. H., Yang, Y., Kilburn, A. E., Lce, W. H., and Elledge, S. J. (1993) The retinoblastoma protein associates with the protein phosphatase type 1 catalytic subunit. *Genes Dev.* **7,** 555–569.
4. Gyuris, J., Golemis, E. A., Chertkov, H., and Brent, R. (1993) Cdi1, a human G1 and S phase protein phosphatase that associates with Cdk2. *Cell* **75,** 791–803.
5. Vojtek, A. B., Hollenberg, S. M., and Cooper, J. A. (1993) Mammalian Ras interacts directly with the serine/threonine kinase Raf. *Cell* **74,** 205–214.
6. Finley, R. and Brent, R. (1994) Interaction mating reveals binary and ternary connections between Drosophila cell cycle regulators. *Proc. Natl. Acad. Sci. USA* **91,** 12,980–12,984.
7. Bartel, P. L., Roecklein, J. A., SenGupta, D., and Fields, S. (1996) A protein linkage map of *Escherichia coli* bacteriophage T7. *Nature Genet.* **12,** 72–77.
8. Fromont-Racine, M., Rain, J.-C., and Legrain, P. (1997) Toward a functional analysis of the yeast genome through exhaustive two-hybrid screens. *Nature Genet.* **16,** 277–282.
9. Serebriiskii, I., Khazak, V., and Golemis, E. A. (1999) A two-hybrid dual bait system to discriminate specificity of protein interactions. *J. Biol. Chem.* **274,** 17,080–17,087.
10. Watson, M. A., Buckholz, R., and Weiner, M. P. (1996) Vectors encoding alternative antibiotic resistance for use in the yeast two-hybrid system. *BioTechniques* **21,** 255–259.

11. Clontech's Yeast Protocols Handbook: <http://www.clontech.com/clontech/ Manuals/ PDF/PT3024-l.pdf>.

12. Harlow, E. and Lane, D. (1988) Antibodies: A Laboratory Manual, Cold Spring Harbor Laboratory, Cold Spring Harbor, NY.

13. Sambrook, J., Fritsch, E. F., and Maniatis, T. (1989) Molecular Cloning: A Laboratory Manual, Cold Spring Harbor Laboratory, Cold Spring Harbor, NY.

14. <http://www.fermentas.com/TechInfo/PCR/DNAamplProtocol.html>.

15. Petermann, R., Mossier, B. M., Aryee, D. N., and Kovar, H. (1998) A recombination based method to rapidly assess specificity of two-hybrid clones in yeast. *Nucleic Acids Res.* **26**, 2252, 2253.

16. Schiestl, R. H., and Gietz, R. D. (1989) High efficiency transformation of intact yeast cells using single stranded nucleic acids as a carrier. *Curr. Genet.* **16**, 339–346.

17. Duttweiler, H. M. (1996) A highly sensitive and non-lethal beta-galactosidase plate assay for yeast. *TIG* **12**, 340, 341.

18. Vidal, M., Brachmann, R. K., Fattaey, A., Harlow, E., and Boeke, J. D. (1996) Reverse two-hybrid and one-hybrid systems to detect dissociation of protein-protein and DNA-protein interactions. *Proc. Natl. Acad. Sci. USA* **93**, 10,315–10,320.

19. Serebriiskii, I. and Golemis, E. A. (1996) http://www.fccc.edu/research/labs/ golemis/InteractionTrapInWork.html.

20. Ruden, D. M., Ma, J., Li, Y., Wood, K., and Ptashne, M. (1991) Generating yeast transcriptional activators containing no yeast protein sequences. *Nature* **350**, 250–252.

21. Brent, R., and Ptashne, M. (1980) The lexA gene product represses its own promoter. *Proc. Natl. Acad. Sci. USA* **77**, 1932–1936.

22. Little, J. W., Mount, D. W., and Yanisch-Perron, C. R. (1981) Purified lexA protein is a repressor of the recA and lexA genes. *Proc. Natl. Acad. Sci. USA* **78**, 4199–4203.

23. Brent, R. and Ptashne, M. (1984) A bacterial repressor protein or a yeast transcriptional terminator can block upstream activation of a yeast gene. *Nature* **312**, 612–615.

27

Methods for Adeno-Associated Virus–Mediated Gene Transfer into Muscle

Terry J. Amiss and Richard Jude Samulski

1. Introduction

Gene therapy vectors based on adeno-associated virus (AAV) are being used to successfully transduce a number of different tissues, including muscle *(1)*. The first demonstration of muscle transduction by recombinant AAV (rAAV) was reported by Xiao et al. *(2)* in 1996. In that report, *LacZ* expression from an AAV vector was established in immunocompetent mice for over 1.5 yr. Since that time, several laboratories have confirmed these observations with direct im injection of rAAV followed by sustained expression of various transgenes such as β-glucuronidase, alpha-1-antitrypsin, erythropoietin, and coagulation factor IX *(3–6)*. Unlike other viral vectors, AAV appears to avoid immune response to the vector transgene, and, therefore, efforts to evaluate this delivery system for human use through testing large animal models have been initiated. Although the initial observations were hailed with success, in 1998 Monohan et al. *(6)* established that trace amounts of adenovirus helper elicit a cellular immune response to the AAV-transduced tissue. Critical to the success of long-term vector expression is the quality of the AAV virus. Soon after this observation, efforts were made to improve the procedure for generating rAAV vectors *(7,8)*. In this chapter, we describe how to produce rAAV free of wild-type adenovirus. In addition, Summerford and Samulski *(9)* recently identified the receptor for AAV, heparan sulfate proteoglycan. This discovery led to a novel purification procedure using affinity chromatography *(10,11)*. The protocol also uses an iodixanol gradient in place of cesium chloride, which has significantly shortened the high-speed centrifugation step and improved the quality of the vector preparations. This method is described in detail. In addition, we discuss methods for

From: *Methods in Molecular Biology, vol. 175: Genomics Protocols*
Edited by: M. P. Starkey and R. Elaswarapu © Humana Press Inc., Totowa, NJ

quantifying the purified vector, im administration, and transgene distribution and expression.

1.1. rAAV Vectors

rAAV vectors are now recognized for their ease of administration and propensity for long-term transgene expression *(1)*. However, the most important characteristic of this virus, which will impact its use as a human gene therapy vector, is its inability to cause disease. After many years of scrutiny, an illness has never been attributed to AAV. For this reason, AAV is the only human viral vector classified as nonpathogenic. Associated with its safety is the inability of the virus to replicate autonomously *(12)*. To propagate, AAV requires the presence of another virus, called a helper virus, which is typically adenovirus *(12–14)*. Initial protocols for AAV production utilized wild-type adenovirus as an integral component. However, new vector production methods (**Fig. 1**) have eliminated the need for adenovirus and any possibility of wild-type viral contamination *(1,7–11)*.

While the production of rAAV has moved closer to clinical grade material, many aspects of the biology of AAV have also proven useful for the vector. For example, AAV has a broad host range and the ability to infect most types of cells whether dividing or nondividing (for a review *see* **ref.** *1*). However, the most exciting characteristic of AAV, yet to be exploited, is its potential to recombine at a specific location on human chromosome 19 *(15–18)*. This characteristic is called site-specific integration, and AAV is the only eukaryotic virus known to have this trait. The obvious benefit of site-specific integration is the reduced risk of random insertional mutation. Currently, all rAAV vectors lack the ability to target chromosome 19, although efforts are continuing to reincorporate this feature back into vectors. Today's version of AAV vectors has the viral Rep and Cap open reading frames removed (96% of the genome) for transgene insertion. The only remaining AAV sequences are the inverted terminal repeats (ITRs). The ITRs are the only *cis*-acting viral structure necessary for replication, packaging, and sustained expression of the transgene *(19)*. Generally, the removal of the *Rep* and *Cap* genes is necessary to avoid recombination and the creation of wild-type AAV during the production of the vector. An rAAV genome size of 4.6 kb or smaller is required for the efficient DNA packaging into viron shells. Although this restricts the transgene size to 4.3 kb or smaller, 80% of all cDNAs fall into this range. Continued success of AAV vectors follows our basic understanding of the biology of this unique human parvovirus. Reviews are available that describe the biology of AAV in more detail *(1,20)*.

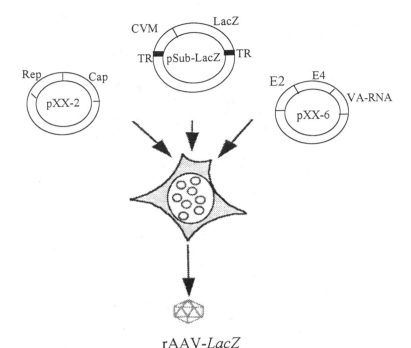

rAAV-*LacZ*

Fig. 1. Generation of adenovirus-free rAAV Three plasmids are used to transfect 293 cells: the plasmid pXX-2 carries the *Rep* and *Cap* genes of AAV but not the terminal repeats (TRs); the plasmid pSub-LacZ carries the AAV TRs and the transgene (in this case *LacZ*); and the plasmid pXX-6 supplies the adenovirus helper genes *E2*, *E4*, and *VA-RNA*. The three plasmids transfected together enable the production of adenovirus-free rAAV.

2. Materials

2.1. Cell Culture

1. Human 293 cells (American Type Culture Collection [ATCC], Rockville, MD; CRL 1573).
2. Phosphate-buffered saline (PBS): 1.0% (w/v) NaCl; 0.25% (w/v) KCl, 0.14% (w/v) Na_2HPO_4; 0.025% (w/v) Na_2HPO_4 (pH 7.2), sterile.
3. Dulbecco's modified Eagle's medium (DMEM) (no. 12440-020; Gibco-BRL Life Technologies).
4. Iscove's modified Dulbecco's medium (IMDM) (12,440-046) (Gibco-BRL Life Technologies).
5. Penicillin G, streptomycin.
6. PBS containing 0.5 mM EDTA.
7. Tissue culture dishes, 10 and 15-cm diameter.
8. Light microscope.

2.2. Plasmids

1. Plasmid psub201 (ATCC 6805), map, and sequence are available on the Internet at http://www.med.unc.edu/genether/.
2. Plasmid pXX2, the AAV helper plasmid (Samulski laboratory); map; and sequence are available on the Internet site.
3. Plasmid pXX6, the adenoviral helper plasmid (Samulski laboratory); map; and sequence are available on the Internet site.

2.3. Adenovirus-Free Production of Recombinant Virus

1. Monolayers of 293 cells at approx 80% confluency.
2. Restriction enzymes *Xba*I and *Hin*dIII.
3. Polystyrene tubes (50 mL) (Falcon).
4. Sure bacteria (Stratagene).
5. 2X HeBS (HEPES-buffered saline): Mix 16.4 g of NaCl, 11.9 g of HEPES, and 0.21 g of Na_2HPO_4, (pH 7.05). Adjust to 1 L and filter sterilize.
6. Nitrocellulose filter sterilization unit (0.45 μm) (Nalgene).

2.4. Purification of Recombinant Virus

1. Centrifuge and rotors GS3 and SS34 (Sorvall).
2. Ultracentrifuge and rotors SW41 and Ti70 (Beckman).
3. Sonicator with 3-mm-diameter probe.
4. EconoPump (Bio-Rad, Hercules, CA).
5. Ethanol/dry ice bath.
6. PBS-MK: Mix 50 mL of 10X PBS, 0.5 mL of 1 M $MgCl_2$, and 0.5 mL of 2.5 M KCl, and adjust to a final volume of 0.5 L with ddH_2O.
7. Optiseal tubes (Beckman).
8. Ultra-Clear tubes (12.5 and 32.4 mL) for SW41 rotor (Beckman).
9. Heparin Sepharose column (1 mL) (HiTrap Heparin, no. 17-0407; Amersham Pharmacia Biotech).
10. Optiprep (Gibco-BRL Life Technologies).
11. 15% Iodixanol with 1 M NaCl: Mix 5 mL of 10X PBS, 0.05 mL of 1 M $MgCl_2$, 0.05 mL of 2.5 M KCl, 10 mL of 5 M NaCl, 0.075 mL of 0.5% stock phenol red, and 12.5 mL of Optiprep. Adjust to a final volume of 50 mL with ddH_2O and filter sterilize.
12. 25% Iodixanol: Mix 5 mL of 10X PBS, 0.05 mL of 1 M $MgCl_2$, 0.05 mL of 2.5 M KCl, 0.1 mL of 0.5% stock phenol red, and 20 mL of Optiprep. Adjust to a final volume of 50 mL with ddH_2O and filter sterilize.
13. 40% Iodixanol: Mix 5 mL of 10X PBS, 0.05 mL of 1 M $MgCl_2$, 0.05 mL of 2.5 M KCl, 33.3 mL of Optiprep. Adjust to a final volume of 50 mL with ddH_2O and filter sterilize.
14. 60% Iodixanol: Mix 0.05 mL of 1 M $MgCl_2$, 0.05 mL of 2.5 M KCl, and 0.025 mL of 0.5% stock phenol red in 50 mL of Optiprep. Filter sterilize.
15. OPTI-MEM I (no. 31985-013; Gibco-BRL Life Technologies).

16. Phenol red (Gibco-BRL Life Technologies).
17. Slide-A-Lyzer 10,000 MWCO (Pierce).
18. Syringes (5 mL) and needles (18 gage).

2.5. Dot-Blot Assay

1. DNase I digestion mixture: 10 mM Tris-HCl, pH 7.5; 10 mM MgCl$_2$, 2 mM CaCl$_2$, 50 U/mL DNase I.
2. Proteinase K digestion mixture: 1 M NaCl, 1% (w/v) Sarkosyl, 200 µg/mL of Proteinase K.
3. Whatman 3MM paper.
4. Dot-blot apparatus.
5. Gene-Screen Plus membrane (New England Nuclear).
6. Random Primer Labelling Kit (Roche).
7. ^{32}P-dCTP (Amersham Pharmacia Biotech).
8. Church buffer: Mix 5 g of BSA, 1 mL of 0.5 M EDTA, 33.5 g of Na$_2$HPO$_4$·7H$_2$O, 1 mL of 85% H$_3$PO$_4$, 35 g of sodium dodecyl sulfate (SDS). Adjust to a final volume of 0.5 L with ddH$_2$O. Heat at 65°C to dissolve. Store on the bench indefinitely.
9. Hybridization low-stringency wash solution: 2X saline sodium citrate (SSC), 2X 0.1% (w/v) SDS.
10. Hybridization medium-stringency wash solution: 0.5X SSC, 1X 0.1% (w/v) SDS.
11. Hybridization high-stringency wash solution: 0.1X SSC, 0.5X 0.1% (w/v) SDS.
12. 2X SSC: Mix 17.5 g of NaCl and 8.8 g of trisodium citrate·2H$_2$O. Adjust the final volume to 1 L and adjust the pH to 7.0.
13. Hybridization bottles (Gibco-BRL Life Technologies).
14. PhosphoImager or scintillation counter.

2.6. Injection of Recombinant Virus into Muscle

1. Swiss Webster mice.
2. 2.5% Avertin.
3. Syringes (1 mL) and needles (30 gage).
4. Leica microtone.
5. Dry ice.

2.7. Detection of LacZ Expression

1. Stain: Mix 0.625 mL of 5-bromo-4-chloro-3-indolyl-β-D-galactopyranoside (X-gal), 0.025 mL of 2 M MgCl$_2$, 1 mL of potassium ferricyanide, and 1 mL of potassium ferrocyanide, and adjust to a final volume of 25 mL with PBS. Warm to 37°C.
2. Fixative solution: Mix 2.7 mL of 37% (v/v) formaldehyde and 0.4 mL of 25% (v/v) glutaraldehyde in a disposable 50-mL tube. Adjust to a final volume of 50 mL with cold PBS.

2.8. Histological Analysis

1. Microscope glass slides and cover slips.
2. Small paintbrush.
3. Mounting medium.
4. Light microscope (e.g., Nikon Eclipse E800).

2.9. Molecular Analysis

1. Lysis buffer: 100 mM NaCl; 10 mM Tris-HCl, pH 8.0; 25 mM EDTA, pH 8.0; 0.5% (w/v) SDS; 0.1 mg/mL of Proteinase K. Add Proteinase K fresh before each use.
2. Phenol/chloroform/isoamyl alcohol (25:24:1).
3. Speed-Vac concentrator.
4. Restriction enzyme *Eco*RV.
5. Gene-Screen Plus membrane (New England Nuclear).

3. Methods

3.1. Ad-Free Production of Recombinant Virus

This section describes the production of rAAV vectors using three plasmids: psub201, pXX2, and pXX6 (**Fig. 1**).

3.1.1. Construction of rAAV Plasmid Vector

Here we will use the *Escherichia coli* β-galactosidase reporter gene (*LacZ*) that harbors a nuclear localization signal and is regulated by the cytomegalovirus (CMV) promoter. The CMV promoter has been shown to produce sustained expression of transgenes after in vivo administration into muscle tissue *(2)*.

1. Modify the plasmid psub201 by digestion with the restriction enzymes *Xba*I and *Hin*dIII (*see* **Note 1**) to remove the *Rep* and *Cap* genes. This produces a 4-kb fragment containing the AAV ITRs.
2. Insert the foreign gene cassette, made of the transgene and its promoter, between the *Xba*I and *Hin*dIII sites (*see* **Notes 2–5**).

3.1.2. Transfection of 293 Cells

1. Grow 293 cells in 15-cm dishes using DMEM + 10% (v/v) fetal bovine serum (FBS) + penicillin G/streptomycin. Generally a total of 20 dishes are transfected for the viral preparation procedure.
2. Split the 293 cells 1 d before transfecting, so that the cells are 70–80% confluent the next day. Three hours before transfection, replace the DMEM with IMDM + 10% (v/v) FBS + penicillin G/streptomycin (*see* **Note 6**).
3. Transfect 293 cells in groups of four 15-cm dishes. Mix in a disposable 50-mL polystyrene tube (*see* **Notes 7** and **8**) 90 µg of pXX6 helper plasmid (provides adenovirus helper genes), 30 µg of rAAV-*LacZ* vector plasmid, 30 µg of pXX2 helper plasmid (provides AAV helper genes), and 0.4 L of 2.5 M CaCl$_2$ Adjust the final volume to 4 mL with ddH$_2$O.

4. Add the 4 mL of plasmid mixture to 4 mL of 2X HeBS in a disposable 50-mL polystyrene tube and mix gently. Incubate for 1–5 min at room temperature, and a very fine precipitate will be apparent (*see* **Note 9**).
5. Add 2 mL of this mixture dropwise, with gentle swirling, to one of the 15 cm dishes containing the 293 cells. Repeat with the remaining three dishes.
6. Repeat **steps 3–5** for the remaining 15-cm dishes of 293 cells.
7. Incubate the cells for 24 h and then change the medium to DMEM + 2% (v/v) FBS + penicillin G/streptomycin. Process each plate individually so that the cells do not dry out (*see* **Note 10**).
8. At 48 h posttransfection, collect the cells and DMEM from the 20 dishes and place in a 250-mL polypropylene centrifuge bottle (*see* **Note 11**).

3.2. Purification of Recombinant Virus

3.2.1. Crude Purification of Recombinant Virus

1. Freeze/thaw the cell suspension using a dry ice–ethanol bath and a 37°C water bath.
2. Repeat the freeze/thaw step two more times.
3. Pellet the 293 cells by centrifuging at 3000*g*. Save the cell pellet and the supernatant. Remove the supernatant (crude lysate containing the rAAV-*LacZ*), and place in a clean 250-mL polypropylene centrifuge bottle.
4. Add 78.5 g of ammonium sulfate per 250 mL of crude lysate. Mix thoroughly to dissolve. Place the mixture in centrifuge tubes and incubate the mixture on ice for 20 min. The ammonium sulfate will precipitate the virus.
5. Collect the rAAV-*LacZ* by centrifuging at 5000*g* in a GS3 rotor at 4°C.
6. Carefully pour off the supernatant and keep the pellet, which contains the rAAV-*LacZ*. Place the pellet on ice. Dispose of the supernatant after autoclaving.
7. Resuspend the pellet from **step 2** in 20 mL of OPTI-MEM and transfer to a disposable 50-mL polypropylene tube.
8. Sonicate this mixture for 40 s (50% duty, power level 2) on ice, in a tissue culture hood dedicated to viral work.
9. Centrifuge the tubes at 3000*g* for 5 min at 4°C. Save the pellet and the supernatant.
10. Transfer the supernatant to a disposable 50-mL polypropylene tube.
11. Resuspend the pellet in 20 mL of OPTI-MEM and repeat **steps 7** and **8**. Then save the supernatant. The pellet can now be discarded.
12. Pool the two supernatants from **steps 8** and **9** Use the pooled supernatants to resuspend the ammonium sulfate pellet from **step 5**.
13. Measure the volume of the supernatant, add 1/3 vol of cold, saturated ammonium sulfate; mix well; and place on ice for 10 min. This will precipitate undesired proteins.
14. Centrifuge at 5000*g* for 10 min at 4°C in an SS34 rotor. Save the supernatant and transfer to a 50-mL high-speed polypropylene tube, leaving a yellow precipitate behind. Discard the precipitate.
15. To the supernatant, add two thirds of the original volume (from **step 11**) of cold, saturated ammonium sulfate; mix well; and place on ice for 20 min. This will

bring the concentration of ammonium sulfate to 50% and precipitate the rAAV-*LacZ*.

16. Centrifuge the mixture at 12,000*g* in an SS34 rotor for 20 min at 4°C. Remove the supernatant and discard after autoclaving. Centrifuge the pellet again and remove any residual liquid. Save the pellet. The pellet can be stored for up to 6 mo at –20°C.

3.2.2. Purification Using an Iodixanol (Optiprep) Gradient

1. Dissolve the pellet from **step 14** in **Subheading 3.2.1.** in 15 mL of PBS-MK. Place half (7.5 mL) of the resuspended rAAV-*LacZ* into each of two Optiseal tubes.
2. A step gradient is made by underlayering and displacing less dense cell suspension with solutions containing increasing amounts of Iodixanol. To both Optiseal tubes successively underlay with 6 mL of 15% Iodixanol (*see* **Notes 12** and **13**), 5 mL of 25% Iodixanol, 5 mL of 40% Iodixanol, and 5 mL of 60% Iodixanol. Carefully remove the tubing without disturbing the gradient layers.
3. Fill the Optiseal tube completely by slowly adding PBS to the viral solution that forms the uppermost layer. Insert a plug and centrifuge at 4°C for 1 h in a Ti70 rotor at 350,000*g*.
4. Carefully remove the Optiseal tubes from the rotor. In a viral hood, remove the plug from the top of the tube. Use a 5-mL syringe with an 18-gage needle to puncture the tube just above the 60% Iodixanol interface. Remove the clear 40% layer containing the purified rAAV-*LacZ* (*see* **Note 14**).

3.2.3. Purification Using a Heparin Column

1. Wash the Bio-Rad EconoPump, tubing, and injector with 20 mL of PBS-MK.
2. Connect the heparin sepharose column (1-mL vol) to the injector and equilibrate the column with 5 vol of PBS-MK at a flow rate of 0.5 mL/min.
3. Reduce the flow rate to 0.2 mL/min, and inject the 40% iodixanol fraction containing the rAAV-*LacZ* from **step 4** in **Subheading 3.2.2.** onto the heparin sulfate column. A viral preparation made from twenty 15-cm dishes of 293 cells can be purified on a 1-mL column with a single injection.
4. Wash the column with five column volumes of PBS-MK. Collect 0.5-mL eluent fractions during each step, including when placing the sample on the column, washing, and the elution (*see* **Note 15**).
5. Elute the rAAV-*LacZ* using a 5-mL linear gradient from 0 to 100% of 1 *M* NaCl in PBS-MK.
6. Wash the heparin column with 2 mL of 1 *M* NaCl in PBS-MK, and then discard the column (*see* **Note 16**).
7. Wash the Bio-Rad EconoPump, tubing, and injector with 20 mL of 0.5 *M* NaOH, followed by 20 mL of 20% (v/v) ethanol.
8. Test the fractions for the presence of virus using the dot-blot hybridization assay (*see* **Subheading 3.3.1.**), and combine the fractions with the highest concentration of virus.

9. Dialyze the virus in an MWCO 10,000 cassette against 1 L of PBS at 4°C. Repeat.
10. Aliquot the virus into smaller fractions and store at −20 to −80°C.

3.3. Delivery of Recombinant Virus In Vitro

3.3.1. Determination of rAAV-LacZ Titer by Dot-Blot Assay

Before infecting a cell line with rAAV virus, it is necessary to determine the titer of the viral preparation. The dot-blot assay *(21)* detects packaged rAAV genomes by using probes specific for the transgene cassette. Although a positive signal in this assay reveals that rAAV virons were produced, it does not indicate whether the virus is infectious or whether the expression cassette is functional. Samples and controls for this assay can easily be prepared directly in a 96-well microtiter plate.

1. Place 5 μL of each fraction collected from the Heparin sulfate column (**step 4, Subheading 3.2.3.**) into a well of a 96-well microtiter plate. Assay duplicate samples of each fraction.
2. Add 50 μL of DNase I digestion mixture and incubate for 1 h at 37°C. This treatment digests any viral DNA that has not been packaged into capsids.
3. Stop the digestion by adding 10 μL of 0.1 M EDTA to each reaction.
4. Add 60 μL of Proteinase K digestion mixture to each sample to release the viral DNA from the capsid. Incubate for 30 min at 50°C.
5. By way of a set of DNA hybridization standards, use plasmid DNA that was used for the transfection, in this case rAAV-*LacZ*. Linearize the plasmid and do serial dilutions in 10 mM Tris-HCl (pH 8.0) and 1 mM EDTA. A volume of 25 μL is convenient for each standard in wells of a 96-well microtiter plate. A suitable standard working range is 500 ng to 10 fg.
6. Denature the samples and control DNAs by adding 100 μL of 0.5 M NaOH to each.
7. Prewet a nylon membrane in 0.4 M Tris-HCl (pH 7.5) and place it between the upper and lower blocks of a dot-blot manifold apparatus.
8. Add the denatured DNAs from the 96-well microtiter plate to the wells of the dot-blot manifold apparatus in the absence of a vacuum. After all the DNA has been transferred into the manifold, apply a vacuum for 5 min.
9. Radiolabel a transgene cassette-specific probe (the probe should not contain plasmid backbone or ITR sequences).
10. In a hybridization bottle, prehybridize the nylon membrane with 5 mL of Church buffer *(22)* for 5 min at 65°C. Discard the prehybridization Church buffer and replace with 5 mL of fresh Church buffer. Place at 65°C.
11. Boil the ^{32}P-dCTP radiolabeled probe for 5 min, place on ice, and add to the hybridization bottle containing the dot-blot. Hybridize overnight at 65°C.
12. Remove the hybridization solution and add 10 mL of low-stringency wash solution. Wash for 10 min at 65°C. Repeat the wash with 10 mL of fresh solution.
13. Wash the dot-blot for 10 min at 65°C with the medium-stringency wash solution and discard the wash solution.

14. Monitor the dot-blot with a Geiger counter. Continue the washes if needed using the high-stringency wash solution (*see* **Note 17**).
15. To quantitate each spot on the dot-blot, expose the filter to a PhosphoImager cassette. Alternatively, employ X-ray film to identify labeled regions on the nylon membrane, excise each sample, and quantitate using a scintillation counter.
16. Plot a standard curve of DNA concentration vs integrated intensity/counts per minute for the DNA standards, and employ the curve to determine the concentration of DNA in the fractions obtained from the Heparin sulfate column (*see* **Notes 18** and **19**).

3.3.2. Determination of rAAV-LacZ Titer by Transgene Expression

The functional titer of rAAV is determined by its ability to transduce cells and express the transgene. Assaying for transgene expression is the most stringent method for determining rAAV titers. Here, we test *LacZ* expression in 293 cells.

1. Plate 293 cells and grow on 6- or 12-well dishes in DMEM + 10% (v/v) FBS + penicillin G/streptomycin.
2. Prepare the rAAV-*LacZ* by serially diluting over several magnitudes in IMDM without serum (*see* **Note 20**).
3. When the cells are 70%–80% confluent, infect the cells in each well with 10 μL of one of the rAAV-*LacZ* serial dilutions.
4. Incubate the cells for 24 h at 37°C and monitor the production of transgene expression (*see* **Subheading 3.3.3.**) over the subsequent days and weeks.

3.3.3. Detection of LacZ Expression

After infection of the 293 cells and X-gal staining, a positive signal indicates that rAAV has successfully infected the cell, and unpackaged and expressed the *LacZ* gene to a level sufficient to allow detection.

1. Prepare fresh stain and warm to 37°C.
2. Immediately before use prepare fixative solution.
3. Twenty-four hours after infection, remove the medium from the 293 cells and add fixative to each well (1 mL/well for a 6-well dish).
4. Incubate for 10 min at room temperature.
5. Discard the fixative solution and rinse the cells thoroughly with cold PBS. Repeat the rinse.
6. Add 0.5 mL of stain to each well. Cover with aluminum foil and incubate at 37°C for 6–24 h.
7. Rinse twice with PBS and count positive (blue) cells.
8. Examine sections for *LacZ* expression. An estimate of the titer can be calculated from the following formula:

$$\text{Infectious units (IU)/mL} = (\text{number of blue colonies/}$$
$$\text{virus volume} \times \text{replication factor} \times \text{number of cells plated})$$

3.4. Delivery of Recombinant Virus In Vivo

Microinjection of rAAV allows one to assess transgene expression in the whole animal. Here we describe the injection of mice with the rAAV-*LacZ*. Successful transduction and expression of the *LacZ* gene with this vector has been monitored for periods up to 1.5 yr *(2)*.

3.4.1. Injection of Recombinant Virus into Muscle

1. Intraperitoneally anesthetize 3-wk to 4-mo old Swiss Webster mice with 2.5% Avertin.
2. Inject 30 μL of rAAV-*LacZ* (approx 3×10^6 IU/mL) percutaneously into the hind leg tibialis anterior muscles.
3. In the following days, euthanize the mice at various time points and harvest muscle tissues. Rapidly freeze tissue in liquid nitrogen.
4. Cryostat section the tissue at 10-μm thickness with a Leica microtone.
5. Stain for *LacZ* expression (see **Subheading 3.4.2.**).

3.4.2. Histologic Analysis

1. Prepare, fix, and stain solutions as in **Subheading 3.3.3.**
2. Fix tissue sections for 1 min and then rinse with PBS. Repeat the wash.
3. Cover tissue sections with stain, place in the dark, and incubate at 37°C for 6–24 h.
4. Wash twice with PBS.
5. Mount sections by placing them in a shallow glass Petri dish set on a dark surface and filled with 0.5X PBS. Using a small paintbrush, gently slide the sections on to glass slides (sections will adhere once out of PBS).
6. Place slides upright to allow PBS to drain and sections to dry until they become translucent (5–10 min depending on thickness).
7. Rinse sections by gently dipping slides in ddH$_2$O several times. Dry slides for 10–30 min.
8. Place a cover slip gently on top of the sections after placing a small amount of mounting medium on a slide. Avoid producing bubbles. Remove excess mounting medium by draining briefly on a paper towel. Allow several minutes for the medium to set.
9. Examine sections for *LacZ* expression by light microscopy.

3.4.3. Molecular Analysis

Both wild-type AAV *(15–18)* and rAAV *(23)* have been shown using in vitro studies to recombine with the host cell chromosome. The most persuasive evidence for AAV integration can be obtained by using polymerase chain reaction to clone host-viral junctions from genomic DNA *(23)*. However, because of the absence of the viral Rep68 or Rep78 proteins in rAAV vectors, the recombination is not targeted to a specific location in chromosome 19. For this reason, the most common method to obtain evidence for rAAV latency is by

Southern analysis of host cell genomic DNA (gDNA). After hybridization using a radiolabeled *LacZ* probe, a positive signal in the DNA from infected cells but not in uninfected cells is an indication that the *LacZ* gene is associated with the high molecular weight of the host cell chromosome and that viral latency has been established.

1. Harvest muscle tissue, mince, and suspend in lysis buffer.
2. Digest overnight at 37°C.
3. Extract with an equal volume of 25:24:1 phenol:chloroform:isoamyl alcohol and repeat until the phenol/aqueous interface is clear. Extract once with an equal volume of chloroform to remove residual phenol.
4. Precipitate the DNA by adding 0.5 vol of 7.5 *M* ammonium acetate and 2 vol of cold 100% (v/v) ethanol. Gently mix the solution to encourage precipitation of the DNA.
5. Centrifuge (3000*g*) and wash the DNA twice with 70% (v/v) ethanol.
6. Remove the 70% (v/v) ethanol and dry the DNA by evaporation at room temperature or by placing in Speed Vac concentrator.
7. Resuspend the DNA in ddH$_2$O and digest with restriction enzyme *Eco*RV at 37°C overnight.
8. Remove restriction enzyme by precipitation of gDNA (as in **steps 4–7**).
9. Run 10 µg of the digested DNA on a 1% (w/v) agarose gel to resolve the digested fragments.
10. Transfer the DNA by Southern transfer to Gene-Screen Plus membrane.
11. Probe for *LacZ* DNA (as described in **Subheading 3.3.1.**, but using a *LacZ*-specific probe).

4. Notes

1. *Hind*III is used in the digest to cut the *rep* and *cap* fragment in half for easy isolation of the plasmid backbone.
2. DNA preparations should be pure. Purify the 4-kb pSub201 fragment by agarose gel separation and running onto Whatman DEAE-8 1 paper or a preparation of equivalent high quality.
3. Alternatively, blunt-end ligation may be used to construct the rAAV vector plasmid.
4. For efficient packaging into AAV capsids, the size of the rAAV construct (including the 190-bp ITRs) must be 4.6 kb or less.
5. Plasmids are grown in the Sure strain of E. *coli*. Even though this is a *RecA* minus strain, it has been observed that the AAV ITRs are unstable in bacteria. To avoid deletion, restrict bacterial growth in the stationary phase. If you still obtain deletions, grow the plasmids at 30°C for only 12 h. The integrity of the plasmids can be assayed by restriction enzyme digests.
6. IMDM contains HEPES and has greater buffering capacity than DMEM.
7. The concentration-dependent, ionic species and ionic strength–dependent aggregates that form adhere to glass and plastic. Polypropylene and glass attract the aggregates more than polystyrene. For this reason, polystyrene mixing containers are preferred for transfections.

8. The total DNA is equal to 37.5 µg/plate and the ratio of rAAV-*LacZ* to the pXX2 and pXX6 is equal to a molar ratio of about 1:1:1.
9. If a coarse precipitate forms, decrease the incubation time.
10. After 24 h, the 293 cells (when viewed through a microscope) should have a rounded appearance owing to viral replication. However, if the cells have detached from the plate, the incubation was too long. If cell detachment has already occurred, discard the plates and redo the transfection.
11. After any of the procedures in **Subheadings 3.1.2.–3.2.3.**, the cells, cell suspensions, or cell precipitates can be stored at –20°C for up to 6 mo.
12. The gradient layers can be placed in an Optiseal tube using a plastic syringe and small-gage plastic tubing or a low-pressure pump, such as the Bio-Rad EconoPump. Be careful not to mix the gradient layers or introduce air bubbles that may disturb the gradient.
13. The NaCl in the 15% Iodixanol layer will separate viral aggregates that may form because of the high concentration of virus.
14. When removing the purified rAAV-*LacZ*, do not contaminate the 40% layer with the 25% layer above; leave approx 0.5 mL of the 40% layer in the tube.
15. Collecting fractions from the flow-through and the washing steps ensures that all the virus was bound to the column and eluted as the salt gradient increased.
16. Using a new Heparin column for each purification ensures that you will not cross-contaminate viral preparations.
17. Do not allow the dot-blot to dry out at this point or the radiolabel probe will permanently adhere to the nylon membrane.
18. The Replication Center Assay is also a useful method to calculate the rAAV titer *(21)*.
19. The rAAV-*LacZ* particle number of each fraction can be calculated. Remember to take into consideration that the plasmid standards are double stranded, whereas the rAAV virions harbor only a single strand.
20. Generally, infecting with an *rAAV-LacZ* particle number to 293 cell number ratios of 1000:1 to 5:1 is sufficient.

References

1. Samulski, R. J., Sally, M., and Muzyczka, N. (1999) Adeno-associated viral vectors, in *The Development of Human Gene Therapy* (Friedmann, T. ed.), Cold Spring Harbor Laboratory, Cold Spring Harbor, NY, pp. 131–172.
2. Xiao, X., Li, J., and Samulski, R. J. (1996) Efficient long-term gene transfer into muscle tissue of immunocompetent mice by adeno-associated virus vector. *J. Virol.* **11,** 8098–8108.
3. Daly, T. M., Okuyama, T., Vogler, C., Haskins, M. E., Muzyczka, N., and Sands, M. S. (1999) Neonatal intramusuclar injection with recombinant adeno-associated virus results in prolonged beta-glucuronidase expression in situ and correction of liver pathology in mucopolysaccharidosis in type VII mice. *Hum. Gene Ther.* **10,** 85–94.
4. Song S., Morgan, M., Ellis, T., Poirier, A., Chesnut, K., Wang, J., Brantly, M., Muzyczka, N., Byrne, B. J., Atkinson, M., and Flotte, T. R. (1998) Sus-

tained secretion of human alpha-1-antitrypsin from murine muscle trans-duced with adeno-associated virus vectors. *Proc. Natl. Acad. Sci. USA* **95,** 14,384–14,388.

5. Bohl, D., Salvetti, A., Moullier, P., and Heard, J. M. (1998) Control of erythropoietin delivery by doxycycline in mice after intramuscular injection of adeno-associated vector. *Blood* **92,** 1512–1517.

6. Monahan, P. E., Samulski, R. J., Tazelaar, J., Xiao, X., Nichols, T. C., Bellinger, D. A., and Read, M. S. (1998) Direct intramuscular injection with recombinant AAV vectors results in sustained expression in a dog model of hemophilia *Gene Ther.* **5,** 40–49.

7. Xiao X., Li, J., and Samulski, R. J. (1998) Production of high-titer recombinant adeno-associated virus vectors in the absence of helper adenovirus. *J. Virol.* **72,** 2224–2232.

8. Ferrari, F. K., Xiao, X., McCarty, D., and Samulski, R. J. (1997) New develop-ments in the generation of Ad-free, high-titer rAAV gene therapy vectors. *Nature Med.* **3,** 1295, 1296.

9. Summerford C. and Samulski, R. J. (1998) Membrane-associated heparan sulfate proteoglycan is a receptor for adeno-associated virus type 2 virions. *J. Virol.* **72,** 1438–1445.

10. Summerford C. and Samulski, R. J. (1999) Viral receptors and vector purification: new approaches for generating clinical-grade reagents. *Nature Med.* **5,** 587, 588.

11. Zolotukhin, S., Byrne, B. J., Mason, E., Zolotuknin, I., Potter, M., Chesnut, K., Summerford, C., Samulski, R. J., and Muzyczka, N. (1999) Recombinant adeno-associated virus purification using novel methods improves infectious titer and yield. *Gene Ther.* **6,** 973–985.

12. Parks, W. P., Melnick, J. L., Rongey, R., and Mayor, H. D. (1967) Physical assay and growth cycle studies of a defective adeno-satellite virus. *J. Virol.* **1,** 171–180.

13. Atchinson, R. W., Casto, B. C., and Hammond, W. M. (1965) Adenovirus-associ-ated defective virus particles. *Science* **149,** 754–756.

14. Hoggan, M. D., Blacklow, N. R., and Row, W. P. (1966) Studies of small DNA viruses found in various adenovirus preparations: physical, biological, and immu-nological characteristics. *Proc. Natl. Acad. Sci. USA* **55,** 1457–1471.

15. Samulski, R. J.,. Zhu, X, Xiao, X., Brook, J. D., Housman, D. E., Epstein, N., and Hunter, L. A. (1991) Targeted integration of adeno-associated virus (AAV) into human chromosome 19. *EMBO J.* **10,** 3941–3950.

16. Samulski, R. J. (1993) Adeno-associated virus: integration at a specific chromo-somal location. *Curr. Opin. Gen. Dev.* **3,** 74–80.

17. Kotin, R. M., Siniscalco, M., Samulski, R. J., Zhu, X., Hunter, L., Laughlin, C. A., McLaughlin, S., Muzyczka, N., Rocchi, M., and Berns, K. L. (1990) Site-specific integration by adeno-assoicated virus. *Proc. Natl. Acad. Sci. USA* **87,** 2211–2215.

18. Kotin, R. M., Linden, R. M., and Berns, K. I. (1992) Characterization of a pre-ferred site on human chromosome 1 9q for integration of adeno-associated virus DNA by non-homologous recombination. *EMBO J.* **11,** 5071–5078.

19. Xiao X., Xiao, W., Li, J., and Samulski, R. J. (1997) A novel 165-base-pair termina repeat sequence is the sole *cis* requirement for the adeno-associated virus life cycle. *J. Virol.* **71,** 941–948.
20. Berns, K. I. and Giraud, C. (1995) Adeno-associated virus (AAV) vectors in gene therapy. *Curr. Topics Microbiol. Immun.* **218,** 1–25.
21. Bartlett, J. S. and Samulski, R. J. (1996) Production of recombinant adeno-associated viral vectors, in *Current Protocols in Human Genetics,* John Wiley & Sons, Philadelphia, pp. 12.1.1–12.1.24.
22. ShiLman, M. I. and Stern, D. G. (1995) A reliable and sensitive method for non-radioactive northern blot analysis of nerve growth factor mRNA from brain tissues. *J. Neurosci. Methods* **59,** 205–208.
23. Yang, C. C., Xiao, X., Zhu, X., Ansardi, D. C., Epstein, N. C., Frey, M. R., Matera, A. G., and Samulski, R. J. (1997) Cellular recombination pathways and viral terminal repeat hairpin structures are sufficient for adeno-associated virus integration *in vivo* and *in vitro. J. Virol.* **71,** 9231–9247.

28

Retroviral-Mediated Gene Transduction

Donald S. Anson

1. Introduction

An obligatory part of the life cycle of retroviruses (**Fig. 1**) is a stable, chromosomally integrated form of the virus, known as the provirus. The existence of the proviral form of retroviruses has provided one of the main driving forces for their use as vectors for gene transfer because, in the instance of a replication-defective retrovirus vector, the proviral form is the end point of the transduction (infection) process of the target cell (**Fig. 2**). The use of (replication) defective retroviral vectors is therefore ideal where the goal is the stable genetic modification of the target cell. The term *transduction* is now used to describe the infection of a cell with such a replication-defective retrovirus. Although replication-competent retroviral vectors have also been made, these are not in general use and offer little to recommend them. In this chapter vector should be taken as referring specifically to replication-defective retroviral vectors.

The archetypal retroviral vectors have been developed from oncogenic retroviruses such as the murine leukemia viruses (MLVs). The proviral form of these MLVs is approx 9 kb long. The first example of these viruses to be cloned and completely sequenced was Moloney murine leukemia virus *(1)*. The genetic structure of MLV is relatively simple (**Fig. 3A**).

The *trans* (i.e., polypeptide coding) genetic functions of the virus consist of three translational reading frames encoded in two RNA molecules. The three translational reading frames encode the viral polyproteins Gag, Pol, and Env. The *gag* gene products are structural proteins found in the virion core; the *pol* gene products are enzymes involved in viral replication, including reverse transcriptase; and the *env* gene product forms the viral envelope protein.

In addition, the virus contains several essential *cis* genetic sequences. The *cis* sequences include the viral long terminal repeats (LTRs) with the 5' LTR

From: *Methods in Molecular Biology, vol. 175: Genomics Protocols*
Edited by: M. P. Starkey and R. Elaswarapu © Humana Press Inc., Totowa, NJ

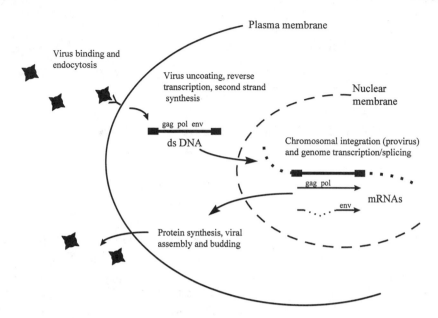

Fig. 1. Retroviral life cycle. Virus particles bind to the cell via specific plasma membrane receptors resulting in endocytosis and virus disassembly. The process of conversion of the single-stranded RNA genome of the virus into double-stranded DNA (dsDNA) via reverse transcription takes place in the cytoplasm. A complex containing dsDNA and retroviral proteins then gains access to the nucleus during cell division and the dsDNA molecule integrates into the chromosome to give the proviral form. This is then transcribed to give mRNAs encoding Gag/Pol and Env proteins. After proteolytic processing, these proteins are assembled into virions along with the viral genomic RNA and virus particles released by budding.

acting as a transcriptional promoter and the 3' LTR as a transcriptional terminator, primer binding sites for first- and second-strand DNA synthesis, and the signals required for efficient incorporation of genomic RNA into the virion (the packaging or psi sequence) and for proviral integration.

To a large extent the *cis* and *trans* functions do not overlap each other although the packaging signal does extend into the 5' end of the *gag* gene. MLV is therefore amenable to the sort of manipulations necessary to produce a safe and effective gene vector. These involve the separation of the *cis* and *trans* genetic functions of the virus into the vector itself and one or more "helper" constructs, respectively (**Fig. 3B**). Retroviral vector/helper systems have been continuously developed and improved over the past two decades, with the result that the latest vector/helper systems (*see* **refs.** *2* and *3*) are now extremely safe and efficient.

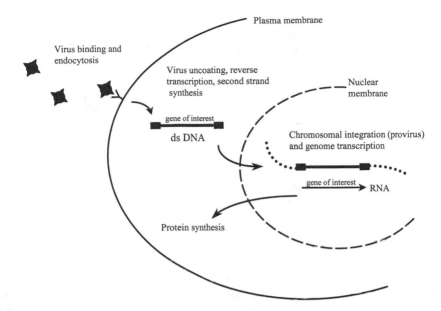

Fig. 2. Recombinant retroviral vector transduction. The initial stages of the process, up to provirus formation, are the same as for wild-type virus (*see* **Fig. 1**). However, because the recombinant vector encodes no functional viral proteins, no virus can be produced. Proviral transcripts simply serve to encode (depending on the exact design of the vector) the gene of interest.

The safety issues associated with the use of retroviral vectors are almost entirely defined by the probability of the production of replication-competent virus by recombination between the vector and helper constructs. The pertinent factors affecting this are the number of recombination events required for this to occur and the degree of homology between the various sequences that are required to recombine. Over the years the situation has improved from a case in which production of helper virus was inevitable to one in which it can, for all practical purposes, be assumed not to occur. However, the routine use of one of the extremely sensitive systems for the detection of helper virus is strongly recommended.

The efficiency of a vector/helper system is most obviously defined by the titer of virus that can be produced. For most MLV-based systems, both for production of viral stocks by transient expression and using stable producer cell lines, titers of between 10^5 and 10^7 NIH3T3 transducing units/mL can be expected. The exact titer will depend on the system and the vector construct being used. In most instances, the use of a retroviral vector allows extremely efficient gene transfer into any cell culture that is growing rapidly, as are most

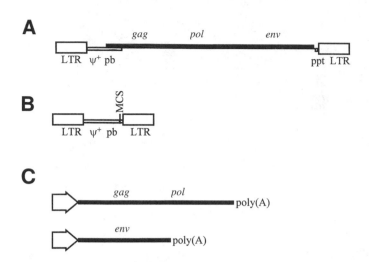

Fig. 3. Structure of wild-type retrovirus and recombinant retroviral vector systems. (A) The structure of a wild-type retrovirus in the proviral form. Sequences active in *cis* are shown as open boxes. LTR, long terminal repeat; ψ+, packaging signal; pb, primer binding site (for first-strand DNA synthesis); ppt, polypurine tract (primer site for second-strand DNA synthesis). Other sequences active in *cis* are splice donor and acceptor sites for generation of the subgenomic message encoding Env. Sequences active in *trans* are shown as a solid line. These are the sequences encoding the viral proteins Gag, Pol, and Env. (B) Minimal recombinant vector. This contains the *cis* active sequences and a multiple cloning site (MCS) for insertion of heterologous sequences. (C) Helper plasmids. These encode the *trans* active sequences under the transcriptional control of heterologous promoters and polyadenylation signals. Normally these constructs are used to generate stable packaging cell lines but can also be used in transient expression systems.

cultured cell lines and many primary cultures, but not into cells that are not actively dividing *(4)*, as are most cells in vivo. Currently, therefore, the use of retroviral vector systems is almost entirely limited to the in vitro transduction of cell populations with a high mitotic index.

The link between the mitotic index of the cell population and the efficiency with which it can be transduced is due to the biology of MLV—the viral preintegration complex that forms in the cytoplasm after transduction cannot access the nucleus, obviously essential for integration to occur, unless the nuclear membrane is absent as occurs during cell division. Although many approaches to gene therapy have been developed in an attempt to negate this limitation, mostly utilizing ex vivo transduction of cells followed by their reimplantation, none of these has proven to be very effective in practice. The title of this chapter, "Retroviral-Mediated Gene Transduction," as opposed to

"Retroviral-Mediated Gene Therapy," reflects the gulf that exists between being able to transduce cell cultures extremely effectively with retroviral vectors and the almost complete lack of ability to use this technology in achieving anything approaching effective gene therapy for a clinical condition. This chapter is therefore limited to describing basic methods for the production of virus and the transduction of cells in culture.

Because of the limitations of MLV-based systems, most importantly an absolute restriction on the ability to transduce noncycling cells, other types of retroviruses have been used to develop vector systems. In recent years, the most notable among these has been the development of vectors from lentiviruses, including human immunodeficiency virus. The attraction of lentiviruses is that they have evolved mechanisms that allow them to transduce nondividing cells. The development of lentiviral vectors has progressed rapidly, and although the technology is still developing, especially regarding the construction of easy-to-use stable packaging cell lines and the range of vectors available, their use should be considered if cells with a low mitotic index are being targeted for transduction. The production of virus by transient expression and their general handling (apart from safety issues) is broadly the same as that described for MLV vectors in **Subheading 3.2.** These vector systems have rapidly been developed using the general principles learned from many years of improvement of MLV-based systems and some useful lentiviral systems produced (*5*). However, the use of lentiviral vectors is not specifically discussed herein. If these are preferred then specific materials and advice should be sought from the laboratories that have actively pursued the development of these vectors.

1.1. Choice of Vector System

Many vectors based on MLV or closely related viruses have been developed. The differences among them can be discussed from two broad perspectives: (1) Does the vector include a selectable marker? (2) What promoter is used to drive transcription of the introduced gene?

The use of vectors with drug-based dominant selectable markers, which enable the selection of transduced cells in culture, has obvious advantages both in making viral producer cell lines and in characterizing and using the virus itself. The most commonly used selectable marker is the neomycin resistance gene (*neo*[r]) that produces resistance to the agent G418. In most cell types, this system is both easy to use and extremely effective, and many vectors incorporating the neomycin resistance gene have been made (**Table 1**). Other drug-based selection systems that have been used in retroviral vectors include puromycin/hygromycin resistance (*6*) and methotrexate resistance (*7*).

Table 1
Retroviral Vectors

Vector	Marker gene	Promoter[a]	Cloning sites	Ref.
LXSN	G418 (*neo*) resistance	LTR	*Eco*RI, *Hpa*I, *Xho*I, *Bam*HI	*11*
LNCX	G418 (*neo*) resistance	CMV	*Hin*dIII, *Cla*I, *Stu*I	*11*
LNSX	G418 (*neo*) resistance	SV40	*Stu*I, *Hin*dIII, *Cla*I	*11*
MFG	None	LTR via splicing	*Nco*I, *Bam*HI	*18*
MSCV*neo* EB	G418 (*neo*) resistance	LTR	*Eco*RI, *Hpa*I, *Xlzo*I, *Bgl*II	*6*
MSCVhph	Hygromycin resistance	LTR	*Bg*/II, *Xho*I, *Hpa*I, *Eco*RI	*6*
MSCVpac	Puromycin resistance	LTR	*Bg*/II, *Xho*I, *Hpa*I, *Eco*RI	*6*
pS2	None	LTR	Numerous	*19*

[a]LTR, long terminal repeat; SV40, simian virus 40 early promoter; CMV, cytomegalovirus immediate early promoter.

However, none of these offer real advantages over the use of neomycin resistance and should not be considered unless neomycin resistance cannot be used for a specific reason (e.g., the cells to be transduced are already G418 resistant). Although the use of a selection gene is of little negative consequence in cell culture systems, there is a general consensus that they may be at least partly responsible for the poor long-term expression seen from many vectors in vivo, although undoubtedly a number of other factors are also involved in this phenomenon. In addition, drug-based selection systems are of little positive use in vivo.

Non-drug-based selection systems are also available. These are generally genes that allow selection via physical means. These may be genes that encode proteins that are expressed on the cell surface allowing detection and isolation via antibody binding (*8,9*) and fluorescence-activated cell sorting (FACS). Alternatively, immunomagnetic bead technology can be used to select cells. This technique is more appropriate for isolating large numbers of transduced cells. More recently, genes that encode proteins that are themselves fluorescent, i.e., green fluorescent protein and its derivatives (*10*), have allowed the direct assay and isolation of transduced cells by FACS. Fluorescent proteins also have the advantages that no processing is required and that they can be analyzed in live cells and in real time. All these selection systems can also be used as marker genes in experiments studying retroviral transduction as an end in itself.

The choice of whether to use a vector containing a selectable marker, and if so which one, depends on the particular project in mind. For projects in which the goal is the transduction of in vitro–cultured cells, a vector containing a marker is highly recommended and a drug resistance marker is usually the easiest to use. If expression and analysis of a marker gene is the aim of the project, then markers such as GFP derivatives that render enhanced sensitivity offer real benefits. However, for the sake of simplicity, this chapter deals only with methods that are based on the use of vectors that carry *neo^r*.

For expression of the gene of interest, two basic choices are available: using the 5' viral LTR to drive transcription or using an internal promoter. The MLV LTR is a robust promoter in many cell types and its use to drive the expression of heterologous genes allows the employment of very simple vectors, although, as with many other promoters, expression is often downregulated in vivo. However, derivatives of the MLV LTR have been made that claim to overcome this effect. Vectors have also been made with LTRs from other viruses, such as myeloproliferative sarcoma virus, which are claimed to offer advantages for expression in specific cell types, in this instance hematopoietic cells. Another approach that has been tried is to incorporate specific regulatory elements from other genes into the LTR to modify its transcriptional regulatory properties. However, although conceptually straightforward this approach has not always been successful. Expression of two gene sequences from a single promoter (either the LTR or an internal promoter) can be achieved by the use of an internal ribosome entry site sequence.

The use of an internal promoter to drive expression of the gene of interest allows the promoter to be carefully selected in the light of criteria such as the specific tissue targeted for transduction or the need for gene regulation. Many examples of the use of tissue-specific promoters have been described, and conspicuous examples include systems designed for expression in muscle and liver cells. More simply, the use of an internal promoter allows the selection of very strong constitutive promoters such as the cytomegalovirus immediate early promoter, which is highly active in many cell types.

In summary, unless specific factors dictate otherwise, a straightforward vector carrying the neomycin resistance gene and allowing expression of the gene from the LTR or a strong internal promoter should be used *(11)*. Some of the many MLV-based vectors available along with pertinent features are given in **Table 1**.

1.2. Vector Construction

Cloning of the gene sequence of interest into the chosen vector is a straightforward molecular biological procedure, and the reader is referred to any of the excellent molecular biology laboratory manuals such as the Maniatis manual *(12)* or *Current Protocols in Molecular Biology (13)*. Specific factors to take into account when using retroviral vectors are size (the total size of the vector should not exceed 8–10 kb) and the presence of RNA processing signals, as retroviruses have a single-stranded RNA genome RNA processing signals (real or cryptic), will be recognized. For example, intron sequences will be unstable, being subject to splicing, and polyadenylation signals will cause premature termination of the retroviral genomic transcript and a lowering of viral titer. Intron-containing sequences can often be stabilized by cloning in the reverse orientation. In all instances it is important to check the integrity of the virus in transduced cells.

Because many of the available retroviral vectors have limited polylinker cloning sequences, insertion of the gene of interest often means using blunt-end cloning, a process that can be inefficient. An alternative is first to customize the polylinker by cloning a short double-stranded oligonucleotide sequence containing convenient restriction enzyme sites for the subsequent cloning of the gene sequence of interest. The sequences of some vectors are available via GenBank, making the choice of restriction enzyme sites straightforward. The DNA preparation of the final construct should be of high purity. Any of the commercial high-quality plasmid purification kits are probably acceptable in this regard. Alternatively, DNA can be prepared on cesium chloride gradients.

1.3. Choice of Packaging System

The main considerations when choosing a packaging system are virus pseudotype, safety, efficiency, and the nature of the vector construct to be packaged. The vector pseudotype is determined by the choice of envelope gene and will define the range of species and cells that can be infected by the recombinant virus. The two most common vector pseudotypes are ecotropic and amphotropic MLV. These generate virus able to transduce only murine cells (ecotropic), or a broad range of species (amphotropic). If only murine cells are to be targeted, the use of ecotropic rather than amphotropic virus adds a significant safety advantage.

Other pseudotypes have been generated by using envelopes from a variety of retroviruses such as the murine virus 10A1; Mus dunni endogenous virus; the cat virus RD114, Gibbon ape leukemia virus (GALV); and, in one instance, an envelope protein from a completely different type of virus, vesicular stomatis virus (VSV)-G protein. In general, none of these seems to offer real advantages with the exception of the VSV-G protein. However, some of these envelopes may provide advantages for the targeting of specific cell types; for example, GALV envelope pseudotyped virus appears more efficient than amphotropic virus in transducing human pluripotent hematopoietic stem cells.

The advantages of the VSV-G protein are twofold. First, being more stable than retroviral envelopes, it facilitates the concentration of virus particles to extremely high titers, and, second, it provides a pantropic pseudotype *(14)*. However, the use of VSV-G protein can also produce artifactual results owing to short-term protein transfer to target cells. In addition, because of the protein's cytotoxicity, VSV-G protein–pseudotyped virus is generally made by transient expression, making large-scale production of virus difficult. However, a stable cell line in which the VSV-G protein is transcriptionally regulated has been constructed to allow the generation of stable virus producer cell lines for VSV-G protein–pseudotyped virus.

In summary, the amphotropic MLV pseudotype is probably the most generally useful and, being the most widely used, provides the greatest choice of packaging systems. Other envelopes should be considered only if there is a definite advantage for the experimental purpose in question. This chapter deals specifically with the production of amphotropic MLV-pseudotyped virus, because it is the most generally useful.

Although some of the early amphotropic packaging cell lines designed for the production of stable viral producer cell lines, such as PA317, are extremely robust and generate high titers of virus, they have now been superseded by more carefully constructed packaging lines. These can be used with the assumption that the probability of replication-competent virus being produced is, for all practical purposes, zero. However, testing for helper virus is still recommended to allow the formal establishment of this fact for each cell line produced, especially if long-term in vitro or any in vivo experiments are being considered. These tests should be repeated at regular intervals. When making virus by transient expression, each batch of virus should be tested. In my experience, the chance of producing replication-competent virus is greater in transient virus production systems than in clonal, stable producer cell lines.

Packaging cell lines based on 293T cells designed for production of virus by transient expression have also been constructed. These are most useful for the rapid production of small amounts of virus (e.g., if many different vector designs are being tested) or production of virus carrying gene sequences that result in cytotoxicity (thus preventing the construction of stable packaging cell lines). These can also be useful in the construction of stable packaging cell lines. Virus can also be produced by transient expression of both vector and helper constructs in a suitable cell line such as the highly transfectable 293T cell line. This is how VSV-G protein–pseudotyped virus is most easily produced.

A list of packaging cell lines and their relevant properties is given in **Table 2**. Some of these are available from the American Type Culture Collection (ATCC). This list is not meant to be exhaustive but includes cell lines for generating most of the available virus pseudotypes.

Table 2
Retroviral Packaging Cell Lines

Cell line	Pseudotype/ basal cell line	Notes	Reference	Availability
PA317	Amphotropic MLV/NIH3T3	One-plasmid system	*20*	ATCC No. CRL-9078
PG13	Gibbon ape leukemia virus/NIH3T3	Two-plasmid system	*21*	ATCC No.: CRL-10686
GP+E-86	Ecotropic MLVINIH3T3	Two-plasmid system	22	ATCC No. CRL-9642
GP-envAm12	Amphotropic/NIH3T3	Two-plasmid system	23	ATCC No. CRL-9641
psiCRE	Ecotropic MLV/NIH3T3	Two-plasmid system	24	Contact author
psiCRIP	Amphotropic MLV/NIH3T3	Two-plasmid system	24	Contact author
FLYA13	Amphotropic MLV/HT 1080	Two-plasmid system	25	Contact author
FLYRD18	RD114/HT1080	Two-plasmid system	25	Contact author
PT67/PT105	10A1/NIH3T3	Two-plasmid system	26	Contact author
293GPG	Vesicular stomatis virus G protein/293	Two-plasmid system	27	Contact author
ProPak-A	Amphotropic MLV	Two-plasmid system	28	Contact author
BOSC 23	Ecotropic MLV/293T	Two-plasmid system[a]	29	Contact author
293T	General transient expression	Not applicable	*30*	Contact author

[a]Suitable for high-titer production of virus by transient expression.

2. Materials

2.1. Cell Culture

1. Dulbecco's modified Eagle's medium supplemented with 10% (v/v) fetal calf serum (Gibco-BRL). The medium base (i.e., without FCS) should be filter sterilized (0.2 μm) into sterile containers and stored at 4°C.
2. Phosphate-buffered saline (PBS) without calcium and magnesium (cat. no. 20012-027; Gibco-BRL).
3. 10X Trypsin solution: 2.5% (w/v) solution (Gibco-BRL cat. no. 15090-046).
4. G418 sulfate (cat. no. 10131-019; Gibco-BRL).

5. T25, T75 tissue culture flasks.
6. Sterile tissue culture dishes (60 and 100 mm).
7. Disposable sterile pipets.
8. Polypropylene centrifuge tubes (10 and 50 mL).
9. Freezing vials.
10. Sterile Eppendorf tubes.
11. Trypan blue vital stain: Mix 0.9% (w/v) NaCl and 1% (w/v) trypan blue in 4:1 ratio. Use within 24 h.
12. Hematocytometer.
13. 100X penicillin-streptomycin solution (Gibco-BRL).
14. Tissue culture grade dimethylsulfoxide (DMSO).
15. Cryo 1°C freezing container (cat. no. 5100-0001; Nalgene).
16. Liquid nitrogen storage system.
17. Glass cloning rings (Bellco Glass).
18. 24-Well tissue culture plates.

2.2. Production of Virus by Transient Expression

1. 2.5 M CaCl$_2$, filter sterilized (0.2 μm).
2. 2X HEPES-buffered saline (HeBS) medium: 50 mM HEPES; 250 mM NaCl; 1.5 mM NaH$_2$PO$_4$, pH 7.1. Filter sterilize. Accurate pH of this solution is critical. It is useful to aliquot and store this solution at –20°C to ensure its stability.
3. Sterile disposable syringes (10–50 mL).
4. Disposable syringe filters (0.22 μm).
5. Sterile polypropylene tubes (10–50 mL).

2.3. Production of Stable Virus Producer Cell Lines

Polybrene (8 mg/mL). Filter sterilize (0.2 μm).

2.4. Assay for Helper (replication-competent) Virus

NIH3T3 cells (ATCC CRL-1658, http://www.atcc.org/).

2.5. Preparation of High-Titer Viral Stocks

Stirred cell ultrafiltration apparatus with ZM500 filters (Amicon, series 8000).

3. Methods

3.1. General Maintenance of Cell Lines

The cell lines that have been developed for packaging retrovirus are all adherent lines, most often derived from NIH3T3 (mouse fibroblast cell line) cells or, more recently, from 293 (human kidney cell line) cells (**Table 2**). In addition, NIH3T3 cells are useful for determining viral titer. On receipt of any cell line, it should be expanded as rapidly as possible and stocks (at least 10 vials) frozen at a low passage number. It is advisable to grow cells in the absence of antibiotics because their use can mask persistent low-grade infections.

3.1.1. Recovery of a Cell Line from a Frozen Stock

1. Thaw the frozen stock as rapidly as possible in a 37°C water bath or incubator. When thawed, make sure the cells are evenly resuspended by pipetting.
2. Transfer the cell suspension into 10 mL of the appropriate complete (i.e., basal medium/FCS) medium in a centrifuge tube and invert to mix.
3. Recover the cells by centrifuging at 1000g for 3 min at room temperature.
4. Remove the supernatant and resuspend the cells in 7 mL of complete medium (25-cm^2 culture flask).
5. Incubate under the appropriate conditions. For most cell lines this will be 37°C in 5% CO_2 in a humidified incubator.
6. Replace with fresh medium every 2–3 d.
7. When the cell monolayer becomes confluent subculture the cells.

3.1.2. Subculturing of Adherent Cell Lines

Adherent cell cultures should be subcultured as they become confluent.

1. Remove the culture medium from the flask and discard.
2. Add 5 mL (for a 25-cm^2 flask) or 10 mL (for a 75-cm^2 flask) of PBS and wash over the cell monolayer by gently rocking the flask.
3. Remove the PBS and add 3–5 mL (for a 25-cm^2 flask) or 5–10 mL (for a 75-cm^2 flask) of 0.25% (w/v) trypsin (in PBS)
4. Incubate at room temperature for 5 min.
5. Examine the cell monolayer using an inverted microscope. The cells should become rounded and start to lift from the substratum. If this is so, proceed to the next step; if not, incubate for a further 5 min and/or replace trypsin solution with a fresh aliquot.
6. Wash the cells from the substratum by pipetting the trypsin solution over the substratum several times. This should also result in a single cell suspension.
7. Aliquot the cells as required into fresh flasks containing complete medium (5–7 mL for a 25-cm^2 flask, 10–15 mL for a 75-cm^2 flask), and incubate under the appropriate conditions (*see* **Note 1**).
8. Replace old medium with fresh medium every 2 to 3 d.

3.1.3. Seeding Cells at a Specific Density

1. Trypsinize and suspend cells as described above and place into a sterile tube.
2. Add an equal volume of complete medium and mix.
3. Dilute a sample of the cell suspension into trypan blue vital stain and count live (cells that exclude trypan blue) and dead (cells that stain with trypan blue) cells using a hematocytometer (*see* **Note 2**).

4. Calculate live cell density in the original cell suspension and adjust if necessary (*see* **Note 3**).
5. Mix the cell suspension well and aliquot as desired.

3.1.4. Picking Colonies with Cloning Rings

Cloning rings are used to isolate colonies to allow them to be individually isolated to produce clonal cell lines. This can only be done with colonies in dishes; flasks do not allow the required access. To facilitate the isolation of colonies using this method, it is best that the dish contain a relatively small number of well-separated colonies.

1. Remove the medium from the dish and carefully rinse once with PBS.
2. Lightly coat one end of a cloning ring with petroleum jelly (Vaseline) and place, coated end down, over a well-separated colony. Repeat for all colonies to be picked.
3. Place 100–200 µL of 0.25% (w/v) trypsin solution in each cloning ring, and leave at room temperature until the cells have dissociated.
4. Pipet the cells into a 24-well tissue culture plate well containing 1 mL of complete medium and then grow/expand as normal.

3.1.5. Freezing Cell Stocks

1. Trypsinize cells as described above from a confluent 75-cm² flask (*see* **Subheading 3.1.2.**) and transfer to a centrifuge tube.
2. Add 2 mL of FCS to neutralize the trypsin.
3. Recover the cells by centrifugation and remove the supernatant.
4. Resuspend the cells in 1 mL of 90% complete medium: 10% DMSO (v/v) and transfer to a freezing vial.
5. Transfer the vial to a Nalgene Cryo 1°C freezing container and place in a –70°C freezer.
6. After 24 h transfer the vial to liquid nitrogen for long-term storage.

3.2. Production of Virus by Transient Expression

The production of virus by transient expression can be either an end in itself or the first step in the construction of a stable producer cell line. It can be achieved by either transfection of the vector construct into a stable packaging cell line or cotransfection of the vector and helper constructs into any suitable (i.e., readily transfectable) cell line (*see* **Note 4**). Calcium phosphate coprecipitation is adequate for this purpose; however, a wide range of equally suitable propriety transfection reagents are available. If transient virus production is being performed as an initial step in the production of a stable producer cell line, it is important that the virus produced by transient expression be of a different pseudotype than the stable packaging line to be used because packaging cell lines are resistant to supertransduction by virus of the same pseudotype. For example, if the aim is to produce stable amphotropic cell lines (as described here), the transiently produced virus should be of an ecotropic or other pseudotype. Packaging cell lines based on NIH3T3 cells, such as PA317, GP+E-86, and GP+envAm12, will produce relatively low titers by this method, probably 10^2–10^3 transducing units/mL. Packaging cell lines specifically designed for production of virus by transient expression, such as Bosc23 cells, or cotransfection of vector and helper plasmids into 293T cells, can be expected to give higher titers, perhaps 10^4–10^6/mL, depending on the particular vector and helper constructs and the cell line used (*see* **Note 5**).

3.2.1. Production of Low-Titer Ecotropic Virus by Transient Expression

The following protocol is for transfection of a 60-mm-diameter dish or 25-cm^2 flask of cells. It can be scaled up or down relative to the surface area of the culture dish/flask to be used. All solutions and procedures should be sterile. DNA solutions can be effectively sterilized by ethanol precipitation in a sterile tube followed by resuspension in sterile water. The solutions to be used for preparing the calcium phosphate precipitate should be at room temperature before use. Generally, the highest titer of virus will be found 2 to 3 d after transfection (*see* **Note 6**). To harvest virus, the conditioned medium is simply collected and passed through a 0.2-μm filter into a sterile container. For small volumes, this is most easily done by harvesting the medium with a syringe and then using a syringe filter. To maximize virus collection, the medium can be collected at 48 h after transfection, and the cells refed with fresh medium (prewarm to 37°C) with subsequent collections made in the same manner after a further 24 and 48 h. The virus can be stored at 4°C for up to a few days or frozen at –70°C for long-term storage. An approximate twofold decrease in titer generally results from the freeze/thaw cycle.

1. Seed 2×10^6 cells of a stable ecotropic packaging cell line such as psiCRE (**Table 2**) in a 60-mm tissue culture dish and incubate for 16–24 h. This should result in an even monolayer that is about 60–80% confluent. The exact number of cells required will depend on the cell line being used.
2. In an Eppendorf tube make up a total of 6 μg of the retroviral construct DNA to be transfected to a final volume of 180 μL of 0.25 M CaCl$_2$ by adding water and 2.5 M CaCl$_2$.
3. Aliquot 180 μL of 2X HeBS into a second Eppendorf tube and then add the DNA/CaCl$_2$ mix dropwise while vortexing at high speed.
4. Continue vortexing for 5–10 s after all the solution has been added.
5. Allow the mixture to stand for 5 min.
6. Add the mixture dropwise to the cells and swirl to mix.
7. Incubate under normal culture conditions for 6–8 h, and then remove the medium from the cells and refeed with fresh complete medium.
8. Incubate again for 48 h.

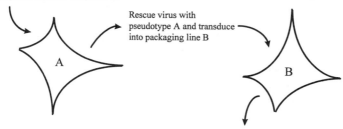

Transfect retroviral construct into
packaging line A/transient expression

Rescue virus with
pseudotype A and transduce
into packaging line B

A

B

Stable cell line producing B pseudotype virus

Fig. 4. Ping-pong method for generating viral producer cell lines. Virus is produced from packaging cell line "A," usually by transient expression and used to transduce a packaging cell line of a different viral pseudotype (line "B"). Introduction of the recombinant virus into the packaging cell by transduction, rather than transfection, facilitates the generation of stable, high-titer producer cell lines.

9. Collect the medium using a sterile disposable syringe, and then pass through a 0.2-μm filter unit into a suitable storage container such as a 10-mL centrifuge tube (*see* **Note 7**).

3.3. Production of Stable Virus Producer Cell Lines

The most efficient way of producing high-titer stable cell lines is to transduce the vector into the packaging cell line of choice. To achieve this, virus of a different pseudotype than the packaging cell line to be used must be made by transient expression (*see* **Subheading 3.2.**). This virus is then used to transduce the packaging cell line being used for production of stable cell lines and clonal cell lines isolated and characterized. This has been termed the ping-pong method of generating producer cell lines (**Fig. 4**). If a vector utilizing a drug-resistance gene is used, isolation of clonal cell lines containing the vector provirus is relatively straightforward. Similarly, if the vector expresses any other gene that enables direct isolation of cells (e.g., cells containing a vector expressing a fluorescent protein can be isolated by FACS), isolation of clonal cell lines is again relatively straightforward. However, if a vector that contains no selectable marker is used, the isolation of clonal cell lines is more problematic but can still be achieved (*see* **Note 8**).

The following protocol assumes that a vector that carries the *neo^r* marker is used and that the amphotropic cell line being used is derived from a murine cell line.

3.3.1. Generation of Amphotropic, Clonal, Stable Producer Cell Lines

1. Produce low-titer ecotropic virus stock by transient expression in a suitable cell line as described in **Subheading 3.2.**

2. Plate the amphotropic packaging cell line of choice in a 60-mm-diameter dish at approx 50% confluence and allow the cells to attach (6–16 h).
3. Aspirate the medium and replace with 2 mL of low-titer ecotropic virus supernatant plus an equal volume of fresh complete medium.
4. Add polybrene to a final concentration of 4–8 µg/mL.
5. Incubate the cells as normal for 8–24 h.
6. Aspirate the medium and feed the cells with fresh medium.
7. Incubate for a further 24 h.
8. Split the cells into 100-mm-diameter dishes of complete medium (10–12 mL) containing G418 (*see* **Note 9**).
9. Feed the cells every 3 or 4 d taking care to add fresh medium slowly to avoid dislodging cells, because this can result in the generation of secondary colonies. The aim is to get several dishes containing 10–30 colonies.
10. After 10–12 d pick individual colonies with cloning rings (*see* **Subheading 3.1.4.**) and expand for characterization (*see* **Subheading 3.4.**).

3.4. Characterization of Producer Clones

Clones should be characterized with respect to viral titer, proviral integrity, and copy number and status with respect to helper virus described as follows.

3.4.1. Determination of Viral Titer as neo^r Colony-Forming Units

There are a number of ways to determine viral titer. Again, the most straightforward instance is where the vector carries a drug-resistance gene or marker gene that can be assayed easily on a cell-by-cell basis. Alternatively, titer can be determined by techniques that directly assay proviral sequences in target cells such as quantitative polymerase chain reaction (PCR) or Southern blot analysis. Extensions of these approaches that may be applied in specific instances would be to assess titer by analysis of target cells by histochemical or immunohistologic means for the gene product expressed by the virus or by use of a specialized technique such as *in situ* hybridization to directly detect proviral sequences. Methods detailing such approaches are not given here, but if such techniques for detecting the gene sequence/gene product of interest are already in use in the laboratory, it should be relatively straightforward to adapt these to measure virus titer.

1. Plate a susceptible cell line (for ecotropic and amphotropic MLV, NIH3T3 cells are a common standard) at 10^6 cells per 60-mm dish, and allow the cells to attach for 6–24 h. The resulting monolayer should be 50–75% confluent.
2. Make dilutions of the viral stock from between 10^0 and 10^{-6} in complete medium. This should be done at room temperature or 4°C, as the virus is relatively stable at these temperatures.

3. Aspirate the medium from the cells and add 1 mL of complete medium containing 16 µg/mL of polybrene. Then add 1 mL of each virus dilution and swirl gently to mix.
4. Incubate as normal for 24 h.
5. Subculture the cells 1:10 into selective medium and grow, feeding when dead cells accumulate or the medium becomes exhausted, again using selective medium, for 10–12 d.
6. After 10–12 d distinct colonies should be apparent. Fix the colonies with 25% acetic acid:75% methanol.
7. Stain with a suitable vital dye such as 1% trypan blue, wash with water to remove excess stain, and enumerate using dilution(s) where the number of colonies is between 10 and 50.
8. Determine the original viral titer as follows: no. of colonies per dish × dilution factor × 10 (the cell subculture factor) = the viral titer of the original stock in *neo^r* colony forming units per milliliter.

3.5. Assay for Helper (replication-competent) Virus in Viral Supernatants

The most straightforward assay for helper virus is horizontal spread of virus. This can be used when the vector being used carries a drug-resistance marker. The viral supernatant to be tested is simply used to transduce a suitable cell line, and the transduced cells are then subcultured and assayed for production of virus carrying the resistance marker. The idea of this assay is that if replication competent virus is present, it will provide the *trans* functions (i.e., act as a helper virus) for packaging the genomic transcript from the vector in the transduced cells, thus generating a titer of virus carrying the drug-resistance marker that can be measured.

3.5.1. Horizontal Virus Spread Assay for Helper Virus

1. Plate NIH3T3 cells at 2 to 3 × 10^6 cells per 100-mm dish or T75 flask. Allow the cells to attach. The resulting monolayer should be approx 50% confluent.
2. Aspirate the medium and add the sample to be tested (if necessary add complete medium to a total volume of 10 mL) and polybrene to a final concentration of 8 µg/mL.
3. Incubate for 16–24 h.
4. Remove the medium and refeed.
5. Grow the cells for 10 d subculturing as they reach confluence (*see* **Note 10**).
6. At the end of d 10, allow the cells to become confluent, aspirate the medium, refeed with fresh medium, and then collect conditioned medium after 24 h. Assay this medium for G418r colony-forming units as described in **Subheading 3.4.**), but when subculturing 1:10 into G418, keep all the cells; that is, set up 10 dishes. This will improve the sensitivity of the assay.

3.6. Southern Blot Analysis of Producer Cell Lines

Southern blot of clonal producer cell lines and target cells is a simple and useful analysis. Using standard methodologies (refer to any molecular biology laboratory manual), Southern analysis should be done with a virus-specific probe (such as the *neo* gene sequence) and a restriction enzyme that cuts twice in the vector, outside of the probe sequence (*see* **Note 11**).

3.7. Preparation of High-Titer Viral Stocks

Viral stocks are simply prepared by collecting conditioned medium from the producer cell line and removing contaminating cells by filtration as described in **Subheading 3.2.1.**). Virus can be concentrated to higher titers by a variety of methods, if required. Because virus pseudotyped with MLV envelope (ecotropic or amphotropic) is relatively labile, care must be taken during concentration to keep the sample cold and to avoid too vigorous agitation (*see* **Notes 12** and **13**). The most useful way of concentrating such virus is by ultrafiltration. The titer can be increased 10- to 50-fold using this approach.

3.7.1. Collection of Viral Supernatant from Stable Producer Cell Lines

1. Subculture cells into the desired number of flasks or dishes. Between 15 and 30 mL of viral supernatant can be collected from a 100-mm dish or T75 flask.
2. Grow the cells to about 80–95% confluency, and then remove the medium and replace with fresh medium.
3. Collect the medium (virus supernatant) after 8–16 h and refeed. This cycle can be repeated for as long as the monolayer remains intact (*see* **Note 14**).

3.7.2. Concentration of Virus by Ultrafiltration

1. Set up a stirred cell ultrafiltration apparatus with a 500,000-kDa cutoff membrane in a 4°C cold room or cold cabinet and rinse thoroughly with water.
2. Add viral supernatant and concentrate 10 to 100-fold (by volume) using a slow stir rate.
3. Collect the concentrated viral supernatant and rinse the apparatus with a small volume of medium and pool.
4. Rinse the membrane well with water, wash in 1 *M* NaCl and store in 10% ethanol.
5. Assay the concentrated virus for viral titer as described in **Subheading 3.4.1.**).

3.8. Transduction of Adherent Cells

The most important criterion for success is to have the target cells growing as rapidly as possible. With most immortalized cell lines this is usually not a problem if care is taken with growing the cells (e.g., regularly exchanging medium, subculturing as cells become confluent rather than allowing cells to sit confluent, making sure the optimal medium is used and that the medium is prepared properly, and screening batches of FCS to identify those optimal for growth of the cell line in question). Sometimes increasing the concentration of serum in the growth medium or adding growth factors can enhance the growth characteristics of a particular cell line. Similarly, newly established cultures of primary cells, such as skin fibroblasts, often grow rapidly. Conversely, primary cells that have been subcultured a significant number of times often divide less rapidly as they approach senescence and thus can become difficult to transduce, even with high-titer viral stocks. Exposing the culture to several cycles of transduction will enhance the overall transduction efficiency. If the growth medium for the target cells is very different from the culture medium in which the viral producer cell line is grown, consideration should be given to collecting virus in target cell medium to ensure optimal growth of the target cells during transduction. Alternatively, virus supernatant can be mixed in a 1:1 ratio with target cell growth medium.

1. Plate an actively growing culture of the cells to be transduced and grow to 25–50% confluency.
2. Remove the growth medium and replace with viral supernatant made to 8 µg/mL polybrene.
3. Culture the cells for 8–16 h, and then remove the medium and either repeat the transduction or add normal growth medium (*see* **Note 15**).
4. Expand the culture and either assess transduction using a suitable assay or select for transduced cells with G418. For most cell lines, 0.5–1 mg (total) of G418/mL is suitable. However, for primary cells it is important to titer the minimum concentration of G418 required to kill nonresistant cells.

3.9. Transduction of Nonadherent Cells

Transduction of nonadherent cells is often more problematic than transduction of adherent cells, but the reason is not entirely clear. There are two basic approaches to transduction of nonadherent cells: supernatant transduction and transduction via cocultivation. In the latter case, the nonadherent cells are cultivated directly on top of virus producer cells. The nonadherent cells can subsequently be recovered by gentle washing (*see* **Note 16**). Contaminating producer cells can be removed from the culture by growing on the cells on tissue culture plastic and allowing them to adhere (*see* **Note 17**).

3.9.1. Supernatant Transduction

1. Recover target cells to be transduced by centrifuging at $1000g$ for 5 min.
2. Resuspend target cells directly in viral supernatant containing 8 µg/mL of polybrene keeping the cells at the optimal density for logarithmic growth. If necessary, add some fresh growth medium to ensure optimal conditions for cell growth during the transduction procedure.

3. Culture for 8–24 h and either repeat or grow out the cells for analysis.
4. Analyze the cells for transduction or select with G418 as described for adherent cells.

3.9.2. Cocultivation Transduction

1. Plate virus producer cells and culture to 50–75% confluency.
2. Add polybrene to 8 μg/mL and nonadherent target cells at a density that will allow continued logarithmic growth for at least 1 to 2 d.
3. At the end of the cocultivation period, resuspend the nonadherent cells by gently washing the monolayer with medium.
4. Recover the cells by centrifugation and plate in tissue culture plastic.
5. After 24 h examine the culture for adherent cells, and if these are present, transfer the culture to a fresh vessel.
6. Repeat this process until no adherent cells are present in the culture.
7. Expand the cells for analysis and apply selection if appropriate.

4. Notes

1. Many cell lines can be subcultured at 1:20 or 1:30 dilutions. However, if in doubt, be conservative: overdilution when subculturing can have serious adverse affects on the cell line's viability.
2. A healthy culture should contain at least 90% viable cells.
3. A more even cell layer often can be obtained by adjusting the cell density such that the required number of cells is contained in the total volume of medium required in the flask/dish, rather than adding small volumes of cells to a larger volume of medium in the flask/dish and then mixing. For example, to plate 2×10^6 cells in a 60-mm dish, adjust the cell suspension to 3.5×10^5/mL and plate 6 mL per dish.
4. For initial experiments it is highly recommended that a vector expressing an easily assayed marker gene such as *neo*[r] be used. This allows rapid and easy identification of problem areas and quick testing of putative solutions to these problems. If it is desired to generate constructs that do not contain selectable markers, this should not be attempted until all procedures have been mastered using a vector carrying a selectable marker gene.
5. When using a vector that does not contain a selectable marker, helper virus can be assayed in a similar manner by using NIH3T3 cells already transduced with a *neo*[r] vector in the assay procedure. In this case, any helper virus in the sample to be tested will result in the mobilization of this virus, which can be detected in the same manner.
6. High-titer virus can be produced by transient expression if a packaging cell line derived from 293T cells (such as Bosc 23) is used. Alternatively, 293T cells can be transfected with both vector and helper plasmids to generate high-titer virus by transient expression. These approaches may be useful if the gene carried in the vector is toxic or for producing VSV-G protein–pseudotyped virus.

7. You may keep this at 4°C for short-term storage (no more than 2 d) or at −70°C for long-term storage.

8. If it is desired to generate amphotropic producer cells in one of the packaging cell lines based on human cells (**Table 2**), then the first half of the ping-pong procedure (production of virus by transient expression) needs to be done in a packaging cell line with a pseudotype other than ecotropic or amphotropic. FLYRD 18 or PT67 would be suitable cell lines.

9. It is best to plate a range of dilutions (1 mL of 10^0–10^{-4} of virus supernatant for ecotropic virus made by transient expression in a stable packaging line) and to have two or three duplicates for each dilution. A concentration of 1 mg (total) G418/mL is suitable for most cell lines.

10. Because the assay is based on viral spread in the culture, and MLV-based viruses can only transduce dividing cells, it is important to keep the culture actively growing rather than confluent. To maintain a large cell number at all times, do not subculture at more than a 1:10 dilution.

11. For instance, use the enzymes that recognize sites in the viral LTR (e.g., *Kpn*I for most MLV-based vectors) and an enzyme that cuts only on one side of the probe sequence within the vector. The first analysis can be used to give a measure of proviral integrity (i.e., the fragment is of the size expected) and the second a measure of the number of proviral sequences present—each provirus, being integrated at a different site in the genome, will give rise to a fragment of different size, one end defined by the enzyme recognition site in the vector, the other by the first site in the adjacent chromosomal sequence.

12. When using a virus that does not carry an easily assessable marker, approximate titers can be obtained by assaying gene transfer at the DNA level by Southern blot analysis or semiquantitative/quantitative PCR. In the first instance, the technique is relatively insensitive and is not easily used unless the viral titer is high and the target cells are readily transduced. This approach can be complicated by signals from normal cellular sequences, such as endogenous gene sequences or proviral sequences, unless a probe specific to the vector can be used. Endogenous gene sequences can be used as a diploid copy number control, if a probe that is contained within a single gene exon/restriction enzyme fragment is used as a probe. Semiquantitative PCR can be achieved by simply doing end-point dilution assays in which the target DNA is serially diluted until no signal is obtained from the PCR. In both these techniques, it is relatively easy to measure comparative titers, but unless a known standard is available, it can be difficult to achieve absolute titers.

13. Virus pseudotyped with VSV-G protein is much more stable and can also be concentrated effectively by ultracentrifugation *(14)*.

14. We find that after a number of collections, the cells detach from the surface and start to roll up. This can be delayed by making sure the medium to be added to the cells is fully prewarmed to 37°C.

15. Some cultures will respond adversely to repeated transduction. If this is the case, alternating virus transduction with short periods of recovery in normal growth medium may be appropriate.

16. Several methodologies, such as spinoculation *(15)* and flow-through transduction *(16)*, have been developed to allow exposure of nonadherent cells to large quantities or high concentrations of virus.

17. If the rate of transduction is low selection of nonadherent cells can be problematic for two reasons: These problems are difficulty of keeping the viable cell density above the critical level required to ensure good growth of the culture, and the accumulation of large numbers of dead cells in the culture that can negatively impact on growth conditions. These two problems are, to a certain extent, linked because if transduction is high enough, the culture will contain fewer dead cells, and these are rapidly lost by dilution of the growing culture. Conversely, if the rate of transduction is low, the culture will contain many dead cells and cannot be expanded rapidly. The use of a vector containing a marker that can allow physical selection of transduced cells is obviously advantageous in this instance. The addition of antioxidants to the medium may also be beneficial *(17)*.

References

1. Shinnick, T. M., Lerner, R. A., and Sutcliffe, J. G. (1981) Nucleotide sequence of Moloney murine leukemia virus. *Nature* **293,** 543–548.
2. Cosset, F.-L., Takeuchi, Y., Battini, J.-L., Weiss, R. A., and Collins, M. K. L. (1995) High-titer packaging cells producing recombinant retroviruses resistant to human serum. *J. Virol.* **69,** 7430–7436.
3. Rigg, R. J., Chen, J., Dando, J. S., Forestell, S. P., Plavec, I., and Bohnlein, E. (1996) A novel amphotropic packaging cell line: high titer, complement resistance, and improved safety. *Virology* **218,** 290–295.
4. Miller, D. G., Adam, M. A., and Miller, A. D. (1990) Gene transfer by retrovirus vectors occurs only in cells that are actively replicating at the time of infection. *Mol. Cell. Biol.* **10,** 4239–4242.
5. Dull, T., Zufferey, R., Kelly, M., Mandel, R. J., Nguyen, M., Trono, D., and Naldini, L. (1998) A third-generation lentivirus vector with a conditional packaging system. *J. Virol.* **72,** 8463–8471.
6. Hawley, R. G., Lieu, F. H. L., Fong, A. Z. C., and Hawley, T. S. (1994) Versatile retroviral vectors for potential use in gene therapy. *Gene Therapy* **1,** 136–138.
7. Miller, A. D., Law, M.-F., and Verma, I. M. (1985) Generation of helper free amphotropic retroviruses that transduce a dominant-acting, methotrexate-resistant dihydrofolate reductase gene. *Mol. Cell. Biol.* **5,** 431–437.
8. Ruggieri, L., Aiuti, A, Salomoni, M., Zappone, E., Ferrari, G., and Bordignon, C. (1997) Cell-surface marking of CD34$^+$-restricted phenotypes of human hematopoietic progenitor cells by retrovirus-mediated gene transfer. *Hum. Gene Ther.* **8,** 1611–1623.
9. Medin, J. A., Migita, M., Pawliuk, R., Jacobson, S., Amiri, M., Kluepfel-Stahl, S., Brady, R. O., Humphries, R. K., and Karlsson, S. (1996) A bicistronic therapeutic retroviral vector enables sorting of transduced CD34$^+$ cells and corrects the enzyme deficiency in cells from Gaucher patients. *Blood* **87,** 1754–1762.

10. Limon, A., Briones, J., Puig, T., Carmona, M., Fornas, O., Cancelas, J. A., Nadal, M., Garcia, J., Rueda, F., and Barquinero, J. (1997) High-titre retroviral vectors containing the enhanced green fluorescent protein gene for efficient expression in hematopoietic cells. *Blood* **90,** 3316–3321.
11. Miller, A. D. and Rosman, G. J. (1989) Improved retroviral vectors for gene transfer and expression. *BioTechniques* **7,** 980–990.
12. Sambrook, J., Fritsch, E. F., and Maniatis, T. (1989) *Molecular Cloning: A Laboratory Manual,* 2nd ed., Cold Spring Harbor Laboratory, Cold Spring Harbor, NY.
13. Ausubel, F. M., Brent, R., Kingston, R. E., Moore, D. D., Seidman, J. G., Smith, J. A., and Struhl, K. (1989) *Current Protocols in Molecular Biology.* Wiley-Interscience, New York.
14. Burns, J. C., Friedmann, T., Driever, W., Burrascano, M., and Yee, J.-K. (1993) Vesicular stomatis virus G glycoprotein pseudotyped retroviral vectors: concentration to very high titer and efficient gene transfer into mammalian and nonmammalian cells. *Proc. Natl. Acad. Sci. USA* **90,** 8033–8037.
15. Su, L., Lee, R., Bonyhadi, M., Matsuzaki, H., Forestell, S., Escaich, S., Bohnlein, E., and Kaneshima, H. (1997) Hematopoietic stem cell-based gene therapy for acquired immunodeficiency syndrome: efficient transduction and expression of RevM10 in myeloid cells in vivo and in vitro. *Blood* **89,** 2283–2290.
16. Chuck, A. S. and Palsson, B. O. (1996) Consistent and high rates of transfer can be obtained using flow-through transduction over a wide range of retroviral titres. *Hum. Gene Ther.* **7,** 743–750.
17. Brielmeier, M., Bechet, J. M., Falk, M. H., Pawlita, M., Polack, A., and Bornkamm, G. W. (1998) Improving stable transfection efficiency: antioxidants dramatically improve the outgrowth of clones under dominant marker selection. *Nucleic Acids Res.* **26,** 2082–2085.
18. Dranoff, G., Jaffee, E., Lazenby, A., Golumbek, P., Levitsky, H., Brose, K., Jackson, V., Hamada, H., Pardoll, D., and Mulligan, R. C. (1993) Vaccination with irradiated tumor cells engineered to secrete murine granulocyte-macrophage colony-stimulating factor stimulates potent, specific, and long-lasting anti-tumor immunity. *Proc. Natl. Acad. Sci. USA* **90,** 3539–3543.
19. Faustinella, F., Kwon, H., Serrano, F., Belmont, J. W., Caskey, C. T., and Aguilar Cordova, E. (1994) A new family of murine retroviral vectors with extended multiple cloning sites for gene insertion. *Hum. Gene Ther.* **5,** 307–312.
20. Miller, A. D. and Buttimore, C. (1986) Redesign of retrovirus packaging cell lines to avoid recombination leading to helper virus production. *Mol. Cell. Biol.* **6,** 2895–2902.
21. Miller, A. D., Garcia, J. V., von-Suhr, N., Lynch, C. M., Wilson, C., and Eiden, M. V. (1991) Construction and properties of retrovirus packaging cells based on gibbon ape leukemia virus. *J. Virol.* **65,** 2220–2224.
22. Markowitz, D., Goff, S., and Bank, A. (1988) A safe packaging line for gene transfer: separating viral genes on two different plasmids. *J. Virol.* **62,** 1120–1124.
23. Markowitz, D., Goff, S., and Bank, A. (1988) Construction and use of a safe and efficient amphotropic packaging cell line. *Virology* **167,** 400–406.

24. Danos, O. and Mulligan, R. C. (1988) Safe and efficient generation of recombinant retroviruses with amphotropic and ecotropic host ranges. *Proc. Natl. Acad. Sci. USA* **85,** 6460–6464.
25. Cosset, F. L., Takeuchi, Y., Battini, J. L., Weiss, R. A., and Collins, M. K. (1995) High-titer packaging cells producing recombinant retroviruses resistant to human serum. *J. Virol.* **69,** 7430–7436.
26. Miller, A. D. and Chen, F. C. (1996) Retrovirus packaging cells based on 10A1 murine leukemia virus for production of vectors that use multiple receptors for cell entry. *J. Virol.* **70,** 5564–5571.
27. Ory, D. S., Neugeboren, B. A., and Mulligan, R. C. (1996) A stable human-derived packaging cell line for production of high titer retrovirus/vesicular stomatis virus G pseudotypes. *Proc. Natl. Acad. Sci. USA* **93,** 11,400–11,406.
28. Rigg, R. J., Chen, J., Dando, J. S., Forestell, S. P., Plavec, I., and Bohnlein, E. (1996) A novel human amphotropic packaging cell line: high titer, complement resistance, and improved safety. *Virology* **218,** 290–295.
29. Pear, W. S., Nolan, G. P., Scott, M. L., and Baltimore, D. (1993) Production of high-titer helper-free retroviruses by transient transfection. *Proc. Natl. Acad. Sci. USA* **90,** 8392–8396.
30. DuBridge, R. B., Tang, P., Hsia, H. C., Leong, P. M., Miller, J. H., and Calos, M. P. (1987) Analysis of mutation in human cells by using an Epstein-Barr virus shuttle system. *Mol. Cell. Biol.* **7,** 379–387.

29

Gene Therapy Approaches to Sensitization of Human Prostate Carcinoma to Cisplatin by Adenoviral Expression of p53 and by Antisense Jun Kinase Oligonucleotide Methods

Ruth Gjerset, Ali Haghighi, Svetlana Lebedeva, and Dan Mercola

1. Introduction

One of the challenges of medical research today is to find ways of bringing our genetic knowledge of cancer to clinical application and to develop improved therapies by exploiting gene-based strategies. By offering increased specificity and reduced toxicity, gene-based approaches promise alternatives when conventional treatments fail. Gene therapy also offers improved responses to conventional treatments when used in combination with gene therapy. Chief among the cancers in urgent need of improved treatment options is prostate cancer—the most commonly diagnosed cancer in men.

Advanced prostate cancer is resistant to most forms of hormone therapy, radiation therapy, and conventional chemotherapy. In fact, many of the most powerful chemotherapeutic drugs commonly used for other cancers are not effective against prostate cancer. Among these agents is cisplatin (also known as *cis*-diamminedichloroplatinum [CDDP], Platinol™, *cis*-platinum), which causes DNA damage in rapidly dividing cells by forming primarily bifunctional intrastrand adducts between adjacent guanines and guanine-adenine dinucleotides. Cisplatin is highly effective against ovarian cancer and bladder cancer and can achieve cures when used against testicular cancer. Cisplatin has also been applied to colon and brain tumors but is not in routine use for these applications *(1,2)*. A method for affecting increased sensitivity to cisplatin and for inhibiting or reversing resistance to cisplatin would provide an extended application for this drug, an important agent with well-known properties.

From: *Methods in Molecular Biology, vol. 175: Genomics Protocols*
Edited by: M. P. Starkey and R. Elaswarapu © Humana Press Inc., Totowa, NJ

The cellular response to stress and DNA damage now appears to be central to the issue of resistance to DNA-damaging chemotherapies such as cisplatin, suggesting that genetic approaches that target these pathways may be effective in reversing resistance and enhancing the benefits of these agents. In this chapter, we describe the potential of reversing drug resistance through gene therapies that target two major stress and DNA damage-response pathways: the Jun NH_2-terminal kinase/stress-activated protein kinase (JNK/SAPK) pathway and the DNA damage-induced apoptotic pathway mediated by the p53 tumor suppressor. There are suggestions that inhibition of the Jun kinase pathway or restoration of the p53 pathway may offer new biologic approaches to therapy sensitization in prostate cancer. These approaches would expand the potential of presently available treatments and offer alternatives when conventional treatment protocols fail. These approaches are illustrated by the use of a p53 adenoviral expression vector and by the use of highly efficient antisense JNK oligonucleotides.

1.1. In Vitro Combination Studies with p53 Adenovirus and Cisplatin

The p53 tumor suppressor has attracted considerable attention, not only for its tumor suppressor properties but also for its ability to sensitize tumor cells to apoptosis following treatment with chemotherapy and radiation *(3–8)*. Recent studies suggest that p53 gene therapy could have a broad application as a therapy sensitizer in cancer, a possibility that greatly expands the clinical application of p53-based approaches. Because many cancers, including prostate cancer, acquire p53 mutations as the disease progresses and becomes resistant to therapy, p53 gene therapy in combination with chemotherapy could have advantageous application for these advanced cancers. Numerous in vitro studies now support the application of p53 gene therapy as a therapy sensitizer for cancer *(3–8)*.

The results of screening tumor cells for sensitivity to various chemotherapeutic agents following exposure of cells to a replication-defective adenovirus encoding wild-type p53 (Adp53) compared to control vector (Ad-β-galactosidase [AD-βgal]) is summarized in **Fig. 1**. The cells were treated under conditions in which some 50–70% of them shows transgene expression, as evidenced by X-gal staining of parallel cultures infected with Ad-βgal. Viability is scored by the methanethiosulfonate (MTS) assay *(9)*. Under these conditions, it was found that growth suppression by Adp53 alone is incomplete and that 7-d viabilities of Adp53-treated cultures were about 60–80% of control vector–treated cultures. In addition, numerous tumor cell types lacking wild-type p53 expression, including the prostate cancer line PC-3, can be sen-

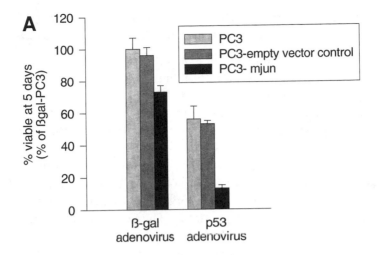

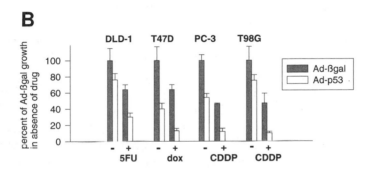

Fig. 1. (**A**) Effect of various chemotherapeutic agents on tumor cells. Ad53 is the wild type whereas Ad-βgal is the control vector. The viability was scored by MTS assay (**B**) Sensitivities of mutant p53-expressing cell lines to Adp53 and chemotherapeutic drugs. Viability assay showing that Adp53 suppresses growth and enhances sensitivity to DNA-damaging chemotherapeutic drugs in p53 mutant–expressing cells (DLD-1 colon carcinoma cells, T47D breast cancer cells, PC-3 prostate cancer cells, and T98G glioblastoma cells). Infection efficiencies were 60–70%, and drug treatments 1 d postinfection were as follows: 5-fluorouracil (5FU), 10 μM 1 h;, doxorubicin (dox) 3.7 μM 1 h, cisplatin (CDDP), 30 μM for 1 h for PC-3 cells and 20 ~M 1 h for T98G cells. Viability was assayed 6 d post drug treatment in all cases except PC-3, in which viability was assayed 4 d post drug treatment and expressed as a percentage of control cells treated with Ad-βgal.

sitized to chemotherapeutic drug treatment following restoration of wild-type p53 activity, consistent with the role of p53 in mediating DNA damage recognition and apoptosis.

1.2. In Vivo Combination Studies Using p53 Adenovirus and Cisplatin in a Nude Mouse Model for Prostate Cancer

Recently it has been shown that p53 is highly effective at suppressing the growth of human prostate xenografts in nude mice but fails to achieve complete tumor eradication by itself *(10,11)*. We have tested the possibility that more complete suppression can be achieved by combining p53 gene therapy with the DNA-damaging chemotherapy, cisplatin. In the experiment shown in **Fig. 2**, with these treatment doses, both Adp53 and cisplatin administered as single agents led to a significant reduction in tumor growth relative to tumors receiving only control vector ($p < 0.001$). When combined, Adp53 and cisplatin led to an even greater reduction in tumor growth, which was significantly better than either agent used alone ($p < 0.02$). The vector doses in this experiment were low (equivalent to about 10–30 plaque-forming units [PFU]/cell) and derive completely without side effects, as judged by periodic weight measurements of the animals and histologic examination of tissues, suggesting that higher doses or more prolonged treatment could have been applied without adverse side effects. This in vivo study therefore confirms the in vitro observations and supports the clinical application of p53 adenovirus combination approaches to tumors expressing mutant p53.

Adenovirus-based approaches are among the most promising for clinical applications of gene therapy. Adenoviruses are relatively easy to prepare, are stable, can be obtained in high titer, and provide high gene-transfer efficiencies. Adenoviruses are also well tolerated in patients and have been used in phase I clinical trials with few side effects even with repeated doses *(12–18)*. Improvements in tissue targeting of adenovirus will extend the application of adenovirus-based approaches to a broad range of clinical situations. Nevertheless, adenovirus-mediated p53 gene transfer has already shown efficacy in clinical trials for lung cancer, hepatocellular carcinoma, and head and neck cancer *(18)*.

1.3. In Vitro Studies Combining Inhibition of the JNK Pathway with Chemotherapy

Another important cellular pathway involved in the DNA damage response is the JNK/SAPK pathway, which is often upregulated in prostate cancer *(19,20)*.

This pathway represents one of the mitogen-activated protein kinase pathways and plays a role in growth factor signaling, oncogene expression, and cellular transformation, as well as the DNA damage response *(9)*.

Numerous reports document the activation of the JNK pathway in cells following treatment with a variety of DNA-damaging agents, including ultravio-

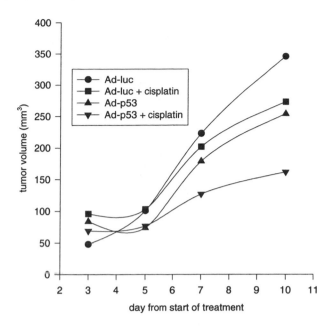

Fig. 2. Suppression of PC-3 prostate tumor growth in nude mice by Adp53 + cisplatin. Vector (Adp53 or control Ad-Luc, 10^8 PFU/tumor) was administered intratumorally on days 3, 5, 7, and 10, and cisplatin was administered intraperitoneal on d 1 and 8.

let (UV) radiation, ionizing radiation, methylethane sulfate, N-nitro-N'-nitroso-guanidine, 1-β-D-arabinofuranosylcytosine), and cisplatin *(19)*. A major substrate of JNK is the transcription factor c-Jun, which is greatly activated on phosphorylation of serine residuals 63 and 73. We have demonstrated that tumor cells that stably express a nonphosphorylatable dominant negative mutant cJun (c-Jun [863A, 573A]) are defective in repair of cisplatin adducts, consistent with their increased sensitivity to cisplatin (**Fig. 3**). The DNA repair assay that we used was based on the observations that cisplatin adducts will inhibit the *Taq* polymerase such that the decrease in yield of the polymerase chain reaction (PCR) product is directly proportional to the degree of platination of the template. The density of adducts can then be calculated based on a Poisson distribution predicted from a random process of platination *(21)*. Thus, (P) the relative PCR signal strength (damaged template relative to undamaged template) is related to the platination level (n), the number of adducts per PCR amplicon-sized fragment by the formula $P = e^{-n}$. In our case, we amplified a 2.7-kb fragment of the HPRTase gene, a fragment providing a sufficiently large target size to enable us to detect significant decreases in PCR

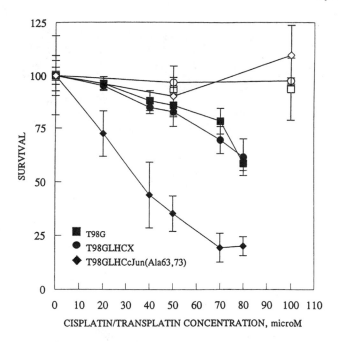

Fig. 3. Cisplatin and Transplatin sensitivity of T98G cells and clones. Cell survival (viability) assay showing that expression of mutant Jun (dnJun) sensitizes clonal T98G cells (■) to cisplatin. As controls, similar viability results are shown for wild-type c-dun overexpressing clonal T98G cells (◆), and empty vector expressing clonal T98G cells (●). Open symbols represent the corresponding experiments with the inactive transplatin control indicating that decreased survival by inhibition of the JNK pathway is specific to cisplatin-generated DNA damage (after **ref. 29**).

signals from templates from cisplatin-treated cells. Amplification of a smaller fragment of 150 bp in length, a fragment too small to register significant levels of platination under our conditions, served as a control for the efficiency of the PCR amplification. **Table 1** summarizes the frequency of adduct formation calculated after quantitating the PCR signal strengths (results of two experiments performed in triplicate). As shown in **Table 1**, cisplatin adducts form at a greater frequency on genomic DNA in mutant Jun-expressing cells than in parental cells. In addition, mutant Jun-expressing cells show no repair of adducts in a 6-h recovery period following a 1-h treatment with cisplatin, whereas parental cells repair about half of the adducts in that time period.

These results have been confirmed using a plasmid recovery DNA repair assay (**Fig. 4**). In this assay, cells are transfected with chloramphenicol acetyltransferase (CAT) reporter plasmids that have been damaged ex vivo by previous treatment with 25 μ*M* cisplatin for 3 h. Reporter gene expression 24

Table 1
Cisplatin-DNA Adducts per 2.7 kb

Treatment	T98G Parental cells	T98G Mutant Jun cells
200 µM cisplatin for 1 h	0.48 ± 0.08	0.63 ± 0.2
200 µM cisplatin for 1 h, 6 h recovery	0.20 ± 0.05	0.55 ± 0.2

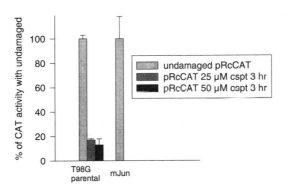

Fig. 4. Plasmid reactivation assay using CAT reporter plasmid damaged ex vivo by treatment with cisplatin (cspt). Reporter gene expression, assayed 24 h post-transfection, indicates that mutant Jun-expressing clonal T98G cells are suppressed in their ability to repair and express the CAT transgene.

and 48 h posttransfection is taken as an indication of DNA repair. As shown in **Fig. 4**, cells that express mutant Jun are suppressed relative to parental cells in their ability to repair the damaged plasmid, consistent with the PCR-based DNA repair assays.

Although the mechanism by which the JNK pathway affects DNA repair is not known, there are several candidate target genes whose roles in DNA synthesis and repair could account for observations that we have made. The promoters of DNA synthesis and repair genes contain the transcript ion factors AP-1 or ATF2/CREB regulatory elements (**Table 2**). These include DNA polymerase β, topoisomerase I, topoisomerase II, uracyl glycosylase, proliferating cell nuclear antigen, and metallothionein. In several cases, such as DNA polymerase β, exposure of cells to UV radiation is known to induce the gene, and ATF2/CREB sites are required for this induction. Thus, a number of genes involved in DNA excision repair may be coordinately upregulated on activation of the JNK pathway following cisplatin damage. Some or all of these could serve as potential targets for gene therapy approaches to drug sensitization of cancer.

Table 2
DNA Repair Associated Genes Containing Potential JNK-Regulated Sequences (after ref. *61*)[a]

Repair Associated Gene	Element	Sequence (consensus sequence)2	LLG Position	Score	Reference for function
DNA polymerase B	AP-1/TRE	CTGACTCA (- t g a c t c a)	337	2.0	It is known to be functional and TPA-activated classic TRE (*30*).
	ATF/CREB	TTACGTAA (t t a c g t c a)	282	2.0	It is known to be genotoxic-activated (*30*,
DNA polymerase a (*32*)	ATF/CREB	CACGTCA (t/g a c g t c a)	−82		The function of ATF/CREB (*32*) is unknown.
		GGGGTCA (t g a g t c a)	−149		AP-1 sites are thought to be significant in DNA repair: DNA polymerase is over expressed in cisplatin-resistant cells and anti-Fos ribozyme sensitizes (27).
Topoisomerase I	AP-1	GGGGGCGG (t g a g t c a)	753	2.0	(*33,34*)
	AP-1	TGACCCA (t g a c t c a)	217	2.0	(*33,34*)
	ATF/CREB	TGACGTCA (t g a c g t c a)	792	2.0	It is known to be functional and stress activated (33, 34).
Topoisomerase IIα	ATF/CREB	TGACGCCG (t g a c g t c a)	286	2.0	(*35,36*); Topo II is UV inducible and functions early in UV-induced DNA damage repair.
Topoisomerase IIβ	AP-1	TGATTGG (t g a g t c a)	337		(*35*)
	AP-1	TGACTCA (t g a c t c a)	3		(*37*)

Gene	Factor	Sequence	Position	Fold	Notes
	AP-1	AGAGTCA (t g a g t c a)	65		(37)
ATF-3	AP-1	TGAGTAA (t g a c g t c a)	-1600		(38,39); ATF-3 is stress-induced, anisomycin (JNK activator)-induced, and induced by ATF-2/c-Jun coexpression suggesting a functional
	AP-1	ATAGTCA (t g a c g t c a)	-1353		role for the ATF/CREB site. ATF-3/c
	AP-1	AGACTAA (t g a c g t c a)	-605		Jun heterodimers bind ATF/CREB sites and activate transcription (40,41)
	AP-1	GAGTCA (t g a c g t c a)	-380		and ATF-3/c-Jun and ATF-3/JunD heterodimers have been shown to bind TTAGTTAC, a ATF/CREB sequence,
	ATF/CRE	TTACGTCA (t g a c g t c a)	-92		which mediates EGF/ras/raf-stimulated transcription (42), however, a role in induction of DNA repair genes is not known.
c-Jun	ATF/CREB	TTACCTCA (t t a c g c a)		2.0	(43–45); The "functional" association with DNA repair is strong induction of c-Jun by genotoxins known to activate JNK/SAPK.
Uracil glycosylase (46)	AP-1	TGGGTCA (t g a g t c a)	141	2.0	Activation regulation is not known.
PCNA	AP-1	TGACTCA (t g a c t c a)	489	2.0	DNA polymerase-A accessory protein function.
PCNA	ATF/CREB	TGAGGTCAGGG (t g a c g t c a - - -)	209	1.64	(47,48); 11-2, a potent JNK/SAPK activator, induces PNCA expression via ATF/CREB promoter sites, which
	ATF/CREB	GTGACGTCAC (- t t a c g t c a - -)	1253	1.60	is blocked by rapamycin.
GADD153 (49)	ATF/CREB	ACTCCTGACCTT (t g/t a c g t c a - - -)	207	1.63	Induction requires phosphorylation-dependent event that is not PKA, PKC (50), or p38 (51) mediated consistent

(continued)

Table 2 (continued)

Repair Associated Gene	Element	Sequence (consensus sequence)2	LLG Position	Score	Reference for function
Growth arrest and DNA-damage-inducible gene	AP-1	TGACTCA (t g a c t c a)	710	2.0	with a role for JNK/SAPK (*50*). Moreover GADD153 is induced by MMS (*50*) and cisplatin (*52,53*). The role of the ATF/CREB site is unknown. GADD153isphoshorylated and activated by p38 in response tostress (*53*).
XRCC1 (*54,55*)	ATF/CREB	ACGTCA (a c g t c a)	1815	2.0	The site at 466 is consistent with c-Jun/ATF-3 vs. ATF-2 (TESS).
X-ray damage repair cross complementing gene product.	ATF/CREB	GGACGTCAA (t a c g t c a)	1814	2.0	Functional roles of these ATF/CREB and AP-1 sites are not known.
	ATF/CREB	CCTGACCTCA (- - t g a c g t c a)	2029	1.64	
	ATF/CREB	GCTGACGTCAG (- - t g a c g t c a -)	466	1.60	
	ATF/CREB	CCAATCA (t g/t a c/g t c a)	93	2.0	
MGMT (*56*)	ATF/CREB	TGCGTCA (t g a c g t c a)	1661	2.0	MGMT is induced by genotoxic agents (*57*). The site at 1674 is consistent with c-Jun/ATF-3 (TESS). The functional significance of these sites is unknown.
06-Methylguanine-DNA-methyl-transferase	ATF/CREB	GTGACATCAT (- t g a c t c a -)	1195	2.0	
	AP-1	TGAGTCA (t g a g t c a)	734	2.0	
	AP-1	TTACTCA (t t a c t c a)	285	1.73	

MSH2 (*58,59*)	ATF/CREB	TGGCGTCA (t g a c t c a)	108	1.62	TESS does not recognize c-Jun participation at 108 site. Role in cisplatin induced repair unknown.
	AP-1	TGAATCA (t g a c/g t c a)	569	2.0	MSH2 has been reported to selectively bind to cisplatin-DNA adducts (*32,58*)
	AP-1	TGATGAAA (t g a c/g t c a)	884	1.62	
MetallothioneinIIA	AP-1	GAGCCGCAAGT (g a g t c a - - - - t GACTTCTAGCG g a c t c a a g t c CGGGGCGTG a - - - - - - t g)	188	2.0	(*60*); It is TPA and UV-light activated.

[1]Repair-associated protein for which only partial promoter sequences are known (i.e., in Genbank) without recognizable AP-1-regulated sites include ADP ribose polymerase, tif2/ref1, SSRP, Ercc1, and thymidylate synthetase.

[a]AP-1: activator protein-1 complex, a Jun and a Fos family member; ATF/CREB, cAMP: response element binding proteins; LLG: log likelyhood score, which is 2 for a perfect match of the candidate response, element with the consensus sequence (TESS criteria) and all ambiguous matches yielding a score of 0. MMS: methyl methar esulfonate; TESS: transcription element search system; PCNA, proliferating cell nuclear antigen; PKA, protein kinase A; PKC, protein kinase C.

[b]AP-1 consensus: TG/TAC/GTCA; CREB/ATF–2 consensus: TG/TACGTCA.

[c]Positions are based on TESS numbering of promoter sequences unless preceded by (–).

1.4. In Vivo Studies Combining Inhibition
of the Jun Kinase Pathway
by Antisense Targeting JNK with Chemotherapy

In a parallel arm of the in vivo study shown in **Fig. 2**, we tested the antitumor efficacy of downregulation of JNK combined with cisplatin. In this study, we downregulated JNK with antisense oligonucleotides targeting either the JNK1 or JNK2 family of JNK isoforms. These compounds were previously developed and characterized as described (22,23).

An important methodological consideration is the use of high affinity antisense oligonucleotides that completely suppress target mRNA and protein at low concentration. In collaborative studies with Isis Pharmaceuticals, we have developed a systematic method that now has been adapted to a multiwell procedure. The salient features are that a large series of phosphorothioate oligonucleotides complementary to 20 nucleotide stretches of JNK1 and JNK2 spaced approximately every 50 bp along the transcribed portion of the gene are prepared on a small scale. Thus, the target gene sequence must be known. These trial oligonucleotides are then tested for the ability to suppress steady-state transcript levels in culture cells 24 h after a 4-h lipid-mediated transfection (22,23). Most of these trial oligonucleotides we tested were not efficient at promoting suppression of target mRNA at low (0.2–0.4 μM) concentration. However, it was readily possible to identify antisense compounds that were >90% efficient at eliminating target mRNA at these low concentrations after a single 4-h transfection. This step is key in avoiding any temptation to use less efficacious antisense compounds by increasing the concentration to high levels (>1 μM) at which many nonspecific interactions leading to aberrant cellular localization and weak membrane-protein complex formation have been observed (24). Moreover, compounds that require >1 μM cannot be considered as potential drugs owing to the generation of nonspecific interactions and to the many drawbacks in attempting to achieve local concentrations on the order of ~1 μM in vivo. These considerations are likely important in understanding the many difficulties some researchers have had in "getting antisense to work."

For the studies summarized here, it was possible to select highly efficient antisense oligonucleotides that are complementary to a sequence that is invariant in all isoforms of JNK1 or JNK2, thereby making it possible to reduce or eliminate all isoforms of JNK1 or JNK2 with a single antisense oligonucleotide. Next, the elapsed time of suppression of target mRNA and target protein was determined (23). These studies showed that a single antisense treatment suppressed target mRNA and protein from approximately 24 h to 72 h, thereby defining a 2-d window in which antisense-mediated effects could be observed ([22,23]; unpublished data). However, for growth studies in which cell numbers are counted or tumor volume is measured, any loss of growth owing to inhibition of a growth-promoting target protein will remain apparent as decreased total growth for at least 3 wk *(22)*.

Because a variety of human tumor cells, including PC-3 cells, were sensitized to the cytotoxic effects of DNA-damaging cisplatin in vitro upon inhibition of the JNK pathway *(9)*, it was decided to test whether xenografts of PC-3 cells could be sensitized to cisplatin. Moreover, because many of the potential JNK-regulated genes encode gene products that facilitate DNA synthesis (**Table 2**), it appeared logical to expect that inhibition of JNK in vivo may affect tumor growth even in the absence of cisplatin *(25)*. This experiment was carried out as a separate arm of the same in vivo study as for the evaluation of Adp53 in **Fig. 2**.

Following inoculation of the mice with the PC-3 cells, the animals were monitored until visible and palpable tumors developed. At this point and for all subsequent observations, tumor volumes were estimated from the length and width of the tumors (*see* **Subheading 3.2.**). Treatment consisted of intraperitoneal injection of oligonucleotide solution (*see* **Subheading 2.2.**) daily for 6 of 7 d/wk. On the d 7, oligonucleotide treatment was omitted and the mice received either vehicle or cisplatin (*see* **Subheading 3.2.**). Treatment (systemic antisense oligonucleotide, 25 mg/kg of an equimolar mixture of antisense JNK1 and antisense JNK2 termed combined-antisense JNK1 + JNK2, or a scrambled-sequence oligonucleotide or vehicle phosphate-buffered saline [PBS] alone) was initiated on development of readily visible and palpable tumors (**Fig. 5**). Every seventh day, antisense treatment was omitted and a subgroup of 15 animals receiving the combined-antisense treatment also received cisplatin, i.e., the same dose of cisplatin and timing as for the p53 treatment regimen. As a control, a separate group of animals received cisplatin alone. To confirm that systemic antisense treatment led to inhibition of JNK activity, JNK activity of tumor extracts was determined 18 h after antisense treatment. These studies demonstrated an 89% reduction in steady-state tumor JNK activity in tumors of antisense-treated animals compared with the activity of PC-3 cells, and an 80% reduction compared with the tumor JNK activity of scrambled sequence oligonucleotide-treated animals (**Fig. 5**).

We observed that treatment with antisense oligonucleotides either antisense JNK2 or combined-antisense treatment—led to marked inhibition of tumor growth, and these results were superior to those for cisplatin alone. When the growth curves in **Fig. 5** were integrated, it was found, e.g., that combined treatment led to 78% inhibition whereas cisplatin treatment led to 47% tumor growth inhibition. These results are significantly less ($p < 0.002$) than those for controls (vehicle alone, scrambled-sequence oligonucleotide) and are significantly different from each other ($p < 0.02$; analysis of variance). The effect of antisense JNK can be attributed largely to antisense JNK2 (**Fig. 5**). The domi-

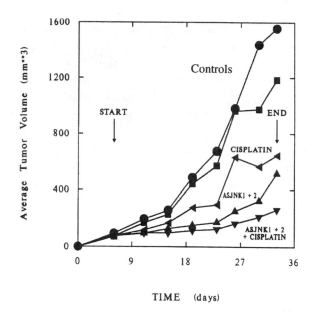

TIME (days)

Fig. 5. Application of antisense JNK and cisplatin chemotherapy to established xenografts of PC-3 human prostate carcinoma cells. Groups of 10–11 or 15 athymic female mice that had been inoculated with PC-3 cells and allowed to develop visible tumors were started on treatment ("start" arrow) of either one of the indicated antisense oligonucleotide solutions by daily IP injection or cisplatin weekly or a control consisting of vehicle alone or a scrambled sequence oligonucleotide. The average size of the tumors for each treatment group is plotted from the time of inoculation to the end of treatment ("end" arrow). The percentage of inhibition of growth was calculated by integrating each curve and expressing the result as $100 \times [1\text{-(growth/growth of control)}]$. These experiments were carried out in parallel with the p53 adenovirus-treated PC-3 tumors.

nance of JNK2 has been observed in human lung carcinoma cells *(22)* and in a series of nine human prostate carcinoma cell lines *(26)*. When antisense cisplatin treatments were combined, growth inhibition was further enhanced to 89% of maximum growth inhibition (**Fig. 5**). Thus, these in vivo studies suggest that it may be possible both to inhibit growth and to sensitize solid tumors to chemotherapy by eliminating the JNK pathway.

1.5. Combined Inhibition of Jun Kinase and Restoration of p53

The approaches described here have implications for therapeutic approaches targeting the DNA damage response in tumor cells. Upregulation of the DNA repair machinery may accompany tumor progression and the development of

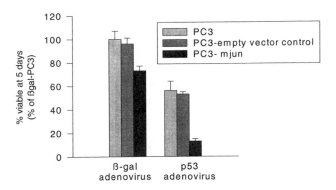

Fig. 6. Cells modified to express mutant jun are sensitized to p53. Relative 4-d growth following Ad p53 treatment or Ad–13gal treatment (control) of PC-3 prostate carcinoma cells (parental), PC-3 empty vector transduced cells, and PC-3 mutant Jun-expressing cells (PC3-mjun). Growth was assayed using the MTT assay.

drug resistance. This process may involve, in part, AP-1 and ATF2/CREB-regulated DNA synthesis and repair genes. In fact, earlier studies by Scanlon et al. *(27)* demonstrated that downregulation of AP-1 activity using a c-fos ribozyme was effective at sensitizing ovarian carcinoma cells to cisplatin, and this correlated with downregulation of DNA polymerase β, topoisomerase I, and thymidylate synthetase, all known to have AP-1 sites in their promoter regions *(27)* (**Table 2**).

Independent of JNK DNA damage response, loss of the p53 tumor suppressor contributes to resistance to DNA-damaging therapies by removing an important component of the DNA damage recognition machinery. Because p53 induces apoptosis in response to the level of DNA damage, it is likely that the success or failure of DNA repair contributes to the suppressive effects of p53. We therefore hypothesized that cells in which the JNK pathway was inhibited would show greater growth inhibition following exposure to p53 adenovirus. As shown in **Fig. 6**, this is indeed the case. In this experiment, PC-3 prostate cancer cells expressing mutant Jun were much more growth suppressed following treatment with p53 adenovirus in 7-d 96-well growth assays than were parental cells or cells modified with empty vector.

These results support the combined application of p53 gene therapy along with antisense therapy to inhibit the JNK pathway, or some downstream target of the pathway. When used in combination with conventional chemotherapies such as cisplatin, the combined approach, which can be foreseen today, may extend the application of conventional treatments to prostate cancer and provide a new strategy for treatment of therapy-resistance advanced disease.

2. Materials

1. Adenoviral vectors (Deborah Wilson, Introgen Therapeutics, Houston, TX) (*see* **Note 1**).
2. Antisense phosphorothiates dexyoligonucleotides (*see* **Note 2**; *see* also **ref. 23**):
   a. JNK1: 5'-CTCTCTGTAGGCCCGCTTGG-3'.
   b. JNK2: 5'-GTCCGGGCCAGGCCAAAGTC-3'.
3. Delbecco's modified minimum medium supplemented with 10% fetal calf serum (Irvine Scientific, Irvine, CA). PC-3 human prostate carcinoma cells, as well as other cell lines used in in vitro assays (T47D breast cancer cells, DLD-1 colon cancer cells, and T98G glioblastoma cells) were grown at 37°C in an environment of 10% CO_2.
4. Animals: 5- to 6-wk athymic female postweaning Harlan Sprague-Dawley mice (Harlan, Indianapolis, IN).
5. 10X PBS: 2 g of anhydrous KH_2PO_4, 11.4 g of anhydrous Na_2HPO_4, 2 g of KCl, 80 g of NaCl. Make up the volume to 1 L with H_2O. Dilute 1:10 before use.
6. X-gal staining solution: 1 mg/mL of 5-bromo-4-chloro-3-indoyl-β-D-galacto-pyrano-side(X-gal), 5 mM potassium ferricyanate, 5 mM potassium ferrocyanate, 2 mM $MgCl_2$ in PBS.
7. *Taq* polymerase (Qiagen).
8. 250 μM dNTPs (Pharmacia Biotech.).
9. PCR Reaction mix: 25-μL reactions contain 0.03–0.25 μg of DNA, 25 pmol each of forward and reverse primer, 250 μM dNTPs (Pharmacia Biotech.), 1.25 U *Taq* polymerase (Qiagen), 1X buffer (Qiagen), Solution Q (Qiagen). The deoxyribonucleotide pruners are 5'-TGGGATTACACGTGTGAACCAACC-3' and 5'-GATCCACAGTCTGCCTGAGTCACT-3', respectively, with a 5' nested primer of 5'-CCTAGAAAGCACATGGAGAGCTAG-3' (*see* **Note 6**).
10. CAT assay reaction mix (per reaction): 70 μL of cell lysate, 30 μL of 5 mM chloramphenicol, 0.4 μL of ^{3}H-acetylCoA (200 mCi/mmol; NEN®Life Science), 0.6 μL (4.4 μg/μL) of nonradioactive acetylCoA (Pharmacia Biotech.).
11. Whole-cell extract (WCE) buffer: 20 mM HEPES, pH 8.0; 75 mM NaCl; 2.5 mM $MgCl_2$, 0.05% (v/v) Triton X-100, 0.5 mM dithiothreitol (DIT); 20 mM β-glycerophosphate; 0.1 mM Na_3VO_4; 2 μg/mL leupeptine, 100 μg/mL paramethylsulfonyl fluoride.
12. JNK assay buffer: 20 mM HEPES, pH 7.7; 20 mM $MgCl_2$, 20 mM β-glycerophosphate; 20 mM *p*-nitrophenyl phosphate; 0.1 mM Na_3VO_4, 2 mM DTT; 20 μM adenosine triphosphate (ATP); 5 μCi of [λ^{32}P] ATP.
13. Oligonucleotide transfection (lipofection) solution: Mix 10 μg/mL of lipofectin (Gibco-BRL, Gaithersburg, MD) reagent in MEM (Gibco-BRL, Gaithersburg, MD) with an equal volume of oligonucleotide solution, incubating this mixture at room temperature for 15 min and diluting it with lipofectin solution to a final oligonucleotide concentration of 0.4 μM.
14. X-gal staining solution: 1 mg/mL 5-bromo-4-chloro-3-indoyl-β-D-galacto-pyranoside, 5 mM potassium ferricyanate, 5 mM potassium ferrocyanate, 2 mM MgCt in PBS.

15. Lipofection solution for plasmid transfection: Prepare a 1 µg/µL stock of DOTAP lipofection reagent (Boehringer Mannheim, Indianapolis, IN). Prepare the mix (per well) of a 24-well tissue culture plate as follows:
    a. Plasmid/HEPES mix: 1.25 µL (1 µg/µL) of plasmid + 11.25 µL 5 mM HEPES, pH 7.8.
    b. DOTAP/HEPES mix: 7.5 µL of DOTAP (1 µg/µL) + 17.5 µL of 5 mM HEPES, pH 7.8.
    Mix the entire contents of (a) and (b) together, and incubate for 30 min at room temperature.
16. Cisplatin (diaminodichloro *cis*-platinum): Aqueous Platinol (Bristol Myers Squibb).

3. Methods
3.1. 96-Well Growth Assay

1. Plate cells in complete medium 1 day prior to vector treatment in 24-well tissue culture plates so that their density at the time of treatment is about 70–80% of confluence.
2. Treat the cells with Adp53 or Ad Egal for 2 to 3 h (100 PFU/cell).
3. Incubate the cells for additional 2 d in one of the Ad-βgal-treated wells.
4. Remove the medium and wash the wells two times with PBS.
5. Fix the cells by overlaying with a solution containing 3.7% parafomaldehyde (v/v) in PBS for mm.
6. Wash the wells with PBS and overlay with X-gal staining solution.
7. Incubate the cells at 37°C overnight to allow development of blue stain in β-galactosidase-expressing cells for estimating the infection efficiency.
8. Following treatment with vector, plate the cells at low density (1000 cells/well) in 96-well plates (*see* **Note 4**). Treat (in triplicate) with drug (e.g., cisplatin) or antisense (*see* **Subheading 3.6.**) for 1–4 h depending on the drug, followed by incubation for an additional 5–7 d (*see* **Note 1**).
9. Incubate the cells for an additional 6 d and score viability by adding the tetrazolium dye MTT for 1 h and determining the A260 of the formazan product as described by the manufacturer (Promega) (*see* refs. **9** and **23**).

3.2. Subcutaneous Tumor Model in Nude Mice

1. Inoculate 5×10^6 PC-3 prostate cancer cells (mutant p53) subcutaneously on the back of nude mice by injecting 100 µL of a cell suspension in PBS at 5×10^7 cells/mL.
2. Allow tumors develop 5 d to a size of 50–100 mm^3.
3. Estimate tumor volume by measuring the length and width of the tumor with a caliper and calculate using the following formula: volume = π/6 (length × width^2).
4. Initiate treatment (designated day 1) and monitor tumor volume every 2 to 3 d (*see* **Note 2**).
5. For oligonucleotide treatment, inject mice intraperitoneally at 25 mg/kg and based on the average weight of all mice by daily ip injection with a solution

at a concentration yielding the total dose in 0.2 mL of PBS. Treat control animals with either vehicle alone or the scrambled-sequence control oligonucleotide.
6. For cisplatin treatment, inject mice intraperitoneally at 0.4 mg/kg once per week. For combined antisense JNK cisplatin treatment, inject antisense JNK oligo-doxynucleotides for 6 d and cisplatin on the day 7.

3.3. Analyses of DNA Repair by PCR Stop Assay

1. Prepare genomic DNA from about 5×10^5 cultured cells using the QlAmp blood kit (Qiagen) essentially following the manufacturer's protocol, except lyse the cells directly on the plate in the presence of PBS, Qiagen protease, and lysis buffer supplied in the kit.
2. Following purification, adjust the DNA concentration to 0.25 mg/mL in sterile water and store at $-20°C$ until use.
3. Carry out quantitative PCR as described *(32)* for the measurement of cisplatin adduct formation on specific regions of DNA (*see* **Notes 3** and **5**). For each primer pair, verify that product formation is directly proportional to input template by performing a pilot experiment with serial twofold dilutions of template, followed by electrophoresis on a 1% agarose gel containing 0.5 μg/mL of ethidium bromide.
4. Quantify bands using a Kodak digital camera and analysis software or an equivalent apparatus for the integration of band intensity from photographic film and determine adduct numbers using $P = e^{-n}$ (*see* **Notes 5** and **10**).
5. For the PCR reaction, use primers at a concentration of 0.03–0.25 μg per 25-μL reaction, depending on the amount of template used in the PCR reaction.
6. Carry out the PCR reaction using the following amplification program: 1 cycle of 94°C for 1 min 30 s; 25 cycles of 94°C for 1 min, 57°C, for 1 min, and 70°C for 2 min 30 s; 1 cycle of 94°C for 1 min; 57°C for 1 min, and 70°C for 7 min.
7. Use two independent templates for each treatment condition and set up each for analysis in triplicate. For such analysis carry out an internal PCR control using primers to generate a 150-bp fragment of the dihydrofolate reductase gene (*see* **Notes 3** and **5**).

3.4. Analysis of DNA Repair Using CAT Reporter Assay

1. Treat 100 μg of CAT reporter plasmid (in which the CAT gene is expressed from the RSV promoter), with 25 μM cisplatin in 300 μL total of PBS on ice for 3 h to create cisplatin-damage reporter DNA.
2. Precipitate the DNA by adding 150 μL of 7.5 M NH$_4$Ac and 450 μL of isopropanol.
3. Leave the mixture at $-20°C$ for 1 h.
4. Centrifuge the DNA at 14,000g for 30 min.
5. Perform two washes with 70% ethanol, followed by a final wash in absolute ethanol.
6. Resuspend the DNA in sterile H$_2$O and use for transfections.
7. Process untreated DNA the same way but without the addition of cisplatin, and use this plasmid preparation as a control.

8. Plate the cells in 24-well plates the day prior to transfection so that their density at the time of transfection is 50% (about 10^5 cells/well).
9. Set up transfections in triplicate wells with either 1–1.25 µg of undamaged plasmid or damaged plasmid for the 24-h time point together with a second set of triplicate wells transfected for the 48-h time point, using the DOTAP liposomal transfection reagent (*see* **Subheading 2.**).
10. Add 500 µL of medium to the entire contents of **step 9** and mix well.
11. Wash the cells in the well of a 24-well plate twice with 1X PBS.
12. Add 537.5 µL of transfection (**step 10**) to the well.
13. Incubate the reaction overnight in the 37°C, 10% CO_2 incubator.
14. Aspirate off the transfection mix and wash the cells twice with 1X PBS.
15. Aspirate off the PBS and replace with 1 mL of fresh complete culture medium.
16. Incubate for 24–48 h at 37°C, 10% CO_2.
17. Remove the medium, wash the cells twice with PBS, and store the plate dry at –70°C until required.

3.5. CAT Assay

1. Thaw the plates from **step 17** in **Subheading 3.4.** for 5 min at 37°C.
2. Add 100 µL of 1X Reporter Lysis Buffer (Promega) to each well of a 24-well plate.
3. Shake the plate vigorously for 15 min.
4. Transfer the entire 100 µL of lysate to microcentrifuge tubes.
5. Spin the lysates for 2 min at 14,000*g* (4°C).
6. Transfer the supernatants to fresh tubes.
7. Heat the supernatants for 10–15 min at 65°C to destroy deacetylase activity. If particulate material is present after this heating step, centrifuge again and collect the supernatants.
8. Measure the protein concentration of each sample using the Bio-Rad Protein Assay (Bio-Rad), following the manufacturer's instructions.
9. Equalize the protein concentration of the samples using 1X Reporter Lysis Buffer (Promega). Add 31 µL of CAT reaction mix to 70 µL of the samples.
10. Incubate the mix at 37°C for 2 h.
11. Add the entire sample to 1 mL of 7 *M* urea.
12. Add 1 mL of toluene:PPO (8 g of PPO [2.5-diphenyloxazole]/mL toluene). Shake well and count using a scintillation counter. The resulting counts are proportional to accumulated CAT expression and, therefore, total CAT activity.

3.6. Antisense Oligonucleotide Transfection

1. Wash 70% confluent cultures (24 h after plating) in tissue culture plates twice with PBS.
2. Incubate the cells with lipofectin-0.4 µM oligonucleotide solution (*see* **Subheading 2**) at 37°C in 10% CO_2 from 4 h to overnight (*see* **Note 7**).
3. Following lipofection, wash the cells once with serum-free MEM and continue the culture in complete medium for 24 h prior to JNK assay (*see* **Subheading 3.7**) or 4 d prior to growth assay (*9*) (*see* **Note 7**).

3.7. JNK Assay

1. Transfect the cells with oligonucleotides as described in **Subheading 3.5.**
2. Wash the cells with ice-cold PBS and suspend in WCE buffer.
3. Determine the protein concentration of the cell extracts by the Bradford dye method (Bio-Rad) (*see* **Note 8**).
4. Carry out the kinase assay as follows *(28,29)*:
   a. Mix 50 μg of WCE with 10 μg of GST-c-Jun (1-223) for 3 h at 4°C (*see* **Note 9**).
   b. Wash four times and incubate the beads with 30 μL of kinase reaction buffer for 20 min at 30°C.
5. Stop the reaction by adding of 20 μL of Laemmli sample buffer.
6. Elute the phosphorylated GST-c-Jun protein by boiling the sample for 5 min.
7. Resolve the components by 10% sodium dodecyl sulfate-polyacrylamide gel electrophoresis (*see* **Note 8**).
8. Quantify the ^{32}P-phosphorylated GST-c-Jun by digitization and integration of the respective "band" values of the autoradiograph of the dried gel (*see* **Note 10**).

4. Notes

1. These vectors are replication-defective adenoviral recombinants in which the early region genes E1A and E1B required for viral replication have been deleted and replaced with an expression cassette containing the transgene of interest. In the case of the p53 adenovirus (Adp53), the expression cassette consisted of the human wild-type p53 coding sequence, flanked by the cytomegalovirus (CMV) promoter, and the simian virus 40 (SV40) polyadenylation signal. In the case of the control adenovirus (Adβgal), the expression cassette consisted of the bacterial β-galactosidase coding sequence flanked by the CMV promoter and SV40 polyadenylation signals. In the case of the control adenovirus (AdLuc), the expression cassette consisted of the firefly luciferase coding sequence flanked by the Rous sarcoma virus promoter and SV40 polyadenylation sequences. Viral stocks were stored at −70° C and repeated freezing and thawing were avoided. The concentrations of the stocks, expressed in plaque-forming units per milliliter were 1 to 2 × 10^{11}.
2. The sequences were determined in preliminary studies utilizing a messenger walk procedure as described (*see* **refs.** *28* and *29*). Since in vivo studies require large amounts of oligonucleotide, a single "scrambled sequence" control sequence was chosen consisting of a scrambled 20-nt sequence previously used as a control in the analysis of antisense protein kinase Ca: 5' TCGCATCGACCCGCCCACTA-3'. Both ASJNK sequences contain a single CpG sequence thought to have potential immunostimulatory properties that, therefore, may influence xenograft growth by immunologic mechanisms. The control oligonucleotide used here has a nucleotide composition closely approximating the average of antisense JNK1 and JNK2 but contains three CpG dinucleotide sequences thereby providing a control for the potential influence of CpG sequences. All three oligonucleotides were prepared and purified as previously described *(34,35)*.

3. The 0.15-kb segment of genomic DNA amplified by use of the nested primer sustains undetectable levels of DNA damage under our conditions and serves as an internal PCR control and the basis for normalization of the amount of amplification of the 2.7-kb fragment. The nested amplification product varies by <5–10% among the various templates that we have used.

4. Wells that do not receive drug serve as a control to which drug-treated wells are compared. Example drug treatments are as follows: 5-fluorouracil (Adrucil™, Pharmacia Biotech.), 10 mM for 1 h; doxorubicin (doxorubicin hydrochloride, Aldrich), 3.7 µM for 1 h, cisplatin (Platinol™, Bristol-Myers Squibb), 30 µM for 1 h for PC-3 and 20 µM for 1 h for T98G.

5. Because *Taq* polymerase is blocked at cisplatin adducts, the relative efficiency of PCR amplification of genomic DNA from cisplatin-treated vs control cells drops in proportion to platination levels. The relative PCR efficiency is equal to the frequency of undamaged strands, P, within a population. P is related to the average number of cisplatin adducts, n, per fragment, by the Poisson formula $P = e^{-n}$, or $-(\ln P) = n$. A drop in the PCR signal to 0.6 of control would therefore reflect an average cisplatin adduct density of $-(\text{in } 0.6) = 0.51$ adducts per fragment. PCR signals ranging from 0.9 to 1.0 of control are generally indistinguishable from the control, owing to standard deviations in the range of ±0.1. Since a PCR signal equal to 0.9 of control reflects an adduct density of 0.1 adduct per fragment, we consider that the assay is not sensitive to adduct densities of <0.1 adduct per fragment. In most cases with genomic DNA from cisplatin-treated cells, the assay requires PCR amplifying a fragment of about 2 to 3 kb long.

6. An example treatment consisted of ip administration if cisplatin (Platinol) on d 1 and 8 at a dose of 4 mg/kg (LD10), i.e., 88 µL/22 g mouse. The dose corresponds to approx 20% of the IC50 of cisplatin for mice and is the maximum tolerable dose for a repeated weekly treatment. Vector (Adp53 or AdLuc) was administered intratumorally at a dose of 10^8 PFU/injection on d 3, 5, and 7 and again on d 10, 12, and 14. Vector was diluted into sterile cold PBS prior to injection so that injection volumes were 100 µL.

7. Generally a 4-h exposure is required for the reduction in target JNK mRNA by >80%. This is observed after 24 h of lipofection as judged by western analysis. Resistant cell types are treated for longer periods, and this approach *is* favored over increasing the oligonucleotide concentration or altering the oligonucleotide:lipofectamine ratio.

8. Typically all preparations yield quite similar protein concentrations, but volumes should be used so as to provide equal amounts of total cellular protein in all samples prior to subsequent analysis.

9. Prepare in advance GST-c-Jun fusion proteins by expression and purification (Qiagen plasmid DNA purification system kit) from *Escherichia coli* and by the addition of Glutathione Sepharose® 4B beads (Pharmacia Biotech).

10. For digitization software that provides interactive designation of the bands by, e.g., drawing boxes around the region to be digitized. If not automated, subtract background by using half-sized boxes placed exactly above and below

the band in question or by subtracting one half of the sum of same-sized boxes placed above and below the band in question. Subtract background values in all cases, thereby yielding "net" band values. Determine the relative JNK activity by normalizing the resulting net band values by division by similar results for control cases such as the scrambled-sequence or mock transfected cell case.

Acknowledgments

This work was supported in part by grants NCI CA69546 (R.A.G.), NCI CA63783 (D.A.M.), and NCI CA76173 (D.A.M.) from the U.S. Public Health Service; by the U.S. Army Breast Cancer Research Program DAMD17-96-1-6038 (R.A.G.); Introgen Therapeutics, Inc. (R.A.G.); and the Fellowship Program of the Sidney Kimmel Cancer Center. We thank Kluwer Academic/Plenum Publishers, Inc. (New York, Boston, Dordrecht, London, Moscow) for permission to reprint Figs. 1 and 2 and Tables 1 and 2 from "Cancer Gene Therapy: Past Achievements and Future Challenges" (Advances in Experimental Medicine and Biology, Vol. 465), N. Habib, ed. (2000).

We thank Angela Narehood for excellent editorial assistance.

References

1. Fischer, D. S., Knobf, M. T., and Durivage, H. J. (1993) *The Cancer Chemotherapy Handbook,* 4th ed, Mosby, St. Louis.
2. Cantrell, J. E., Hart, R. D., Taylor, R. F., and Harvey, J. H. Jr. (1987) Pilot trial of prolonged continuous-infusion 5-fluorouracil and weekly cisplatin in advanced colorectal cancer. *Cancer Treat. Rep.* **71,** 615–618.
3. Clarke, A. R., Purdie, C. A., Harrison, D. J., Morris, R. G., Bird C. C., Hooper M. L., and Wyllie, A. H. (1993) Thymocyte apoptosis induced by pS3-dependent and independent pathways. *Nature* **362,** 849–852.
4. Gjerset, R. A., Turla, S. T., Sobol, R. E., Scalise, J. J., Mercola, D. M., Collins, H., and Hopkins, P. J. (1995) Use of wild-type pS3 to achieve complete treatment sensitization of tumor cells expressing endogenous mutant p35. *Mol. Carcinog.* **14,** 275–285.
5. Dorigo, O., Turla, S. T., Lebedeva, S., and Gjerset, R. A. (1998) Sensitization of rat glioblastoma multiforme to cisplatin *in vivo* following restoration of wild-type pS3 function. *J. Neurosurg.* **88,** 535–540.
6. Lotem, J. and Sachs, L. (1993) Hematopoietic cells from mice deficient in wild-type pS3 are more resistant to induction of apoptosis by some agents. *Blood* **82,** 1092–1096.
7. Lowe, S. W., Bodis, S., McClatchy, A., Remington, L., Ruley, H. E., Fisher, D. E., Housman, D. E., and Jacks, T. (1994) p53 status and the efficacy of cancer therapy *in vivo. Science* **266,** 807–810.
8. Lowe, S. W., Ruley, H. E., Jacks, T., and Housman, D. E. (1993) p53-mediated apoptosis modulates the cytotoxicity of anti-cancer agents. *Cell* **74,** 957–967.

9. Potapova, O., Haghighi, A., Bost, F., Liu, C., Birrer, M. J., Gjerset, R., and Mercola, D. (1997) The Jun kinase/stress-activated protein kinase pathway functions to regulate DNA repair and inhibition of the pathway sensitizes tumor cells to cisplatin. *J. Biol. Chem.* **30,** 14,041–14,044.

10. Asgari, K., Sesterhenn, I. A., McLeod, D. G., Cowan, K., Moul, J. W., Seth, P., and Srivastava, S. (1997) Inhibition of the growth of pre-established subcutaneous tumor nodules of human prostate cancer cells by single injection of the recombinant adenovirus p53 expression vector. *J. Cancer* **71,** 377–382.

11. Ko, S. C., Gotoh, A., Thalmann, G. N., Zhau, H. E., Johnston, D. A., Zhang, W. W., Kao, C., and Chung, L. W. (1996) Molecular therapy with recombinant p53 adenovirus in an androgen-independent, metastatic human prostate cancer model. *Hum. Gene Ther.* **7,** 1683–1691.

12. Swisher, S. G., Roth, J. A., Nemunaitis, et al. (1999) Adenovirus-mediated pS3 gene transfer in advanced non-small cell lung cancer. *J. Natl. Cancer Inst.* **91,** 763–771.

13. Kauczor, H. U., Schuler, M., Heussel, C. P., von Weymarn, A., Bongartz, G., Rochlitz, C., Huber, C., and Thelen, M. (1999) CT-guided intratumoral gene therapy in non-smallcell lung cancer. *Eur. Radiol.* **9,** 292–296.

14. Roth, J. A. (1998) Restoration of tumor suppressor gene expression for cancer. *Forum* **8,** 368–376.

15. Schuler, M., Rochlitz, C., Horowitz, J. A., Schelgel, J., Perruchoud, A. P., Kommoss, F., Bolliger, C. T., Kauzor, H. U., Dalquen, P., Fritz, M. A., Swanson, S., Herrmann, R., and Huber, C. (1998) A phase I study of adenovirus-mediated wild-type pS3 gene transfer in patients with advanced non-small cell lung cancer. *Hum. Gene Ther.* **9,** 2075–2082.

16. Roth, J. A., Swisher, S. G., Merritt, J. A., et al. (1998) Gene therapy for non-small cell lung cancer: a preliminary report of a phase I trial of adenoviral p53 gene replacement. *Oncology* **25,** 33–37.

17. Zwaka, R. M. and Dunlop, M. G. (1998) Gene therapy for colon cancer. *Hematol. Oncol. Clin. North Am.* **12,** 595–615.

18. Clayman, G. L., el-Naggar, A. K., Lippmann, S. M., et al. (1998) Adenovirus-mediated p53 gene transfer in patients with advanced recurrent head and neck squamous cell carcinoma. *J. Clin. Oncol.* **16,** 2221–2232.

19. Bost, F., Potapova, O., Liu, C., Zhang, Y.-M., Charbono, W., Dean, N., McKay, R., and Mercola, D. (1999) High frequency regression of established human prostate carcinoma PC-3 xenografts by systemic treatment with antisense Jun kinase. *The Prostate* **38,** 320, 321.

20. Loda Magi-Galluzzi, C., Mishra, R., Fiorentino, M., Montironi, R., Yao, H., Capodieci, P., Wishnow, K., Kaplan, I., Stork, P. J., and Loda, M. (1997) Mitogen-activated protein kinase phosphatase 1 is overexpressed in prostate cancers and is inversely related to apoptosis. *Lab. Invest.* **76,** 61–70.

21. Jennerwein, M. M. and Eastrman, A. (1991) A polymerase chain reaction-based method to detect cisplatin adducts in specific genes. *Nucleic Acids Res.* **19,** 6209–6214.

22. Bost, F., McKay, R., Bost, M., Potapova, O., Dean, N., and Mercola, D. (1999) Jun Kinase–2 isoform is preferentially required for epidermal growth factor-induced proliferation of human A549 lung carcinoma cells. *Mol. Cell. Biol.* **19,** 1938–1949.

23. Bost, F., McKay, R., Dean, N., and Mercola, D. (2000) Antisense methods for the discrimination of phenotypic properties of closely related gene products: the Jun kinase Family. *Methods Enzymol.* **314,** 541, 542.

24. Stein, C. A. (1995) Does antisense exist? *Nature Med.* **1,** 1119–1121.

25. Bost, F., Dean, N., McKay, R., and Mercola, D. (1999) Activation of the jun kinase/stress-activated protein kinase pathway is required for EGF-autocrine stimulated growth of human A549 lung carcinoma cells. *J. Biol. Chem.* **272,** 33,422–33,429.

26. Yang, Y. M., Bost, F., Liu, C., and Mercola, D. (1998) The Jun Kinase pathway promotes growth of prostate carcinoma cell lines. *Cancer Gene Ther.* **5,** S31 (abstract PD–96).

27. Scanlon, K., Jiao, L., Funato, T., Wang, W., Tone, T., Rossi, J., and Kashani-Sabet, M. (1991) Ribozyme-mediated cleavage of *c-fos* MRNA reduces gene expression of DNA synthesis enzymes and metallothionein. *Proc. Natl. Acad. Sci. USA* **88,** 10,591.

28. Binétury, B., Smeal, T., and Karin, M. (1991) Ha-Ras augments c-dun activity and stimulates phosphorylation of its activation domain. *Nature* **351,** 22–27.

29. Gjerset, R. A., Lebedeva, S., Haghighi, A., Turla, S. T., and Mercola, D. (1999) Inhibition of the Jun kinase pathway blocks DNA repair, enhances p53-mediated apoptosis and promotes gene amplification. *Cell Growth Differ.* **10,** 545–554.

30. Srivastava, D. K., Rawson, T. Y., Showalter, S. D., and Wilson, S. H. (1995) Phorbol ester abrogates up-regulation of DNA polymerase by DNA-alkylating agents in Chinese hamster ovary cells. *J. Biol. Chem.* **270,** 16,402–16,408.

31. Kedar, P. S., Widen, S. G., Englander, E. W., Fornace, A. J. Jr., and Wilson, S. H. (1991) The ATF/CREB transcription factor-binding site in the polymerase beta promoter mediates the positive effect of N-methyl-N'-nitro-N-nitrosoguanidine on transcription. *Proc. Natl. Acad. Sci. USA* **88,** 3729–3733.

32. Mu, D., Tursun, M., Duckett, D. R., Drummond, J. T., Modrich, P., and Sancar, A. (1997) Recognition and repair of compound DNA lesions (base damage and mismatch) by human mismatch repair and excision repair systems. *Mol. Cell. Biol.* **17,** 760–769.

33. Baumgartner, B., Heiland, S., Kunze, N., Richter, A., and Knippers, R. (1994) Conserved regulatory elements in the type I DNA topoisomerase gene promoters of mouse and man. *Biochem. Biophys. Acta* **1218,** 123–127.

34. Heiland, S., Knippers, R., and Kunze, N. (1993) The promoter region of the human typeI-DNA-topoisomerase gene: protein-binding sites and sequences involved in transcriptional regulation. *Eur. J. Biochem.* **217,** 813–822.

35. Hochhauser, D., Stanway, C. A., Harris, A. L., and Hickson, I. D. (1992) Cloning and characterization of the 5'-flanking region of the human topoisomerase II alpha gene. *J. Biol. Chem.* **267,** 18,961–18,965.

36. Popanda, O. and Thielmann, H. W. (1992) The function of DNA topoisomerases in IV-induced DNA excision repair: studies with specific inhibitors in permeabilized human fibroblasts. *Carcinogenesis* **12,** 2321–2328.
37. Institute of Genomics Ressearch (1995) Genebank Accession no. T29334.
38. Liang, G., Wolfgang, C. D., Chen, B. P., Chen, T. H., and Hai, T. (1996) ATF3 gene: genomic organization, promoter, and regulation. *J. Biol. Chem.* **271,** 1695–1701.
39. Nilsson, M., Ford, J., Bohm, S., and Toftgard, R. (1997) Characterization of a nuclear factor that binds juxtaposed with ATF3/Jun on a composite response element specifically mediating induced transcription in response to an epidermal growth factor/Ras/Raf signaling pathway. *Cell Growth Dev.* **8,** 913–920.
40. Hsu, J. C., Bravo, R., and Taub, R. (1992) Interactions among LRF-1, JunB, c-Jun, and c-Fos define a regulatory program in the G1 phase of liver regeneration. *Mol. Cell. Biol.* **12,** 4654–4665.
41. Kharbanda, S., Rubin, E., Gunji, H., Hinz, H., Giovanella, B., Pantazis, P., and Kule, D. (1991) Camptothecin and its derivatives induce expression of the cjun protooncogene in human myeloid leukemia cells. *Cancer Res.* **51,** 6636–6642.
42. Pearson, B. E., Nasheuer, H. P., and Wang, T. S. (1991) Human DNA polymerase alpha gene: sequences controlling expression in cycling and serum-stimulated cells. *Mol. Cell. Biol.* **11,** 2081–2095.
43. Kharbanda, S. M., Sherman, M. L., and Kute, D. W. (1990) Transcriptional regulation of cjun gene expression by arabinofuranosylcytosine in human myeloid leukemia cells. *J. Clin. Invest.* **86,** 1517–1523.
44. Haug, T., Skorpen, F., Kvaloy, K., Eftedal, I., Lund, H., and Krokan, H. E. (1996) Human uracil-DNA glycosylase gene: sequence organization, methylation pattern, and mapping to chromosome 12q23-q24.1. *Genomics* **36,** 408–416.
45. Scanlon, K. J., Ishida, H., and Kashani-Sabet, M. (1994) Ribozyme-mediated reversal of the multidrug-resistant phenotype. *Proc. Natl. Acad. Sci. USA* **91,** 11,123–11,127.
46. Lee, W., Haslinger, A., Karin, M., and Tijan, R. (1987) Activationof transcription by two factors that bind promoter and enhancer sequences of the human methallothionein gene and SV40. *Nature* **325,** 368–372.
47. Feuerstein, N., Huang D., and Prystowsky M. B. (1995) Rapamycin selectively blocks interleukin-2-induced proliferating cell nuclear antigen gene expression in T lymphocyte. *J. Biol. Chem.* **270,** 9454–9458.
48. Huang, D., Shipman-Appasamy, P. M., Orten, D. J., Hinrichs, S. H., and Prystowsky, M. B. (1994) Promoter activity of the proliferating-cell nuclear antigen gene is associated with inducible CRE-binding proteins in interleukin 2-stimulated T lymphocytes. *Mol. Cell. Biol.* **14,** 4233–4338.
49. Park, J. S., Luethy, J. D., Wang, M. G., Fargnoli, J., Fornace, A. J. Jr., McBride, O. W., and Holbrook, N. J. (1992) Isolation, characterization and chromosomal localization of the human GADD153 gene. *Gene* **116,** 259–267.
50. Luethy, J. D. and Holbrook, N. J. (1994) The pathway regulating GADD153 induction in response to DNA damage is independent of protein kinase C and tyrosine kineses. *Cancer Res.* **54,** 1902–1906.

51. Gately, D. P., Jones, J. A., Christen, R., Barton, R. M., Los, G., and Howell, S. B. (1994) Induction of the growth arrest and DNA damage-inducible gene GADD153 by cisplatin in vitro and in vivo. *Br. J. Cancer* **70,** 1102–1106.
52. Delmastro, D. A., Li, J., Vaisman, A., Solle, M., and Chaney, S. G. (1997) DNA damage inducible-gene expression following platinum treatment in human ovarian carcinoma cell lines. *Cancer Chemother. Pharmacol.* **39,** 245–253.
53. Kolodner, R. D., Hall, N. R., Liptord, J., Kane, M. F., Rao, M. R., Morrison, P., Wirth, L., Finan, P. J., Burn, J., and Chapman, P. (1994) Structure of the human MSH2 locus and analysis of two Muir-Torre kindreds for msh2 mutations. *Genomics* **3,** 516–526.
54. Lamerdin, J. E., Montgomery, M. A., Stilwagen, S. A., Scheidecker, L. K., Tebbs, R. S., Brookman, K. W., Thompson, L. H., and Carrano, A. V. (1995) Genomic sequence comparison of the human and mouse XRCC1 DNA repair gene regions. *Genomics* **25,** 547–554.
55. Leach, F. S., Nicolaides, N. C., Papadopoulos, N., et al. (1993) Mutations of a mutS homologin hereditary nonpolyposis colorectal cancer. *Cell* **75,** 1215–1225.
56. Iwakuma, T., Shiraishi, A., Fukuhara, M., Kawate, H., and Sekiguchi, M. (1996) Organization and expression of the mouse gene for DNA repair methyltransferase. *DNA Cell Biol.* **15,** 863–872.
57. Lefebvre, P., Zak, P., and Laval, F. (1993) Induction of 06-methylguanine-DNA methyltransferase and N3-methyladenine-DNA-glycosylase in human cells exposed to DNA-damaging agents. *Cell Biol.* **12,** 233–241.
58. Scherer, S. J., Seib, T., Seitz, G., Dooley, S., and Welter, C. (1996) Isolation and characterization of the human mismatch repair gene hMSH2 promoter region. *Hum. Genet.* **97,** 114–116.
59. Mello, J. A., Acharya, S., Fishel, R., and Essigmann, J. M. (1996) The mismatch-repair protein hMSH2 binds selectively to DNA adducts of the anticancer drug cisplatin. *Chem. Biol.* **3,** 579–589.
60. Dalton, T. P., Li, Q., Bittel, D., Liang, L., and Andrews, G. K. (1996) Oxidative stress activates metal-responsive transcription factor–1 binding activity: occupancy *in vivo* of metal response elements in the metallothionein-I gene promoter. *J. Biol. Chem.* **271,** 26,233–26,241.
61. Gjerset, R. and Mercola, D. (2000) Sensitization of tumors to chemotherapy through gene therapy, in *Advances in Experimental Medicine and Biology* (Habib, N., ed.), Plenum, New York, pp. 273–292.

30

Ribozyme Gene Therapy

Leonidas A. Phylactou

1. Introduction

The completely unexpected discovery that the RNA molecule has catalytic properties *(1,2)* has led to a plethora of interest in the identification and utilization of a variety of catalytic RNA molecules, or ribozymes, that occur in nature. Among others, hammerhead ribozyme is a small catalytic RNA molecule whose catalytic activity resides in a core of less than 40 ribonucleotides *(3)*. In its naturally occurring form, the hammerhead ribozyme has the ability to cut itself in a base-specific way. Hammerhead ribozymes can be designed in the laboratory to act in a *trans*-acting fashion, i.e., to have their catalytic effect on other RNA molecules *(4)*. This ability to cleave target RNA molecules can be applied to downregulate unwanted gene expression, a form of genetic therapy. The aim of this chapter is to describe how hammerhead ribozyme activity can be tested in a cell-free environment prior to cell culture and animal experiments. This is an important step in identifying functional ribozymes for use in gene therapy. The following procedures describe the synthesis and testing of hammerhead ribozymes against labeled versions of target RNA molecules.

2. Materials

1. *Hind*III and *Eco*RI and reaction buffers (New England Biolabs).
2. Phenol:chloroform (1:1), pH 8.0.
3. T4 DNA ligase (1 U/μL) (Gibco-BRL Life Technologies).
4. pGEM-4Z cloning vector (Promega UK).
5. *Escherichia coli* competent cells, DH5α (Gibco-BRL Life Technologies).
6. LB medium: 1% (w/v) Bacto-tryptone, 0.5% (w/v) Bacto-yeast extract, 0.5% (w/v) NaCl.
7. LB/ampicillin agar: LB medium + 1.5% (w/v) agar, 100 μg/μL of ampicillin.

From: *Methods in Molecular Biology, vol. 175: Genomics Protocols*
Edited by: M. P. Starkey and R. Elaswarapu © Humana Press Inc., Totowa, NJ

8. Reagents for small-scale minipreparation of DNA—Miniprep lysis buffer:
   a. Solution I: 25 m*M* Tris-HCl, pH 8.0; 10 m*M* EDTA; 50 m*M* glucose.
   b. Solution II: 0.1 *M* NaOH, 1% (w/v) sodium dodecyl sulfate.
   c. Solution III (per 100 mL): 60 mL of 5 *M* potassium acetate, 11.5 mL of gla-
      cial acetic acid, 28.5 mL of H$_2$O.
9. Dideoxy sequencing reagents: T7 Sequenase 2.0 DNA Sequencing kit (Amersham
   Pharmacia Biotech).
10. In vitro transcription reagents: MAXIscript kit (Ambion Inc.).
11. Ribonuclease inhibitor (Roche).
12. T7 RNA polymerase (Roche).
13. [α-^{32}P UTP] (800 Ci/mmol) (Amersham Pharmacia Biotech).
14. RNase-free DNase I (Roche).
15. *Taq* DNA polymerase and reagents for PCR (Qiagen).
16. RNA extraction reagent: TRIZOL (Gibco-BRL Life Technologies).
17. cDNA synthesis reagents (Gibco-BRL Life Technologies).
18. Scintillation counter.

3. Methods

3.1. Design of Hammerhead Ribozymes

The hammerhead ribozyme is a small catalytic RNA molecule whose catalytic activity resides in a core of less than 40 ribonucleotides. This core consists of three base-paired helices connected by two single-stranded regions
(**Fig. 1**). In general, the single-stranded regions, which contain the catalytic
domain, are largely invariant, unlike the stems, which do not contain conserved
nucleotides *(5)*. This lack of conserved sequence allows stems I and III to be
designed to bind to any desired target sequence. Thus, potential hammerhead
ribozymes possess an invariant catalytic domain and flanking sequence (stems
I and III) complementary to a target mRNA molecule. Stems I and III will
surround the selected cleavage site in the target molecule. The ribozyme is thus
designed to cleave *in trans* at the selected target sequence within that mRNA.
Although in nature the most commonly found cleavage site is the GUC triplet,
mutagenesis studies have revealed that cleavage triplets of the type XUY are
tolerated, in which X is any nucleotide and Y is any nucleotide except G *(6)*.
In-depth analysis of the hammerhead ribozyme cleavage reaction has revealed
a hierarchy of preferred cleavage sites, which depends on the relative concentrations of ribozyme and substrate. Stems I and III of the ribozyme need to
provide sufficient stability of the ribozyme:substrate complex. They need to
ensure that there is an adequate association rate of ribozyme and target and that
the ribozyme is not displaced from its target before cleavage has occurred.
It is important to select ribozyme cleavage sites in the target mRNA that are
likely to be accessible to the ribozyme. There are very different activities

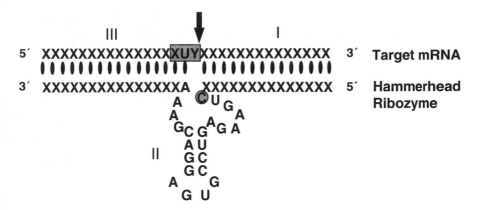

Fig. 1. A *trans*-acting hammerhead ribozyme. The hammerhead ribozyme (bottom strand) is shown in a typical three-stem structure (I, II, and III) bound to its target RNA (top strand). The cleavage site XUY is shown in a rectangular frame and the actual position of cleavage is denoted by a vertical arrow. The encircled base shows one of the sites that can be mutated to create the inactive versions of hammerhead ribozymes.

of ribozymes targeted to different sites on an mRNA because, at least in part, RNA folds readily into complex secondary structures that can interfere with binding of a ribozyme. It is difficult to select efficient ribozyme-cleavage sites on long RNA molecules. Generally, cleavage-susceptible sequences are determined either by trial and error or by predictions of the secondary structure of the target. Programs such as MFold and RNAstructure can also help predict RNA secondary structure. These programs are user friendly, and entry of the RNA sequence will provide an output of the pre dicted RNA structure.

3.2. In Vitro Ribozyme Synthesis by Cloning

Ribozymes can be cloned into vectors and then used as templates for in vitro transcription (**Fig. 2**). Alternatively, a synthetic DNA fragment can be used directly as template for ribozyme synthesis (*see* **Note 1**).

Having chosen the appropriate RNA target sites and designed the RNA catalytic molecules, the DNA equivalent of ribozyme sequences is synthesized in a DNA synthesizer. Both sense and antisense ribozyme oligonucleotides are made. For easier cloning of ribozymes, it is advisable to include restriction sites at the 5' end of the oligonucleotides. During experiments with ribozymes, it is necessary to include an inactive version of the ribozyme to prove that cleavage is ribozyme specific (**Fig. 1**). It is possible to clone active and inactive versions of ribozymes in a single ligation reaction. One of the ribozyme

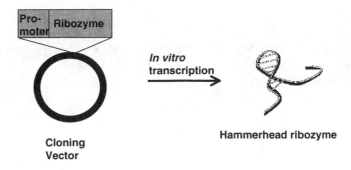

Fig. 2. Hammerhead ribozymes can be cloned into vectors containing prokaryotic promoters and synthesized by in vitro transcription.

oligonucleotide strands can include a degenerate base so that both active and inactive molecules can be present in the ligation reaction *(7)*.

3.2.1. Annealing and Digestion of Ribozyme Oligonucleotides

1. Mix 4 pmol of both ribozyme strands in 10 m*M* Tris-HCl; 10 m*M* MgCl$_2$; 10 m*M* NaCl; and 50 m*M* dithiothreitol (DTT), pH 7.9.
2. Incubate at 95°C for 5 min, then at 65°C for 10 min, followed by gradual cooling to room temperature.
3. Concentrate the annealed oligonucleotides by ethanol precipitation.
4. Perform sequential digests of the double-stranded oligonucleotides using appropriate restriction enzymes, e.g., *Hin*dIII and *Eco*RI (for pGEM-4Z).
5. Following digestion, extract the restriction endonucleases with phenol/chloroform and precipitate the digested double-stranded oligonucleotides with ethanol.
6. Sequentially digest 1 µg of pGEM-4Z with *Hin*dIII and *Eco*RI (as described in **steps 4** and **5**).

3.2.2. Construction of Hammerhead Ribozymes

1. Perform an overnight ligation at 6°C of 0.1 pmol of double-digested double-stranded ribozyme oligonucleotides and the linearized vector by using 3–5 *M* excess of the former in a total volume of 10 µL.
2. Transform competent *E. coli* cells with 3 µL of the ligation mix, and select recombinant clones.
3. Extract plasmid DNA from individual colonies, and identify active and inactive ribozyme clones by restriction digestion and dideoxy sequencing.
4. Linearize the ribozyme-containing constructs by restriction digestion. Choose an appropriate restriction endonuclease (i.e., *Eco*RI for a ribozyme cloned in the appropriate orientation between the *Hin*dIII and *Eco*RI sites of pGEM-4Z) so that the construct is linearized at the end of the cloned ribozyme sequence (*see* **Note 2**).

3.2.3. Ribozyme Synthesis by In Vitro Transcription

1. Mix 33 nmol of linearized plasmid with all four ribonucleotide triphosphates (ATP, CTP, UTP, and GTP), at a final concentration of 5 mM, in the presence of 1 5 mM MgCl$_2$; 2 mM spermidine; 50 mM Tris-HCl, pH 7.5; 5 mM DTT; 25 U of ribonuclease inhibitor; and 20 U of T7 RNA polymerase (for a ribozyme cloned in the appropriate orientation between the *Hin*dIII and *Eco*RI sites of pGEM-4Z) in a total volume of 50 µL. Add all the reagents (*see* **Note 3**) at room temperature to avoid precipitation of DNA.
2. Incubate the reaction at 37°C for 2–4 h and stop the reaction by adding of 4 U of RNase-free DNase I and further incubating at 37°C for 15 min.
3. Remove enzymes by phenol/chloroform extraction and recover the newly synthesized transcript by ethanol precipitation.
4. Check the quality and amount of ribozymes by reading their absorbance at 260 nm and or by denaturing (7 M urea) polyacrylamide gel electrophoresis (PAGE) alongside markers of known concentration (*see* **Note 4**).

3.3. Production of RNA Target

A labeled target RNA can be synthesized by in vitro transcription. As template, a PCR product can be used that contains the T7 promoter upstream of the target cDNA. The T7 promoter can be incorporated into the PCR fragment by a second PCR reaction. The first PCR product is generated from cDNA synthesized from total RNA extracted from cells or tissue expressing the target gene (**Fig. 3**).

3.3.1. Target Synthesis by Direct Template Production

The method used to synthesize labeled RNA target in our laboratory uses a PCR product as the template for in vitro transcription The PCR product used for transcription is the result of two rounds of amplification reaction *(7)* (**Fig. 3**). During the first, the target cDNA, containing the ribozyme binding site, is amplified, and in the second round of amplification, a T7 promoter is added to the 5' end of the PCR product. Target RNA is then synthesized by in vitro transcription, using T7 RNA polymerase. Alternatively, target RNA can be constructed and synthesized by cloning the first PCR product followed by linearization of the target cDNA-containing construct and in vitro transcription (*see* **Note 5**).

1. Extract total RNA from cells or tissue, expressing the target gene, using TRIZOL according to the manufacturer's instructions.
2. Carry out a reverse transcription with either an oligo(dT) primer or a primer specific for the RNA of interest.
3. Set up a PCR amplification of the newly synthesized cDNA using upstream and downstream primers designed to amplify the part of the target cDNA, that con-

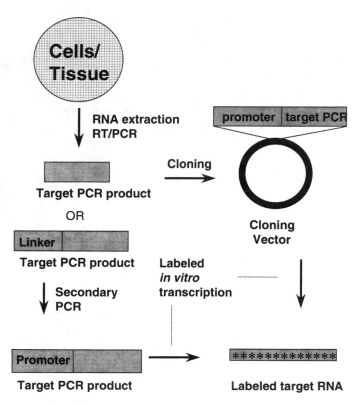

Fig. 3. Construction and synthesis of labeled target RNA used for in vitro ribozyme testing. Template for in vitro transcription can be in the form of either linearized plasmid or a PCR product. Target can be cloned into the vector of choice in the form of a PCR-amplified cDNA, derived from total RNA extracted from target-expressing cells. Alternatively, a T7 promoter can be added to the PCR product by a second PCR amplification, thus creating a template for target synthesis by in vitro transcription.

      tains the ribozyme cleavage site. Ensure that the PCR reaction has been successful by checking a small sample by agarose or PAGE.

4. Use 5 ng of the first-round PCR product as a template for the second round of amplification. Employ the same downstream primer as in the first round of PCR, but the upstream primer should be a universal primer composed of the T7 promoter (*see* **Note 6**). Ensure that the PCR reaction has been successful by checking a small sample by agarose or PAGE.

3.3.2. In Vitro Target RNA Synthesis

    RNA targets are synthesized by in vitro transcription. Our standard protocol uses [α-^{32}P UTP] to incorporate labeled nucleotide. The method used is similar to that used for synthesizing ribozyme.

1. Mix 33 nmol of the second PCR product (**Subheading 3.31., step 4**) with ATP, CTP, and GTP at a final concentration of 0.5 mM; 50 μCi of [α-^{32}P UTP] (800 Ci/mmol); 1 5 mM MgCl$_2$; 2 mM spermidine; 50 mM Tris-HCl, pH 7.5; 5 mM DTT; 12.5 U of ribonuclease inhibitor; and 10 U of T7 RNA polymerase in a total volume of 20 μL. Add all reagents at room temperature to avoid precipitation of DNA.
2. Incubate the reaction at 37°C for 60 min, and halt by adding 4 U of RNase-free DNase I and further incubating at 37°C for 15 min.
3. Remove all the enzymes by phenol/chloroform extraction, and then recover the newly synthesized transcript by ethanol precipitation.
4. Determine the specific activity of the labeled target by precipitation with trichloroacetic acid followed by liquid scintillation counting (*see* **Note 7**).

3.4. In Vitro Ribozyme Cleavage Assay

In vitro synthesized ribozymes can then be tested for their ability to cleave the target RNA prior to cell culture experiments. This can be done by incubating the ribozyme with the labeled mini-target under optimum conditions (*see* **Note 8**) *(8)*.

1. Mix the hammerhead ribozyme (active or inactive) with the labeled target RNA in the presence of 50 mM Tris-HCl, pH 7.5, and 20 mM MgCl$_2$ in a total volume of 20 μL. Incubate the samples at either 37°C (physiologic temperature) or at 50°C (cleavage being more efficient at the higher temperature.
2. Halt the reaction by adding of 20 mM EDTA.
3. Separate the labeled cleavage products from the target RNA by denaturing (7 M urea) PAGE and detect by autoradiography (**Fig. 4**).

4. Notes

1. To avoid the time and expense of cloning the ribozyme sequence adjacent to a prokaryotic promoter, an alternative approach is to produce hammerhead ribozymes directly off a synthetic DNA template *(7)*. The template can contain the ribozyme sequence and the promoter. The annealing of the oligonucleotides is performed as in **Subheading 3.2.1.**, followed by in vitro transcription as described in **Subheading 3.2.3.**
2. Restriction enzymes that create a 3' overhang should be avoided since the transcription will be inefficient.
3. Particular care should be taken to prepare ribonuclease-free solutions since contamination will result in degradation of both target and ribozyme. All commercially available reagents used for RNA work are prepared with ribonuclease-free solutions. Solutions made in the laboratory that will be used for RNA work should be prepared with diethylpyrocarbonate (DEPC) treated water (0.5% [v/v] DEPC in dH$_2$O). Mix vigorously and leave at room temperature overnight. Autoclave to break down the DEPC to CO$_2$ and H$_2$O.

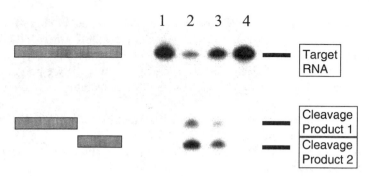

Fig. 4. Example of hammerhead ribozyme-mediated cleavage of a target RNA. Labeled target RNA has been incubated with a hammerhead ribozyme at different time intervals (lanes 2 and 3), or with its catalytically inactive version (lane 4) at 37°C. Lane 1 shows incubation of the labeled target in the absence of ribozyme. Labeled target and cleavage products have been detected by denaturing PAGE.

4. A combination of the two methods is advised, because neither of them alone can provide a very accurate calculation of the ribozyme concentration.
5. An alternative way to synthesize labeled target RNA is by cloning the first PCR product described in **Subheading 3.3.1.** If the PCR primers include restriction sites at their 5' ends, the PCR product can be cloned as described in **Subheading 3.2.2.** The target-containing vector can be linearized by restriction digest as described in **Subheading 3.2.2.** In vitro transcription is then used to produce the labeled target RNA in the same way as described in **Subheading 3.3.2.**
6. The T7 RNA polymerase promoter sequence 5'-CTCACTATAGCC is incorporated at the 5' end of the universal upstream primer (5'-AATTTAATACGACT CACTATAG-3') used in the second PCR amplification. The conditions for both PCR reactions are standard, with an appropriate annealing temperature that depends on the GC content of the PCR primers complementary to the target cDNA sequence.
7. We usually find that the radioactive ribonucleotide is not limiting during transcription when an RNA target of <400 bases is used. For synthesis of longer labeled target RNAs, it may be necessary to supplement the reaction with unlabeled UTP followed by gel purification in order to synthesize full-length transcripts.
8. The ribozyme-to-target RNA molar ratio can be determined depending on the ribozyme cleavage efficiency during initial assays.

Acknowledgments

This work in the author's laboratory is supported by the A. G. Leventis Foundation, the Association for International Cancer Research, Human Frontier Science Program Organization, the Association Française Contre les Myopathies, and the Muscular Dystrophy Campaign UK.

References

1. Cech, T. R., Zaug, A. J., and Grabowski, P. J. (1981) *In vitro* splicing of the ribosomal RNA precursor of Tetrahymena: involvement of a guanosine nucleotide in the excision of the intervening sequence. *Cell* **27,** 487–496.
2. Guerrier-Takada, C., Gardiner, K., Marsh, T., Pace, N., and Altman, S. (1983) The RNA moiety of ribonuclease P is the catalytic subunit of the enzyme. *Cell* **35,** 849–857.
3. Symons, R. H. (1992) Small catalytic RNAs. *Annu. Rev. Biochem.* **61,** 641–671.
4. Haseloff, J., and Gerlach, W. L. (1988) Simple RNA enzymes with new and highly specific endoribonuclease activities. *Nature* **334,** 585–591.
5. Birikh, K. R., Heaton, P. A., and Eckstein, F. (1997) The structure, function and application of the hammerhead ribozyme. *Eur. J. Biochem.* **245,** 1–16.
6. Shimayama, T., Nishikawa, S., and Taira, K. (1995) Generality of the NUX rule: kinetic analysis of the results of systematic mutations in the trinucleotide at the cleavage site of hammerhead ribozymes. *Biochemistry* **34,** 3649–3654.
7. Phylactou, L. A., Tsipouras, P., and Kilpatrick, M. W. (1998) Hammerhead ribozymes targeted to the FBN1 mRNA can discriminate a single base mismatch between ribozyme and target. *Biochem. Biophys. Res. Commun.* **249,** 804–810.
8. Kilpatrick, M. W., Phylactou, L. A., Godfrey, M., Wu, C. H., Wu, G. Y., and Tsipouras, P. (1996) Delivery of a hammerhead ribozyme specifically down-regulates the production of fibrillin–1 by cultured dermal fibroblasts. *Hum. Mol. Genet.* **5,** 1939–1944.

Index

A

Adenovirus, 496, 498, 514
Adeno–associated virus, 455–457
  adenovirus helper virus, 456, 457
  delivery into a cell line, 463, 464
  intramuscular administration, 465
  mediated gene transfer, 455–469
  production of wild–type free
      recombinant adeno–associated
      virus, 455, 456, 460, 461
  purification of recombinant adeno–
      associated virus, 455, 456, 461–
      463
Antisense
  oligonucleotides, 506, 507, 513
  protein kinase, 514
  treatment, 507
Apoptosis, 497
Arrays
  cDNA, 42, 284, 285
Automation, 162

B

BAC, *see* Bacterial artificial
      chromosome
Bacterial artificial chromosome, 57, 66,
      68, 80, 113, 123, 129, 136, 192,
      206–208,251,259

Bacterial artificial chromosome *(cont.)*
  DNA, 65, 207, 208, 253, 254, 258
  preparation, 223, 224
  library, 57, 67, 71
  preparation, 65, 80
  sequencing, 217–234
  subcloning, 217, 224–226
  vector, 57, 58, 60, 64–66
Biotin labeling, 51
BMD, *see* Mineral density of the bone

C

Cancer
  bladder, 495
  breast, 497
  ovarian, 495
  pancreatic, 283
  prostate, 495, 497, 498
  testicular, 495
Cat reporter
  assay, 512
  plasmids, 500
cDNA
  arrays, 169, 284
    hybridization screening of, 292
  colony filters, 277
  filters, 185
  hybridization, 201
    subtractive, 279–281, 284, 289, 291

From: *Methods in Molecular Biology, vol. 175, Genomics Protocols*
Edited by: M. P. Starkey and R. Elaswarapu © Humana Press Inc., Totowa, NJ